The Diabetic Kidney

CONTEMPORARY DIABETES

ARISTIDIS VEVES, MD
SERIES EDITOR

The Diabetic Kidney, edited by *Pedro Cortes,* MD *and Carl Erik Mogensen,* MD, *2006*
The Diabetic Foot, *Second Edition,* edited by *Aristidis Veves,* MD, *John M. Giurini,* DPM, *and Frank W. LoGerfo,* MD, *2006*
Obesity and Diabetes, edited by *Christos S. Mantzoros,* MD, *2006*

THE DIABETIC KIDNEY

Edited by

PEDRO CORTES, MD

Henry Ford Hospital, Detroit, MI

CARL ERIK MOGENSEN, MD

Aarhus University Hospital, Aarhus, Denmark

HUMANA PRESS
TOTOWA, NEW JERSEY

999 Riverview Drive, Suite 208
Totowa, New Jersey 07512

www.humanapress.com

Production Editor: Robin B. Weisberg

Cover design by Patricia F. Cleary

Cover Illustration: From Fig. 4, Chapter 13, "Hepatocyte Growth Factor: *Physiological and Therapeutic Ligand to Attenuate Diabetic Nephropathy,*" by Shinya Mizuno and Toshikazu Nakamura

For additional copies, pricing for bulk purchases, and/or information about other Humana titles, contact Humana at the above address or at any of the following numbers: Tel.: 973-256-1699; Fax: 973-256-8341, E-mail: orders@humanapr.com; or visit our Website: www.humanapress.com

This publication is printed on acid-free paper. ∞
ANSI Z39.48-1984 (American National Standards Institute) Permanence of Paper for Printed Library Materials.

Printed in the United States of America. 10 9 8 7 6 5 4 3 2 1

e-ISBN 1-59745-153-3

Library of Congress Cataloging-in-Publication Data

The diabetic kidney / edited by Pedro Cortes, Carl Erik Mogensen.
p. ; cm. -- (Contemporary diabetes)
Includes bibliographical references and index.
ISBN 1-58829-624-5 (alk. paper)
1. Diabetic nephropathies. 2. Diabetes. I. Cortes, Pedro.
II. Mogensen, Carl Erik. III. Series.
[DNLM: 1. Diabetic Nephropathies--physiopathology. 2. Diabetes
Mellitus--diagnosis. 3. Diabetes Mellitus--therapy. WK 835 D5358
2006]
RC918.D53D522 2006
616.6'1--dc22 2005034845

Dedication

This book is dedicated to Dr. Nathan W. Levin and the late Dr. Knud Lundbaek,
our mentors and friends.
They have been a great inspiration to us.

SERIES EDITOR'S INTRODUCTION

Diabetes is becoming a pandemic that affects not only developed countries but developing countries as well. As a result, there is also a dramatic increase in long-term diabetes complications, including diabetic nephropathy. The fact that 50% of the patients undergoing dialysis also have diabetes is further proof of the seriousness of the situation.

In *The Diabetic Kidney*, we are honored to collaborate with two distinguished clinicians and researchers, Drs. Pedro Cortes and Carl Eric Mogensen, who have edited an excellent book on diabetic nephropathy that greatly increases the scientific impact of the "Contemporary Diabetes" series. Drs. Cortes and Mogensen have assembled a stellar group of contributors who discuss the pathophysiology and clinical aspects of diabetic kidney disease. Readers can achieve a clear understanding of the progress that has been made regarding the pathogenesis of the disease along with the therapeutic interventions to prevent its development or to treat clinical diabetic nephropathy.

I have no doubt that *The Diabetic Kidney* will be of value not only to practicing clinicians but also to researchers in this field. Therefore, I sincerely thank the editors for their efforts to produce this book and also the contributors for the excellent chapters. I have no doubt that *The Diabetic Kidney* can become a reference text that has a major impact on our efforts to improve the lives of diabetic patients with kidney disease.

Aristidis Veves, MD
Series Editor

PREFACE

Renal abnormalities in diabetes were first recorded in the 19th century, where French and German clinicians described the renal hypertrophy and proteinuria in diabetes. A breakthrough in the understanding of the diabetic renal disease came with Kimmelstiel and Wilson's description of glomerular lesions and diabetes in 1936. The area remained very silent until the late 1960s, when the seriousness of diabetic nephropathy became extremely clear. Since that time, there has been an increase in the number of patients with diabetes, especially type 2 diabetes, and subsequent renal disease, ending up in advanced renal disease with need for dialysis. Since the 1980s, there has been a tremendous input of diabetic patients in the dialysis and transplantation units. We are finally beginning to see a decline in the number of patients in the dialysis unit, at least in Europe. It is no secret that about 50% of the patients in the dialysis unit in most countries are patients with diabetes.

In the last few years, there has been a steady increase in the scientific activity regarding both the basic and clinical side of the problem. This is reflected in *The Diabetic Kidney*, where the background, biochemically and biologically speaking, for diabetic renal disease is described in many chapters focusing on the multiple abnormalities.

The clinical section also reflects a great level of activity within the area. Presently, there is greater focus on early detection of nephropathy by screening for microalbuminuria, and on early treatment. The main basis for developing diabetic renal disease still constitutes problems of the improving glycemic control. Despite the DCTT and UKPDS studies, many patients with both type 1 and type 2 diabetes have far from optimal glycemic control, and in many centers, the mean A1c is between 8.5 and 9% in unselected populations with type 1 and type 2 diabetes. Obviously, there are also good examples of extremely well-controlled patients, but on the other hand, there are a large number of poorly controlled patients, sometimes explained by noncompliance or often difficulties in controlling the diabetic state.

The editors of *The Diabetic Kidney* are sure that the activity described by many of the authors will further increase the understanding of the basis for abnormalities in diabetic renal disease as well as better understanding of the diagnosis and treatment in patients with diabetes.

It has been the editors' pleasure to select many of the top scientists within the diabetic renal disease field who have equally worked effectively on the chapters and submitted them in due time for an up-to-date status of our still severe problem of diabetic nephropathy.

***Pedro Cortes,* MD**
***Carl Erik Mogensen,* MD**

Contents

CONTRIBUTORS

JOSEPH P. BAST, MD • *Department of Medicine, Loyola University Stritch School of Medicine, Chicago, IL*

GEOFFREY BONER, MBBCh • *Department of Internal Medicine, Sackler Faculty of Medicine, Tel Aviv University, Tel Aviv, Israel and Danielle Alberti Memorial Centre for Diabetes Complications, Vascular Division, Wynn Domain, Baker Medical Research Institute, Melbourne, Australia*

ERWIN BOTTINGER, MD • *Division of Nephrology, Department of Medicine, Mount Sinai School of Medicine, Dorrace Hamilton Research Laboratories, New York, NY*

PAMELA K. CARMINES, MD • *Department of Cellular and Integrative Physiology, University of Nebraska College of Medicine, Omaha, NE*

QING CHEN, MD • *Department of Internal Medicine, Washington University School of Medicine, St. Louis, MO*

SHELDON CHEN, MD • *Renal-Electrolyte and Hypertension Division, Department of Medicine and the Penn Center for the Molecular Studies of Kidney Diseases, University of Pennsylvania, Philadelphia, PA*

ELLIE CHUANG, MD • *Division of Endocrinology, Metabolism and Molecular Medicine, Northwestern University Feinberg School of Medicine, Chicago, IL*

MARK E. COOPER, MD • *Danielle Alberti Memorial Centre for Diabetes Complications, Vascular Division, Wyann Domain, Baker Medical Research Institute, Melbourne, Australia*

PEDRO CORTES, MD • *Division of Nephrology and Hypertension, Department of Medicine, Henry Ford Hospital, Detroit, MI*

PATRICIA A. CRAVEN, PhD • *Department of Medicine, VA Pittsburgh Healthcare System, University of Pittsburgh School of Medicine Pittsburgh, PA*

VIVETTE D'AGATI, MD • *Department of Pathology, Columbia University, College of Physicians & Surgeons, New York, NY*

LAURA DE PETRIS, MD • *Department of Pediatrics, Washington University School of Medicine, St. Louis, MO*

FREDERICK R. DERUBERTIS, MD • *Department of Medicine, VA Pittsburgh Healthcare System, University of Pittsburgh School of Medicine, Pittsburgh, PA*

I. GEORGE FANTUS, MDCM • *Department of Medicine, Mount Sinai Hospital/University Health Network and Banting and Best Diabetes Centre, University of Toronto, Toronto, Ontario Canada*

DENIS FELIERS, PhD • *Department of Medicine, University of Texas Health Science Center, San antonio, TX*

ALESSIA FORNONI, PhD, MD • *The Division of Nephrology and Hypertension, University of Miami School of Medicine, Miami, FL*

THERESA GEURS, BS • *Department of Pediatrics, Washington University School of Medicine, St. Louis, MO*
HOWARD J. GOLDBERG, MD • *Department of Medicine, Mount Sinai Hospital/University Health Network and Banting and Best Diabetes Centre, University of Toronto, Toronto, Ontario, Canada*
MASAKAZU HANEDA, MD, PhD • *Second Department of Medicine, Asahikawa Medical College, Asahikawa, Hokkaido, Japan*
CHARLES W. HEILIG, MD • *Division of Nephrology, University of Chicago Hospitals, Chicago, IL*
RAIMUND HIRSCHBERG, MD • *Los Angeles Biomedical Research Institute at Harbor-UCLA Medical Center, Torrance, CA*
NIELS HOLMARK ANDERSEN, MD, PhD • *Department of Internal Medicine M (Diabetes & Endocrinology), Aarhus University Hospital, Aarhus, Denmark*
ALFONS J.H.M. HOUBEN, PhD • *Department of Medicine, Divisions of General Internal Medicine and Endocrinology, Maastricht University and University Hospital, Maastricht, The Netherlands*
KEITH A. HRUSKA, MD • *Departments of Pediatrics and Internal Medicine, Washington University School of Medicine, St. Louis, MO*
MAYA S. P. HUIJBERTS, MD, PhD • *Department of Medicine, Divisions of General Internal Medicine and Endocrinology, Maastricht University and University Hospital, Maastricht, The Netherlands*
NAOHITO ISHII, PhD • *Department of Hematological Informatics, Kitasato University School of Allied Health Sciences, Kanagawa, Japan*
KEIJI ISSHIKI, MD, PhD • *Department of Medicine, Shiga University of Medical Science, Otsu, Shiga, Japan*
GEORGE JERUMS, MD, MBBS, FRACP • *Endocrine Unit and Department of Medicine, University of Melbourne, Melbourne, Australia*
SUJATHA KAROOR, PhD • *Renal Division, Baxter Health Care, McGaw, IL*
BALAKUNTALAM S. KASINATH, MD • *Department of Medicine, University of Texas Health Science Center, South Texas Veterans Health Care System, San Antonio, TX*
RONALD KLEIN, MD, MPH • *Department of Ophthalmology and Visual Sciences, University of Wisconsin School of Medicine and Public Health, Madison, WI*
DAISUKE KOYA, MD, PhD • *Department of Endocrinology and Metabolism, Kanazawa Medical University, Uchinada, Kahoku, Ishikawa, Japan*
ANDRZEJ S. KROLEWSKI, MD, PhD • *Research Division, Joslin Diabetes Center and Department of Medicine, Harvard Medical School, Boston, MA*
MYUNG JA LEE, PhD • *Department of Medicine, University of Texas Health Science Center, San Antonio, TX*
DAVID J. LEEHEY, MD • *Department of Medicine, Veterans Affairs Hospital, Hines, IL and Loyola University Stritch School of Medicine, Maywood, IL*
TINGTING LI, MD • *Department of Internal Medicine, Washington University School of Medicine, St. Louis, MO*
HELEN LIAPIS, MD • *Department of Pathology, Washington University, St. Louis, MO*
RICHARD MACISAAC, MD, PhD, FRACP • *Endocrine Unit, Department of Medicine, University of Melbourne, Melbourne, Australia*
MICHAEL MAUER, MD • *Division of Pediatric Nephrology, Department of Pediatrics, University of Minnesota Medical School, Minneapolis, MN*

SHINYA MIZUNO, PhD • *Division of Molecular Regenerative Medicine, Department of Molecular Regenerative Medicine, Osaka University Graduate School of Medicine, Suita Osaka, Japan*
CARL ERIK MOGENSEN, MD • *Department of Internal Medicine M (Diabetes and Endocrinology), Aarhus University Hospital, Aarhus, Denmark*
MARK E. MOLITCH, MD • *Division of Endocrinology, Metabolism and Molecular Medicine, Northwestern University Feinberg School of Medicine, Chicago, IL*
BEHZAD NAJAFIAN, MD • *Department of Pediatrics and Department of Laboratory Medicine and Pathology, University of Minnesota Medical School, Minneapolis, MN*
TOSHIKAZU NAKAMURA, PhD • *Division of Molecular Regenerative Medicine, Department of Molecular Regenerative Medicine, Osaka University Graduate School of Medicine, Suita Osaka, Japan*
ROBERT G. NELSON, MD, PhD • *Phoenix Epidemiological and Clinical Research Branch, National Institute of Diabetes and Digestive and Kidney Diseases, Phoenix, AZ*
DIMITRIOS G. OREPOULOS, MD • *The Toronto Hospital Western, Toronto, Ontario, Canada*
SIANNA PANAGIOTOPOULOS, PhD • *Endocrine Unit and Department of Medicine, Austin Health and University of Melbourne, Melbourne, Australia*
PLOUMIS S. PASSADAKIS, MD • *The Toronto Hospital Western, Toronto, Ontario, Canada*
GRZEGORZ PLACHA, MD, PhD • *Research Division, Joslin Diabetes Center and Department of Medicine, Harvard Medical School, Boston, MA and Department of Internal Medicine and Hypertension, The Medical University of Warsaw, Warsaw, Poland*
BRUCE L. RISER, PhD • *Baxter Health Care, Renal Division, McGaw, IL; and Rosalind Franklin University of Medicine and Science, North Chicago, IL*
EBERHARD RITZ, MD • *Department of Internal Medicine, Ruperto Carola University, Heidelberg, Germany*
Nicolaas C. Schaper, MD, PhD • *Department of Medicine, Maastricht University and University Hospital Maastricht, Maastricht, The Netherlands*
ANN MARIE SCHMIDT, MD • *Department of Surgery, Columbia University, College of Physicians & Surgeons, New York, NY*
KUMAR SHARMA, MD • *Center for Diabetic Kidney Disease, Dorrance Hamilton Research Laboratories and Division of Nephrology, Department of Medicine, Jefferson University, Philadelphia, PA*
ASHOK K. SINGH, PhD • *Hektoen Institute for Medical Research, Chicago, IL*
REKHA SINGH, PhD • *Research Service, Veterans Affairs Hospital, Hines, IL*
NAHUM SONENBERG, PhD • *Department of Biochemistry, McGill University, Montreal, Canada*
JAMES R. SOWERS, MD • *Department of Internal Medicine, University of Missouri-Columbia School of Medicine and Divisions of Endocrinology and Nephrology, Harry S. Truman VA Medical Center, Columbia, MO*
KURT SOWERS, MD • *Department of Internal Medicine, University of Missouri-Columbia School of Medicine and Divisions of Endocrinology and Nephrology, Harry S. Truman VA Medical Center, Columbia, MO*
COEN D. A. STEHOUWER, MD, PhD • *Department of Medicine, Maastricht University and University Hospital Maastricht, Maastricht, The Netherlands*

FRANK STREBECK, BS • *Department of Pediatrics, Washington University School of Medicine, St. Louis, MO*
KATALIN SUSZTAK, PhD, MD • *Division of Nephrology, Department of Medicine, Albert Einstein College of Medicine, Bronx, NY*
BALAZS SZAMOSFALVI, MD • *Division of Nephrology and Hypertension, Department of Medicine, Henry Ford Hospital, Detroit, MI*
MERLIN THOMAS, MB, ChB, PhD • *Baker Medical Research Institute, Melbourne, Australia*
VISITH THONGBOONKERD, MD, FRCPT • *Medical Molecular Biology Unit, Office for Research and Development, Faculty of Medicine at Siriraj Hospital, Mahidol University, Bangkok, Thailand*
DELILAH TOPIC, MD • *Department of Medicine, Mount Sinai Hospital/University Health Network and Banting and Best Diabetes Centre, University of Toronto, Toronto, Ontario Canada*
KATHERINE R. TUTTLE, MD • *Providence Medical Research Center, Sacred Heart Medical Center, University of Washington School of Medicine, Spokane, WA*
SONG WANG, MD • *Third Hospital of Beijing Medical University, Beijing, China*
E. JENNIFER WEIL, MD • *Phoenix Epidemiological and Clinical Research Branch, National Institute of Diabetes and Digestive and Kidney Diseases, Phoenix, AZ*
ADAM WHALEY-CONNELL, DO • *Department of Internal Medicine, University of Missouri-Columbia School of Medicine and Divisions of Endocrinology and Nephrology, Harry S. Truman VA Medical Center, Columbia, MO*
CATHARINE I. WHITESIDE, MD, PhD • *Department of Medicine, Mount Sinai Hospital/ University Health Network and Banting and Best Diabetes Centre, University of Toronto, Toronto, Ontario Canada*
GUNTHER WOLF, MD • *Zentrum Innere Medizin, Medizinische Klinik IV, Universitätsklinikum Hamburg—Eppendorf, Hamburg Germany*
JERRY YEE, MD • *Division of Nephrology and Hypertension, Department of Medicine, Henry Ford Hospital, Detroit, MI*
FUAD N. ZIYADEH, MD • *Renal-Electrolyte and Hypertension Division, Department of Medicine and the Penn Center for the Molecular Studies of Kidney Diseases, University of Pennsylvania , Philadelphia, PA and Faculty of Medicine, American University of Beirut, Beirut, Lebanon*

I

Basic Pathophysiology and Biochemistry of Diabetic Nephropathy

A. Pathophysiology

1 Angiotensin II and Its Receptors in the Pathogenesis of Diabetic Nephropathy

David J. Leehey, MD, *Ashok K. Singh,* PhD, *and Rekha Singh,* PhD

CONTENTS

INTRODUCTION

Diabetic nephropathy (DN) is characterized by accumulation of extracellular matrix (ECM) in the kidney. Glomerular mesangial expansion and tubulo-interstitial fibrosis eventually leads to renal failure. The mediators of renal injury in this disease have not been fully identified. The peptide angiotensin (Ang) II has many hemodynamic and biochemical effects that could contribute to DN (Table 1). A prominent role for Ang II has been suggested by experimental and clinical evidence indicating that angiotensin-converting enzyme (ACE) inhibitors and angiotensin receptor blockers (ARBs) have renoprotective effects and that these agents can attenuate the progression of glomerulosclerosis *(1)*. In clinical studies, as well as studies conducted in experimental diabetic animals, it is difficult to separate hemodynamic from nonhemodynamic effects of Ang II. On the other hand, in vitro studies using cultured cells allow study of the specifically nonhemodynamic effects of Ang II and its inhibition *(2)*. These nonhemodynamic effects of Ang II include stimulation of transforming growth factor (TGF)-β_1, activation of matrix protein synthesis, and inhibition of matrix degradation *(3,4)*. Ang II also increases generation of reactive oxygen species (ROS) in mesangial cells (MCs) *(5)* and may contribute to oxidant-induced renal injury.

THE RENIN–ANGIOTENSIN SYSTEM IN DIABETES

The classical components of the renin–angiotensin system (RAS) include the renin substrate angiotensinogen, and the enzymes renin and ACE that participate in the

From: *Contemporary Diabetes: The Diabetic Kidney*
Edited by: P. Cortes and C. E. Mogensen © Humana Press Inc., Totowa, NJ

Table 1
Proposed Mechanisms of Ang II Effects in Diabetic Nephropathy

Hemodynamic effects	*Nonhemodynamic effects*
Systemic hypertension	Induction of renal hypertrophy and cell proliferation
Systemic and renal vasoconstriction	Stimulation of extracellular matrix synthesis
Stimulation of other vasoconstrictors (endothelin) and inhibition of vasodilators (nitric oxide and atrial natriuretic peptide)	Inhibition of extracellular matrix degradation
Increased glomerular capillary pressure and permeability	Increased tubular uptake of proteins
Mesangial cell contraction leading to reduction in filtration surface area	Stimulation of cytokine (e.g., TGF-β, vascular endothelial growth factor, endothelin) production
	Stimulation of superoxide production
	Activation of nuclear factor-κB
	Reduction in podocyte nephrin expression

formation of Ang II (Fig. 1). Angiotensinogen is a heterogeneous glycoprotein and the only known substrate for renin. Inactive renin or prorenin has a prosegment of 43 amino acid residues attached to the N-terminus of active renin and cleavage of this prosegment (by a trypsin-like-activating enzyme) results in the formation of active renin. The prorenin molecule can also undergo nonproteolytic activation to an enzymatically active state (*see* "Renin and ACE"). Active renin cleaves the first 10 amino acids from the N-terminus of angiotensinogen to form the decapeptide Ang I. Ang II is converted from Ang I by removal of the two amino acids at the carboxy terminus by ACE and is further degraded into Ang III, Ang IV, and other Ang fragments by amino peptidases and carboxy peptidases. Among all the peptides originating from angiotensinogen, Ang II is the most studied because it exerts a variety of actions on cell functions.

Systemic RAS

The beneficial effects of ACE inhibitors and ARBs in attenuation of proteinuria and glomerulosclerosis in both experimental and clinical DN suggest that either the systemic RAS and/or the RAS within the kidney is activated in diabetes. However, studies on the systemic RAS in experimental diabetes have generally shown suppression of the system. In streptozotocin (STZ)-induced diabetes in rats (a model of type 1 diabetes), plasma renin activity (PRA) and angiotensinogen levels were significantly decreased *(6,7)*. No significant changes in plasma Ang II levels in STZ diabetic rats were observed *(8)*. Studies in the Zucker diabetic fatty (ZDF) rat (a model of type 2 diabetes), have also shown PRA to be decreased as compared with lean controls *(9)*. Variable findings have been reported in clinical diabetes. Early in the disease, PRA has been reported to be elevated *(10)*, yet it is generally suppressed in patients with DN *(11)*. However, diabetic patients with nephropathy have a heightened renal hemodynamic response to ARBs in the face of low PRA, suggesting that intrarenal Ang II production may be increased; this may in part explain the therapeutic effectiveness of interrupting the RAS in DN. Thus, high

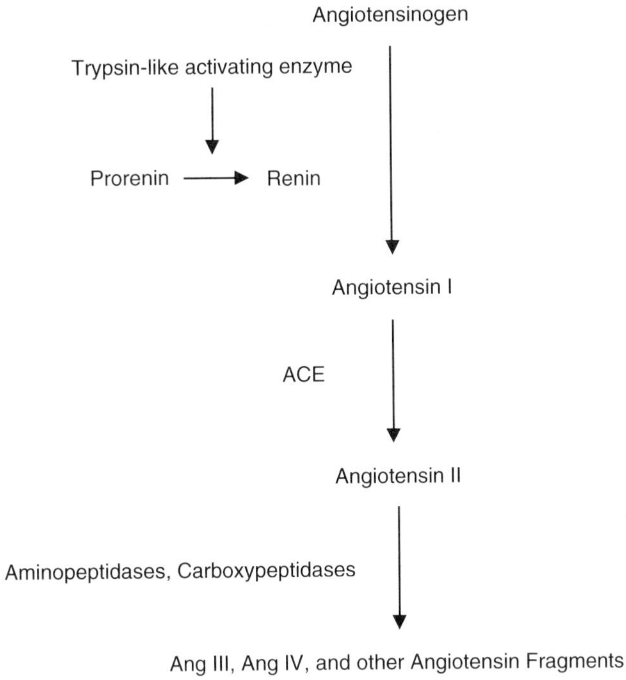

Fig. 1. The classical components of the renin–angiotensin system (RAS). ACE, angiotensin-converting enzyme.

glucose/diabetes may stimulate the local RAS within the kidney or the "intrarenal" RAS. This chapter focuses on the intrarenal RAS in cell culture and animal models of diabetes.

Intrarenal RAS

In recent years, the role of the intrarenal RAS in the pathophysiology of renal diseases such as DN has been the subject of extensive investigation. Cultured glomeruli and mesangial cells contain all of the elements of the RAS, including the substrates and the enzymes required for Ang II generation *(12–14)*. Indirect evidence for the presence of a locally regulated RAS within the kidney is also provided by the studies showing much higher concentrations of Ang II in several intrarenal compartments than those found in the systemic circulation *(15–17)*. The effects of high glucose/diabetes on various components of the intrarenal RAS are reviewed here.

Angiotensinogen

In cultured MCs, high glucose increases angiotensinogen mRNA expression accompanied by an increase in angiotensinogen protein levels *(18)*. Also, in the STZ-induced diabetic rat, an increase in angiotensinogen mRNA expression in the whole kidney *(19)* and angiotensinogen protein levels in the glomeruli *(20)* have been observed. The mechanism(s) by which high glucose increases angiotensinogen mRNA and protein levels has not been fully elucidated. In rat proximal tubular cells, the effects of high glucose on angiotensinogen gene transcription are mediated by the p38 mitogen-activated protein kinase (MAPK) *(21)*, ROS *(22)*, and by activation of the hexosamine pathway *(23)*. Our preliminary studies in cultured MCs have shown that high glucose-induced increase in angiotensinogen levels is mediated via the p38 MAPK pathway.

Renin and ACE

MCs secrete both forms of the renin enzyme, that is, active renin and inactive prorenin *(24)*, and contain receptors for prorenin and renin *(25)*. Prorenin can be converted into active renin by proteolytic enzymes including cathepsin B, which act on the pro-segment of prorenin *(26)*. In cultured MCs, high glucose increased renin activity by stimulating prorenin gene transcription and conversion of prorenin to active renin *(27)*. In recent studies, a prorenin/renin receptor was identified in human MCs, which showed renin- and prorenin-specific binding *(28)*. The binding of renin to this receptor resulted in increased catalytic efficiency of the enzyme, leading to increased conversion of angiotensinogen to Ang I, and the binding of prorenin to this receptor caused a conformational change of the prorenin molecule to an enzymatically active state (termed nonproteolytic activation of prorenin) *(28)*. Recently, it has been shown that the nonproteolytic activation of prorenin can be blocked by a decoy peptide with an amino acid sequence corresponding to the "handle" region of the prorenin prosegment *(29)*. Infusion of this peptide into STZ diabetic rats decreased the renal content of Ang I and Ang II and completely inhibited the development of DN *(29)*. Thus, peptides that can inhibit activation of prorenin at the cellular level may be useful in suppressing enhanced RAS activity in the diabetic kidney.

ACE is a dipeptidyl carboxypeptidase enzyme that converts the inactive decapeptide Ang I to the active octapeptide Ang II by removing two amino acids at the carboxyl terminus. MCs in culture express ACE mRNA and synthesize this enzyme *(14)*. ACE is also present in proximal tubular cells mainly localized to the brush border and thus plays a regulatory role by generating Ang II, which in turn affects tubular reabsorption of sodium *(30)*. Studies in cultured MCs in our laboratory have demonstrated that high glucose does not affect ACE activity or levels *(18)*, although a recent study has reported a stimulatory effect of high glucose on ACE gene transcription and activity *(27)*; thus this issue needs further investigation. Few studies have examined the effects of diabetes on ACE in the kidney. In the STZ diabetic rat, total renal ACE activity was decreased although ACE immunostaining was enhanced in glomeruli and reduced in proximal tubules *(19)*. However, ACE protein levels in glomeruli were similar in STZ diabetic and nondiabetic rats *(20)*.

Angiotensin II

Studies from our laboratory have demonstrated that high glucose increases Ang II levels in rat mesangial cell lysates in a concentration-dependent fashion *(4)* (Fig. 2). High glucose also increased Ang II levels in human MCs *(31)*. Ang II is increased due to both an increase in the substrate angiotensinogen as well as increased conversion of Ang I to Ang II via ACE-independent mechanisms *(18)*. When the conversion of *exogenous* Ang I to Ang II was studied in MC extracts by high-performance liquid chromatography (HPLC), there was significant formation of the intermediate peptide angiotensin(1–9) [Ang(1–9)] *(18)*. MC extracts incubated with *exogenous* Ang(1–9) converted it to Ang II (Fig. 3), indicating the presence of an enzyme that can convert Ang(1–9) to Ang II. Also, the conversion of Ang(1–9) to Ang II was increased in high glucose-treated MC extracts (Fig. 3), suggesting that the activity of this pathway is increased under high-glucose conditions *(18)*. In support of this hypothesis, increased Ang II levels were observed in glomeruli from STZ diabetic rats, which may also

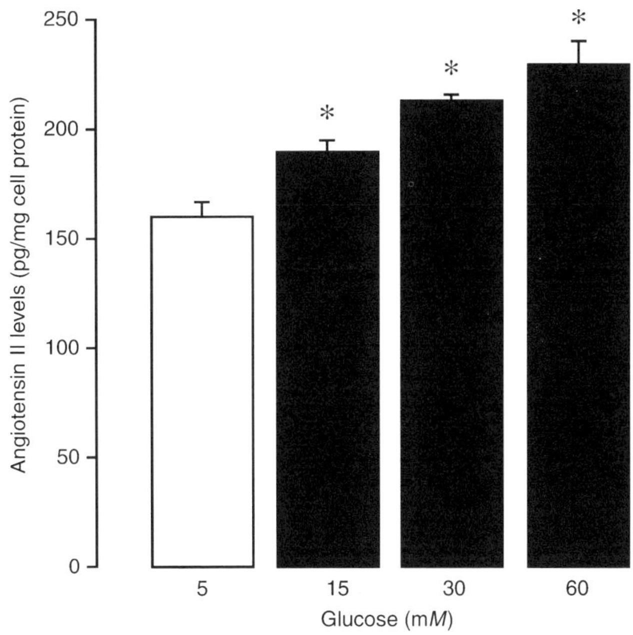

Fig. 2. Ang II levels in mesangial cell lysates after incubation of cells with varying concentrations of glucose (5–60 m*M*) for 24 h. Ang II levels were measured by ELISA. Data shown are the means ± SEM of four experiments. Glucose loading increased Ang II production in a concentration-dependent manner. The asterisk denotes $p < 0.05$ vs 5 m*M* glucose. (From ref. *4* with permission.)

involve increased conversion of Ang(1–9) to Ang II *(20)*. Because inhibitors of ACE or chymase did not block conversion of Ang(1–9) to Ang II, this may be one of the non-ACE mechanisms for enhanced formation of Ang II in diabetes *(20)*.

There are various other enzymes besides ACE that are involved in the formation of Ang II. These include tonin, trypsin, kallikrein, cathepsin G, and chymase *(32)*. In the heart, much of Ang II formation is the result of chymase *(33)*, but in the kidney, the role of chymase in Ang II formation is not fully established. A recent study has shown that the chymase-dependent Ang II generation is upregulated in the human diabetic kidney *(34)*. In ACE knockout mice, local Ang II generation in kidney is unchanged owing to a 14-fold increase in chymase activity *(35)*. Thus, it appears that the chymase enzyme may constitute one of the non-ACE pathways for enhanced formation of Ang II in the diabetic condition.

Increased Ang II levels in tissues could be due to increased formation and/or decreased degradation. Ang II is known to be degraded by aminopeptidases to Ang III and Ang IV by sequential removal of aminoterminal amino acids *(36)*. A specific carboxypeptidase that can remove a C-terminal amino acid from various Ang peptides was identified from a human heart failure ventricle cDNA library *(37)* and from a human lymphoma cDNA library *(38)*. This enzyme has been termed ACE2 and although having a similar catalytic domain to ACE, it is present in only heart, kidney, and testis. Although ACE2 can convert Ang I to Ang(1–9), it is 400 times more active in degrading Ang II to Ang(1–7) *(39)*. In ACE2 knockout mice, Ang II levels are increased in the kidney and heart suggesting that ACE2 is important in the degradation of Ang II *(40)*. ACE2 mRNA expression is reduced in renal tubules of STZ diabetic rats *(41)*. In a preliminary study, we have also found decreased ACE2 activity in

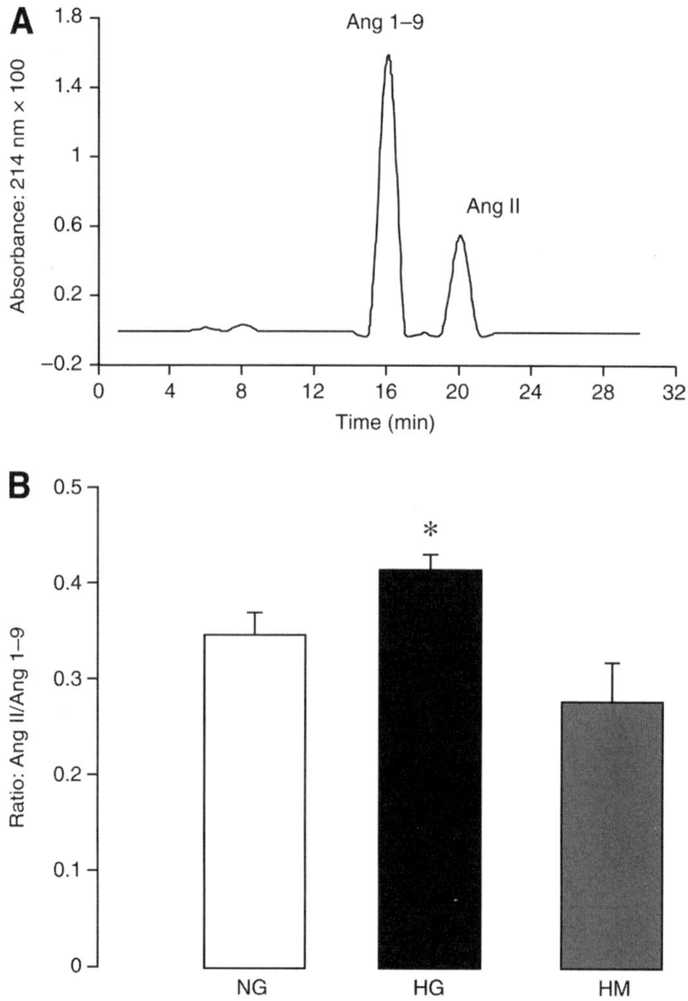

Fig. 3. (A) A sample chromatograph showing formation of Ang II from exogenously added Ang(1–9) ($10^{-4}M$) in mesangial cell extracts. **(B)** The effect of 30 m*M* glucose (HG) on formation of Ang II from Ang(1–9) in mesangial cell extracts. The peak absorbance for Ang II or Ang(1–9) was calculated from the respective peak height. A significant increase in Ang II/Ang(1–9) peak ratio was observed in HG suggesting that formation of Ang II from exogenously added Ang(1–9) is increased in mesangial cells incubated in HG. NG, normal (5 m*M*) glucose; HM, osmotic control (5 m*M* glucose + 25 m*M* mannitol). Values presented are mean ± SEM of three experiments. The asterisk denotes $p < 0.05$ vs NG and HM. (From ref. *18* with permission.)

glomerular extracts of STZ diabetic rats (Fig. 4). Further studies are needed to establish the role of ACE2 in the regulation of Ang II levels in the diabetic kidney.

Angiotensin(1–7)

Ang(1–7) can be formed from Ang II (via ACE2), Ang(1–9) (via ACE), or from Ang I via neutral endopeptidases (Fig. 5). Of the various metabolites of Ang II, this peptide has generated the most interest because it has important physiological functions that are often opposed to those of Ang II *(42)*. Ang(1–7) has antiproliferative effects *(43)*, acts as an endogenous ACE inhibitor *(44)*, and may also downregulate AT_1 receptors *(45)*. Additionally, Ang(1–7) attenuates Ang II-induced vasoconstriction *(46)* and dilates rabbit-afferent arterioles *(47)*. The latter effect is blocked by A-779, a selective

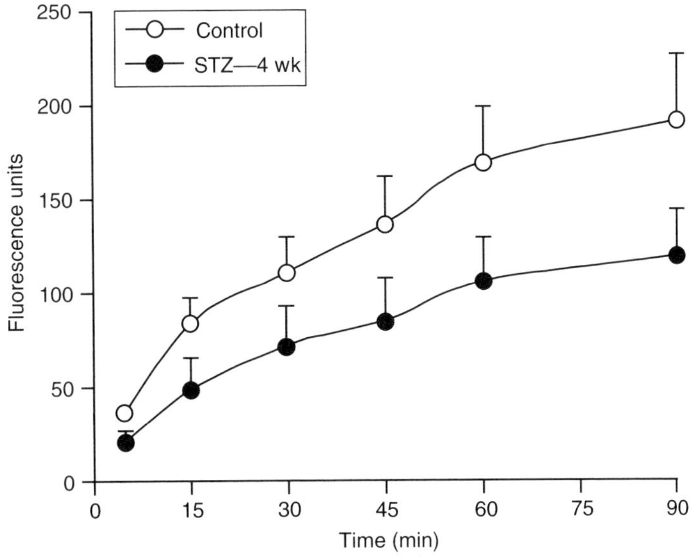

Fig. 4. ACE2 activity in control and STZ diabetic rat glomeruli. The figure depicts the time-course of conversion of a fluorogenic substrate to product. ACE2 activity was reduced in STZ diabetic rat glomerular extracts. Values are mean ± SEM ($n = 3$ rats for each group).

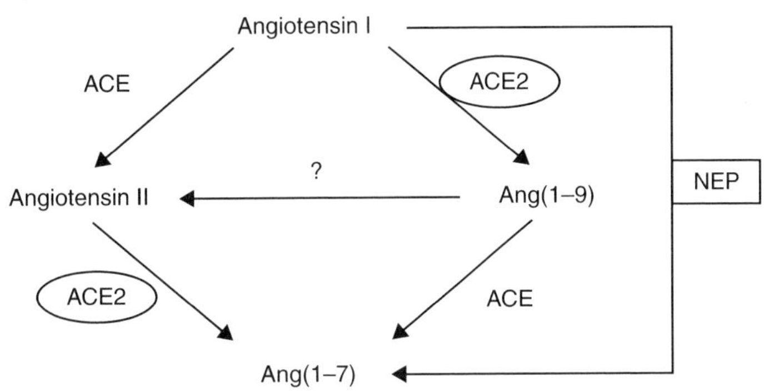

Fig. 5. Metabolic pathways leading to formation of Ang(1–7) from Ang I and other Ang peptides. NEP, neutral endopeptidase; ?, unknown carboxypeptidase.

Ang(1–7) antagonist, but not by AT_1 and AT_2 receptor antagonists *(47)*, suggesting that a specific receptor may exist for Ang(1–7). The effects of Ang(1–7) on matrix accumulation in diabetes requires further study.

ANG II RECEPTORS

Ang II Receptor Subtypes

Ang II is known to mediate its various effects by binding to two specific receptors, AT_1 and AT_2, and both have been shown to belong to the G protein-coupled receptor superfamily. In some species, such as rats and mice, there are two subtypes of AT_1 receptors: AT_{1a} and AT_{1b}. Most of the known effects of Ang II in glomerular MCs are mediated via activation of AT_1 receptors *(48)*. Although AT_2 receptors are also described for rat mesangial cells *(49)*, their role in Ang II-mediated effects in kidney are not fully understood.

AT_1 receptors are seven-transmembrane domain receptors and their primary structures have been described by molecular cloning *(50)*. The activation of signaling mechanisms due to binding of Ang II to the AT_1 receptor depends on many factors, including the rate of transcription, stability, and translational efficiency of the receptor mRNA as well as degradation of the receptor protein, because these factors regulate the availability of the receptors. A direct relationship between AT_1 receptor mRNA levels and Ang II-binding sites has been shown in glomeruli and MCs *(51)*. Whereas exposure to Ang II resulted in downregulation of AT_1 receptor mRNA and protein expression in MCs *(51)*, AT_1 receptor mRNA was upregulated in proximal tubular cells *(52)*. Upregulation of AT_2 receptors by Ang II has been noted in rat cerebral cortical neuronal cultures, but it is not clear if this also occurs in the kidney *(53)*.

Ang II binding to its receptors at the cell membrane is followed by translocation of the Ang II–AT_1 receptor complex to the intracellular vesicles *(54)* with internalization occurring with a half-life of less than 2 min *(55)*. In contrast to AT_2 receptors, which are not internalized, AT_1 receptors are recycled from endosomal vesicles to the plasma cell membrane. The internalized Ang II is either degraded or it may be translocated to the nucleus, where it may directly affect gene transcription as shown in the case of hepatic cells *(56)*. Alternatively, Ang II may activate intracellular kinases, which subsequently activate nuclear transcription factors. Although receptor-ligand internalization is an accepted mechanism by which Ang II gains access inside the cell, the generation of locally synthesized Ang II and its interaction with intracellular Ang II receptors cannot be excluded (discussed in the following subsection).

In the kidney, AT_2 receptors are known to increase nitric oxide release and cyclic-guanosine-monophosphate (cGMP) levels and binding of Ang II to these receptors induces vasodilation *(57)*. The role of AT_2 receptors in mediating growth- and matrix-promoting effects of Ang II is not well understood, but appears to counteract the effects of the AT_1 receptor *(58)*. A reduction in glomerular AT_2 receptor protein expression has been observed in STZ diabetes *(59)*. Whether or not this is beneficial is not clear, since the activated AT_2 receptor may also mediate adverse events such as stimulation of proinflammatory pathways by induction of nuclear factor-κB *(60,61)*.

Activation of AT_1 receptors by Ang II initiates stimulation of signal transduction pathways including activation of phospholipases A_2 and C, inositol triphosphate, intracellular calcium release, activation of protein kinase C (PKC), and inhibition of adenylate cyclase activity *(62)*. In addition, Ang II-mediated growth effects are carried out by the activation of cellular tyrosine kinase pathways such as p21 ras, C-Src, the Janus-activated kinase/signal transducer and activator of transcription pathway, and MAPKs *(62)*. Recent studies have also shown that Ang II stimulates the activation of an MAPK termed extracellular signal-regulated kinase *(63)* and that extracellular signal-regulated kinase, through activation of transcription factor activator protein-1, is involved in Ang II-induced increase in TGF-β_1 mRNA expression *(64)*. Ang II also increases generation of ROS via activation of the reduced form of NAD(P)H oxidase *(5)*, whereby ROS act as a signaling pathway for transduction of Ang II effects. The stimulatory effect of Ang II on ROS is mediated via AT_1 receptor-linked activation of NAD(P)H because this effect of Ang II is blocked by AT_1 antagonist, losartan, as well as by the flavoprotein inhibitor diphenylene iodoinium (DPI) *(31)*. Also, AT_1 receptors stimulate expression of the cell cycle-dependent kinase inhibitors (such as $p27^{kip1}$) which plays an important role in Ang II-mediated cell hypertrophy *(65)*.

The signaling pathways linked with AT_2 receptor activation are not fully understood. However, AT_2 receptor activation has been shown to cause decreased MAPK activity *(66)*, which may be associated with antiproliferative effects in non-renal cells *(67)*.

Autocrine/Paracrine vs Intracrine Effects of Ang II

The *de novo* tissue generation of Ang II and its binding to Ang II receptors present either on the same or adjacent cell membranes results in activation of signaling mechanisms leading to autocrine or paracrine effects, respectively. Recently, it has been proposed that Ang II may exert "intracrine" effects by binding to receptors present on intracellular organelles *(68)*. Possible modes of intracellular action include binding to receptors in endoplasmic reticulum, intracellular vesicles after internalization, nuclear membrane, nucleolar components, or chromatin *(68)*. The binding of Ang II to these intracellular receptors may also activate intracellular second messengers, eventually leading to biological effects, whereas Ang II binding to nuclear receptors could directly stimulate gene transcription. For example, Ang II binding to hepatic nuclear receptors resulted in increased mRNA gene expression for renin and angiotensinogen *(56)*. These intracrine actions of Ang II may mediate the effects of glucose/diabetes on cell metabolism and matrix synthesis (*see* next section).

MECHANISMS OF ACTION OF ANG II

Glucose Transport

Among the six glucose transporters described, glucose transporter 1 (GLUT1) is the predominant form expressed in mesangial cells *(69)*. Ang II increases glucose uptake by upregulation of GLUT1 mRNA expression in mesangial cells *(70)*. Overexpression of GLUT1 has been shown to result in increased synthesis of extracellular matrix proteins *(71,72)*. Also, TGF-β_1 that is stimulated by Ang II has been shown to increase GLUT1 expression and glucose uptake in MCs *(73)*. Single-nucleotide polymorphisms (SNPs) at the GLUT1 locus have been reported to enhance susceptibility to diabetic nephropathy in type 1 diabetes mellitus, suggesting that a hereditary disposition to increased cellular uptake could be of pathogenic importance in patients with diabetic nephropathy *(74,75)*.

Glucose flux through the hexosamine pathway has been implicated in some of the adverse effects of glucose *(76)* via changes in the final product, uridine diphosphate *N*-acetylglucosamine (UDP-GlcNac) which participates in the *O*-glycosylation of transcription factors *(77)*. Under physiological conditions, a small percentage of glucose entering cells is shunted through the hexosamine pathway, which is regulated by the rate-limiting enzyme, glutamine:fructose-6-phosphate amidotransferase (GFAT; *77)*. Ang II has been shown to activate the GFAT promoter in mesangial cells *(78)*, thus increasing glucose shunting into the hexasoamine pathway in addition to increasing cellular uptake of glucose.

TGF-β_1 and Extracellular Matrix Accumulation

The major matrix proteins expressed in mesangial cells are fibronectin, collagen I, collagen IV, and laminin *(79)*. Ang II has been shown to stimulate synthesis of matrix proteins in MCs via induction of TGF-β_1 *(3)*. In addition to increased synthesis, accumulation of ECM in the presence of high glucose can also result from decreased degradation of matrix proteins *(80)*. The enzymes involved in the degradation of matrix proteins are known as matrix metalloproteinases (MMPs) *(81)*, of which MMP-2 is predominant in MCs. Mesangial matrix is degraded by MMP-2; in addition, the protease plasmin both activates MMPs and itself degrades matrix. Activity of MMPs is also regulated by specific protein inhibitors called tissue inhibitors of metalloproteinases (TIMPs), TIMP-2 being the specific inhibitor of MMP-2 *(81)*. Plasmin activity is regulated by the plasminogen activators (PA) and their inhibitors (PAI-1,2) *(82)*. In rat MCs, the inhibitory effects of Ang II on matrix degradation are mediated via decreased MMP-2 activity *(4)* and increased production of PAI-1 *(82)*. Also, Ang II decreased MMP-2 levels in MCs and this effect of Ang II was accompanied by an increase in TGF-β_1 secretion *(4)* (Fig. 6). As TGF-β_1 also inhibits MMP-2 activity and increases TIMP-2 levels in a concentration-dependent fashion *(83)*, it is likely that the effects of Ang II on MMP-2 and TIMP-2 are mediated by TGF-β_1. Ang II-induced upregulation of PAI-1 gene transcription is also mediated in part through induction of TGF-β_1 *(82)*.

Reactive Oxygen Species

ROS include superoxide anion, hydrogen peroxide (H_2O_2), and free hydroxyl radical. At low levels, ROS function as redox signaling molecules but increased generation or accumulation of ROS and/or oxidative products may cause oxidative injury. ROS can be produced by mitochondrial oxidative phosphorylation *(84)* and cytoplasmic oxidative enzymes such as NAD(P)H oxidase *(85)*. Among the two types of NAD(P)H oxidases, the non-phagocytic NAD(P)H oxidases, as opposed to phagocytic oxidases, generate constitutive low levels of superoxide in a predominantly intracellular location. Both types of NADPH oxidases express p22phox, p47phox, rac1, and the p67phox subunits and both possess a catalytic moiety (gp91phox or a nox isoform, either nox 1-5), which is inhibited by DPI.

Ang II increases superoxide production by activating NAD(P)H oxidase probably via a PKC-dependent pathway *(5)*. Activation of NAD(P)H oxidase occurs via translocation of p47 phox from the cytoplasm to the membrane, as endothelial cells from p47 phox knockout mice do not produce superoxide from Ang II *(86,87)*. Also, recent studies have suggested that Ang II-induced increased H_2O_2 production is mediated by the activation of the p22 phox subunit of NAD(P)H because transfection of cells with antisense p22 phox reduced NAD(P)H oxidase activity and H_2O_2 production *(88)*. Additionally, Gorin et al. *(89)* found that Ang II-induced increased protein synthesis was absent in MCs transfected with antisense nox4, suggesting that activation of nox4 subunit of NAD(P)H oxidase may also be involved in Ang II-linked superoxide generation and cell proliferation. The effect of Ang II on NAD(P)H oxidase activity is mediated via AT1 receptor activation because both superoxide and H_2O_2 production were blocked by AT1 receptor antagonists *(31,88)*.

ROS are scavenged by antioxidant enzymes such as catalase, glutathione peroxidase, and superoxide dismutase (SOD). Mostly, H_2O_2 is derived by dismutation of the free radical superoxide by SOD and is converted to H_2O by catalase or scavenged by glutathione peroxidase. Recent studies have shown that neither SOD activity *(31,88)* nor catalase activity *(88)* was affected by Ang II. However, upregulation of heme oxygenase-1, an antioxidant enzyme, ameliorated Ang II-induced oxidant injury in proximal tubules *(90)*.

Interrelationships Between Glucose, Ang II, ROS, TGF-β_1, and Matrix Accumulation

In recent years, oxidative stress has been proposed as the cause of diabetic complications *(84)*. NAD(P)H oxidase activity is significantly enhanced in diabetic glomeruli,

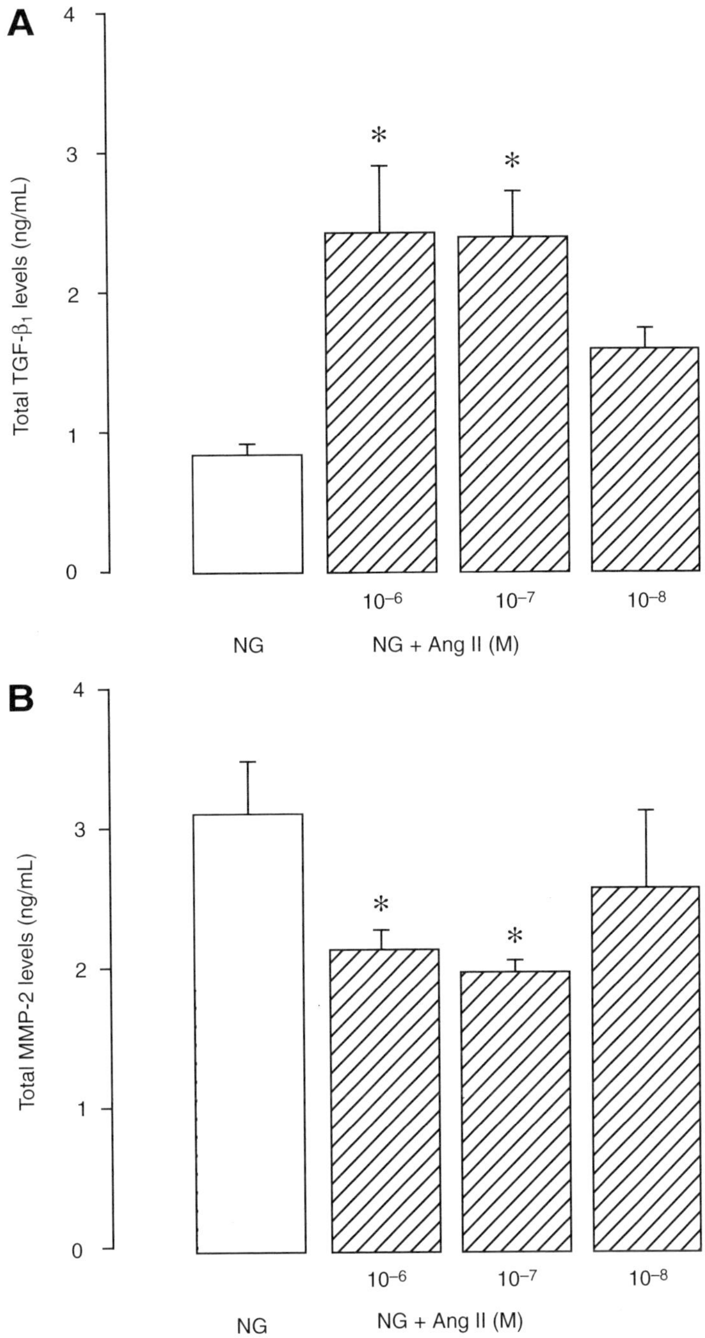

Fig. 6. Effect of Ang II on TGF-β_1 and MMP-2 levels in mesangial cells incubated in NG plus various concentrations of Ang II for 24 h. Cell media were analyzed for total TGF-β_1 and MMP-2 levels by ELISA. Ang II significantly increased TGF-β_1 secretion and decreased MMP-2 secretion at the higher concentrations of Ang II. Values are mean ± SEM of three experiments. The asterisk denotes $p < 0.05$ compared with NG. (From ref. *4* with permission.)

and its activity is decreased by treatment with the PKC-β inhibitor ruboxistaurin, which prevents membranous translocation of glomerular p47 phox (as well as p67phox) *(91)*.

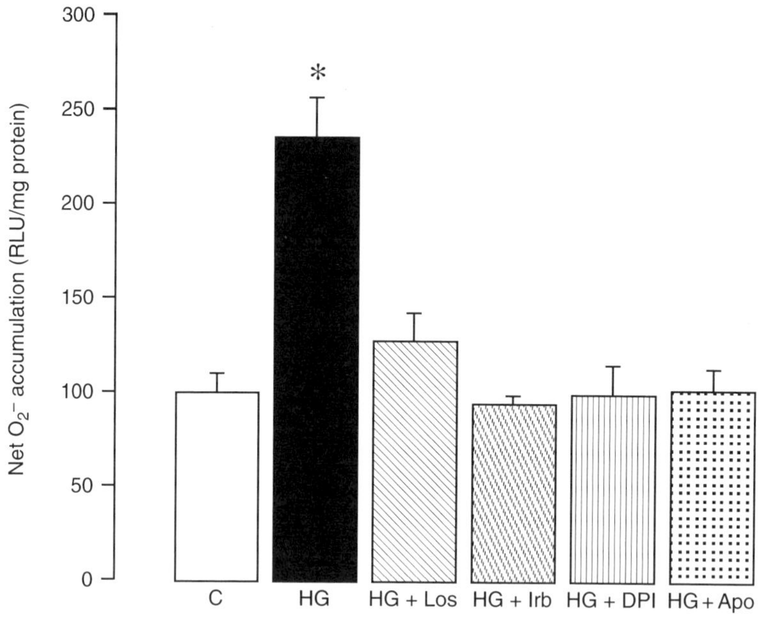

Fig. 7. Effect of high glucose on net superoxide (O_2^-) accumulation in human mesangial cells. Cells were incubated in 10 m*M* glucose (C), HG, or HG with either AT_1 antagonists [losartan (Los) or irbesartan (Irb)] or NAD(P)H oxidase inhibitors [DPI or apocynin (Apo)] (all $10^{-4}M$) for 24 h. O_2^- accumulation was measured using the chemiluminescence of lucigenin and represented as relative light units (RLU)/mg protein. The HG-induced increase in O_2^- accumulation was prevented by both AT_1 antagonists and NAD(P)H oxidase inhibitors. Values are mean ± SEM of five experiments. The asterisk denotes $p < 0.01$ compared with the other five groups. (From ref. *31* with permission.)

Because Ang II also stimulates NAD(P)H oxidase activity (*see* "Reactive Oxygen Species" section), it is possible that oxidative stress in high glucose/diabetes may be due to stimulation of the Ang II-NAD(P)H oxidase system. Indeed, our recent studies have demonstrated that high glucose-induced superoxide accumulation was blocked by the AT_1 antagonists losartan and irbesartan as well as by NAD(P)H oxidase inhibitors apocynin and DPI *(31)* (Fig. 7). Studies in STZ diabetic rats have further characterized the link between Ang II, NAD(P)H oxidase, and ROS. Increased expression of NAD(P)H oxidase subunits nox4 and p22phox and reversibility by insulin treatment have been observed in 4- and 8-wk STZ diabetic rats *(92)*. Also, STZ-induced diabetes is associated with increased lipid peroxidation and protein carbonylation in renal cortex which were improved with insulin, antioxidants, and ACE/ARBs *(93,94)*. These data suggest that Ang II-induced ROS formation may be a critical mediator of the deleterious effects of high glucose.

To summarize, data from our laboratory and others indicate that high glucose/diabetes increases intracellular Ang II levels. The role of Ang II in increased TGF-β_1 secretion and matrix accumulation has been well established. However, studies from our laboratory using ARBs have demonstrated that Ang II inhibition prevents high glucose-induced increase in TGF-β_1 secretion (Fig. 8) and collagen accumulation (Fig. 9) in mesangial cells *(4)*. In addition, intracellular Ang II production in response to high glucose leads to ROS generation via NAD(P)H oxidase *(31)*. ROS may subsequently stimulate TGF-β_1 secretion, which in turn may activate NAD(P)H

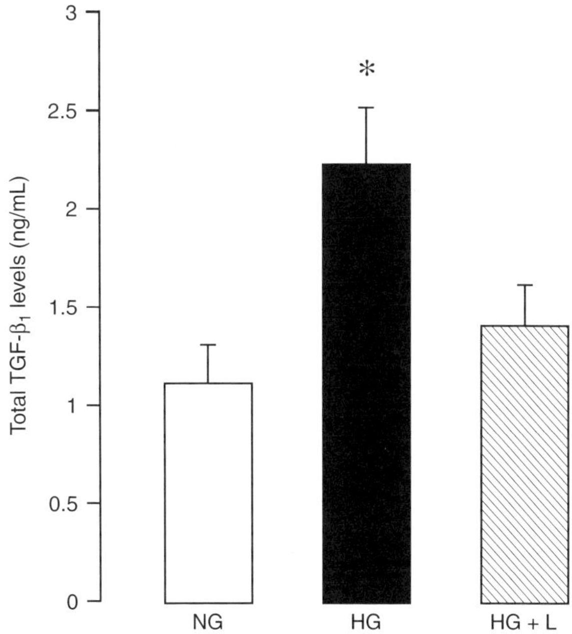

Fig. 8. Total TGF-β_1 levels in media from mesangial cells incubated in NG, HG, or HG + $10^{-4}M$ of the AT_1 receptor antagonist losartan (HG + L). Losartan prevented the glucose-induced increase in TGF-β_1. Values are mean ± SEM of six experiments. The asterisk denotes $p < 0.05$ vs NG and HG + L. (From ref. *4* with permission.)

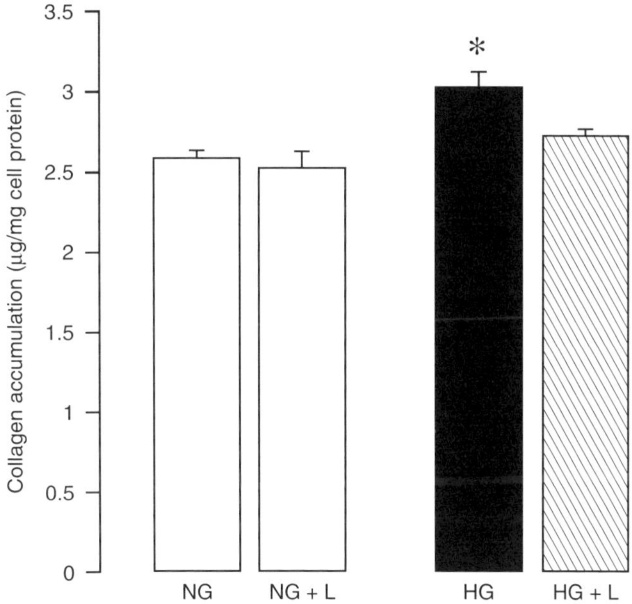

Fig. 9. Mesangial cell collagen accumulation in response to NG or HG in the presence or absence of $10^{-4}M$ L. The glucose-induced increase in collagen accumulation was prevented by losartan. Values are mean ± SEM of 10 experiments. The asterisk denotes $p < 0.05$ vs NG, NG + L, and HG + L. (From ref. *4* with permission.)

oxidase activity, leading to more ROS production *(85)*. The stimulatory effect of TGF-β_1 on matrix protein gene expression via Smad pathways is also well established *(95)*.

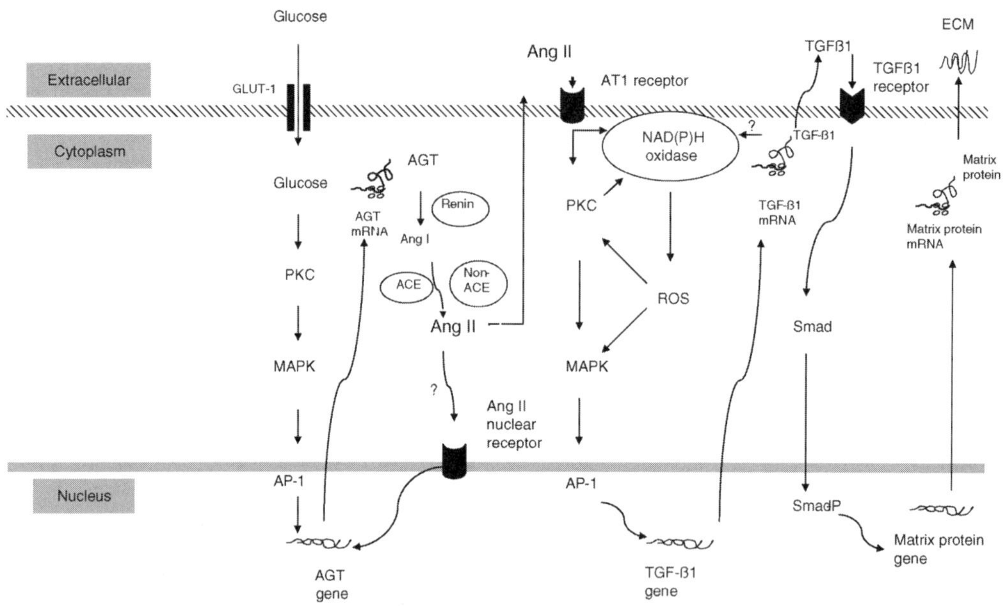

Fig. 10. Postulated interrelationships between glucose, Ang II, ROS, transforming growth factor (TGF)-β_1, and extracellular matrix (ECM) protein accumulation in renal mesangial cells. GLUT1, mesangial glucose transporter; PKC, protein kinase C; MAPK, mitogen-activated protein kinase; AP-1, activated protein-1 (transcription factor); AGT, angiotensinogen; Ang I, angiotensin I; AT1, Ang type 1; ROS, reactive oxygen species; Smad, nuclear transcription factor for TGF-β_1.

Our hypothesis that high glucose increases Ang II levels, which in turn stimulates ROS production via NAD(P)H oxidase activation leading to enhanced production of TGF-β_1 and matrix accumulation is depicted in Fig. 10.

FUTURE DIRECTIONS

The importance of Ang II in matrix remodeling in glomerular mesangium has become increasingly evident. Recent studies have established the presence of a functional RAS within the glomerulus that includes MCs and proximal tubules. Glucose stimulates RAS activity in these tissues, specifically by increasing angiotensinogen and Ang II production. The effects of Ang II occur in autocrine, paracrine, or intracrine fashion, the latter being a relatively new concept that remains to be explored in the future. However, intracrine (intacellular) actions of Ang II suggest that Ang II may act as a signaling peptide. For example, Ang II produced locally inside the cell can either stimulate other intracellular signaling pathways or bind to nuclear receptors to initiate transcriptional changes for particular genes. Indeed, at least in the hepatic cells, Ang II has been shown to regulate angiotensinogen and renin gene transcription and expression by binding to nuclear receptors. In view of these findings, it is important to explore the localization of nuclear Ang II receptors and their role in the regulation of gene transcription and expression of matrix proteins in glomerular MCs.

Future work related to the local RAS also should be focused on some of the newly discovered members of the RAS, such as prorenin/renin receptors, ACE2, and Ang(1–7). Recently, renin and prorenin have been shown to bind to receptor-binding proteins causing cell hypertrophy and increased conversion of angiotensinogen to

Ang I and Ang II within the cell. Thus, a study of the functional role of the prorenin/renin receptor in tissue Ang II production may provide useful explanations for the increased RAS activity in diabetes mellitus and lead to new approaches to prevent this enhanced activity. In addition, ACE2 has emerged as a regulator of Ang II levels in the heart and kidney by converting or inactivating Ang II to Ang(1–7). The study of ACE2 in diabetes should prove useful in understanding the mechanisms by which glucose increases Ang II accumulation in glomeruli. Indeed, preliminary work from our laboratory has shown that ACE2 activity is decreased in glomerular extracts from STZ diabetic rats compared with controls, suggesting that inhibition of ACE2 activity may be one of the mechanisms by which Ang II levels are increased in the glomeruli from STZ diabetic rats. Future studies are also warranted on understanding the role of Ang(1–7) in matrix remodeling in the glomerular mesangium because this peptide has been shown to counterbalance the effects of Ang II in the heart, blood vessels, and kidneys, probably via an unknown receptor that has yet to be identified.

It is clear that our understanding of the intrarenal RAS is still rudimentary, but in the past few decades much progress has been made. Few now doubt the existence and importance of the intrarenal RAS. Further research on the intracellular effects of Ang II and related peptides should advance our knowledge on the role of intrarenal RAS in the development of diabetic nephropathy.

REFERENCES

1. Mogensen CE, Cooper ME. Diabetic renal disease: from recent studies to improved clinical practice. Diabet Med 2004;21(1):4–17.
2. Leehey DJ, Singh AK, Alavi N, Singh R. Role of angiotensin II in diabetic nephropathy. Kidney Int 2000;58(77):S93–S98.
3. Kagami S, Border WA, Miller DE, Noble NA. Angiotensin II stimulated extracellular matrix protein synthesis through induction of transforming growth factor-β expression in rat glomerular cells. J Clin Invest 1994;93:2431–2437.
4. Singh R, Alavi N, Singh AK, Leehey DJ. Role of angiotensin II in glucose-induced inhibition of mesangial matrix degradation. Diabetes 1999;48:2066–2073.
5. Jaimes EA, Galceran JM, Raij L. Angiotensin II induces superoxide anion production by mesangial cells. Kidney Int 1998;54(3):775–784.
6. Cassis LA. Downregulation of the renin-angiotensin system in streptozotocin-diabetic rats. Am J Physiol 1992;262:E105–E109.
7. Brown L, Wall D, Marchant C, Sernia C. Tissue-specific changes in angiotensin II receptors in streptozotocin-diabetic rats. J Endocrinol 1997;154:355–362.
8. Vallon V, Mead LM, Blantz RC. Renal hemodynamics and plasma and kidney angiotensin II in established diabetes mellitus in rats: effects of sodium and salt restriction. J Am Soc Nephrol 1995;5:1761–1767.
9. Harker CT, O'Donnell MP, Rossetti RG, Guberski DL, Like AA. The renin-angiotensin II system in the type II diabetic obese Zucker rat. J Am Soc Nephrol 1993;4:1354–1361.
10. Miller JA, Floras JS, Zinman B, Skorecki KL, Logan AG. Effect of hyperglycemia on arterial pressure, plasma renin activity, and renal function in early diabetes. Clin Sci 1996;90:189–195.
11. Price DA, Porter LE, Gordon M, et al. The paradox of the low-renin state in diabetic nephropathy. J Am Soc Nephrol 1999;10:2382–2391.
12. Atiyeh BA, Arant BS Jr, Henrich WL, Seikaly MG. In vitro production of angiotensin II by isolated glomeruli. Am J Physiol 1995;268:F266–F272.
13. Becker BN, Yasuda T, Kondo S, Vaikunth S, Homma T, Harris RC. Mechanical stretch/relaxation stimulates a cellular renin-angiotensin system in cultured rat mesangial cells. Exp Nephrol 1998; 6:57–66.
14. Andrade MC, Quinto BM, Carmona AK, et al. Purification and characterization of angiotensin I-converting enzymes from mesangial cells in culture. J Hypertens 1998;16(12 Part 2):2063–2074.

15. Seikaly MG, Arant BS Jr, Seney FD Jr. Endogenous angiotensin concentrations in specific intrarenal fluid compartments in the rat. J Clin Invest 1990;86:1352–1357.
16. Nishiyama A, Seth DM, Navar LG. Renal interstitial fluid concentrations of angiotensins I and II in anesthetized rats. Hypertension 2002;39:129–134.
17. vanKats JP, Schalekamp MA, Verdouw PD, et al. Intrarenal angiotensin II: interstitial and cellular levels and site of production. Kidney Int 2001;60:2311–2317.
18. Singh R, Singh AK, Alavi N, Leehey DJ. Mechanism of increased angiotensin II levels in glomerular mesangial cells cultured in high glucose. J Am Soc Nephrol 2003;14:873–880.
19. Anderson S, Jung FF, Inglefinger JR. Renin-angiotensin system in diabetic rats: functional, immunohistochemical, and molecular biologic correlations. Am J Physiol 1993;265:F477–F486.
20. Singh R, Singh AK, Leehey DJ. A novel mechanism for angiotensin II formation in streptozotocin-diabetic rat glomeruli. Am J Physiol Renal Physiol 2005;288:F1183–1190.
21. Zhang SL, Tang SS, Chen X, Filep JG, Inglefinger JR, Chan JSD. High levels of glucose stimulate angiotensinogen gene expression via the p38 mitogen-activated protein kinase pathway in rat kidney proximal tubular cells. Endocrinology 2000;141(12):4637–4646.
22. Hsieh TJ, Zhang SL, Filep JG, Tang SS, Ingelfinger JR, Chan JS. High glucose stimulates angiotensinogen gene expression via reactive oxygen species generation in rat kidney proximal tubular cells. Endocrinology 2002;143(8):2975–2985.
23. Hsieh TJ, Fustier P, Zhang SL, et al. High glucose stimulates angiotensinogen gene expression and cell hypertrophy via activation of the hexosamine biosynthesis pathway in rat kidney proximal tubular cells. Endocrinology 2003;144:4338–4349.
24. Andrade AQ, Casarini DE, Schor N, Boim MA. Characterization of renin mRNA expression and enzyme activity in rat and mouse mesangial cells. Braz J Med Biol Res 2002;35:17–24.
25. Nguyen G, Delarue F, Berrou J, Rondeau E, Sraer JD. Specific receptor binding of renin on human mesangial cells in culture increases plasminogen activator inhibitor-1 antigen. Kidney Int 1996;50:1897–1903.
26. Neves FAR, Duncan KG, Baxter JD. Cathepsin B is a prorenin processing enzyme. Hypertension 1996;27:514–517.
27. Vidotti DB, Casarini DE, Cristovam PC, Leite CA, Schor N, Boim MA. High glucose concentration stimulates intracellular renin activity and angiotensin II generation in rat mesangial cells. Am J Physiol Renal Physiol 2004;286(6):F1039–F1045.
28. Nguyen G, Delarue F, Burckle C, Bouzhir L, Giller T, Sraer JD. Pivotal role of the renin/prorenin receptor in angiotensin II production and cellular responses to renin. J Clin Invest 2002; 109(11):1417–1427.
29. Ichihara A, Hayashi M, Kaneshiro Y, et al. Inhibition of diabetic nephropathy by a decoy peptide corresponding to the "handle" region for nonproteolytic activation of prorenin. J Clin Invest 2004;114:1128–1135.
30. Casarini DE, Boim MA, Stella RCR, Krieger-Azzolini MH, Krieger KE, Schor N. Angiotensin I-converting enzyme activity in tubular fluid along the rat nephron. Am J Physiol 1997;272:F405–F409.
31. Leehey DJ, Isreb MA, Marcic S, Singh AK, Singh R. Effect of high glucose on superoxide in human mesangial cells: role of angiotensin II. Nephron Exp Nephrol 2005;100:46–53.
32. Akasu M, Urata H, Kinoshita A, Sasaguri M, Ideishi M, Arakawa K. Differences in tissue angiotensin II-forming pathways by species and organs in vitro. Hypertension 1998;32(3):514–520.
33. Urata H, Kinoshita A, Misono KS, Bumpus FM, Husain A. Identification of a highly specific chymase as the major angiotensin II-forming enzyme in the human heart. J Biol Chem 1990;265(36): 22,348–22,357.
34. Huang XR, Chen WY, Truong LD, Lan HY. Chymase is upregulated in diabetic nephropathy: implications for an alternative pathway of angiotensin II-mediated diabetic renal and vascular disease. J Am Soc Nephrol 2003;14(7):1952–1954.
35. Wei CC, Tian B, Perry G, et al. Differential Ang II generation in plasma and tissue of mice with decreased expression of the ACE gene. Am J Physiol Heart Cir Physiol 2002;282:H2254–H2258.
36. Ardaillou R, Chansel D. Synthesis and effects of active fragments of angiotensin II. Kidney Int 1997;52(6):1458–1468.
37. Donoghue M, Hsieh F, Baronas E, et al. A novel angiotensin-converting enzyme-related carboxypeptidase (ACE2) converts angiotensin I to angiotensin 1-9. Circ Res 2000;87:e1–e9.
38. Tipnis SA, Hooper NM, Hyde R, Karran E, Christie G, Turner AJ. A human homolog of angiotensin-converting enzyme. J Biol Chem 2000;275:33,238–33,243.

39. Vickers C, Hales P, Kaushik V et al. Hydrolysis of biological peptides by human angiotensin-converting enzyme-related carboxypeptidase. J Biol Chem 2002;277:14,838–14,843.
40. Crackower MA, Sarao R, Oudlt GY, et al. Angiotensin-converting enzyme 2 is an essential regulator of heart function. Nature 2002;417:822–828.
41. Tikellis C, Johnston CI, Forbes JM, et al. Characterization of renal angiotensin-converting enzyme 2 in diabetic nephropathy. Hypertension 2003;41(3):392–397.
42. Ferrario CM, Iyer SN. Angiotensin-(1–7): a bioactive fragment of the rennin-angiotensin system. Reg Peptides 1998;78:13–18.
43. Freeman EJ, Chisolm GM, Ferrario CM, Tallant EA. Angiotensin(1–7) inhibits vascular smooth muscle cell growth. Hypertension 1996;28:104–108.
44. Deddish PA, Marcic B, Jackman HL, Wang HZ, Skidgel AR, Erdos EG. N-domain specific substrate and C-domain inhibition of angiotensin-converting enzyme: angiotensin(1–7) and keto-ACE. Hypertension 1998;31:912–917.
45. Clark MA, Diz DI, Tallant EA. Angiotensin-(1–7) downregulates the angiotensin II type 1 receptor in vascular smooth muscle cells. Hypertension 2001;37:1141–1146.
46. Santos RAS, Campagnole-Santos MJ, Andrade SP. Angiotensin-(1–7): an update. Regul Pept 2000;91:45–62.
47. Ren Y, Garvin JL, Carretero OA. Vasodilator action of angiotensin-(1–7) on isolated rabbit afferent arterioles. Hypertension 2002;39(3):799–802.
48. Ardaillou R, Chansel D, Chatziantoniou C, Dussaule J. Mesangial AT_1 receptors: expression, signaling, and regulation. J Am Soc Nephrol 1999;10:S40–S46.
49. Goto M, Makoyama M, Suga S, et al. Growth-dependent induction of angiotensin type 2 receptor in rat mesangial cells. Hypertension 1997;30:358–362.
50. Murphy TJ, Alexander RW, Griendling KK, Runge MS, Bernstein KE. Isolation of a cDNA encoding the vascular type-1 angiotensin II receptor. Nature 1991;351:233–236.
51. Makita N, Iwai N, Inagami T, Badr KF. Two distinct pathways in the down-regulation of type-1 angiotensin II receptor genes in rat glomerular mesangial cells. Biochem Biophys Res Commun 1992;185:142–146.
52. Cheng H-F, Becker BN, Burns KD, Harris RC. Angiotensin II upregulates type-1 angiotensin II receptors in renal proximal tubule. J Clin Invest 1995;77:1993–2000.
53. Gallinat S, Busche S, Raizada MK, Sumners C. The angiotensin II type 2 receptor: An enigma with multiple variations. Am J Physiol 2000;278:E357–E374.
54. Sasamura H, Hein L, Saruta T, Pratt RE. Evidence for internalization of both type 1 angiotensin receptors subtypes (AT_{1a}, AT_{1b}) by a protein kinase C independent mechanism. Hypertens Res 1997;20:295–300.
55. Anderson KM, Murahashi T, Dostal DE, Peach MJ. Morphological and biochemical analysis of angiotensin II internalization in cultured rat aortic smooth muscle cells. Am J Physiol 1993;264: C179–C188.
56. Eggena P, Zhu JH, Clegg K, Barrett JD. Nuclear angiotensin receptors induce transcription of renin and angiotensinogen mRNA. Hypertension 1993;22:496–501.
57. Siragy HM, Carey RM. The subtype 2 (AT2) angiotensin receptor mediates renal production of nitric oxide in conscious rats. J Clinc Invest 1997;100:264–269.
58. Nakajima M, Hutchinson HG, Fujinaga M, et al. The angiotensin II type 2 (AT2) receptor antagonizes the growth effects of the AT1 receptor: gain of function study using gene transfer. Proc Natl Acad Sci USA 1996;92:10,663–10,667.
59. Wehbi GJ, Zimpelmann J, Carey RM, Levine DZ, Burns KD. Early streptozotocin-diabetes mellitus downregulates rat kidney AT2 receptors. Am J Physiol Renal Physiol 2001;280(2):F254–F265.
60. Wolf G, Wenzel U, Burns KD, et al. Angiotensin II activates nuclear transcription factor-kappaB through AT1 and AT2 receptors. Kidney Int 2002;61:1986–1995.
61. Cao Z, Bonnet F, Candido R, et al. Angiotensin type 2 receptor antagonism confers renal protection in a rat model of progressive renal injury. J Am Soc Nephrol 2002;13:1773–1787.
62. Burns KD. Angiotensin II and its receptors in the diabetic kidney. Am J Kidney Dis 2000;36:449–467.
63. Griendling KK, Ushio Fukai M, Lassegue B, Alexander RW. Angiotensin II signaling in vascular smooth muscle: new concepts. Hypertension 1997;29:366–373.
64. Hamaguchi A, Kim S, Izumi Y, Zhan Y, Yamanaka S, Iwao H. Contribution of extracellular signal-regulated kinase to angiotensin II-induced transforming growth factor-β1 expression in vascular smooth muscle cells. Hypertension 1999;34:126–131.
65. Wolf G, Wenzel UO. Angiotensin and cell cycle regulation. Hypertension 2004;43:693–698.

66. Bedecs K, Elbaz N, Sutren M, et al. Angiotensin II type 2 receptors inhibition of mitogen-activated protein kinase cascade and functional activation of SHP-1 tyrosine phosphatase. Biochem J 1997;325:449–454.
67. Stoll M, Steckelings UM, Paul M, et al. The angiotensin AT2 receptor mediates inhibition of cell proliferation in coronary endothelial cells. J Clin Invest 1995;95:651–657.
68. Re R. The nature of intracrine peptide hormone action. Hypertension 1999;34:534–538.
69. Klip A, Tsakiridis T, Marette A, Ortiz PA. Regulation of expression of glucose transporters by glucose: a review of studies in vivo and in cell cultures. FASEB J 1994;8:43–53.
70. Nose A, Mori Y, Uchiyama-Tanaka Y, et al. Regulation of glucose transporter (GLUT1) gene expression by angiotensin II in mesangial cells: involvement of HB-EGF and EGF receptor transactivation. Hypertens Res 2003;26(1):67–73.
71. Heilig CW, Conception LA, Riser BL, Freytag SO, Zhu M, Cortes P. Overexpression of glucose transpoters in rat mesangial cells cultured in a normal glucose milieu mimics the diabetic phenotype. J Clin Invest 1995;96:1802–1814.
72. Weigert C, Brodbeck K, Brosius FC III, et al. Evidence for a novel TGF-b1-independent mechanism of fibronectin production in mesangial cells overexpressing glucose transporters. Diabetes 2003; 52:527–535.
73. Inoki K, Haneda M, Maeda S, Koya D, Kikkawa R. TGF-beta 1 stimulates glucose uptake by enhancing GLUT1 expression in mesangial cells. Kidney Int 1999;55:1704–1712.
74. Hodgkinson AD, Millward BA, Demaine AG. Polymorphisms of the glucose transporter (GLUT1) gene are associated with diabetic nephropathy. Kidney Int 2001;59:985–989.
75. Ng DP, Canani L, Araki S, et al. Minor effect of GLUT1 polymorphisms on susceptibility to diabetic nephropathy in type 1 diabetes. Diabetes 2002;51:2264–2269.
76. Hebert LF Jr, Daniels MC, Zhou J, et al. Overexpression of glutamine:fructose-6-phosphate amidotransferase in transgenic mice leads to insulin resistance. J Clin Invest 1996;98:930–936.
77. Marshall S, Bacote V, Traxinger RR. Discovery of a metabolic pathway mediating glucose-induced desensitization of the glucose transport system. Role of hexosamine biosynthesis in induction of insulin resistance. J Biol Chem 1991;266:4706–4712.
78. Leighton RJ, Ingram A, Ly H, Thai K, Cai L, Scholey JW. Angiotensin II activates the GFAT promoter in mesangial cells. Am J Physiol Renal Physiol 2001;281:F151–F162.
79. Ayo SH, Radnik RA, Glass WF II, et al. Increased extracellular matrix synthesis and mRNA in mesangial cells grown in high-glucose medium. Am J Physiol 1991;260:F185–F191.
80. Leehey DJ, Song RH, Alavi N, Singh AK. Decreased degradative enzymes in mesangial cells cultured in high glucose media. Diabetes 1995;44:929–935.
81. Birkedal-Hansen H. Role of matrix metalloproteinases in human periodontal diseases. J Periodontol 1993;64:474–484.
82. Kagami S, Kuhara T, Okada K, Kuroda Y, Border WA, Noble NA. Dual effects of angiotensin II on the plasminogen/plasmin system in rat mesangial cells. Kidney Int 1997;51(3):664–671.
83. Singh R, Song RH, Alavi N, Pegoraro AA, Singh AK, Leehey DJ. High glucose decreases matrix metalloproteinase-2 activity in rat mesangial cells via transforming growth factor-b1. Exp Nephrol 2001;9:249–257.
84. Nishikawa T, Edelstein D, Du XL, et al. Normalizing mitochondrial superoxide production blocks three pathways of hyperglycaemic damage. Nature 2000;404:787–790.
85. Lee HB, Yu M-R, Yang Y, Jiang Z, Ha H. Reactive oxygen species-regulated signaling pathways in diabetic nephropathy. J Am Soc Nephrol 2003,4:S241–S245.
86. Li J, Shah AM. Mechanism of endothelial cell NADPH oxidase activation by angiotensin II: Role of the p47phox subunit. J Biol Chem 2003;278:12,094–12,100.
87. Landmesser U, Cai H, Dikalov S, et al. Role of p47phox in vascular oxidative stress and hypertension caused by angiotensin II. Hypertension 2002;40:511–515.
88. Zafari AM, Ushio-Fukai M, Akers M, et al. Role of NADH/NADPH oxidase-derived H_2O_2 in angiotensin II-induced vascular hypertrophy. Hypertension 1998;32:488–495.
89. Gorin Y, Ricono JM, Kim H-N, Bhandari B, Choudhury GG, Abboud HE. Nox4 mediates angiotensin II-induced activation of Akt/protein kinase B in mesangial cells. Am J Physiol Renal Physiol 2003;285:F219–F229.
90. Quan S, Yang L, Shnouda S, et al. Expression of human heme oxygenase-1 in the thick ascending limb attenuates angiotensin II-mediated increase in oxidative injury. Kidney Int 2004;65(5): 1628–1639.

91. Kitada M, Koya D, Sugimoto T, et al. Translocation of glomerular p47phox and p67phox by protein kinase C-beta activation is required for oxidative stress in diabetic nephropathy. Diabetes 2003;52: 2603–2614.
92. Etoh T, Inoguchi T, Kakimoto M, et al. Increased expression of NAD(P)H oxidase subunits, nox4 and p22phox, in the kidney of streptozotocin-induced diabetic rats and its reversibility by interventive insulin treatment. Diabetologia 2003;46:1428–1437.
93. Koo JR, Vaziri ND. Effects of diabetes, insulin and antioxidants on NO synthase abundance and NO interaction with reactive oxygen species. Kidney Int 2003;63(1):195–201.
94. Onozato ML, Tojo A, Goto A, Fujita T, Wilcox CS. Oxidative stress and nitric oxide synthase in rat diabetic nephropathy: effects of ACEI and ARB. Kidney Int 2002;61:186–194.
95. Schnaper HW, Hayashida T, Hubchak SC, Poncelet AC. TGF-beta signal transduction and mesangial cell fibrogenesis. Am J Physiol Renal Physiol 2003;284:F243–F252.

2

Altered Renal Microvascular Function in Early Diabetes

Pamela K. Carmines, PhD, *Joseph P. Bast,* MD, *and Naohito Ishii,* PhD

CONTENTS

INTRODUCTION

The early stage of type 1 diabetes (T1D) is characterized by glomerular hyperfiltration that arises as the result of preglomerular (primarily afferent arteriolar) vasodilation. Although hyperglycemia is the trigger for this process, the mechanism linking hyperglycemia to reduced afferent arteriolar tone remains an area of active debate. It is well established that diabetic hyperglycemia provokes a condition of oxidative stress in many organs including the kidney. In this chapter, we consider the possible role of oxidative stress in producing a defect in afferent arteriolar electromechanical coupling that involves K^+ channel activation, membrane hyperpolarization, and a consequent decrease in Ca^{2+} influx through voltage-gated channels. As voltage-dependent Ca^{2+} influx is a primary determinant of afferent (but not efferent) arteriolar tone and vasoconstrictor responsiveness, this scenario offers a potential mechanism whereby hyperglycemia results in the preglomerular vasodilation that underlies diabetic hyperfiltration.

TIME-COURSE OF RENAL FUNCTIONAL ALTERATIONS IN T1D

The renal functional complications of T1D are complex and evolve markedly with duration of the disease. The early stage of T1D is characterized by substantial increases in renal blood flow and glomerular filtration rate (GFR). In humans, diabetic hyperfiltration persists for 5–10 yr, before waning to a normal and eventually subnormal GFR. The onset of diabetic nephropathy (DN) is heralded by the appearance of

From: *Contemporary Diabetes: The Diabetic Kidney*
Edited by: P. Cortes and C. E. Mogensen © Humana Press Inc., Totowa, NJ

microalbuminuria and albuminuria. Advanced DN is characterized by proteinuria, further deterioration of renal function and GFR, glomerulosclerosis, and interstitial fibrosis. This progression is exacerbated by hypertension, underscoring the vascular basis of the process. Maneuvers that limit or prevent development of diabetic hyperfiltration (e.g., by decreasing efferent arteriolar resistance, as provided by angiotensin-converting enzyme (ACE) inhibitors) delay or prevent onset of DN, suggesting that the hyperfiltration occurring early in T1D engenders eventual development of DN.

LOCALIZATION OF THE RENAL MICROVASCULAR DYSREGULATION IN EARLY T1D

Diabetic hyperfiltration is evident not only in humans with T1D, but also in rodent models of T1D. Most experimental studies of renal hemodynamic and glomerular function in diabetes have utilized the streptozotocin (STZ)-treated rat. Renal cross-transplantation studies have established that STZ exerts minimal direct nephrotoxic effects, such that the renal functional changes evident in the STZ rat arise as a consequence of the induction of T1D *(1)*. Within 3 d after STZ injection, renal and glomerular hypertrophy are evident *(2)*, whereas hyperfiltration arises within 1 wk and remains evident for weeks to months (probably dependent on the magnitude of the hyperglycemia). The hyperfiltration can be substantial, as exemplified by our observation of an 80% increase in inulin clearance in Sprague-Dawley rats studied 2 wk after STZ treatment *(3)*. Hence, although there are some limitations in the utility of the STZ rat in studying the processes occurring during advanced DN *(2)*, the STZ rat provides a useful tool for studying the mechanisms underlying diabetic hyperfiltration.

During the 1980s, micropuncture studies in the STZ rat provided the first documentation that diabetic hyperfiltration results from a reduction in preglomerular vascular resistance, with the ultrafiltration coefficient and efferent arteriolar resistance usually unaffected *(4,5)*. This situation increases glomerular plasma flow and capillary hydrostatic pressure, thereby spawning the substantial increase in GFR. The glomerular capillary hypertension in STZ rats is an acutely reversible consequence of insulin deficiency and the resulting hyperglycemia *(4)*. Indeed, acute restoration of euglycemia also restores GFR to normal values in humans with recent onset T1D *(6)*. Hyperfiltration in STZ rats is evident not only at the whole kidney level and in superficial nephrons accessible by standard in vivo micropuncture methods, but also occurs in juxtamedullary nephrons *(3)*. Data obtained through the use of videomicroscopy in concert with the in vitro blood-perfused juxtamedullary nephron technique have confirmed that the increase in GFR can be attributed to a significantly greater afferent arteriolar lumen diameter in STZ kidneys, compared with kidneys from Sham (vehicle-treated) rats, whereas efferent arteriolar diameter is unaffected *(3)*. In addition to the reduced basal arteriolar tone, afferent (but not efferent) arterioles from moderately hyperglycemic STZ rats display attenuated vasoconstrictor responsiveness to norepinephrine *(3)*. Over the course of several studies, we have observed a bell-shaped relationship between blood glucose levels and juxtamedullary afferent arteriolar diameter (Fig. 1). This observation is in accord with previous reports that hyperfiltration occurs in moderately hyperglycemic STZ rats, whereas severe hyperglycemia evokes a reduction in GFR *(5)*.

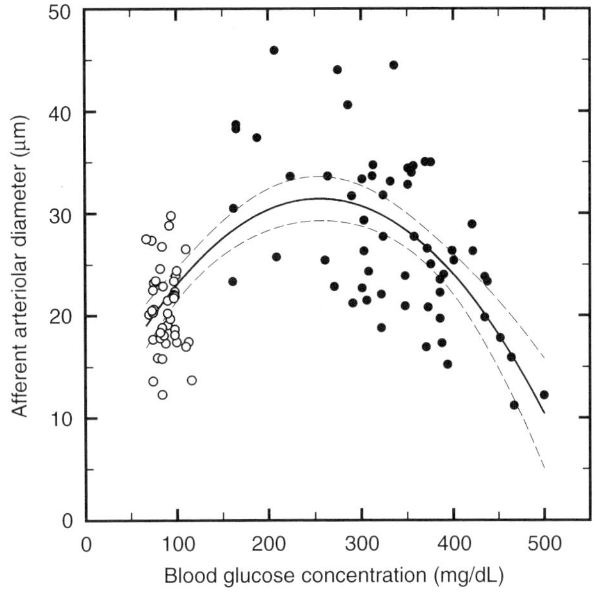

Fig. 1. Relationship between blood glucose concentration and juxtamedullary afferent arteriolar lumen diameter in kidneys from nondiabetic rats (Sham, ◦) and rats with STZ-induced T1D (λ). The second-order regression line (solid) with 95% confidence intervals (•) is also provided.

ETIOLOGY OF THE AFFERENT ARTERIOLAR DILATION UNDERLYING DIABETIC HYPERFILTRATION

Results from the Diabetes Control and Complications Trial *(7,8)* established that intensive insulin therapy aimed at near normalization of blood glucose levels reduces the occurrence of microalbuminuria and albuminuria by 39 and 54%, respectively, compared with conventional insulin therapy. These benefits were greatest when intensive therapy was initiated soon after onset of T1D, underscoring the importance of early hyperglycemia-induced processes in leading to development of DN. Whereas it seems likely that hyperglycemia triggers or promotes the development of diabetic hyperfiltration, the events linking hyperglycemia to impaired preglomerular microvascular function in T1D have not been definitively established. Indeed, intensive investigation of many different pathophysiological sequelae proposed to underlie diabetic hyperfiltration (renal prostaglandins, sorbitol, growth hormone, atrial natriuretic peptide, nitric oxide, glucagon, kallikrein–kinin system, the renin–angiotensin system (RAS), etc.) has failed to unveil the undisputed key insult. In this chapter, we consider the possibility that altered electromechanical regulation of vascular smooth muscle tone and renal oxidative stress act in concert to promote the afferent arteriolar dilation underlying diabetic hyperfiltration.

Renal Oxidative Stress in T1D

One widespread consequence of hyperglycemia in T1D is oxidative stress reflecting net accumulation of reactive oxygen species (ROS), which encompass a variety of partially reduced metabolites oxygen. At the forefront of the array of ROS lies superoxide anion ($O_2^{\cdot -}$), which is formed in biological systems as the result of a one-electron reduction

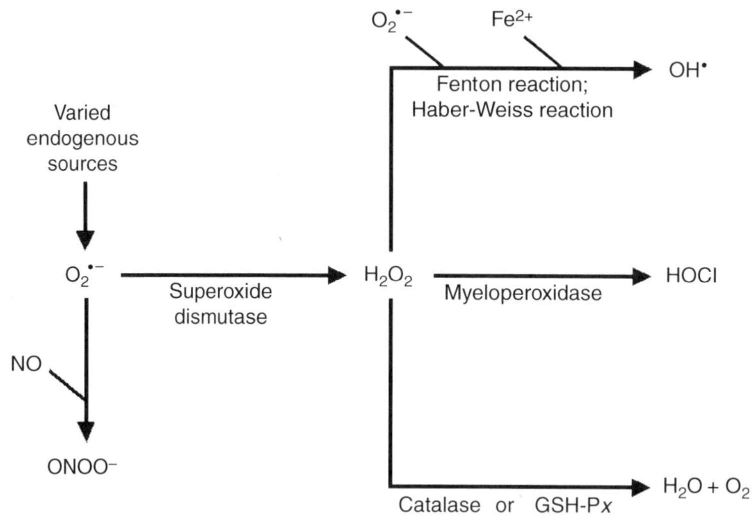

Fig. 2. Cascade of endogenous ROS formation. $O_2^{\bullet-}$, superoxide anion; NO, nitric oxide; $ONOO^-$, peroxynitrite; H_2O_2, hydrogen peroxide; $OH^{\cdot}$, hydroxyl radical; HOCl, hypochlorous acid; GSH-Px, glutathione peroxidase.

of molecular oxygen by oxidases and auto-oxidation processes. As summarized in Fig. 2, $O_2^{\bullet-}$ formation leads to production of several ROS. The initial fate of $O_2^{\bullet-}$ is either dismutation to form hydrogen peroxide (H_2O_2) or reaction with nitric oxide (NO) to form peroxynitrite ($ONOO^-$). Spontaneous dismutation of $O_2^{\bullet-}$ is accelerated more than 30,000-fold by superoxide dismutase (SOD), a reaction that proceeds at approx 60% of the rate of $ONOO^-$ formation *(9)*. Significant amounts of H_2O_2 are produced that, in turn, can be degraded to H_2O and O_2 by antioxidant enzymes. Alternatively, H_2O_2 can serve as a precursor of other damaging substances such as hypochlorous acid (HOCl) and hydroxyl radical ($OH^{\cdot}$).

Whereas net accumulation of one or more ROS can result from excess formation and/or inadequate degradation mechanisms (enzymatic and nonenzymatic scavengers and so on), the initiating event in this cascade is $O_2^{\bullet-}$ production. The cellular sources of $O_2^{\bullet-}$ include the mitochondrial electron transport chain, NAD(P)H oxidase, NO synthase (NOS), xanthine oxidase, cyclooxygenase, and the oxygenated form of cytochrome P450 *(9)*. $O_2^{\bullet-}$ production by the mitochondrial electron transport chain has been proposed to represent a common element that triggers glucose-induced activation of several processes implicated in the vascular complications of T1D *(10,11)*; however, NAD(P)H oxidase and NOS have also been implicated as a sources of excess $O_2^{\bullet-}$ production in T1D *(12,13)*. Activation of one or more of these oxidant pathways during T1D drives an increase in $O_2^{\bullet-}$ formation in the vasculature and in the renal cortex *(14)*. Moreover, compensatory increases in renal antioxidant enzyme activities are evident *(15–17)*. A consequence of accelerated $O_2^{\bullet-}$ production is the formation of $ONOO^-$ and/or H_2O_2. $ONOO^-$ can react with tyrosine residues on proteins, a process presumed to underlie the increase in renal cortical protein tyrosine nitration in T1D *(14,18)*. The possibility of increased renal H_2O_2 production in T1D has received little attention, although this situation can be expected to result from the increases in both $O_2^{\bullet-}$ production and SOD activity *(14)*. In recent preliminary studies, we found that STZ rats exhibit increased urinary H_2O_2 excretion, which could reflect

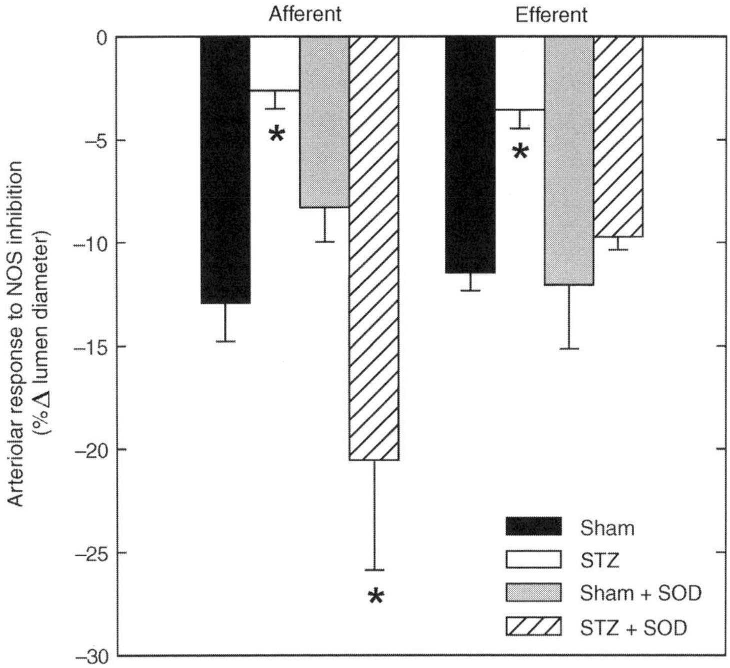

Fig. 3. Suppressed influence of NOS inhibition (100 μ*M* Nitro-L-arginine) on juxtamedullary afferent and efferent arteriolar diameter in STZ kidneys is restored by exogenous SOD (150 U/mL of blood perfusate). $p < 0.05$ vs Sham; $n = 7–10$ arterioles. (Data from Ohishi and Carmines *[27]*.)

net increases in systemic and/or renal H_2O_2 production. H_2O_2 is relatively stable and easily crosses cell membranes; hence, any accumulation of H_2O_2 in the kidney could influence the function of a variety of cell types *(19)*. Alternatively, H_2O_2 could be degraded by catalase or glutathione peroxidase, or it could serve as a substrate for formation of $OH^{\cdot}$ and/or HOCl. Winiarska et al. *(20)* have reported accelerated $OH^{\cdot}$ generation by renal cortical tubules from rabbits with alloxan-induced T1D. Because $OH^{\cdot}$ is highly reactive, it is very short-lived and thus assumed to exert its effects locally. An unexplored possibility is that $OH^{\cdot}$ is produced by (and subsequently influences the function of) the renal microvasculature in T1D. It is also possible that infiltration and activation of leukocytes (the only cells that express myeloperoxidase) leads to HOCl production in the kidney during the early stage of T1D. Indeed, although glomerular infiltration by leukocytes and monocytes/macrophages is evident within 1 wk of STZ injection in rats *(21)*, no attempts have been made to determine if renal HOCl production occurs in diabetes.

Microvascular Impact of Renal Oxidative Stress in T1D

The best-documented vascular consequence of oxidative stress in T1D is a decreased half-life of NO (accelerated degradation as a result of $ONOO^-$ formation). The resulting impairment of agonist-induced NO-dependent relaxation in aorta and other vascular beds is normalized by antioxidant maneuvers *(22–24)*. Agonist-induced endothelium-dependent relaxation is impaired in small intrarenal arteries from STZ rats, apparently as a result of $O_2^{\cdot -}$, $OH^{\cdot}$, and prostaglandin endoperoxide opposition of the effects of NO *(25)*. $O_2^{\cdot -}$-dependent processes are also implicated in impaired endothelium-dependent relaxation of afferent arterioles isolated from diabetic rabbits *(26)*. As illustrated in Fig. 3, renal arteriolar constrictor responses to NOS inhibition are attenuated in kidneys from STZ rats, but restored by acute exposure to SOD *(27)*. This observation indicates that $O_2^{\cdot-}$ production diminishes the tonic dilator influence of endogenous NO on the renal microvasculature. The $O_2^{\cdot-}$-dependent decrease in NO bioavailability is evident in both afferent and efferent arterioles; thus, it is difficult to envision this phenomenon as contributing to diabetic hyperfiltration. In fact, the decrease in NO bioavailability in early T1D actually increases pre- and postglomerular vascular resistance, rather than producing the selective decline in preglomerular resistance that engenders diabetic hyperfiltration.

$O_2^{\cdot-}$ may also alter renal vascular function via NO-independent mechanisms. In non-renal vascular beds, $O_2^{\cdot-}$ generally promotes vasoconstriction via effects on intracellular Ca^{2+} homeostasis and signaling events *(28–33)*, although a few studies indicate attenuated contractile responsiveness *(34,35)*. $O_2^{\cdot-}$ has also been variably reported to influence K^+ channels and L-type voltage-gated Ca^{2+} channels (VGCCs) *(31,36)*, which are particularly critical to regulation of renal preglomerular microvascular function *(37–39)*. However, no studies have examined the possibility that $O_2^{\cdot-}$ exerts an NO-independent influence on the renal vasculature.

Systemic infusion of $ONOO^-$ evokes renal, hindquarter and mesenteric vasodilation possibly via a mechanism involving ATP-sensitive K^+ channels (K_{ATP} channels) *(40,41)*. $ONOO^-$ also dilates cerebral arterioles by activating K_{ATP} channels *(35)*. In contrast, $ONOO^-$ contracts rat cerebral artery *(42,43)* and diminishes currents through voltage-sensitive K^+ channels (K_v channels), as well as reducing the dilator influence of these channels in rat small coronary arteries *(44)*. This phenomenon may result from nitration of tyrosine residues in the pore-forming α-subunit of the K_v channel *(44)*. As $ONOO^-$ appears to activate K_{ATP} channels and inhibit K_v channels in vascular smooth muscle, the resulting change in vascular tone may reflect the relative prominence of these channel subtypes in a particular vascular bed. It is intriguing note that K_{ATP} channels have increased functional impact on afferent arteriolar function in T1D (*see* pp. 30–31), thus raising the possibility that this phenomenon might arise via a $ONOO^-$-dependent mechanism.

A survey of literature concerning the vasoactive effects of H_2O_2 yields a mixed bag of constrictor *(31,45)* and dilator effects *(46–48)*. In some cases, contraction is evident at low concentrations with higher concentrations provoking a transient contractile response followed by a sustained dilation *(49,50)*. Most studies indicating vasodilator responses to H_2O_2 have implicated increased K^+ channel activity in the response *(49,51–53)*. Renal medullary interstitial infusion of H_2O_2 decreases medullary blood flow *(54)*; however, our preliminary data unveiled a concentration-dependent, NOS-independent afferent arteriolar dilator response to H_2O_2 *(55)*. Although we do not know if this phenomenon is endothelium dependent or if it reflects vasoactive effects of H_2O_2 metabolism products ($OH^\cdot$ and HOCl), this observation suggests that increased H_2O_2 production in the renal cortex during T1D might contribute to the afferent arteriolar dilation and hyperfiltration.

Little information exists concerning the potential renal vascular effects of $OH^\cdot$, except for one report indicating that $OH^\cdot$ contributes to impaired endothelium-dependent dilation of small intrarenal arteries from STZ rats *(25)*. A similar effect of $OH^\cdot$ has been described in the basilar artery of STZ rats *(56)*. Thus, it appears likely that $OH^\cdot$ impairs NO-dependent dilator events, possibly by oxidizing NO *(57)*.

However, conflicting reports regarding the effects of OH˙ on vascular tone include a vasodilator impact on cerebral arterioles *(58)*, but an endothelium-independent constrictor influence on rat aorta *(59)*.

Among the ROS, the vasoactive effects of HOCl are the most poorly characterized. HOCl increases vascular resistance in the perfused rat liver *(60)*. In isolated pulmonary arteries from sheep, HOCl produces vasoconstriction under resting force and vasodilation when the pulmonary arteries are precontracted *(61)*. HOCl also appears capable of impairing NO-dependent vasodilation *(62,63)*. Moreover, a recent report indicates that exposure of rat aortic rings to 20 m*M* glucose for 5 h sensitizes the vessel to myeloperoxidase-induced endothelial dysfunction *(64)*, an observation that underscores the potential for a vascular effect of HOCl if even only modest renal leukocyte infiltration/activation occurs during the early stage of T1D. However, nothing is known about the effects of HOCl on renal hemodynamics, even in inflammatory states in which increased renal myeloperoxidase activity and HOCl-oxidized protein have been documented *(65–67)*. It is interesting to note that immunosuppressant/anti-inflammatory therapy is beneficial in preventing glomerular injury in uninephrectomized STZ rats (which display accelerated development of diabetic nephropathy), although this phenomenon appeared to arise independent of the hemodynamic changes associated with diabetic hyperfiltration *(68)*.

In addition to direct effects on the renal vasculature, ROS production in T1D may elicit tubuloglomerular feedback-dependent alterations in afferent arteriolar tone. A complex interaction exists between $O_2^{\cdot -}$ and NO in determining tubuloglomerular feedback regulation of afferent arteriolar tone *(69)*. Moreover, ROS can influence Na^+ transport by various segments of the nephron. For example, in the medullary thick ascending limb, $O_2^{\cdot -}$ increases net NaCl reabsorption, $ONOO^-$ inhibits Na^+-K^+-ATPase activity, and H_2O_2 has no effect on Na^+ transport *(70)*. The possibility that HOCl and OH˙ might influence renal Na^+ transport has not been explored. The pluripotential effects of the various ROS on Na^+ transport might change solute delivery to the macula densa, thereby indirectly altering afferent arteriolar resistance. Obviously, this phenomenon could represent a mechanism through which ROS influence the magnitude of diabetic hyperfiltration.

Summary of the Potential Role of Oxidative Stress in Diabetic Hyperfiltration

Oxidative stress in T1D is implicated in multiple complications of the disease, including diabetic nephropathy, which has its origin in dysregulation of renal preglomerular microvascular tone. Intense investigative effort has established several pathways through which ROS production results from hyperglycemia. However, it is not clear which renal cells produce excess ROS in T1D, nor is it clear which ROS predominates in the kidney (and in the renal microvasculature) under these conditions. Even less well understood are the functional effects of the various ROS—information that is critical for understanding the mechanisms through which these substances contribute to the deleterious effects of T1D. Each ROS has the potential to influence renal microvascular tone via direct effects on the resident vascular smooth muscle cells, through effects on NO bioavailability (as documented for $O_2^{\cdot -}$), or indirectly via effects on tubular transport that evoke tubuloglomerular feedback-mediated vascular responses. Any or all of these events can be expected to influence the magnitude of diabetic hyperfiltration.

Disrupted Electromechanical Regulation of Preglomerular Microvascular Resistance in STZ-Induced T1D

Basal tone and contractile responsiveness of the preglomerular microvasculature are highly dependent on Ca^{2+} influx through voltage-gated channels, whereas efferent arteriolar function seems much less reliant on this process *(37)*. Accordingly, alterations in electromechanical coupling events would have a functional impact on a variety of processes in the preglomerular microvasculature, with little impact on the efferent arteriole *(71)*. In light of the fact that multiple aspects of afferent arteriolar function are impaired in T1D, with relative preservation of efferent arteriolar function, we have proposed that T1D provokes a functional defect in electromechanical regulation of afferent arteriolar function.

Functional Impairment of Afferent Arteriolar Voltage-Gated Ca^{2+} Channels in T1D

Bank and colleagues *(72)* first suggested that insulinopenia in T1D might impair Ca^{2+} movement through VGCCs in the renal vasculature. Subsequently, Williams and Schrier *(73)* found that cultured rat aortic vascular smooth muscle cells exposed to high extracellular glucose concentrations for 12 h exhibited suppressed voltage-sensitive and agonist-induced [$^{45}Ca^{2+}$] uptake responses. In recent preliminary studies, we confirmed that culture of renal preglomerular microvascular smooth muscle cells for 3–5 d in high-glucose media significantly impaired $[Ca^{2+}]_i$ responses to depolarization *(74)*. These observations link hyperglycemia with depressed VGCC activation. We have reported attenuation of afferent arteriolar contractile responses to BAY K 8644 (a dihydropyridine activator of L-type VGCCs) in kidneys from STZ rats. Moreover, the EC_{50} for KCl-induced afferent arteriolar contraction was 40% greater in STZ kidneys than in kidneys from Sham rats *(75)*. We also found that afferent arterioles from STZ rats isolated and studied in media containing 20 m*M* glucose exhibited blunted $[Ca^{2+}]_i$ responses to K^+-induced depolarization (Fig. 4) *(75)*. Although afferent arterioles from Sham rats were unaffected by bath glucose concentration, $[Ca^{2+}]_i$ responsiveness to depolarization in arterioles from STZ rats was restored within 10 min of exposure to normal bath glucose values. The rapid reversibility of this phenomenon is reminiscent of the ability of acute restoration of euglycemia to normalize GFR in STZ rats, as noted earlier *(4)*, and also makes it unlikely that a decrease in VGCC expression in afferent arteriolar smooth muscle cells is responsible. Rather, these observations suggest that hyperglycemia in T1D provokes altered regulation of afferent arteriolar VGCCs, probably representing a diminished sensitivity to membrane potential. This phenomenon can be expected to result in reduced responses to a variety of stimuli that normally rely on depolarization-dependent Ca^{2+} influx to evoke increases in preglomerular vascular resistance—including autoregulatory and tubuloglomerular feedback responses, as well as contractile responses to AngII, vasopressin, norepinephrine, and other agonists *(37,76–78)*. Accordingly, the impaired afferent arteriolar responsiveness to depolarization in T1D should promote afferent arteriolar dilation and diabetic hyperfiltration *(71)*.

Exaggerated Impact of ATP-Sensitive K^+ Channels on Afferent Arteriolar Tone in T1D

Studies from our laboratory have also explored the possibility that K^+ channel regulation of afferent arteriolar function is altered in T1D. In particular, we have focused on

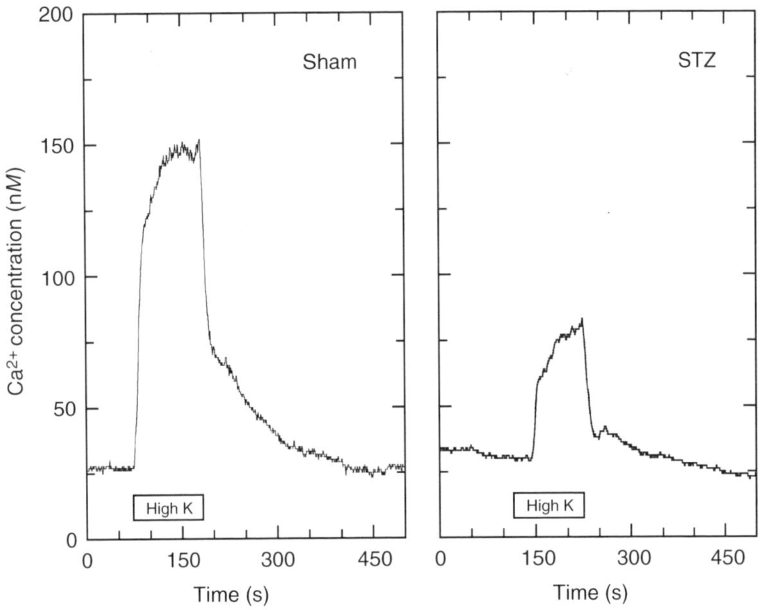

Fig. 4. Typical $[Ca^{2+}]_i$ responses to depolarization (40 mM K^+ bath) of isolated afferent arterioles from Sham and STZ rats. (Data from Carmines et al. *[75]*.)

the K_{ATP} channel *(79)*, the activation of which may reflect the cellular metabolic state. Several studies have provided functional evidence of K_{ATP} channel expression in the renal microcirculation *(80–83)*. We confirmed that potassium channel openers (pinacidil or PCO-400; both specific for K_{ATP}) evoke concentration-dependent afferent arteriolar dilation in kidneys from nondiabetic rats (Fig. 5), indicating the functional expression of K_{ATP} channels; however, the normal afferent arteriole is minimally responsive to glibenclamide (a sulfonylurea K_{ATP} inhibitor). Thus, the normal afferent arteriole possesses a recruitable pool of K_{ATP} channels having a low open probability in the absence of pharmagological activators and in the presence of physiologic intracellular ATP levels. In contrast, afferent arterioles from STZ rats contracted significantly in response to glibenclamide (Fig. 5), indicating the emergence of a K_{ATP} channel-dependent component of afferent arteriolar tone in T1D. Indeed, as the afferent arteriole is typically vasodilated in the hyperfiltering kidney of the STZ rat, glibenclamide-induced contraction of these vessels restored arteriolar diameter to values that did not differ significantly from arterioles in Sham kidneys *(79)*. Afferent arterioles from STZ rats also exhibited an exaggerated vasodilator response to pinacidil and PCO-400, consistent with an increased functional expression of K_{ATP} channels and/or an enhanced impact of these channels on membrane potential (and hence arteriolar tone). As opening of K_{ATP} channels promotes afferent arteriolar dilation, this phenomenon can be expected to contribute to the etiology of diabetic hyperfiltration *(71)*.

Summary of the Potential Role of Impaired Afferent Arteriolar Electromechanical Coupling in Diabetic Hyperfiltration

Increased functional availability and basal activation of K_{ATP} channels in T1D should result in dysregulation of membrane potential (favoring hyperpolarization). Moreover, this situation should be exacerbated by impaired VGCC responsiveness

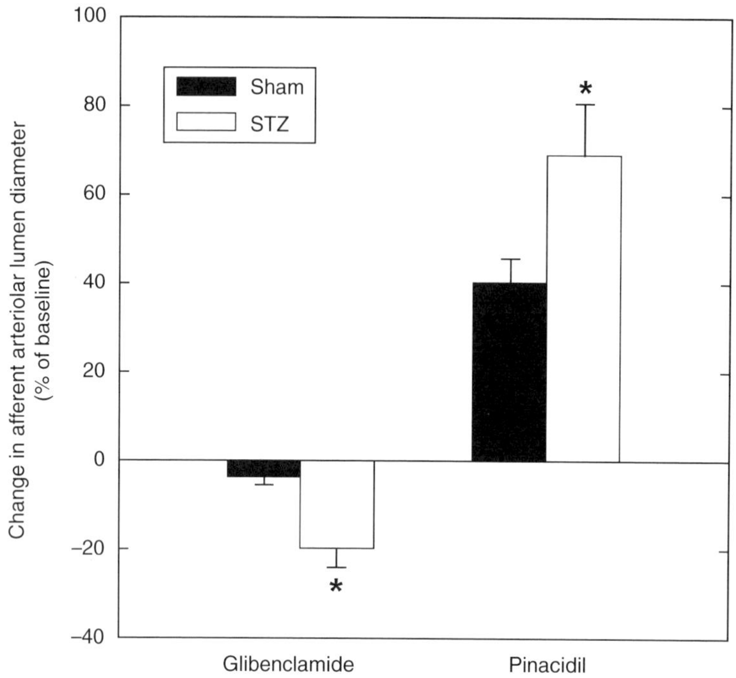

Fig. 5. Impact of K_{ATP} channels on juxtamedullary afferent arteriolar lumen diameter in kidneys from Sham and STZ rats. Responses to 100 μM glibenclamide (K_{ATP} blocker) and 100 μM pinacidil (K_{ATP} opener) are illustrated. $p < 0.05$ vs Sham; $n = 7–9$ arterioles. (Data from Ikenaga et al. *[79]*.)

to membrane depolarization. These synergistic effects of T1D on K_{ATP} channels and VGCCs would tend to diminish afferent arteriolar responsiveness to myriad constrictor stimuli, thus promoting the characteristic afferent arteriolar dilation that evokes diabetic hyperfiltration. However, the events that underlie altered electromechanical coupling in the preglomerular microvasculature during T1D have not been elucidated.

Could Oxidative Stress in T1D Underlie the Alterations in Afferent Arteriolar Electromechanical Coupling?

In considering the potential roles of renal oxidative stress and impaired afferent arteriolar electromechanical coupling in the etiology of diabetic hyperfiltration, it is intriguing to note a potential link between these phenomena. Indeed, many of the direct vasoactive effects of ROS arise via changes in K^+ channels that regulate membrane potential or Ca^{2+} channels that respond to changes in membrane potential. These channels play prominent roles in the electromechanical regulation of afferent arteriolar tone (and are much less prominent in the efferent arteriole). Thus, as illustrated in Fig. 6, it is conceivable that renal oxidative stress in T1D might activate K^+ channels (perhaps the K_{ATP} channel) in afferent arteriolar smooth muscle cells, resulting in hyperpolarization and diminished Ca^{2+} influx through VGCCs, thus engendering afferent arteriolar dilation and hyperfiltration. These events may occur in parallel with effects of ROS that reduce NO bioavailability (tempering hyperfiltration) and/or ROS-stimulated changes in tubular transport that evoke tubuloglomerular feedback-dependent responses (which could either favor or blunt hyperfiltration). This complex scenario of factors impacting the magnitude of diabetic hyperglycemia awaits validation through detailed experimental scrutiny.

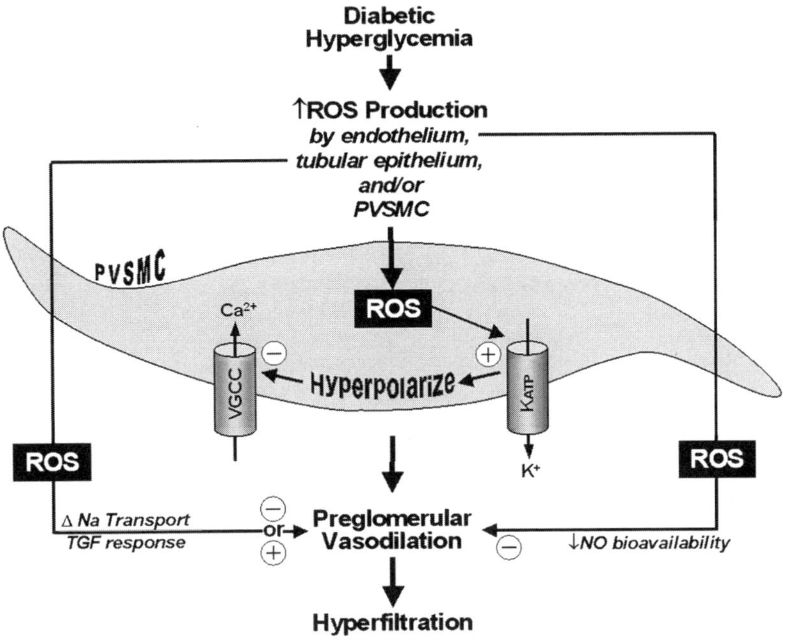

Fig. 6. Putative means through which renal oxidative stress in T1D might evoke hyperfiltration by impairing electromechanical coupling in preglomerular microvascular smooth muscle cells (PVSMCs). Also indicated are the potential indirect effects of ROS on afferent arteriolar function arising via reduced NO bioavailability and tubuloglomerular feedback.

REFERENCES

1. Churchill P, Churchill M, Bidani A, Dunbar J Jr. Streptozotocin-induced renal hemodynamic changes in isogenic Lewis rats: a transplant study. Am J Physiol Renal Fluid Electrolyte Physiol 1993;264: F100–F105.
2. Hirose K, Østerby R, Nozawa M, Gundersen HJ. Development of glomerular lesions in experimental long-term diabetes in the rat. Kidney Int 1982;21:889–895.
3. Ohishi K, Okwueze MI, Vari RC, Carmines PK. Juxtamedullary microvascular dysfunction during the hyperfiltration stage of diabetes mellitus. Am J Physiol Renal Fluid Electrolyte Physiol 1994;267:F99–F105.
4. Scholey JW, Meyer TW. Control of glomerular hypertension by insulin administration in diabetic rats. J Clin Invest 1989;83:1384–1389.
5. Hostetter TH, Troy JL, Brenner BM. Glomerular hemodynamics in experimental diabetes mellitus. Kidney Int 1981;19:410–415.
6. Mogensen CE. Kidney function and glomerular permeability to macromolecules in early juvenile diabetes. Scand J Clin Lab Invest 1971;28:91–100.
7. Diabetes Control and Complications Trial/Epidemiology of Diabetes Interventions and Complications Research Group. Retinopathy and nephropathy in patients with type 1 diabetes four years after a trial of intensive therapy. N Engl J Med 2000;342:381–389.
8. Diabetes Control and Complications Trial Research Group. The effect of intensive treatment of diabetes on the development and progression of long-term complications in insulin-dependent diabetes mellitus. N Engl J Med 1993;329:977–986.
9. Wolin MS, Gupte SA, Oeckler RA. Superoxide in the vascular system. J Vasc Res 2002;39:191–207.
10. Brownlee M. Biochemistry and molecular cell biology of diabetic complications. Nature (London) 2001;414:813–820.
11. Nishikawa T, Edelstein D, Du XL, et al. Normalizing mitochondrial superoxide production blocks three pathways of hyperglycaemic damage. Nature (London) 2000;404:787–790.
12. Hink U, Li H, Mollnau H, et al. Mechanisms underlying endothelial dysfunction in diabetes mellitus. Circ Res 2001;88:e14–e22.

13. Sonta T, Inoguchi T, Tsubouchi H, et al. Evidence for contribution of vascular Nad(P)H oxidase to increased oxidative stress in animal models of diabetes and obesity. Free Radic Biol Med 2004;37: 115–123.
14. Ishii N, Patel KP, Lane PH, et al. Nitric oxide synthesis and oxidative stress in the renal cortex of rats with diabetes mellitus. J Am Soc Nephrol 2001;12:1630–1639.
15. Kakkar R, Mantha SV, Radhi J, Prasad K, Kalra J. Antioxidant defense system in diabetic kidney: A time course study. Life Sci 1997;60:667–679.
16. Kakkar R, Kalra J, Mantha SV, Prasad K. Lipid peroxidation and activity of antioxidant enzymes in diabetic rats. Mol Cell Biochem 1995;151:113–119.
17. Sechi LA, Ceriello A, Griffin CA, et al. Renal antioxidant enzyme mRNA levels are increased in rats with experimental diabetes mellitus. Diabetologia 1997;40:23–29.
18. Griendling KK, Sorescu D, Lasségue B, Ushio-Fukai M. Modulation of protein kinase activity and gene expression by reactive oxygen species and their role in vascular physiology and pathophysiology. Arterioscler Thromb Vasc Biol 2000;20:2175–2183.
19. Baud L, Ardaillou R. Reactive oxygen species: production and role in the kidney. Am J Physiol Renal Fluid Electrolyte Physiol 1986;251:F765–F776.
20. Winiarska K, Drozak J, Wegrzynowicz M, Fraczyk T, Bryla J. Diabetes-induced changes in glucose synthesis, intracellular glutathione status and hydroxyl free radical generation in rabbit kidney-cortex tubules. Mol Cell Biochem 2004;261:91–98.
21. Sugimoto H, Shikata K, Hirata K, et al. Increased expression of intercellular adhesion molecule-1 (ICAM-1) in diabetic rat glomeruli: glomerular hyperfiltration is a potential mechanism of ICAM-1 upregulation. Diabetes 1997;46:2075–2081.
22. Tesfamariam B. Free radicals in diabetic endothelial cell dysfunction. Free Radic Biol Med 1994; 16:383–391.
23. Hattori Y, Kawasaki H, Abe K, Kanno M. Superoxide dismutase recovers altered endothelium-dependent relaxation in diabetic rat aorta. Am J Physiol Heart Circ Physiol 1991;261:H1086–H1094.
24. Mayhan WG. Superoxide dismutase partially restores impaired dilatation of the basilar artery during diabetes mellitus. Brain Res 1997;760:204–209.
25. Dai F-X, Diederich A, Skopec J, Diederich D. Diabetes-induced endothelial dysfunction in streptozotocin-treated rats: Role of prostaglandin endoperoxides and free radicals. J Am Soc Nephrol 1993;4:1327–1336.
26. Schnackenberg CG, Wilcox CS. The SOD mimetic tempol restores vasodilation in afferent arterioles of experimental diabetes. Kidney Int 2001;59:1859–1864.
27. Ohishi K, Carmines PK. Superoxide dismutase restores the influence of nitric oxide on renal arterioles in diabetes mellitus. J Am Soc Nephrol 1995;5:1559–1566.
28. Suzuki YJ, Ford GD. Superoxide stimulates IP_3-induced Ca^{2+} release from vascular smooth muscle sarcoplasmic reticulum. Am J Physiol Heart Circ Physiol 1992;262:H114–H116.
29. Katusic ZS, Vanhoutte PM. Superoxide anion is an endothelium-derived contracting factor. Am J Physiol Heart Circ Physiol 1989;257:H33–H37.
30. Wu L, De Champlain J. Superoxide anion-induced formation of inositol phosphates involves tyrosine kinase activation in smooth muscle cells from rat mesenteric artery. Biochem Biophys Res Commun 1999;259:239–243.
31. Tabet F, Savoia C, Schiffrin EL, Touyz RM. Differential calcium regulation by hydrogen peroxide and superoxide in vascular smooth muscle cells from spontaneously hypertensive rats. J Cardiovasc Pharmacol 2004;44:200–208.
32. Zhang AY, Yi F, Teggatz EG, Zou AP, Li PL. Enhanced production and action of cyclic ADP-ribose during oxidative stress in small bovine coronary arterial smooth muscle. Microvasc Res 2004;67: 159–167.
33. Suzuki YJ, Ford GD. Inhibition of Ca^{2+}-ATPase of vascular smooth muscle sarcoplasmic reticulum by reactive oxygen intermediates. Am J Physiol Heart Circ Physiol 1991;261:H568–H574.
34. Kimura C, Cheng W, Hisadome K, et al. Superoxide anion impairs contractility in cultured aortic smooth muscle cells. Am J Physiol Heart Circ Physiol 2002;283:H382–H390.
35. Wei EP, Kontos HA, Beckman JS. Mechanisms of cerebral vasodilation by superoxide, hydrogen peroxide, and peroxynitrite. Am J Physiol Heart Circ Physiol 1996;271:H1262–H1266.
36. Liu YP, Terata K, Rusch NJ, Gutterman DD. High glucose impairs voltage-gated K^+ channel current in rat small coronary arteries. Circ Res 2001;89:146–152.
37. Navar LG, Inscho EW, Majid DSA, Imig JD, Harrison-Bernard LM, Mitchell KD. Paracrine regulation of the renal microcirculation. Physiol Rev 1996;76:425–536.

38. Gebremedhin D, Kaldunski M, Jacobs ER, Harder DR, Roman RJ. Coexistence of two types of Ca^{2+}-activated K^+ channels in rat renal arterioles. Am J Physiol Renal Fluid Electrolyte Physiol 1996;270:F69–F81.
39. Roman RJ, Harder DR. Cellular and ionic signal transduction mechanisms for the mechanical activation of renal arterial vascular smooth muscle. J Am Soc Nephrol 1993;4:986–996.
40. Benkusky NA, Lewis SJ, Kooy NW. Peroxynitrite-mediated attenuation of α- and β-adrenoceptor agonist-induced vascular responses in vivo. Eur J Pharmacol 1999;364:151–158.
41. Benkusky NA, Lewis SJ, Kooy NW. Attenuation of vascular relaxation after development of tachyphylaxis to peroxynitrite in vivo. Am J Physiol 1998;275:H501–H508.
42. Brzezinska AK, Gebremedhin D, Chilian WM, Kalyanaraman B, Elliott SJ. Peroxynitrite reversibly inhibits Ca^{2+}-activated K^+ channels in rat cerebral artery smooth muscle cells. Am J Physiol Heart Circ Physiol 2000;278:H1883–H1890.
43. Elliott SJ, Lacey DJ, Chilian WM, Brzezinska AK. Peroxynitrite is a contractile agonist of cerebral artery smooth muscle cells. Am J Physiol 1998;275:H1585–H1591.
44. Li H, Gutterman DD, Rusch NJ, Bubolz A, Liu Y. Nitration and functional loss of voltage-gated K^+ channels in rat coronary microvessels exposed to high glucose. Diabetes 2004;53:2436–2442.
45. Gonzalez-Pacheco FR, Caramelo C, Castilla MA, et al. Mechanism of vascular smooth muscle cells activation by hydrogen peroxide: role of phospholipase Cγ. Nephrol Dial Transplant 2002; 17: 392–398.
46. Thengchaisri N, Kuo L. Hydrogen peroxide induces endothelium-dependent and -independent coronary arteriolar dilation: role of cyclooxygenase and potassium channels. Am J Physiol Heart Circ Physiol 2003;285:H2255–H2263.
47. Ellis A, Pannirselvam M, Anderson TJ, Triggle CR. Catalase has negligible inhibitory effects on endothelium-dependent relaxations in mouse isolated aorta and small mesenteric artery. Br J Pharmacol 2003;140:1193–1200.
48. Fujimoto S, Asano T, Sakai M, et al. Mechanisms of hydrogen peroxide-induced relaxation in rabbit mesenteric small artery. Eur J Pharmacol 2001;412:291–300.
49. Cseko C, Bagi Z, Koller A. Biphasic effect of hydrogen peroxide on skeletal muscle arteriolar tone via activation of endothelial and smooth muscle signaling pathways. J Appl Physiol 2004;97:1130–1137.
50. Gao YJ, Hirota S, Zhang DW, Janssen LJ, Lee RM. Mechanisms of hydrogen-peroxide-induced biphasic response in rat mesenteric artery. Br J Pharmacol 2003;138:1085–1092.
51. Hattori T, Kajikuri J, Katsuya H, Itoh T. Effects of H_2O_2 on membrane potential of smooth muscle cells in rabbit mesenteric resistance artery. Eur J Pharmacol 2003;464:101–109.
52. Barlow RS, White RE. Hydrogen peroxide relaxes porcine coronary arteries by stimulating BK_{Ca} channel activity. Am J Physiol Heart Circ Physiol 1998;44:H1283–H1289.
53. Hayabuchi Y, Nakaya Y, Matsuoka S, Kuroda Y. Hydrogen peroxide-induced vascular relaxation in porcine coronary arteries is mediated by Ca^{2+}-activated K^+ channels. Heart Vessels 1998;13:9–17.
54. Chen YF, Cowley AW Jr, Zou AP. Increased H_2O_2 counteracts the vasodilator and natriuretic effects of superoxide dismutation by tempol in renal medulla. Am J Physiol Regul Integr Comp Physiol 2003;285:R827–R833.
55. Carmines PK, Fallet RW, Pollock JS. Effect of H_2O_2 on afferent arteriolar diameter in normal rat kidney. FASEB J 2005;19:A1145 (Abstract).
56. Mayhan WG, Patel KP. Treatment with dimethylthiourea prevents impaired dilatation of the basilar artery during diabetes mellitus. Am J Physiol Heart Circ Physiol 1998;274:H1895–H1901.
57. Marshall JJ, Wei EP, Kontos HA. Independent blockade of cerebral vasodilation from acetylcholine and nitric oxide. Am J Physiol Heart Circ Physiol 1988;255:H847–H854.
58. Wei EP, Christman CW, Kontos HA, Povlishock JT. Effects of oxygen radicals on cerebral arterioles. Am J Physiol Heart Circ Physiol 1985;248:H157–H162.
59. Shen J-Z, Zheng X-F, Kwan C-Y. Differential contractile actions of reactive oxygen species on rat aorta: selective activation of ATP receptor by H_2O_2. Life Sci 2000;66:291–296.
60. Bilzer M, Lauterburg BH. Effects of hypochlorous acid and chloramines on vascular resistance, cell integrity, and biliary glutathione disulfide in the perfused rat liver: modulation by glutathione. J Hepatol 1991;46:84–89.
61. Turan NN, Demiryurek AT, Kanzik I. Hypochlorous acid-induced responses in sheep isolated pulmonary artery rings. Pharmacol Res 2000;41:589–596.
62. Stocker R, Huang A, Jeranian E, et al. Hypochlorous acid impairs endothelium-derived nitric oxide bioactivity through a superoxide-dependent mechanism. Arterioscler Thromb Vasc Biol 2004;24: 2028–2033.

63. Jaimes EA, Sweeney C, Raij L. Effects of the reactive oxygen species hydrogen peroxide and hypochlorite on endothelial nitric oxide production. Hypertension 2001;38:877–883.
64. Zhang C, Yang J, Jennings LK. Leukocyte-derived myeloperoxidase amplifies high glucose-induced endothelial dysfunction through interaction with high glucose-stimulated, vascular non-leukocyte-derived reactive oxygen species. Diabetes 2004;53:2950–2959.
65. Malle E, Woenckhaue C, Waeg G, Esterbauer H, Grone EF, Grone HJ. Immunological evidence for hypochlorite-modified proteins in human kidney. Am J Pathol 1997;150:603–615.
66. Maruyama Y, Lindholm B, Stenvinkel P. Inflammation and oxidative stress in ESRD—the role of myeloperoxidase. J Nephrol 2004;17(8):S72–S76.
67. Porubsky S, Schmid H, Bonrouhi M, et al. Influence of native and hypochlorite-modified low-density lipoprotein on gene expression in human proximal tubular epithelium. Am J Pathol 2004;164: 2175–2187.
68. Utimura R, Fujihara CK, Mattar AL, Malheiros DMAC, Noronha ID, Zatz R. Mycophenolate mofetil prevents the development of glomerular injury in experimental diabetes. Kidney Int 2003;63:209–216.
69. Wilcox CS. Redox regulation of the afferent arteriole and tubuloglomerular feedback. Acta Physiol Scand 2003;179:217–223.
70. Garvin JL, Ortiz PA. The role of reactive oxygen species in the regulation of tubular function. Acta Physiol Scand 2003;179:225–232.
71. Carmines PK, Fujiwara K. Altered electromechanical coupling in the renal microvasculature during the early stage of diabetes mellitus. Clin Exp Pharmacol Physiol 2002;29:143–148.
72. Bank N, Lahorra MA, Aynedjian HS. Acute effect of calcium and insulin on hyperfiltration of early diabetes. Am J Physiol Endocrinol Metab 1987;252:E13–E20.
73. Williams BW, Schrier RW. Effect of elevated extracellular glucose concentrations on transmembrane calcium ion fluxes in cultured rat VSMC. Kidney Int 1993;44:344–351.
74. Bast JP, Singaravelu K, Ehlers CJ, Fallet RW, Carmines PK. Impaired renal preglomerular responses to depolarization in diabetes: potential roles of extracellular glucose and oxidative stress. FASEB J 2004;18:A293 (Abstract).
75. Carmines PK, Ohishi K, Ikenaga H. Functional impairment of renal afferent arteriolar voltage-gated calcium channels in rats with diabetes mellitus. J Clin Invest 1996;98:2564–2571.
76. Carmines PK, Fowler BC, Bell PD. Segmentally distinct effects of depolarization on intracellular [Ca^{2+}] in renal arterioles. Am J Physiol Renal Fluid Electrolyte Physiol 1993;265:F677–F685.
77. Fallet RW, Ikenaga H, Bast JP, Carmines PK. Relative contributions of Ca^{2+} mobilization and influx in renal arteriolar contractile responses to arginine vasopressin. Am J Physiol Renal Physiol 2005;288:F551.
78. Salomonsson M, Sorensen CM, Arendshorst WJ, Steendahl J, Holstein-Rathlou NH. Calcium handling in afferent arterioles. Acta Physiol Scand 2004;181:421–429.
79. Ikenaga H, Bast JP, Fallet RW, Carmines PK. Exaggerated impact of ATP-sensitive K^+ channels on afferent arteriolar diameter in diabetes mellitus. J Am Soc Nephrol 2000;11:1199–1207.
80. Loutzenhiser RD, Parker MJ. Hypoxia inhibits myogenic reactivity of renal afferent arterioles by activating ATP-sensitive K^+ channels. Circ Res 1994;74:861–869.
81. Reslerova M, Loutzenhiser R. Divergent mechanisms of ATP-sensitive K^+ channel-induced vasodilation in renal afferent and efferent arterioles: Evidence of L-type Ca^{2+} channel-dependent and -independent actions of pinacidil. Circ Res 1995;77:1114–1120.
82. Reslerova M, Loutzenhiser R. Renal microvascular actions of calcitonin gene-related peptide. Am J Physiol Renal Physiol 1998;274:F1078–F1085.
83. Lorenz JN, Schnermann J, Brosius FC, Briggs JP, Furspan PB. Intracellular ATP can regulate afferent arteriolar tone via ATP-sensitive K^+ channels in the rabbit. J Clin Invest 1992;90:733–740.

I

Basic Pathophysiology and Biochemistry of Diabetic Nephropathy

B. Interstitial Disease

3 Proteinuria and Interstitial Fibrogenesis in Diabetic Nephropathy

Raimund Hirschberg, MD

CONTENTS

INTRODUCTION

In chronic renal glomerular diseases the degree of interstitial fibrosis determines renal failure and the rate of progression toward end-stage renal disease. This relationship between renal insufficiency and interstitial fibrosis has also emerged in the most common single disease entity causing renal failure with the need for chronic renal replacement therapy, namely diabetic nephropathy (DN) *(1,2)*.

Clinical studies have demonstrated that proteinuria is a risk factor for the rate of progression of renal failure *(3,4)*. Even small rates of proteinuria (≤1–3 g/d) impose an increased risk *(3)*. In combination, the histopathological and clinical observations give rise to the hypothesis that ultrafiltered proteins interact with tubular cells and, indirectly, with cells in the interstitium promoting fibrogenesis and, hence, accelerating renal disease progression. This hypothesis does not exclude important contributions of metabolic abnormalities to tubulo-interstitial injury in DN. Nevertheless, a causative role of glomerular protein ultrafiltration has recently emerged from experimental study and is supported by clinical observations.

GLOMERULAR PROTEINURIA AND THE RENAL INTERSTITIUM

The nephrotic syndrome in ouvert DN is associated with nonselective proteinuria (i.e., 50–60% of the urinary protein excretion consists of albumin with the balance including proteins of lower as well as high molecular weights). Diabetic microalbuminuria

From: *Contemporary Diabetes: The Diabetic Kidney*
Edited by: P. Cortes and C. E. Mogensen © Humana Press Inc., Totowa, NJ

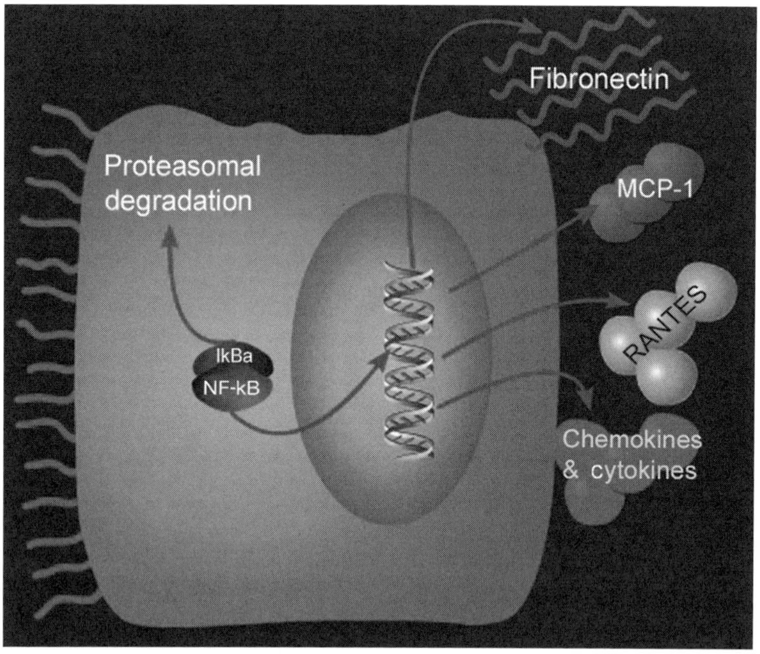

Fig. 1. Activation of nuclear factor (NF)-κB by proteasomal degradation of its inhibitor, I-κB, in tubular cells occurs in response to various modes of cell injury including the exposure to large concentrations of albumin, other proteins and some cytokines such as transforming growth factor-β. NF-κB upregulates expression of some ECM proteins (fibronectin) and C–C chemokines.

is clinically defined by but not limited to albumin excretion. In diabetic microalbuminuria there is also increased urinary excretion of IgG and β_2-macroglobulin indicative of nonselective glomerular proteinuria, albeit at low rates *(5,6)*. Although the most abundant protein that is translocated into tubular fluid in micro- as well as macroproteinuric states of DN is albumin, it is not the only ultrafiltered protein.

Albumin as a Tubular Toxin

Given the preponderance of albumin in glomerular protein ultrafiltration in DN (and other proteinuric glomerular diseases), several laboratories tested the hypothesis that albumin is the culprit for tubular cell injury, which subsequently entertains interstitial fibrogenesis. This conclusion is largely derived from in vitro experimental observations *(7–10)*. Incubation of cultured tubular cells with albumin activates the transcription factor nuclear factor (NF)-κB *(8–10)*. Activation of this transcription factor occurs as a general response to many modes of injury including exposure to several cytokines in many cell types and is not specific to the exposure with albumin *(11,12)*. NF-κB transcriptionally activates the C–C chemokines monocyte chemoattractant protein (MCP)-1, Regulated on Activation, Normal T Expressed and Secreted (RANTES), and fractalkine, and possibly other chemokines (Fig. 1). These molecules may attract mononuclear cells (macrophages) into the peritubular interstitium, which release fibrogenesis-promoting factors such as transforming growth factor (TGF)-β, endothelin-1, angiotensin II, and plasminogen activator inhibitor-1, which can act on tubular cells as well as on interstitial fibroblasts. In this model, albumin in tubular fluid directly and by itself initiates a cascade of events that promotes interstitial fibrogenesis. In this sense, albuminuria would not only be a risk factor for interstitial fibrosis but also causatively involved.

Although this "albumin hypothesis" appears to provide an attractive model of interstitial fibrogenesis in DN, several other clinical observations and experimental findings remain unexplained and in fact at odds. In the minimal change nephrotic syndrome, despite severe (selective) albuminuria, there is no evidence of progressive interstitial fibrosis, and peritubular macrophage infiltrates are generally not seen. Moreover, other investigators were not able to demonstrate tubular cell toxicity by purified albumin *(13–15)*. Its polyanionic nature gives rise to binding of various compounds to plasma albumin, which include fatty acids and other metabolites or drugs. Schreiner and his associates provided experimental evidence that metabolites of certain albumin-bound fatty acids are released intracellularly and are toxic to proximal tubular cells *(16)*. Indeed, a potentially toxic role of albumin-bound fatty acids (but not albumin *per se*) is further supported by experimental findings by Arici and coworkers *(17–19)*.

The minimal concentration of albumin that is required for activation of NF-κB (5–10 mg/mL) far exceeds the albumin levels in glomerular ultrafiltrate and proximal tubular fluid in vivo in the nephrotic syndrome, perhaps by two orders of magnitude, and even more so in subnephrotic proteinuria or microalbuminuria of early DN *(20)*. Burton and associates performed experimental studies that help to explain a predictive but not necessarily causative relationship between albuminuria, interstitial fibrogenesis, and rate of progression of renal failure in DN. Incubation of proximal tubular cells with purified albumin (1 mg/mL) does not raise the secretion of MCP-1 but equivalent concentrations of the 40–100 kDa fraction of heat-inactivated serum increases the secretion of this C–C chemokine as well as of platelet-derived growth factor (PDGF) *(14)*. Similarly, this fraction (but not albumin) also raises the basolateral secretion of fibronectin in apically stimulated cells *(13)*.

In the aggregate, experimental findings favor an alternative hypothesis that apical tubular cell exposure to ultrafiltered compounds of molecular sizes, similar, or greater than albumin are causative in interstitial fibrogenesis, and the presence of albuminuria is indicative of the translocation of such bioactive molecules into tubular fluid.

Glomerular Ultrafiltration of Growth Factor: Cytokines

Glomerular proteinuria does not only translocate albumin but also highly bioactive growth factors and cytokines into tubular fluid. In plasma, these molecules are usually present in bioinactive, high molecular weight precursor forms that are normally excluded from glomerular utrafiltration because of their molecular size. In proteinuric glomerulopathies ultrafiltration has been demonstrated for insulin-like growth factor (IGF)-I, hepatocyte growth factor (HGF), and TGF-β, and their potential contributions to tubular cell "activation" and in the context of interstitial fibrogenesis in DN has been examined.

ULTRAFILTERED IGF-I

IGF-I (7.6 kDa) is present in circulating plasma at considerably high levels (20–40 n*M*) but almost exclusively in high-molecular-weight-binding protein (BP) complexes. Approximately 75% are bound to IGFBP-3 that forms together with an acid-labile subunit a complex of 150 kDa. Most of the remaining IGF-I is bound to IGFBP-1, -2, or -4 in molecular complexes of 45–50 kDa. This molecular size distribution of plasma

IGF-I explains its exclusion from glomerular ultrafiltration in physiological states. However, in the experimental nephrotic syndrome, IGF-I undergoes translocation into proximal tubular fluid together with (some of its) BPs, perhaps primarily as 45–50 kDa complexes *(20)*, and estimated tubular fluid levels are 1.3 n*M*, which is probably two orders of magnitude above its lowest level of bioactivity. In tubular fluid, IGF-I becomes bioactive as demonstrated by the ability of nephrotic rat proximal tubular fluid to phosphorylate the IGF-I receptor β-subunit and to increase ^{3}H-thymidine incorporation in cultured tubular cells which is inhibitable by IGF-I neutralizing antibodies *(20)*.

The fractional urinary excretion of IGF-I in the nephrotic syndrome in rats has been estimated at 0.1% and the nephron clearance of IGF-I, is on an average threefold greater than that of albumin. These experimental observations demonstrate the presence of considerably great levels of IGF-I in proximal tubular fluid in proteinuric states. This data also suggests that ultrafiltration of IGF-I may reach biologically meaningful tubular fluid levels even in moderate degrees of glomerular proteinuria such as in early DN.

IGF-I transmits its activity through specific IGF-I receptors which have been demonstrated in basolateral but also in apical membranes of some nephron segments *(21)* and biological activity can be transduced through apical tubular membrane receptors *(22,23)*. Thus, IGF-I undergoes glomerular ultrafiltration in high-molecular-weight complexes in proteinuric glomerulopathies and can act through apical tubular receptors. Among its documented actions in tubular cells is cell growth, and this may contribute to growth in nephron size and length that has been described in early experimental DN *(24,25)*. Other biological actions of ultrafiltered IGF-I include moderately increased rates of tubular cell secretions of extracellular matrix (ECM) proteins, specifically collagens type I and IV, which could contribute to the interstitial accumulation of ECM proteins and hence interstitial fibrosis *(20)*.

Ultrafiltered HGF

HGF is also present in plasma, albeit at lesser concentrations compared with IGF-I, including both the bioinactive, monomeric precursor form of HGF (97 kDa) and mature, bioactive, heterodimeric HGF (80–92 kDa). In streptozotocin (STZ)-induced diabetes in rats, serum levels of pro-HGF as well as mature HGF tend to increase in comparison with controls *(26)*. Diabetic but not normal rats excrete the bioactive form of HGF in urine. Moreover, early proximal tubular fluid obtained by nephron micropuncture from diabetic rats contains mature HGF, which is absent in normal controls *(26)*. Thus, similar to IGF-I, HGF is also translocated from plasma into tubular fluid by glomerular ultrafiltration in rats with DN but not in control animals.

HGF exerts biological activity through its specific receptor, the $p190^{met}$ protein. HGF receptors are expressed in several nephron segments in basolateral membranes and in apical membranes. Proximal tubular $p190^{met}$ expression is increased in DN *(26)*. This increase in tubular HGF-receptor expression seems to be mediated by TGF-β. The *c-met* gene contains a *cis*-acting smad-responsive element adjacent to a Sp1-site, and TGF-β transcriptionally upregulates $p190^{met}$ smad dependently with additional requirement of Sp1 *(27)*.

Although some experimental findings are supportive of a contributory role of ultrafiltered HGF to interstitial fibrogenesis in DN, other evidence is less supportive or even opposing such a role. Glomerular ultrafiltrate from diabetic (but not from control) rats as well as recombinant human HGF (rhHGF) increase fibronectin expression in cultured proximal tubular cells and induce other profibrogenic molecules (chemokines and

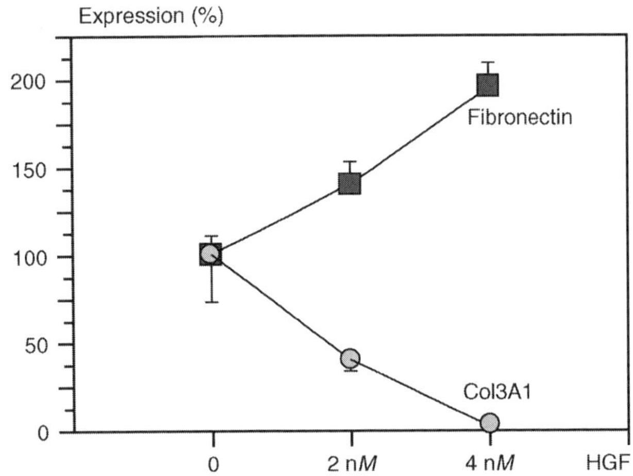

Fig. 2. Dual actions of rhHGF in tubular cells. Although HGF moderately raises the expression of some matrix proteins such as fibronectin, the expression of the A1 chain of collagen type III is almost quantitatively blocked.

PDGF-BB). In contrast, HGF concentration dependently downregulates expression of Col3A1, a subunit of collagen type III *(28)*. Thus, the contribution of ultrafiltered HGF to interstitial fibrogenesis in DN remains questionable (Fig. 2).

Ultrafiltered TGF-β

TGF-β is also present in serum at considerable levels and large amounts are stored in platelets and released on degranulation *(29)*. Ninety-nine percent or more of serum TGF-β is bound to latency-associated protein and TGF-β-latency-associated protein is actually the transcriptional and translational product of the *TGF*-β gene. This protein is largely bound to latent TGF-β BP forming a complex of about 220 kDa or to β_2-macroglobulin (900 kDa). Thus, TGF-β is normally effectively excluded from glomerular ultrafiltration except in glomerular proteinuria.

Indeed, in DN TGF-β is found in early proximal tubular fluid at biologically significant levels (800 pg/mL). Approximately 10% is directly bioactive, and the reminder appears to undergo activation by proteolytic enzymes, thrombospondin-1, progressive acidification, and increasing urea levels that occur with downstream travel of tubular fluid. TGF-β that is present in tubular fluid may be plasma-derived, and/or may originate from increased expression in glomeruli, or from degranulating platelets. TGF-β receptors are also expressed in several nephron segments, including expression in apical membranes *(26,30)*.

The validity of these findings in experimental animals is also supported by clinical observations. In patients with membranous nephropathy, urinary excretion of TGF-β is increased and levels are predictive of the rate of progression of renal failure *(31)*. Urinary excretion of TGF-β has also been shown specifically in patients with DN *(32,33)*. There is compelling evidence for a major profibrogenic role for ultrafiltered TGF-β in DN.

BIOLOGICAL RESPONSES TO ULTRAFILTERED GROWTH FACTORS

Although three growth factors have been shown to undergo glomerular ultrafiltration in proteinuric glomerulopathies in general and specifically in DN, it is possible,

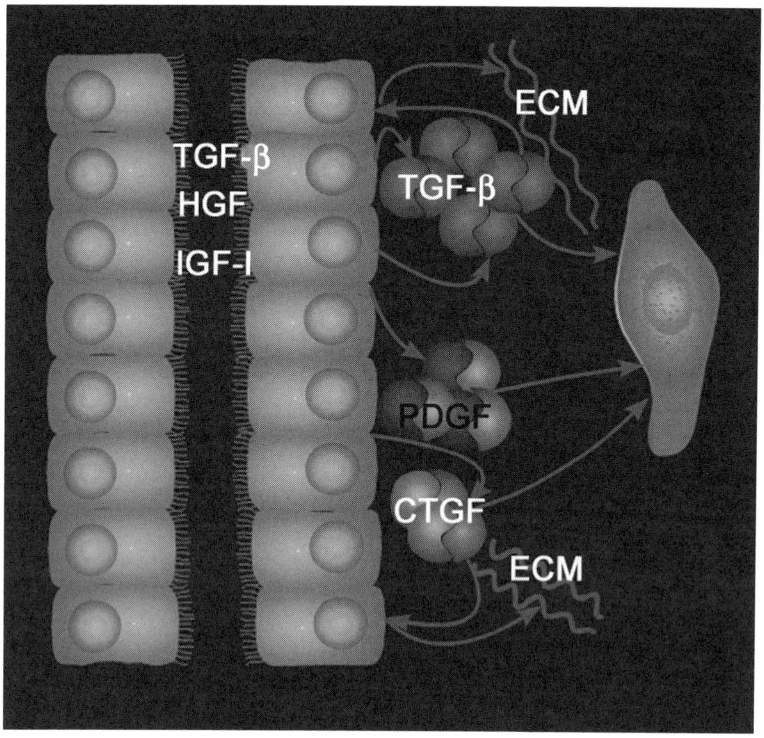

Fig. 3. Ultrafiltered TGF-β, HGF, and IGF-I interact with apical membrane receptors in tubules and raise the expression of some ECM-proteins as well as of PDGF, CTGF, and possibly TGF-β. These latter cytokines may act in autocrine/paracrine modes on tubular cells but important targets are renal interstitial fibroblasts.

perhaps likely, that several other bioactive proteins take similar routes. Demonstrated bioactivity data are only available for ultrafiltered IGF-I, HGF, and TGF-β, and most data on the latter two proteins.

Direct Profibrogenic Responses by Tubular Cells

Ultrafiltered IGF-I increases the secretion of collagen type I and IV *(20)*, and TGF-β increases col3A1 expression, albeit moderately in proximal tubular cells *(28)*. In contrast, HGF appears to be a negative regulator for this latter protein chain (Fig. 2) *(28)*. Both, HGF and TGF-β raise fibronectin expression in proximal tubular as well as inner medullary collecting duct cells, and this can be reproduced by incubating cells with diluted proximal tubular fluid from rats with DN but not from control animals (Fig. 3). These ECM proteins contribute to interstitial fibrosis in DN, and the findings suggest that tubular cells when stimulated with ultrafiltered IGF-I and TGF-β (and perhaps HGF) contribute directly to interstitial fibrosis. However, tubular cells express minimally, if at all, col1A2, and this is not much increased by TGF-β or HGF. This indicates that collagen type I, which substantially contributes to interstitial fibrosis, is not of tubular origin (but derived from interstitial myofibroblasts).

Incubation of proximal tubular cells with early tubular fluid that was collected by micropuncture from rats with DN also induces PDGF-BB expression (Fig. 3) *(28)*. Both ultrafiltered HGF and TGF-β contribute to increased tubular cell PDGF-BB and coincubation in the presence of a mixture of TGF-β- and HGF-neutralizing antibodies ameliorates this activity of tubular fluid. Moreover, rhHGF as well as rhTGF-β each raise PDGF-BB expression in proximal tubular cells substantially with TGF-β being more powerful in an equimolar comparison *(28)*. PDGF-BB is an important proliferative regulator for interstitial renal fibroblasts *(34,35)* and may contribute modestly to the expression of some ECM-proteins (col3A1) but not of others (col1A2 and fibronectin) in these cells *(28)*. Thus, apical exposure to ultrafiltered cytokines is translated by tubular cells into another cytokine signal (PDGF-BB) that has specific actions on interstitial cells.

Connective Tissue Growth Factor

On its discovery, connective tissue growth factor (CTGF) was thought to be exclusively expressed in (myo) fibroblasts downstream of the TGF-β receptor *(36–38)*. However, more recently it was determined that CTGF is widely expressed in varying cell types including epithelial cells in the distal nephron and in mesangial cells. Moreover, it is not exclusively induced by TGF-β but also by other cytokines *(39)*. CTGF raises the expression of ECM-proteins and other matrix-promoting regulators in myofibroblasts (and other cell types).

Early proximal tubular fluid from rats with DN moderately increases CTGF in cultured tubular cells which is mainly driven by the TGF-β content of early proximal tubular fluid (Fig. 3) *(39)*. Interestingly, CTGF binds to IGF-I, albeit with lesser affinity in comparison with the "classic" IGFBPs *(40,41)*. This may be of major functional importance, given that a specific signaling receptor for CTGF has not (yet) been identified. Although, a very high molecular weight, probably nonspecific cell surface BP has been described, it appears that it functions perhaps as a scavenger rather than a signaling receptor *(42)*. The lack of a defined receptor-signaling model for CTGF gives rise to an alternative hypothesis of action of this profibrogenic protein, namely binding to IGF-I and amplifying the activity of the latter through the IGF-I receptor. Indeed, CTGF amplifies the effects of IGF-I on the expression of collagen type III (col3A1) and thrombospondin-1 *(39)*. Further evidence on collaboration between CTGF and IGF-I has more recently been described in fibroblasts specifically in the context of diabetes *(43)*.

Proinflammatory Responses to Ultrafiltered Cytokines

Renal fibrogenesis may be compared with skin-wound healing. In this setting, inflammatory infiltrates are required for subsequent scarring and even large fetal wounds, which lack inflammation, heal without scars *(44)*. Similarly, renal interstitial fibrogenesis is thought to require inflammatory cells (mainly macrophages), which express important cytokines in the interstitium. Although early DN is thought by some scholars to completely lack the interstitial accumulation of macrophages, quantitative histological analysis indicates increased numbers of renal interstitial macrophages *(45)*. Experimental evidence suggests that ultrafiltered HGF and TGF-β are causative in inducing tubular basolateral chemokine secretion including MCP-1 and RANTES, which then regulate and activate interstitial macrophages (Fig. 4).

Tubular Secretion of MCP-1

Exposure of cultured tubular cells to glomerular ultrafiltrate from rats with DN raises the expression of MCP-1 *(26)*. There are two observations suggesting a major contribution

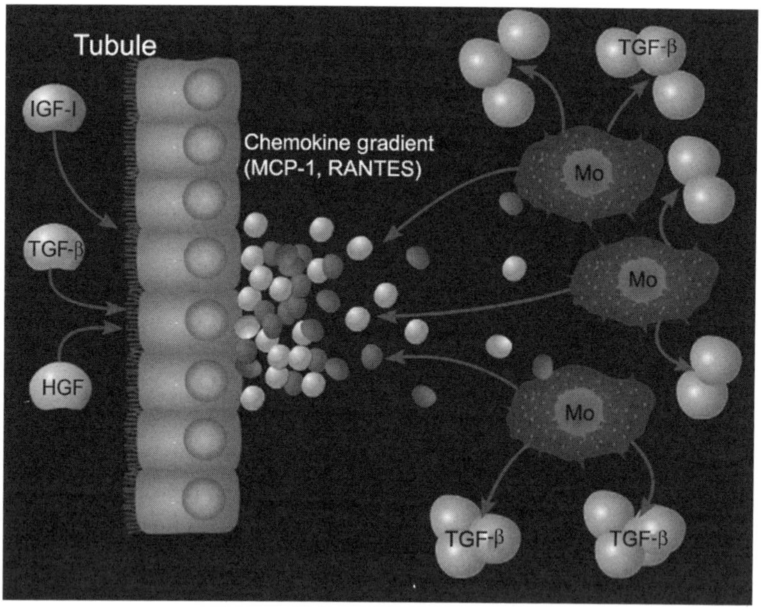

Fig. 4. Cytokines in tubular fluid induce a chemokine gradient in the peritubular interstitium which is recognized by CCR2 receptors on macrophages as a homing signal. MCP-1 also raises TGF-β secretion by macrophages, which appear to be an important source for this fibrogenic cytokine in the renal interstitium.

of TGF-β and HGF to the induction of MCP-1 in tubular cells: First, incubation with recombinant HGF or TGF-β each raises MCP-1; second, coincubation with early proximal tubular fluid and neutralizing antibodies suppressing HGF and TGF-β activity blocks MCP-1 secretion.

The effect of the glomerular ultrafiltrate can also be shown in inner medullary collecting duct cells suggesting that several nephron segments respond to apical, ultrafiltered TGF-β and HGF. Two-thirds of the MCP-1 is secreted through the basolateral membrane and one third is secreted apically and can undergo urinary excretion *(26)*. Indeed, increased urinary MCP-1 excretion has been demonstrated in patients with DN *(45–48)*. In addition, moderately increased urinary MCP-1 excretion occurs already with diabetic microalbuminuria *(48)*.

Tubular Secretion of RANTES

The C–C chemokine RANTES is also induced in tubular cells on apical stimulation with TGF-β or HGF. The vast majority is secreted basolaterally and a minor portion leaves the cell through the apical membrane and would be expected to undergo urinary excretion *(26)*.

In concert, these experimental observations give rise to a pathophysiological paradigm that glomerular ultra filterer of growth factors in early DN interact with apical tubular cell receptors, "activate" tubular cells, and induce basolateral secretion of chemokines (Fig. 4). But is there evidence for this paradigm in vivo in patients with DN? Mezzano and associates demonstrated increased tubular expression and levels of MCP-1 and RANTES in renal biopsy specimens from patients with DN. The tubular levels of both chemokines correlated tightly with the degree of proteinuria in these subjects and were colocalized with activated NF-κB *(49)*.

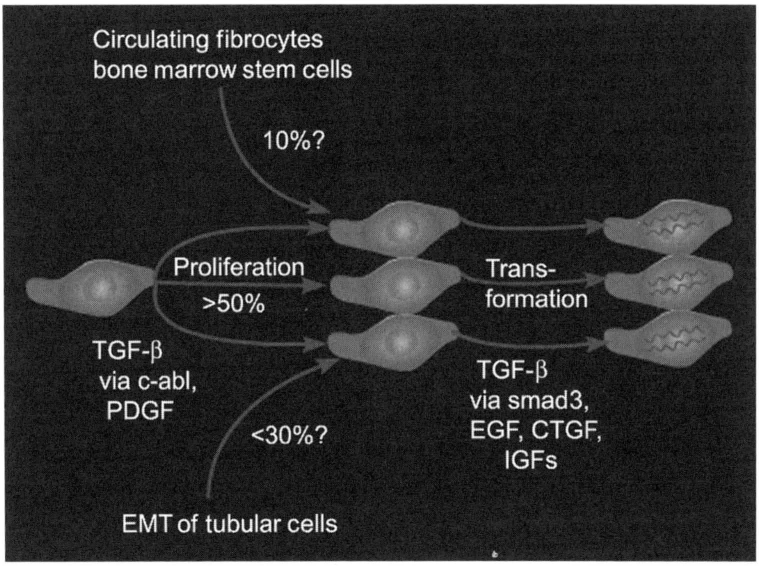

Fig. 5. Multiplication of renal interstitial fibroblasts and their subsequent transition to myofibroblasts are important events in renal fibrogenesis as only myofibroblasts are very efficient ECM-producing cells. Proliferation of residential fibroblasts is mainly regulated by TGF-β (utilizing a pathway that is unique to fibroblasts and involves *c*-abl) and PDGF. Additional recruitment of fibroblasts may occur by epithelial–mesenchymal transition (EMT) and from bone marrow stromal stem cells, although these mechanisms may contribute only in very advanced renal fibrosis. Multiple growth factors participate in the phenotype transition to myofibroblasts.

Macrophage Response to Tubular Chemokines

MCP-1 and RANTES, which are basolaterally secreted form chemokine gradients in the peritubular interstitium, are recognized by specific receptors (CCR2) on monocytes/macrophages causing a homing response (Fig. 4). Although DN is not associated with severe interstitial inflammation, increased numbers of renal interstitial macrophages have been found in STZ-induced DN in rodents as well as in human diabetes *(26,45,49)*. CCR2 receptors do not only serve as homing devices for macrophages but their interactions with specific ligands such as MCP-1 also cause macrophage activation. In response to MCP-1, macrophages increase their expression of TGF-β dose dependently (Fig. 4) *(26)*. Macrophages are the most prominent source of TGF-β in the renal interstitium in chronic renal diseases, including DN. Interstitial TGF-β is an important proliferation activator for fibroblasts and raises the profibrogenic activity in myofibroblasts.

FIBROBLASTS AND MYOFIBROBLASTS IN DIABETIC NEPHROPATHY

In the normal renal interstitium, fibroblasts are found only scarcely. These cells have a very modest capacity to produce ECM proteins. On stimulation with PDGF or TGF-β, fibroblasts proliferate. Given that TGF-β has either no effect on cell growth or induces apoptosis in several other cell types, its proliferative response in fibroblasts suggests involvement of unique signaling pathways (Fig. 5). TGF-β-induced proliferation of fibroblasts involves activation of the nonreceptor tyrosine kinase ableson (*c-abl*) *(50)*. An inhibitor of both, the PDGF-receptor kinase and *c*-abl, imatinib mesylate, reduces the increase in fibroblast number that precedes interstitial fibrosis and retards the development and progression of DN *(50,51)*.

Fibroblasts are precursor cells for myofibroblasts (Fig. 5). These latter cells express efficiently various ECM-proteins and are the most powerful matrix generators in the renal interstitium. The fibroblast–myofibroblast transition is regulated by CTGF and (macrophage-derived) TGF-β and is enhanced by collaboration with other cytokines, notably IGF-I and -II or epithelial growth factor (EGF) *(36,52)*. Increased numbers of interstitial myofibroblasts have been found in renal biopsy specimens from patients with DN *(53)*.

The transition to the myofibroblast phenotype is associated with new onset expression of motor proteins such as α-smooth muscle actin and myosin providing locomotion. Myofibroblasts are highly differentiated, lost much of their ability to proliferate but produce ECM proteins. In addition to *in situ* proliferation, additional fibroblasts may be recruited by transformation of severely injured tubular epithelial cells in a process termed epithelial–mesenchymal transition (EMT), which can be regulated by TGF-β in association with EGF. The mechanisms have been recently reviewed extensively *(54,55)*. This process appears to occur only in very advanced stages of interstitial fibrosis and has not yet been demonstrated specifically in DN. Fibroblasts may also be recruited from circulating fibrocytes and/or bone marrow stromal stem cells. The contribution of this latter mechanism to DN, if any, is not known *(56,57)*.

A MECHANISTIC MODEL FOR PROTEINURIA-DEPENDENT RENAL INTERSTITIAL FIBROGENESIS IN DIABETIC NEPHROPATHY

The glomerular ultrafiltrate in DN contains growth factor cytokines including IGF-I, TGF-β, and HGF, which are ultrafiltered in high-molecular-weight forms, become bioactive in tubular fluid and act on tubular epithelial cells through apical membranes. The cells respond with the secretion of modest amounts of ECM-proteins (fibronectin) and various mediators including PDGF-BB and CTGF as well as the C–C chemokines MCP-1 and RANTES. These latter molecules attract and activate macrophages into the interstitium, which are the major source for TGF-β in this renal compartment with important profibrogenic activity in fibroblasts and myofibroblasts. TGF-β (via a non-smad pathway involving *c*-abl) and PDGF induce proliferation of residential fibroblasts. TGF-β and CTGF in collaboration with IGFs and/or EGF induce phenotype transition to myofibroblasts, the major ECM-producing cell in the renal interstitium. Transcription of ECM proteins is also accelerated by these cytokines in myofibroblasts together with the provision of other profibrogenic, matrix-regulating enzymes and proteins from macrophages and myofibroblasts. These interactions that can be triggered by growth factors that are translocated into tubular fluid by glomerular ultrafiltration in proteinuric DN give rise to tested and novel therapies; the latter have, at present, mainly experimental and academic interest as they still require testing in patients with diabetic renal disease.

CURRENT AND NOVEL THERAPEUTIC APPROACHES AND TARGETS

Therapies to reduce tubulo-interstitial fibrogenesis in DN may be directed toward preventing the glomerular ultrafiltration of growth factors and other proteins into tubular fluid or to inhibit downstream interactions with tubular cells; or to modify the tubulo-interstitial responses. At present, generally accepted preventative therapies are aimed at reducing proteinuria/glomerular protein ultrafiltration. Several other interventions and therapeutic targets have been tested experimentally and some may give rise to clinical therapies in the future.

Antiproteinuric Therapies in Diabetic Nephropathy

Mechanistic experimental studies support that proteinuria is a risk factor but growth factor cytokines that are present in proteinuric glomerular ultrafiltrate are culprits in entertaining tubulo-interstitial fibrogenesis. Thus, the goal is to reduce glomerular macromolecule filtration. To this end angiotensin-converting enzyme (ACE) inhibitors have become the standard of care in DN. Substantial reductions in proteinuria can also be achieved with angiotensin receptor blockers (ARBs). In the Reduction of Endpoints in NIDDM with the Angiotensin II Antagonist Losartan (RENAAL) study, the level of proteinuria in type 2 diabetic patients with nephropathy who were treated with losartan decreased, on an average by 35% *(58)*. Losartan has also been shown to reduce urinary TGF-β excretion without affecting TGF-β serum levels *(59)*. With irbesartan, proteinuria can be reduced by approx 60% in type 2 diabetics with nephropathy and microalbuminuria as demonstrated in the Irbesartan in Microalbuminuria (IRMA)-2 study *(60)*. A review of multiple clinical trials indicates that ACE inhibitors or ARBs are beneficial in patients with DN and reduce the rates of proteinuria as well as of the progression of renal failure *(61)*.

ACE inhibitors, even at maximum dosages, do not completely block angiotensin II generation. Some angiotensin II persists, perhaps through parallel, ACE-independent pathways. Thus, theoretically, combination therapies with an ACE inhibitor and an ARB may provide additive benefits. This question has undergone only very limited clinical study thus far. Further reductions in proteinuria and urinary excretion of TGF-β with combined therapy using ramipril or candesartan in comparison with ramipril alone was demonstrated in a small trial in patients with IgA-nephropathy, but this benefit was not achieved in patients with DN *(33)*. The COOPERATE trial demonstrated added benefit of combination therapy with losartan and trandolapril in patients with nondiabetic renal diseases but similar studies in DN are presently not available *(62)*. Moreover, combinations of ACE inhibitors and ARBs may increase the risk for serious complications such as symptomatic hyperkalemia.

Emerging Novel Therapeutic Targets and Strategies

Better understanding of events that are mediated and perpetuated by glomerular proteinuria and "activation" of tubular cells by ultrafiltered growth factor cytokines gives potentially rise to several targeted interventions (Fig. 6). Their possible therapeutic utility in DN is merely inferential from experimental observations at present, and there are almost no studies in humans yet that would indicate benefit and/or safety. Nevertheless, some of these therapeutic principles may find their way into the clinic in the future.

Inhibition of the Interstitial Inflammatory Response and Macrophage Activation

One of the initial tubular cell responses to ultrafiltered proteins and growth factors is the basolateral secretion of C–C chemokines (MCP-1, and RANTES), which attract and activate macrophages. The latter are thought to be the primary source for profibrogenic

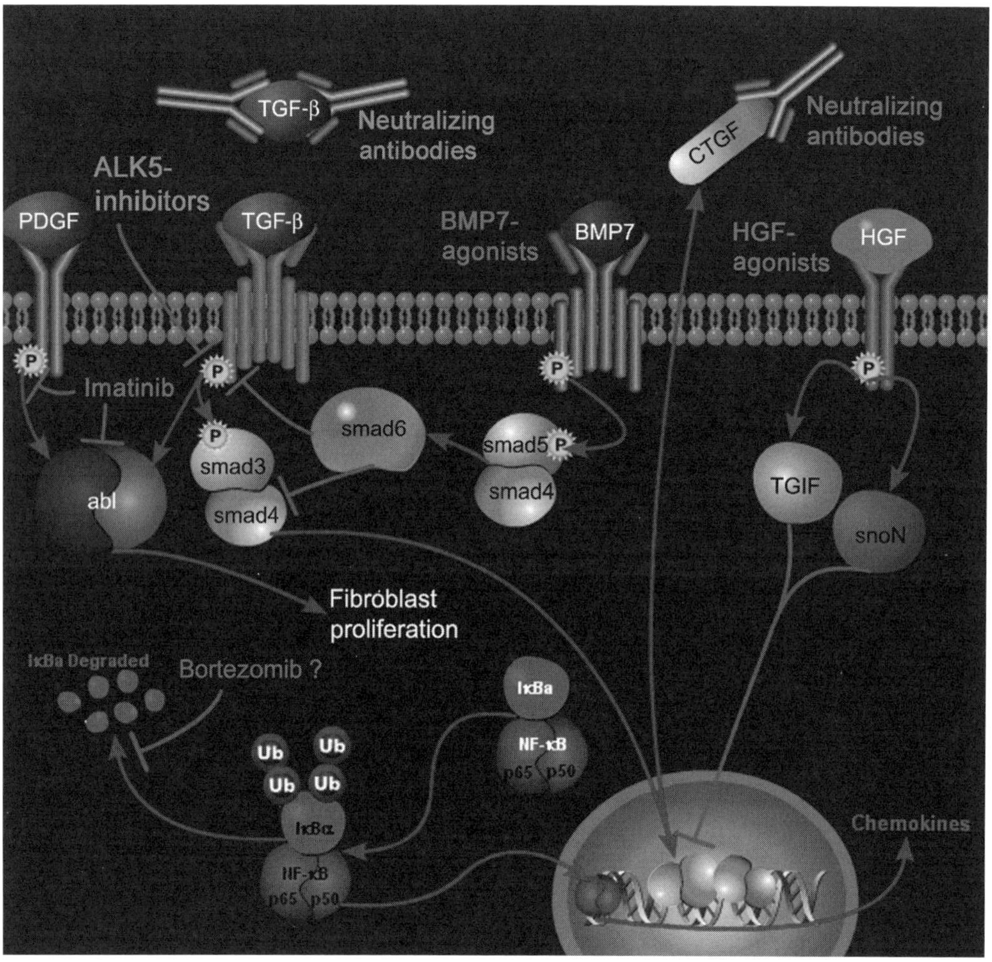

Fig. 6. Summary of novel therapeutic targets in DN. Potentially useful therapeutic principles are depicted in light gray lettering. *See* text in "Emerging, Novel Therapeutic Targets and Strategies" Section for explanations.

TGF-β in the renal interstitium, and fibroblasts are the primary target. Transcriptional upregulation of C–C chemokines appears to be NF-κB-dependent which, in turn, is activated by proteasomal degradation of its endogenous inhibitor, I-κB. Indeed, inhibition of MCP-1 with 7ND by means of renal overexpression of a 7ND expression plasmid reduces interstitial fibrogenesis *(63)*. Similarly, renal overexpression of IκB with an adenoviral vector reduces the MCP-1 response and the macrophage infiltrate and lessens interstitial fibrosis *(64)*. These experiments provide proof of concept but are perhaps therapeutically not feasable in patients. Prolongation of the half-life of endogenous I-κB with a specific proteasomal inhibitor, bortezomib (PS-341, Velcade®, Millenium Pharmaceuticals, Cambridge, MA), which is approved for the treatment of multiple myeloma by regulatory agencies, could provide a testable therapeutic avenue for the management of renal interstitial fibrogenesis in DN (Fig. 6) but neither experimental nor clinical data are currently available in this setting *(65,66)*.

Recombinant Human HGF

rhHGF is present in glomerular ultrafiltrate in rats with DN and acts through apical membranes on tubular epithelial cells. As discussed earlier, some of the cells' responses, but not others, suggest contributions to renal fibrogenesis. However, in the renal interstitium, rhHGF appears to inhibit profibrogenic TGF-β signals. Cell culture studies indicate that HGF induces the smad transcriptional corepressor snoN and reduces the catabolism of the smad corepressor TGIF (Fig. 6) *(67–69)*. This reduces TGF-β-induced ECM production as well as TGF-β-driven CTGF transcription *(70)*. Systemic administration of rhHGF or of a HGF-expression plasmid ameliorate DN in mice *(69,71)*. Thus, systemically administered rhHGF or (small molecule) HGF agonists may be beneficial in DN (Fig. 6).

Bone Morphogenetic Protein 7

Bone morphogenetic protein (BMP)7 is a member of the TGF-β superfamily of cysteine knot cytokines and plays pivotal roles during renal and eye development. In adult mammalian organisms, expression of BMP7 is retained very selectively and the kidney is among the sites of prominent expression, primarily in selective tubular segments and in glomerular podocytes. In bone, BMP7 promotes osteoblast function, giving rise to the hypothesis that renal BMP7 functions as an osteotrophic hormone. In STZ diabetes in rats, renal BMP7 expression decreases predating other renal pathologies *(72)*. Several experimental observations support the notion that renal BMP7 opposes TGF-β actions and has antifibrogenic activity. In vitro studies demonstrate that coincubation of mesangial cells with BMP7 lessens TGF-β-driven expression of ECM-proteins and profibrogenic regulators *(73)*. Its mechanisms of action have been partially delineated and include smad6, which is induced by BMP7 smad5 dependently (Fig. 6). Smad6 reduces effective nuclear translocation of TGF-β-induced smad3/4 complexes without involvement of smad corepressors *(74)*. BMP7 also opposes TGF-β-dependent epithelial–mesenchymal transition in vitro and in vivo *(75)*. Systemic administration of rhBMP7 reduces renal fibrogenesis in rodents with DN *(76)*. At present, there are no studies in humans with diabetic renal disease involving rhHGF or rhBMP7.

TGF-β Receptor Kinase Inhibitors

Given the pivotal contribution of ultrafiltered as well as interstitial TGF-β in renal fibrogenesis in DN, it is no surprise that inhibition of this cytokine such as with neutralizing antibodies ameliorates renal fibrosis (Fig. 6) *(77)*. Small molecule derivatives of imidazole inhibitors of p38 mitogen-activated protein kinase selectively inhibiting the TGF-β-receptor I kinase (activin-like kinase [ALK]-5) have recently been developed and tested in in vitro experiments and found to block many or all actions of TGF-β *(78–82)*. These compounds also inhibit ALK-4 and -7 but not the BMP-activated type-I receptors (ALK-2, -3, or -6). Unfortunately, no in vivo experimental studies with these ALK-5 inhibitors in animal models of renal diseases, especially DN, have yet been published. Because TGF-β knockout mice develop systemic lymphoma-like illnesses with accelerated mortality (indicating a role of this cytokine in immune surveillance), systemic therapy with a global TGF-β antagonist in humans could be risky *(83)*.

CTGF Antagonists

CTGF is induced, although not exclusively, by TGF-β and is involved in the upregulation of ECM-expression in several cell types. Moreover, this growth factor also contributes to the phenotype transition of fibroblasts to myofibroblasts. Antisense oligonucleotides that reduce CTGF have been shown to lessen renal fibrogenesis *(84)*. An anti-CTGF human monoclonal antibody is presently examined in phase Ib clinical trials in patients with DN *(85)*.

Imatinib Mesylate

Imatinib mesylate (Gleevec®, Novartis, New Hanover, NJ) has been developed for the treatment of Philadelphia+ acute myelogenous leukemia expressing B-cell receptor-abl and for tumors that grow *c*-kit dependently. In addition to these two oncogene products, this compound inhibits abelson and the PDGF-receptor kinase (Fig. 6). There are two reasons why imatinib could be a useful antifibrogenic therapeutic agent in renal diseases such as DN. First, PDGF is an important proliferative agent for renal fibroblasts *(35)*. Second, recent observations indicate a dual function of TGF-β in (renal) fibroblasts. TGF-β-dependent fibroblast proliferation utilizes the ableson nonreceptor tyrosine kinase (*c*-abl) but other fibrogenic functions of this cytokine such as promoting transition to myofibroblasts and upregulation of matrix expression in these latter cells appears to be mainly smad3-dependent *(50)*. In vivo studies in a rat model demonstrate that imatinib ameliorates TGF-β-driven renal interstitial fibrosis by reducing fibroblast proliferation *(50,51)*. Thus, although data in DN in humans are not available, imatinib mesylate or newer drugs with similar functions could be useful in the therapy of DN pending further (especially human) studies *(86)*.

SUMMARY

The degree of interstitial fibrosis determines severity and progression of chronic renal failure in DN, and glomerular protein ultrafiltration appears to be causatively involved. Ultrafiltered albumin and, importantly, ultrafiltered growth factor cytokines (IGF-I, TGF-β, HGF, and potentially others) activate the transcription factor NF-κB and transcriptionally activate a number of genes with profibrogenic effects in tubular cells. This leads to basolateral formation of chemokine gradients causing macrophage attraction and activation. These latter cells in peritubular spaces are perhaps the major source of interstitial TGF-β, the most important, single fibrogenesis regulator. Through its antiproliferative effects in epithelial cells TGF-β may contribute to tubular atrophy whereas it has proliferative activity on resting interstitial fibroblasts (through non-smad passways) and transforms fibroblasts to the myofibroblast phenotype (through smad2/3 passways). Myofibroblasts are the predominant source of interstitially accumulating ECM proteins. Some of the profibrogenic actions of TGF-β are mediated by CTGF whereas BMP7 is a TGF-β smad-signal inhibitor. Other cytokines such as PDGF-BB, which are also secreted by tubular cells in glomerular proteinuria also contribute to interstitial fibrogenesis such as by contributing to fibroblast proliferation.

These complex interactions between different cell types through intercellular cytokine and chemokine signals give rise to several, potential therapeutic interventions in addition to classical therapies aimed at reducing glomerular proteinuria with ACE inhibitors and ARBs with the goal to reduce interstitial fibrogenesis and hence the rate of progression of renal failure in DN.

REFERENCES

1. Bohle A, Wehrmann M, Bogenschutz O, Batz C, Muller CA, Muller GA. The pathogenesis of chronic renal failure in diabetic nephropathy. Investigation of 488 cases of diabetic glomerulosclerosis. Pathol Res Pract 1991;187:251–259.
2. Taft JL, Nolan CJ, Yeung SP, Hewitson TD, Martin FI. Clinical and histological correlations of decline in renal function in diabetic patients with proteinuria. Diabetes 1994;43:1046–1051.
3. Peterson JC, Adler S, Burkart JM, et al. Blood pressure control, proteinuria, and the progression of renal disease. The Modification of Diet in Renal Disease Study. Ann Int Med 1995;123:754–762.

4. Ruggenenti P, Perna A, Mosconi L, et al. Proteinuria predicts end-stage renal failure in non-diabetic chronic nephropathies. The "Gruppo Italiano di Studi Epidemiologici in Nefrologia" (GISEN). Kidney Int Suppl 1997;63:S54–S57.
5. Narita T, Koshimura J, Suzuki K, et al. Effects of short-term glycemic control, low protein diet and administration of enalapril on renal hemodynamics and protein permselectivity in type 2 diabetic patients with microalbuminuria. Tohoku J Exp Med 1999;189:117–133.
6. Narita T, Sasaki H, Hosoba M, et al. Parallel increase in urinary excretion rates of immunoglobulin G, ceruloplasmin, transferrin, and orosomucoid in normoalbuminuric type 2 diabetic patients. Diabetes Care 2004;27:1176–1181.
7. Zoja C, Morigi M, Remuzzi G. Proteinuria and phenotypic change of proximal tubular cells. J Am Soc Nephrol 2003;14(1):S36–S41.
8. Donadelli R, Abbate M, Zanchi C, et al. Protein traffic activates NF-kB gene signaling and promotes MCP-1-dependent interstitial inflammation. Am J Kidney Dis 2000;36:1226–1241.
9. Donadelli R, Zanchi C, Morigi M, et al. Protein overload induces fractalkine upregulation in proximal tubular cells through nuclear factor kappaB- and p38 mitogen-activated protein kinase-dependent pathways. J Am Soc Nephrol 2003;14:2436–2446.
10. Zoja C, Donadelli R, Colleoni S, et al. Protein overload stimulates RANTES production by proximal tubular cells depending on NF-kappa B activation. Kidney International 1998;53:1608–1615.
11. Hanada T, Yoshimura A. Regulation of cytokine signaling and inflammation. Cytokine Growth Factor Rev 2002;13:413–421.
12. Miyajima A, Kosaka T, Seta K, Asano T, Umezawa K, Hayakawa M. Novel nuclear factor kappa B activation inhibitor prevents inflammatory injury in unilateral ureteral obstruction. J Urol 2003;169:1559–1563.
13. Burton CJ, Combe C, Walls J, Harris KP. Fibronectin production by human tubular cells: the effect of apical protein. Kidney Int 1996;50:760–767.
14. Burton CJ, Combe C, Walls J, Harris KP. Secretion of chemokines and cytokines by human tubular epithelial cells in response to proteins. Nephrol Dial Transplant 1999;14:2628–2633.
15. Thomas ME, Brunskill NJ, Harris KP, et al. Proteinuria induces tubular cell turnover: A potential mechanism for tubular atrophy. Kidney Int 1999;55:890–898.
16. Schreiner GF. Renal toxicity of albumin and other lipoproteins. Curr Opin Nephrol Hypertens 1995;4:369–373.
17. Arici M, Brown J, Harris K, Walls J, Brunskill N. Albumin induced changes in human proximal tubular cell function are dependent on its fatty acid content. J Am Soc Nephrol 1999;10:654 "abstract."
18. Arici M, Brown J, Williams M, Harris KP, Walls J, Brunskill NJ. Fatty acids carried on albumin modulate proximal tubular cell fibronectin production: a role for protein kinase C. Nephrol Dial Transplant 2002;17:1751–1757.
19. Arici M, Chana R, Lewington A, Brown J, Brunskill NJ. Stimulation of proximal tubular cell apoptosis by albumin-bound fatty acids mediated by peroxisome proliferator activated receptor-gamma. J Am Soc Nephrol 2003;14:17–27.
20. Hirschberg R. Bioactivity of glomerular ultrafiltrate during heavy proteinuria may contribute to renal tubulo-interstitial lesions: evidence for a role for insulin-like growth factor I. J Clin Invest 1996;98:116–124.
21. Hammerman MR, Rogers S. Distribution of IGF receptors in the plasma membrane of proximal tubular cells. Am J Physiol 1987;253:F841–F847.
22. Quigley R, Baum M. Effects of growth hormone and insulin-like growth factor I on rabbit proximal convoluted tubule transport. J Clin Invest 1991;88:368–374.
23. Hirschberg R, Kaysen GA. Insulin-like growth factor I and its binding proteins in the experimental nephrotic syndrome. Endocrinology 1995;136:1565–1571.
24. Nyengaard JR, Flyvbjerg A, Rasch R. The impact of renal growth, regression and regrowth in experimental diabetes mellitus on number and size of proximal and distal tubular cells in the rat kidney. Diabetologia 1993;36:1126–1131.
25. Rasch R. Tubular lesions in streptozotocin-diabetic rats. Diabetologia 1984;27:32–37.
26. Wang S, LaPage J, Hirschberg R. Role of glomerular ultrafiltration of growth factors in progressive interstitial fibrosis in diabetic nephropathy. Kidney Int 2000;57:1002–1014.
27. Zhang X, Yang J, Li Y, Liu Y. Both Sp1 and Smad participate in mediating TGF-beta1-induced HGF receptor expression in renal epithelial cells. Am J Physiol Renal Physiol 2005;288:F16–F26.
28. Wang S, Hirschberg R. Growth factor ultrafiltration in experimental diabetic nephropathy contributes to interstitial fibrosis. Am J Physiol 2000;278:F554–F560.

29. Roberts AB. Molecular and cell biology of TGF-beta. Miner Electrolyte Metab 1998;24:111–119.
30. Ando T, Okuda S, Yanagida T, Fujishima M. Localization of TGF-beta and its receptors in the kidney. Miner Electrolyte Metab 1998;24:149–153.
31. Honkanen E, Teppo AM, Tornroth T, Groop PH, Gronhagen-Riska C. Urinary transforming growth factor-beta 1 in membranous glomerulonephritis. Nephrol Dial Transplant 1997;12:2562–2568.
32. Sato H, Iwano M, Akai Y, et al. Increased excretion of urinary transforming growth factor beta 1 in patients with diabetic nephropathy. Am J Nephrol 1998;18:490–494.
33. Song JH, Lee SW, Suh JH, et al. The effects of dual blockade of the renin-angiotensin system on urinary protein and transforming growth factor-beta excretion in 2 groups of patients with IgA and diabetic nephropathy. Clin Nephrol 2003;60:318–326.
34. Johnson DW, Saunders HJ, Baxter RC, Field MJ, Pollock CA. Paracrine stimulation of human renal fibroblasts by proximal tubule cells. Kidney Int 1998;54:747–757.
35. Tang WW, Ulich TR, Lacey DL, et al. Platelet-derived growth factor-BB induces renal tubulointerstitial myofibroblast formation and tubulointerstitial fibrosis. Am J Pathol 1996;148:1169–1180.
36. Grotendorst GR, Rahmanie H, Duncan MR. Combinatorial signaling pathways determine fibroblast proliferation and myofibroblast differentiation. FASEB J 2004;18:469–479.
37. Bradham DM, Igarashi A, Potter RL, Grotendorst GR. Connective tissue growth factor: a cysteine-rich mitogen secreted by human vascular endothelial cells is related to the SRC-induced immediate early gene product CEF-10. J Cell Biol 1991;114:1285–1294.
38. Grotendorst GR, Okochi H, Hayashi N. A novel transforming growth factor beta response element controls the expression of the connective tissue growth factor gene. Cell Growth Differ 1996;7:469–480.
39. Wang S, Denichilo M, Brubaker C, Hirschberg R. Connective tissue growth factor in tubulointerstitial injury of diabetic nephropathy. Kidney Int 2001;60:96–105.
40. Yang DH, Kim HS, Wilson EM, Rosenfeld RG, Oh Y. Identification of glycosylated 38-kDa connective tissue growth factor (IGFBP-related protein 2) and proteolytic fragments in human biological fluids, and up-regulation of IGFBP-rP2 expression by TGF-beta in Hs578T human breast cancer cells. J Clin Endocrinol Metab 1998;83:2593–2596.
41. Kim HS, Nagalla SR, Oh Y, Wilson E, Roberts CT Jr, Rosenfeld RG. Identification of a family of low-affinity insulin-like growth factor binding proteins (IGFBPs): characterization of connective tissue growth factor as a member of the IGFBP superfamily. Proc Natl Acad Sci USA 1997;94:12,981–12,986.
42. Segarini PR, Nesbitt JE, Li D, Hays LG, Yates JR 3rd, Carmichael DF. The low density lipoprotein receptor-related protein/alpha2-macroglobulin receptor is a receptor for connective tissue growth factor. J Biol Chem 2001;276:40,659–40,667.
43. Lam S, van der Geest RN, Verhagen NA, et al. Connective tissue growth factor and igf-I are produced by human renal fibroblasts and cooperate in the induction of collagen production by high glucose. Diabetes 2003;52:2975–2983.
44. Martin P. Wound healing—aiming for perfect skin regeneration. Science 1997;276:75–81.
45. Wada T, Furuichi K, Sakai N, et al. Up-regulation of monocyte chemoattractant protein-1 in tubulointerstitial lesions of human diabetic nephropathy. Kidney Int 2000;58:1492–1499.
46. Amann B, Tinzmann R, Angelkort B. ACE inhibitors improve diabetic nephropathy through suppression of renal MCP-1. Diabetes Care 2003;26:2421–2425.
47. Rovin BH, Doe N, Tan LC. Monocyte chemoattractant protein-1 levels in patients with glomerular disease. Am J Kidney Dis 1996;27:640–646.
48. Morii T, Fujita H, Narita T, et al. Association of monocyte chemoattractant protein-1 with renal tubular damage in diabetic nephropathy. J Diabetes Complications 2003;17:11–15.
49. Mezzano S, Aros C, Droguett A, et al. NF-kappaB activation and overexpression of regulated genes in human diabetic nephropathy. Nephrol Dial Transplant 2004;19:2505–2512.
50. Wang S, Wilkes MC, Leof EB, Hirschberg R. Imatinib mesylate blocks a non-Smad TGF-beta pathway and reduces renal fibrogenesis in vivo. FASEB J 2005;19:1–11.
51. Lassila M, Jandeleit-Dahm K, Seah KK, et al. Imatinib attenuates diabetic nephropathy in apolipoprotein E-knockout mice. J Am Soc Nephrol 2005;16:363–373.
52. Massague J, Kelly B, Mottola C. Stimulation by insulin-like growth factors is required for cellular transformation by type beta transforming growth factor. J Biol Chem 1985;260:4551–4554.
53. Essawy M, Soylemezoglu O, Muchaneta-Kubara EC, Shortland J, Brown CB, el Nahas AM. Myofibroblasts and the progression of diabetic nephropathy. Nephrol Dial Transplant 1997;12:43–50.
54. Kalluri R, Neilson EG. Epithelial-mesenchymal transition and its implications for fibrosis. J Clin Invest 2003;112:1776–1784.

55. Lan HY. Tubular epithelial–myofibroblast transdifferentiation mechanisms in proximal tubule cells. Curr Opin Nephrol Hypertens 2003;12:25–29.
56. Hashimoto N, Jin H, Liu T, Chensue SW, Phan SH. Bone marrow-derived progenitor cells in pulmonary fibrosis. J Clin Invest 2004;113:243–252.
57. Iwano M, Plieth D, Danoff TM, Xue C, Okada H, Neilson EG. Evidence that fibroblasts derive from epithelium during tissue fibrosis. J Clin Invest 2002;110:341–350.
58. Brenner BM, Cooper ME, de Zeeuw D, et al. Effects of losartan on renal and cardiovascular outcomes in patients with type 2 diabetes and nephropathy. N Engl J Med 2001;345:861–869.
59. Park HC, Xu ZG, Choi S, et al. Effect of losartan and amlodipine on proteinuria and transforming growth factor-beta1 in patients with IgA nephropathy. Nephrol Dial Transplant 2003;18:1115–1121.
60. Andersen S, Brochner-Mortensen J, Parving HH. Kidney function during and after withdrawal of long-term irbesartan treatment in patients with type 2 diabetes and microalbuminuria. Diabetes Care 2003;26:3296–3302.
61. Ruilope LM, Segura J. Losartan and other angiotensin II antagonists for nephropathy in type 2 diabetes mellitus: a review of the clinical trial evidence. Clin Ther 2003;25:3044–3064.
62. Nakao N, Yoshimura A, Morita H, Takada M, Kayano T, Ideura T. Combination treatment of angiotensin-II receptor blocker and angiotensin-converting-enzyme inhibitor in non-diabetic renal disease (COOPERATE): a randomised controlled trial. Lancet 2003;361:117–124.
63. Shimizu H, Maruyama S, Yuzawa Y, et al. Anti-monocyte chemoattractant protein-1 gene therapy attenuates renal injury induced by protein-overload proteinuria. J Am Soc Nephrol 2003;14: 1496–505.
64. Takase O, Hirahashi J, Takayanagi A, et al. Gene transfer of truncated IkappaBalpha prevents tubulointerstitial injury. Kidney Int 2003;63:501–513.
65. Rajkumar SV, Richardson PG, Hideshima T, Anderson KC. Proteasome inhibition as a novel therapeutic target in human cancer. J Clin Oncol 2005;23:630–639.
66. Hideshima T, Chauhan D, Richardson P, et al. NF-kappa B as a therapeutic target in multiple myeloma. J Biol Chem 2002;277:16,639–16,347.
67. Liu Y. Hepatocyte growth factor in kidney fibrosis: therapeutic potential and mechanisms of action. Am J Physiol Renal Physiol 2004;287:F7–F16.
68. Dai C, Liu Y. Hepatocyte growth factor antagonizes the profibrotic action of TGF-beta1 in mesangial cells by stabilizing Smad transcriptional corepressor TGIF. J Am Soc Nephrol 2004;15:1402–1412.
69. Dai C, Yang J, Bastacky S, Xia J, Li Y, Liu Y. Intravenous administration of hepatocyte growth factor gene ameliorates diabetic nephropathy in mice. J Am Soc Nephrol 2004;15:2637–2647.
70. Inoue T, Okada H, Kobayashi T, et al. Hepatocyte growth factor counteracts transforming growth factor-beta1, through attenuation of connective tissue growth factor induction, and prevents renal fibrogenesis in 5/6 nephrectomized mice. FASEB J 2003;17:268–270.
71. Cruzado JM, Lloberas N, Torras J, et al. Regression of advanced diabetic nephropathy by hepatocyte growth factor gene therapy in rats. Diabetes 2004;53:1119–1127.
72. Wang S, LaPage J, Hirschberg R. Loss of tubular bone morphogenetic protein-7 (BMP7) in diabetic nephropathy. J Am Soc Nephrol 2001;12:2392–2399.
73. Wang S, Hirschberg R. BMP7 antagonizes TGF-beta -dependent fibrogenesis in mesangial cells. Am J Physiol Renal Physiol 2003;284:F1006–F1013.
74. Wang S, Hirschberg R. Bone morphogenetic protein-7 signals opposing transforming growth factor beta in mesangial cells. J Biol Chem 2004;279:23,200–23,206.
75. Zeisberg M, Hanai J, Sugimoto H, et al. BMP-7 counteracts TGF-beta1-induced epithelial-to-mesenchymal transition and reverses chronic renal injury. Nat Med 2003;9:964–968.
76. Wang S, Chen Q, Simon TC, et al. Bone morphogenic protein-7 (BMP-7), a novel therapy for diabetic nephropathy. Kidney Int 2003;63:2037–2049.
77. Ziyadeh FN, Hoffman BB, Han DC, et al. Long-term prevention of renal insufficiency, excess matrix gene expression, and glomerular mesangial matrix expansion by treatment with monoclonal anti-transforming growth factor-beta antibody in db/db diabetic mice (see comments). Proc Natl Acad Sci USA 2000;97:8015–8020.
78. Callahan JF, Burgess JL, Fornwald JA, et al. Identification of novel inhibitors of the transforming growth factor beta1 (TGF-beta1) type 1 receptor (ALK5). J Med Chem 2002;45:999–1001.
79. DaCosta Byfield S, Major C, Laping NJ, Roberts AB. SB-505124 is a selective inhibitor of transforming growth factor-beta type I receptors ALK4, ALK5, and ALK7. Mol Pharmacol 2004;65:744–752.
80. Hjelmeland MD, Hjelmeland AB, Sathornsumetee S, et al. SB-431542, a small molecule transforming growth factor-beta-receptor antagonist, inhibits human glioma cell line proliferation and motility. Mol Cancer Ther 2004;3:737–745.

81. Inman GJ, Nicolas FJ, Callahan JF, et al. SB-431542 is a potent and specific inhibitor of transforming growth factor-beta superfamily type I activin receptor-like kinase (ALK) receptors ALK4, ALK5, and ALK7. Mol Pharmacol 2002;62:65–74.
82. Laping NJ. ALK5 inhibition in renal disease. Curr Opin Pharmacol 2003;3:204–208.
83. Letterio JJ, Bottinger EP. TGF-beta knockout and dominant-negative receptor transgenic mice. Miner Electrolyte Metab 1998;24:161–167.
84. Yokoi H, Mukoyama M, Nagae T, et al. Reduction in connective tissue growth factor by antisense treatment ameliorates renal tubulointerstitial fibrosis. J Am Soc Nephrol 2004;15:1430–1440.
85. Fibrogen Inc. URL: www.fibrogen.com/pipeline/chart/diabetes.html#mid, March 2005.
86. Shah NP, Tran C, Lee FY, Chen P, Norris D, Sawyers CL. Overriding imatinib resistance with a novel ABL kinase inhibitor. Science 2004;305:399–401.

I

Basic Pathophysiology and Biochemistry of Diabetic Nephropathy

C. Podocytes

4 Podocytes and Diabetic Nephropathy

George Jerums, MBBS, MD,
Sianna Panagiotopoulos, PhD,
and Richard MacIsaac, PhD, MD

CONTENTS

INTRODUCTION

The glomerular capillary wall comprises three major components: the fenestrated endothelium surrounded by glycocalyx, the glomerular basement membrane, and the podocyte layer. Podocytes are specialized epithelial cells that form a network of interdigitating foot processes. The predominant filtration pathway for macromolecules is through slit diaphragms bounded by podocyte foot processes. Nephrin is a key component of the slit diaphragm in association with other intracellular proteins, including CD2-associated protein (CD2AP), podocin, and α-actinin IV (Fig. 1). Together, these proteins contribute to the role of the slit diaphragm as the major size-selective filtration barrier.

Recent studies using electron tomography have shown that the slit diaphragm consists of extracellular nephrin strands with pores of similar size to albumin, approx 40 nm wide *(1)*. Genetic studies have revealed abnormalities in nephrin expression that result in severe proteinuria accompanied by abnormalities of the slit diaphragm. For

From: *Contemporary Diabetes: The Diabetic Kidney*
Edited by: P. Cortes and C. E. Mogensen © Humana Press Inc., Totowa, NJ

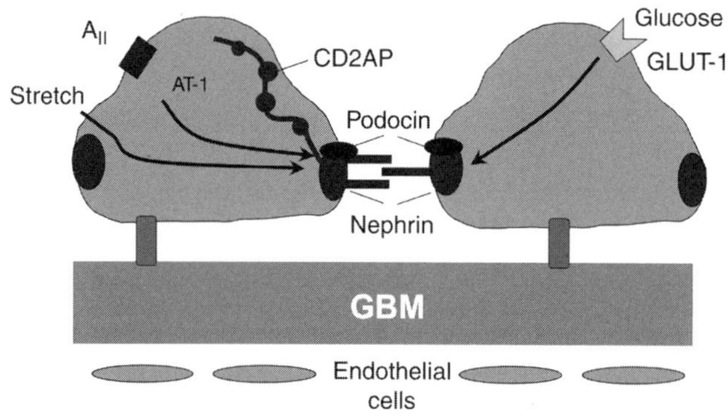

Fig. 1. The normal glomerular filtration barrier, indicating the slit diaphragm composed of overlapping nephrin strands.

instance, congenital nephrotic syndrome of the Finnish type is caused by various mutations in the nephrin gene (*NPH S*1), which result in different phenotypes *(2)*. Mutations of the gene encoding podocin, which connects nephrin to the cytoskeleton, have been found in steroid-resistant congenital nephrotic syndrome *(3)*. Mice lacking the gene for CD2-associated protein also develop a congenital nephrotic syndrome *(4)*. Apart from their role in protecting against massive or lethal proteinuria, the podocytes and nephrin constitute the major cellular and molecular modulators of protein filtration by the glomerulus.

The above discoveries have diminished the importance of the basement membrane endothelium in glomerular protein filtration even though the permeability of the basement membrane to albumin is less than 1% of a layer of water of equal thickness. The placement of the glomerular basement membrane upstream to the slit diaphragm means that its size selectivity for proteins is likely to be completely masked *(5)*. Deletion of heparan sulphate, which is a major negatively charged constituent of the glomerular basement membrane, does not lead to proteinuria *(6)*. Nevertheless, the glomerular basement membrane is the major determinant of glomerular hydraulic permeability. Although the fenestrae of the endothelium are too large to sieve proteins, there is evidence that the endothelial glycocalyx contributes to glomerular sieving function *(7)*.

The present review of the role of podocytes in diabetic nephropathy will focus, first, on podocyte ultrastructure, followed by assessment of nephrin expression in experimental and human studies, and then the regulation of podocyte function in diabetes. Finally, it will analyze the role of the podocyte in initiating increases in albuminuria in diabetic nephropathy (DN) and its possible contribution to the progression of DN. The components, constituents, products, functions, and changes in DN of the glomerular filtration barrier and its associated mesangial cells (MCs) are summarized in Table 1.

PODOCYTE ULTRASTRUCTURE IN TYPE 1 DIABETES

There have been several studies of glomerular ultrastructure in patients with type 1 diabetes spanning the spectrum from normoalbuminuria through microalbuminuria to overt nephropathy (Table 2). Using light microscopy, comparisons of renal ultrastructural changes in microalbuminuric patients and healthy controls have focused on basement membrane thickening and matrix/glomerular volume fraction. In some studies, microalbuminuric patients were shown to have significantly increased glomerular

Table 1
The Glomerular Filtration Barrier in Diabetes

Component	*Constituents*	*Products*	*Regenerative potential*	*Functions*	*Changes in diabetic nephropathy*
Podocyte	Nephrin Podocin GLUT-1 GLUT-4 CD-2 associated protein Local RAS VEGF R-1	TGF-β VEGF	Absent	Size-selective filter of macromolecules at level of slit diaphragm, formed by extracellular nephrin strands	↓ podocyte density and foot process flattening Nephrin redistribution and ↓ expression Loss of slit diaphragm
Basement membrane	Collagen IV, laminin Fibronectin HSPG		N/A	Major site of hydraulic resistance and solute filter	GBM thickening
Mesangial cell	Local RAS	TGF-β	Present	Control of intraglomerular pressure in association with afferent and efferent glomerular arterioles	Extracellular matrix accumulation eventually contributing to ↓ GFR in association with nephron dropout
Endothelial cell Glycocalyx	Local RAS VEGFR-1 VEGFR-2	I-CAM V-CAM Selectins VWF	Present	Endothelial glycocalyx modulates glomerular permeability in response to VEGF	Endothelial dysfunction at glomerular and systemic level

RAS, renin–angiotensin system; VEGF, vascular endothelial growth factor; TGF-β, transforming growth factor-β; HSPG, heparan sulphate proteoglycan; GBM, glomerular basement membrane; GFR, glomerular filtration rate.

Table 2
Ultrastructure of Podocytes in Type 1 Diabetes

Study	*Subjects*	*Stage of nephropathy*	*Findings*
Ellis (1987) *(13)*	28 diabetic 28 nondiabetic	15 N 5 micro 8 overt	1. FPW in micro equal to FPW in N 2. ↑ FPW in micro patients c/w control subjects 3. ↑ FPW with overt DN
Bjorn (1995) *(75)*	27 diabetic 11 nondiabetic	9 N 9 micro 9 overt	1. Overall trend to ↑ FPW with ↑ AER 2. Widening of filtration slits does not explain ↑ AER 3. Filtration slit width ↓ as GFR ↓
Berg (1998) *(76)*	36 diabetic (adolescents)	36 N (8 transient micro at time of biopsy)	1. Negative correlation between FPW and AER 2. Negative correlation between filtration slit length density and AER 3. ↑ FPW suggests glomeruli are enlarged and/or exposed to ↑ intraglomerular pressure
Steffes (2001) *(14)*	46 diabetic 36 nondiabetic	Varied (AER data not shown)	1. Podocyte density did not change with duration of diabetes or severity of DN 2. Podocyte number in diabetes c/w controls, even in short duration diabetes
White (2002) *(15)* Esprit Study	50 diabetic (all normotensive) 10 nondiabetic	32 Micro 18 overt Enalapril vs nifedipine vs placebo	1. Overall no significant ↓ in podocyte number in normotensive patients with raised AER 2. In subgroup with overt DN: podocyte number correlated negatively with ↑ AER 3. In placebo-treated patients: decrease in podocyte density over 3 yr correlated with final AER 4. Association between podocyte loss and AER may be response to, cause of, or concomitant with, progression of DN

DN, diabetic nephropathy; N, normoalbuminuria; micro, microalbuminuria; FPW, foot process width; AER, albumin excretion rate; c/w, compared with.

basement membrane thickness and matrix/glomerular volume fraction when compared with normoalbuminuric patients *(8–10)*. However, other studies using different methodology, did not confirm these findings *(11,12)*. None of these studies, which were performed in the 1990s, addressed podocyte ultrastructure by electron microscopy.

Using electron microscopy, alterations in podocytes have been described even in normoalbuminuric patients. In a mixed group of type 1 diabetic patients with microalbuminuria and overt nephropathy, the first observations of glomerular epithelial cell structure were reported in 1987 *(13)*. This showed increased foot process width in patients with either microalbuminuria or overt nephropathy compared with control subjects. Another study in nine normoalbuminuric and nine microalbuminuric patients as well as nine patients with overt nephropathy also showed a trend for increased foot process width with increasing albuminuria *(14)*. Widening of filtration slits did not correlate with increases in albuminuria, but a decrease in filtration slit width was associated with a decrease in glomerular filtration rate *(14)*. In a study of 36 adolescent patients with normoalbuminuria, 8 of whom had transient microalbuminuria at the time of biopsy, a positive correlation was found between foot process width and albumin excretion rate and a negative correlation between filtration slit length density and albumin excretion rate *(15)*. The authors of this study concluded that increased foot process width suggests that glomeruli are enlarged and/or exposed to increased intraglomerular pressure resulting in adaptive change by the podocytes. A subsequent study by Steffes in 2001 found that podocyte density did not change with duration of diabetes or severity of diabetic nephropathy *(14)*. However, decrease in podocyte number was found in patients with type 1 diabetes compared with controls, even in those with a relatively short duration of diabetes. Unfortunately, albumin excretion data were not shown, which makes it difficult to compare this study with others.

A more recent study of 32 patients with type 1 diabetes and microalbuminuria and 18 patients with overt nephropathy showed that when these patients were analyzed as a group, there was no significant decrease in podocyte number *(15)*. However, in the subgroup with overt nephropathy, podocyte number correlated negatively with an increase in albumin excretion rate. Serial biopsies in normotensive patients showed that a decrease in podocyte density over 3 yr correlated with final albumin excretion rate. The authors concluded that the association between podocyte loss and albumin excretion rate may be a response to, rather than a cause of, progression of nephropathy. The importance of serial ultrastructural studies was emphasized.

PODOCYTE ULTRASTRUCTURE IN TYPE 2 DIABETES

The main findings of studies examining podocyte ultrastructure in type 2 diabetes are summarized in Table 3. The first two studies of podocyte ultrastructure in type 2 diabetes were performed in Pima Indians. In the first, 51 patients with a range of albumin excretion rates from normo- to macroalbuminuria were studied *(16)*. Microalbuminuria could not be distinguished from normoalbuminuria on structural grounds. Broadening of foot processes was associated with enlarged glomeruli and a decrease in podocyte numbers was found in patients with overt nephropathy. It was concluded that podocyte loss contributes to progression of nephropathy. The second study focussed on 16 Pima Indians with microalbuminuria and found that a decrease in podocyte density predicted progression of albumin excretion rate over 4 yr *(17)*.

Table 3
Ultrastructure of Podocytes in Type 2 Diabetes

Study	*Subjects*	*Stage of nephropathy*	*Findings*
Pagtalunan (1997) *(16)*	51 diabetic (Pimas) Eight nondiabetic	10 N-early 12 N-late 17 micro 12 overt	1. Micro could not be distinguished from N on structural grounds 2. Broadening of foot processes associated with large glomeruli and ↓ podocyte number in overt DN 3. Podocyte loss contributes to progression of DN
Meyer (1999) *(17)*	16 diabetic (Pimas)	micro	1. Podocyte density predicts AER ↑ over 4 yr 2. Podocytes important in development and progression of DN
Dalla Vestra (2003) *(18)*	67 diabetic (Caucasian) 20 nondiabetic	21 N 23 micro 23 overt	1. Podocyte density ↓ in all diabetic c/w controls 2. Podocyte density and filtration slit length density ↓ as AER ↑ 3. Foot process width ↑ as AER ↑ 4. Podocyte density may be more relevant than absolute number
White (2004) *(19)*	16 diabetic (Caucasian) (hypertensive) 28 nondiabetic	16 overt	1. Podocyte number ↓ in diabetic c/w controls 2. Glomerular volume ↑ in diabetic c/w controls 3. Negative correlation between proteinuria and podocyte number and podocyte density per glomerulus 4. Longitudinal studies are required to determine sequence of events leading to podocyte loss

DN, diabetic nephropathy; N, normoalbuminuria; Micro, microalbuminuria; AER, albumin excretion rate; c/w, compared with.

Subsequently, two studies were performed in Caucasian patients with type 2 diabetes. In the first, a group of 67 patients with an approximately equal proportion of normo-, micro-, and macroalbuminuric subjects was studied *(18)*. Podocyte density was decreased in all diabetic patients regardless of albuminuria status compared with controls. Podocyte density and filtration slit length density decreased as albuminuria increased and foot process width increased as albuminuria increased. It was concluded that podocyte density may be more relevant to nephropathy than absolute podocyte number. A second study in 16 hypertensive Caucasian diabetic patients with overt nephropathy was performed recently *(19)*. This showed that podocyte number was decreased whereas glomerular volume was increased in diabetic subjects compared with controls. There was a negative correlation between proteinuria and podocyte number and between proteinuria and podocyte density per glomerulus. It was pointed out that longitudinal studies are required to determine the sequence of events leading to podocyte loss. As in their previous study in type 1 patients, these authors raised the possibility that podocyte loss may be part of the disease process rather than a causal factor. This would be consistent with the concept that albuminuria is a marker but not the culprit in the progression of renal disease *(20)*.

PODOCYTE AND NEPHRIN EXPRESSION IN EXPERIMENTAL DIABETES

Nephrin is a 130-kDa transmembrane protein of the immunoglobulin superfamily of cell adhesion molecules, which is specifically expressed in podocytes *(21)*. Studies in experimental diabetes have generally demonstrated a biphasic expression of nephrin with increasing albuminuria (Table 4). Four studies from Melbourne have assessed nephrin gene expression in rats with streptozotocin-induced diabetes. In a 24-wk study, glomerular nephrin gene expression was increased at 8 wk followed by a decrease at 16 and 24 wk in hypertensive diabetic rats *(22)*. By comparison, in normotensive diabetic rats, there was an increase in nephrin gene expression at 8 wk but no significant decrease at 16 or 24 wk despite an increase in albumin excretion rate *(22)*. Irbesartan therapy prevented the decrease in glomerular nephrin gene expression and nephrin immunostaining and attenuated albumin excretion in hypertensive diabetic rats *(23)*.

In normotensive diabetic rats assessed at 1 and 24 wk, decreased nephrin gene expression was found in the late proteinuric phase but not in the preproteinuric phase *(24)*. Perindopril therapy attenuated changes in nephrin gene expression and also albuminuria. By contrast, aminoguanidine therapy attenuated albuminuria but not nephrin gene expression *(24)*. An electron microscopic study in normotensive diabetic rats demonstrated a decrease in the number of slit pores per unit length of glomerular basement membrane after 24 wk, consistent with podocyte foot process broadening *(25)*. These changes were attenuated by treatment with either ramipril or valsartan and were consistent with results obtained later in human studies.

NEPHRIN EXPRESSION IN HUMAN DIABETES

Two studies have assessed nephrin expression in human diabetic nephropathy (Table 5). In the first, 14 patients with type-2 diabetes and overt nephropathy were randomized to 2-yr treatment with perindopril or placebo as part of the diabiopsies study *(26)*. Similar degrees of proteinuria were noted in the perindopril and placebo groups at the time of biopsy performed 2 yr after randomization. In the placebo group, decreased nephrin

Table 4
Podocyte and Nephrin Expression in Diabetic Nephropathy (Animal Studies)

Study	*Model*	*Intervention*	*Duration*	*Findings*
Forbes (2002) *(22)*	HTN and NT diabetic and nondiabetic rats	Nil	8, 16, 24 wk	1. HT diabetic rats: glomerular NGE ↑ at 8 wk, followed by ↓ at 16 and 24 wk in association with ↑ AER 2. NT diabetic rats: ↑ NGE at 8 wk, but no significant decrease in NGE at 16 or 24 wk
Bonnet (2001) *(23)*	HTN diabetic rats	Irbesartan vs placebo	32 wk	1. ↓ glomerular NGE and nephrin immunostaining in diabetic SHR 2. Normalised by irbesartan, in parallel with prevention of AER increase
Mifsud (2001) *(25)*	NT diabetic rat	Control Diabetic Diabetic + ramipril Diabetic + valsartan	24 wk	1. ↓ in number of slit pores per unit length of GBM, corrected for glomerular volume, indicating podocyte foot process broadening in diabetic rats 2. Attenuated by ramipril and valsartan
Kelly (2002) *(24)*	NT diabetic rat	Perindopril vs aminoguanidine vs placebo	1, 24 wk	1. ↓ NGE in late proteinuric phase but not in pre-proteinuric phase 2. Perindopril attenuated ↓ NGE and ↑ AER 3. Aminoguanidine attenuated ↑ AER but not NGE

HTN, hypertensive; NT, normotensive; NGE, nephrin gene expression.

Table 5
Nephrin Expression in Diabetic Nephropathy (Human Studies)

Study	*Subjects*	*Intervention*	*Duration*	*Findings*
Langham (2002) *(26)* Diabiopsies study	Type 2 diabetes + overt DN	Perindopril (n = 7) Placebo (n = 7)	Renal biopsy 2 yr after randomization	1. Similar proteinuria in perindopril and placebo groups at time of biopsy 2. Placebo: ↓ NGE c/w nondiabetic subjects 3. Perindopril: NGE same as in nondiabetic subjects 4. Close inverse correlation between NGE and proteinuria in both perindopril and placebo groups
Doublier (2003) *(27)*	Normal subjects *(10)* Diabetic + micro (1 type 1, 5 type 2) Diabetic + overt DN (7 type 1, 10 type 2)	Nil	Cross-sectional study	1. ↓ nephrin immunostaining in both micro and overt DN groups 2. ↓ nephrin immunostaining on exposure to angiotensin II or glycated albumin, acting via RAGE in cultured human podocytes

Micro, microalbuminuria; DN, diabetic nephropathy; NGE, nephrin gene expression.

gene expression was found compared with a nondiabetic control group, whereas in perindopril-treated patients nephrin gene expression was the same as in the control group. A close inverse relationship was found between nephrin gene expression and proteinuria in both the perindopril (n = 7) and placebo (n = 7) groups.

In the second study, nephrin immunostaining was assessed in a mixed group of type 1 and type 2 diabetic patients. Ten normal subjects were compared with 6 diabetic patients with microalbuminuria and 17 diabetic patients with overt nephropathy *(27)*. Decreased nephrin immunostaining was observed in both diabetic groups. In the same report, studies in cultured human podocytes showed a decrease in nephrin immunostaining after exposure to angiotensin II or glycated albumin acting via the receptor for advanced glycation endproducts (RAGE).

The above studies indicate that there is a strong inverse relationship between nephrin gene expression and proteinuria in experimental and human diabetes. In the human studies, the numbers are too small to differentiate between any specific changes in nephrin expression in type 1 as opposed to type 2 diabetes. The question of whether changes in nephrin expression precede, follow, or are part of the process of proteinuria is not yet resolved.

Despite the small number of studies to date, current evidence suggests that modulation of nephrin expression may regulate glomerular permeability to proteins and that blockade of the renin–angiotensin system (RAS) may exert a direct intrarenal effect on angiotensin action at the glomerular filtration barrier. This is supported by evidence that angiotensin II receptors are found in isolated intact glomeruli *(28)*. The renoprotective effects of RAS blockade may, therefore, include a local action on podocyte number and structure and nephrin expression as suggested by Tryggvason *(29)*. By contrast, the antiproteinuric effects of aminoguanidine, which inhibits advanced glycation, may depend on alterations of lysosomal albumin-processing mechanisms in the renal tubules *(24,30)*.

ALTERATIONS OF PODOCYTE FUNCTION IN DIABETES

Both metabolic (hyperglycemia) and hemodynamic (stretch and systemic hypertension) mechanisms are important mediators of podocyte dysfunction in diabetic nephropathy. Podocytes are the principal cell type involved in the formation of the glomerular basement membrane *(31)*. Podocytes also secrete matrix metalloproteinases (MMPs) that modulate matrix remodeling *(32)*. Recent studies in cultured human podocytes have shown that glucose decreases MMP activity and enhances tissue inhibitor of matrix metalloproteinase (TIMP)-2 expression, thereby reducing extracellular matrix (ECM) degradation *(33)*. These results are similar to earlier reports of the effects of glucose on MMP activity in mesangial cells (MCs) *(34)*.

In diabetes, podocytes can be stimulated by hyperglycemia to produce several cytokines and growth factors that may mediate both functional and structural alterations in the glomerular filtration barrier *(35)*. Glucose influx is modulated by GLUT-1 in both podocytes and MCs and GLUT-4 in podocytes *(36)*. Transgenic experiments have shown that overexpression of GLUT-1 in MCs cultured in a normal glucose milieu mimics the diabetic phenotype *(37,38)*. Both insulin and transforming growth factor (TGF)-β_1 stimulate glucose uptake by enhancing GLUT-1 expression in podocytes and MCs, and it has been hypothesized that resistance to insulin action at the level of the podocyte may explain the occurrence of microalbuminuria in patients with type 2 diabetes *(39,40)*. Endogenous TGF-β_1, platelet-derived growth factor, and connective tissue growth factor play important roles as mediators of sclerosis and fibrosis at both glomerular and tubular levels *(41)*.

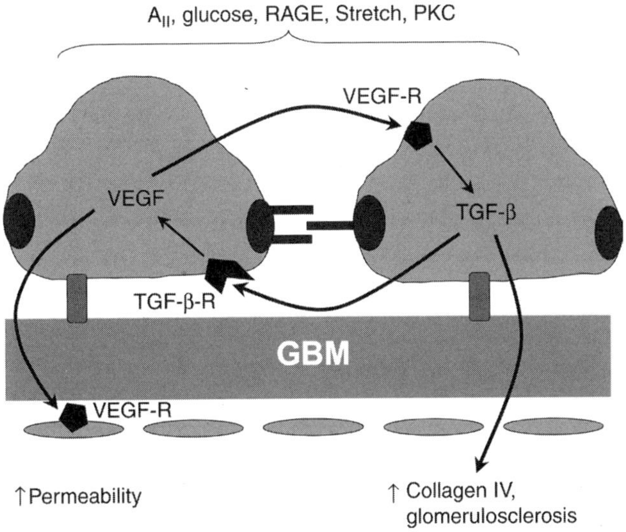

Fig. 2. The autocrine effects of VEGF and TGF-β on the podocoyte, induced by metabolic and/or hemodynamic stimuli.

PODOCYTES AND TGF-β

Several studies have linked TGF-β to both functional and structural changes in DN. TGF-β gene expression and protein levels are significantly increased in glomeruli and the tubulo-interstitium, in human and experimental diabetes *(41)*. However, the interaction between high glucose levels and TGF-β_1 expression in podocytes is indirect. High glucose does not induce TGF-β_1 expression in podocytes but it enhances podocyte responsiveness to TGF-β_1 by increasing the expression of the TGF-β_1 type-2 receptor *(42)*. Angiotensin II is an additional factor that stimulates renal cells to produce TGF-β_1. In vitro studies have shown that cyclic stretch of MCs and podocytes stimulates TGF-β_1 gene expression and protein secretion *(43)* and enhances the expression of TGF-β receptors *(44)*.

A recent study has made it possible to dissociate glomerulosclerosis and tubulo-interstitial fibrosis from albuminuria using anti-TGF-β antibodies *(45)*. In this study, long-term administration of monoclonal anti-TGF antibody to genetically diabetic db/db mice prevented the development of glomerular mesangial matrix expansion and renal insufficiency, but failed to prevent an increase in albuminuria. By contrast, blockade of vascular cadothelial growth factor (VEGF) by administration of neutralizing antibodies to diabetic rats abolished hyperfiltration and partially suppressed urinary albumin excretion *(46)*. These studies suggest that activation of distinct VEGF and TGF-β axes may contribute to the functional and morphological alterations in DN *(47)*.

PODOCYTES AND VEGF

Apart from increasing the expression of TGF-β type-2 receptors, high glucose levels stimulate podocytes to produce VEGF (Fig. 2). Interestingly, although podocytes are the major site of VEGF production in the kidney, glomerular endothelial cells constitutively express VEGF receptors *(48)*. VEGF increases vascular permeability but also has a role in cytoprotection and in maintaining normal glomerular function *(49)*. For instance, VEGF is implicated in both protection and regeneration of the glomerular endothelium *(50)*. In experimental diabetes, podocyte exposure to VEGF prevents podocyte apoptosis by inducing nephrin phosphorylation *(51)*. These results would argue for a renoprotective role for VEGF.

In contrast to the evidence that VEGF is renoprotective, antibodies against VEGF have been shown to improve early renal dysfunction in experimental diabetes *(46)*. Recently, a study in mouse podocytes showed that in addition to actions on the glomerular endothelium, VEGF may be involved in an autocrine loop and act on the podocyte itself, because mouse podocytes possess a VEGF receptor *(52)*. This study showed that VEGF signaling proceeds through activation of the phosphatidyl inositol 3-kinase pathway to stimulate α-3 (IV) collagen production. It was concluded that endogenous VEGF, stimulated by TGF-β_1, may contribute to glomerular basement membrane thickening and altered macromolecular permeability *(52)*.

Glucose induces changes in cytokine and growth factor expression in both podocytes and MCs, with a major focus on VEGF in podocytes and TGF-β in MCs. Studies in isolated MCs have shown that glucose induces expression and activation of TGF-β. High glucose also induces TGF-β receptor expression and magnifies TGF-β intracellular signaling in MCs *(53)*. In addition, TGF-β blockade prevents glucose-induced MC hypertrophy and ECM production in diabetes, indicating the presence of an autocrine mechanism *(45)*.

Clinical studies have shown that VEGF is increased in podocytes and in distal tubular cells in biopsies from patients with early DN *(54)*. In contrast, VEGF expression was decreased or absent in sclerotic glomeruli in patients with advanced DN *(53)*. These findings were supported by another study of patients with DN, which showed that glomerular VEGF expression was highest in patients with milder sclerotic changes and decreased or absent with increasing sclerosis *(55)*.

In addition to stimulation by high glucose, advanced glycation endproducts (AGE) and stretch also induce VEGF expression in podocytes *(47)*. In experimental diabetes, increased VEGF gene expression has been demonstrated in the glomerulus *(56)* and two studies have examined the effects of antiglycation therapies on VEGF expression in podocytes. As discussed in detail later in this chapter, podocytes isolated from diabetic db/db mice were found to have elevated levels of the receptor for advanced glycation endproducts (RAGE) as well as increased levels of VEGF *(47)*. Treatment of these mice with soluble RAGE led to a reduction in VEGF and improvements in albuminuria and glomerulosclerosis. In a second study performed in Otsuka Long-Evans Tokushima Fatty (OLETF) rats, long-term treatment with the AGE inhibitor OPB/9195 was renoprotective and abolished the enhanced renal VEGF immunoreactivity *(57)*. In this study, OPB-9195 also suppressed TGF expression in parallel with its effects on VEGF.

PODOCYTES AND RAGE

Expression of RAGE is enhanced in the diabetic kidney both in animals and in man *(58)*. In the glomerulus, RAGE is expressed especially at the base of podocytes but not in mesangium or endothelium *(58)*. As mentioned, a recent study tested the hypothesis that activation of RAGE contributed to increased excretion of urinary albumin and attraction of mononuclear phagocytes to diabetic glomeruli, driven by enhanced expression of podocyte VEGF and expansion of mesangial matrix mediated by TGF-β *(47)*. It showed that RAGE expression was increased in podocytes in spontaneously diabetic db/db mice by an age of 13 wk and that RAGE-bearing podocytes expressed high levels of VEGF.

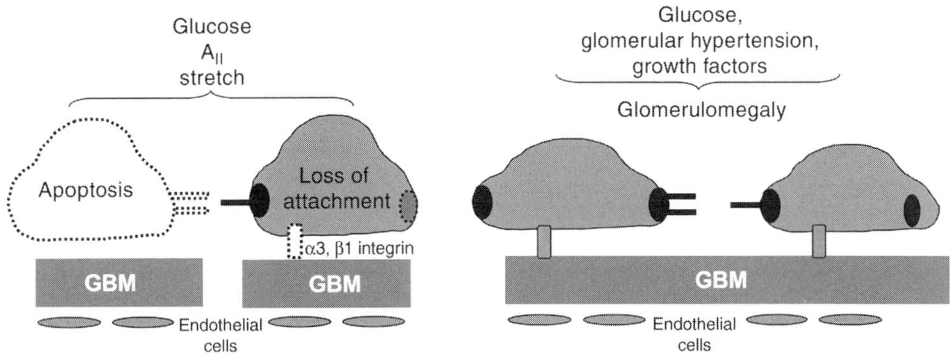

Podocyte density	↓	↓	↓
Podocyte number	↓	↓	→

Fig. 3. The proposed mechanisms leading to a decrease in podocyte density in diabetes: apoptosis, loss of podocyte attachment to the glomerular basement membrane (GBM) and glomerulomegaly.

Treatment with soluble RAGE, which blocks RAGE receptors, resulted in decreased albuminuria and glomerulosclerosis at 27 wk and improved renal function *(47)*. In other experiments, the same investigators showed that diabetic homozygous RAGE null mice failed to develop increased mesangial matrix expansion or thickening of the glomerular basement membrane *(47)*. These results indicate that activation of RAGE contributes to the expression of VEGF and enhanced attraction of inflammatory cells in the glomerulus, thereby setting the stage for mesangial activation and TGF-β production *(47)*. In summary, the data support the concept that RAGE-mediated proteinuria and glomerulosclerosis rely on podocyte VEGF as a primary mediator with increased generation of TGF-β as a secondary component leading to glomerulosclerosis.

The above hypothesis separates the consequences of RAGE activation into a hyperpermeability mechanism that is linked to albuminuria and a mesangial activation mechanism linked to glomerulosclerosis and a decrease in glomerular filtration rate. An independent pathogenetic role for albuminuria in renal and cardiovascular disease has also been identified in recent clinical studies. Albuminuria is an independent risk factor for progression of nephropathy in type 2 diabetes as well as being an independent predictor of cardiovascular events in patients with type 2 diabetes and nephropathy *(59)*.

PODOCYTE DENSITY IN DIABETIC NEPHROPATHY

At least three processes may explain a decrease in podocyte density in patients with DN (Fig. 3). First, it is possible that glomerular enlargement caused by glucose, intraglomerular hypertension, and/or growth factors leads to separation of podocyte foot processes without a decrease in podocyte number. As the podocyte is a terminally differentiated cell, any acquired increase in glomerular size induced by diabetes result in increases in endothelial cell and MC number but not in podocyte number. Increases in glomerular size have been reported in association with diabetes especially in non-Caucasian patients. For instance, glomerulomegaly has been reported in the inhabitants of the Tiwi Islands but not in other studies of glomerular size in indigenous Australian patients with diabetes *(60)*.

The response of the podocyte to acquired glomerular enlargement includes foot process widening as an adaptive response to maintain normal glomerular slit pore function. It is possible that albuminuria and the associated changes in nephrin distribution and function develop once the adaptive changes in podocyte density prove to be inadequate to compensate for the glomerulomegaly.

There are two other mechanisms for a decrease in podocyte density, which involve a decrease in podocyte number. The first is apoptosis (Fig. 1). It is well established that podocytes are unable to undergo regenerative proliferation to compensate for an increase in the surface area of the glomerular basement membrane *(61)* and apoptosis is a candidate mechanism to explain the decrease in the number of podocytes per glomerulus in diabetes. In isolated podocytes, stretch activates the local RAS to release angiotensin II, which then induces apoptosis by binding to the AT-1 receptor *(62)*. Stretch also enhances the apoptotic response by inducing TGF-β formation in podocytes. Other workers have shown that TGF-β_1 and the TGF-β signaling molecule SMAD7 also promote apoptosis in podocytes *(63)*.

Another mechanism, which may explain a decrease in podocyte density in association with a decrease in podocyte numbers per glomerulus, relates to matrix podocyte interactions. The integrins and $\alpha_3\beta_1$ dystroglycans are specific matrix receptors that anchor podocyte foot processes to the glomerular basement membrane *(64)*. The basal surface of podocyte foot processes is connected to the glomerular basement membrane mainly by $\alpha_3\beta_1$ integrin. Studies in cultured podocytes have shown that high glucose levels and stretch induce a decrease in $\alpha_3\beta_1$ integrin expression. Also, in vivo reduction in $\alpha_3\beta_1$ integrin expression has been reported in both human and experimental DN *(65)*. Furthermore, studies by Tsilibary's group have shown that podocyte binding to nonenzymatically glycated matrix leads to alterations in podocyte phenotype *(66)*. This evidence implies that loss of attachment of podocytes in patients with DN would lead to increased podocyte excretion in the urine. One study has shown that treatment with thiazolidinediones can reduce the number of podocytes in the urine of patients with diabetes *(67)*.

Whereas the major focus of ultrastructural studies of podocyte density in diabetes has been on glucose as the initiating stimulus, it is likely that systemic hypertension when transmitted to the glomerulus may start a similar process leading to mechanical stress and loss of podocytes followed by exposure of bare glomerular basement membrane, protein leakage, and ultimately to glomerulosclerosis and loss of nephrons *(61)*.

INTERACTION OF PROTEINS AND OTHER PLASMA FACTORS WITH PODOCYTES AND TUBULES IN DIABETIC NEPHROPATHY

Although the glomerular slit diaphragm is the major site for size-selective filtration of proteins, several studies indicate that additional cellular processing of proteins occurs during their renal passage through the glomerulus and renal tubules. In the proximal tubule, albumin is reabsorbed by endocytosis, mediated by two receptors, cubilin and megalin, acting in concert *(68)*. In human diabetes, filtered albumin is subject to lysosomal degradation and albumin-derived fragments are returned to the tubular lumen *(69)*. This means that urinary albumin-derived material consists mainly of peptide fragments, which cannot be detected by immunoassay but can be measured by labeling tracer amounts of albumin with tritium. However, as albuminuria increases, lysosomal degradation is attenuated *(69)*.

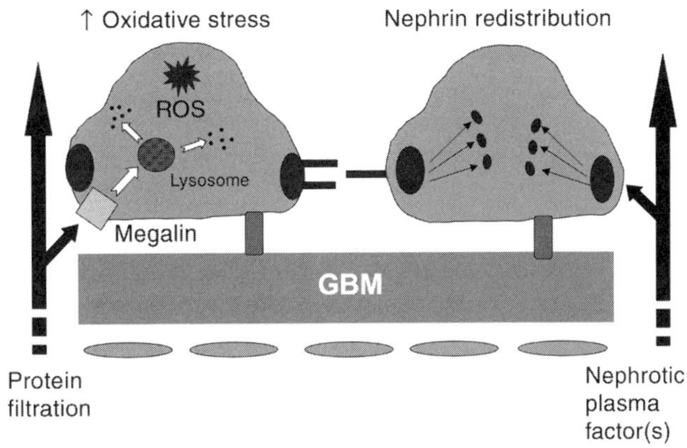

Fig. 4. Two proposed mechanisms describing the interaction of filtered plasma proteins leading to protein degradation and reactive oxidative stress (ROS) in podocytes (left-hand side) and the effects of postulated plasma factors from patients with nephrotic syndrome on nephrin redistribution in podocytes (right-hand side). GBM, glomerular basement membrane.

Interventions in experimental diabetes have shown that agents that reduce proteinuria also induce parallel changes in the renal tubules. For instance, in experimental diabetes, ramipril and aminoguanidine both prevent diabetes-related increases in albumin excretion rate and restore renal tubular lysosomal processing to normal levels *(30)*. Intervention with an angiotensin receptor blocker as well as an angiotensin-converting enzyme inhibitor also ameliorates the endocytosis of urinary albumin and restores renal tubular megalin expression to normal while preventing increases in diabetes-related albuminuria *(70)*. It is likely that receptor-mediated endocytosis also occurs in the podocyte because podocytes also contain megalin receptors *(71)*. Megalin is a 600-kDa transmembrane protein belonging to the low-density lipoprotein receptor gene family and is identified in rat podocytes as the target for immune deposit-forming antibodies in Heymann nephritis *(72)*. Studies in isolated rat podocytes have shown that megalin acts as an endocytic receptor that contributes to the uptake of lipoproteins as well as proteins *(73)*. The binding of albumin and other proteins to megalin initiates several intracellular processes *(67)* including lysosomal degradation of protein and generation of reactive oxygen species (ROS) (Fig. 4). The above evidence suggests that the process of renal handling of plasma proteins at the glomerulus is not purely an extracellular event regulated by slit diaphragms but also involves intracellular protein processing in the podocyte. To what degree the podocyte contributes to renal protein processing of proteins compared with the renal tubules remains to be defined.

A recent study has added a novel concept to podocyte slit diaphragm functioning *(74)*. Using human podocytes in cell culture, it was shown that exposure to normal and non-nephrotic human plasma leads to the concentration of nephrin, podocin, CD2AP, and actin at the cell surface (Fig. 4). By contrast, when podocytes are exposed to nephrotic plasma, nephrin, podocin, and CD2AP assume a cytoplasmic distribution. Furthermore, the relocation of nephrin induced by nephrotic plasma can be reversed by coincubation with non-nephrotic plasma. The changes induced by nephrotic plasma involve intracellular calcium signaling mediated by tyrosine kinase phosphorylation. Furthermore, using nephrin mutant human cell lines, it was shown that the nephrin translocation response with normal plasma is nephrin-dependent. The authors concluded that nephrotic plasma is deficient in factors acting via the podocyte slit diaphragm complex that are essential for maintaining its physiological function. The study was performed in six patients with focal and segmental glomerulosclerosis, one patient with lupus nephritis, and one control non-nephrotic patient. Because a proportion of patients with focal segmental glomerulosclerosis respond to plasma exchange, this suggests that removal of a pathogenetic plasma factor acting on podocytes may help to attenuate proteinuria. These results raise the possibility that the podocyte in normal conditions is constantly maintained by a milieu of circulating factors and that disruption of this process leads to loss of slit diaphragm stability, reorganization of associated actin filaments and subsequent foot process effacement *(74)*. However, it is not known whether a similar process operates in diabetic patients.

SUMMARY

The podocyte and its processes containing nephrin strands represent the major size selective barrier in the glomerulus. Changes in podocyte structure and function are closely related to increases in albuminuria in a variety of renal disorders including diabetic nephropathy. Metabolic (hyperglycaemia and RAGE activation) and hemodynamic (intraglomerular hypertension and glomerular stretch) derangements in diabetes lead to a finite number of pathological changes in the podocyte. The earliest signs of damage involve loss of the normal pattern of podocyte foot processes which leads to a decrease in podocyte density and eventually to a reduction in podocyte number. The processes mediating this include apoptosis, detachment of podocytes from the glomerular basement membrane, and alterations in intracellular microfilaments in association with an increase in generation of ROS.

The podocyte is a dynamic functional cell that is under the influence of vasoactive peptides including angiotensin, cytokines including VEGF and TGF-β, and as yet unidentified circulating factors that determine the intracellular distribution of nephrin. As a consequence of being involved in the filtration and processing of proteins, the podocyte contributes to glomerular damage, with the loss of podocytes being a major potential starting point for glomerular injury *(61)*.

In type 1 diabetes, predominantly glucose-mediated stimuli produce similar ultrastructural effects in the podocyte as the combination of raised blood pressure and glucose do in older patients with type 2 diabetes. Nephrin expression at the genetic and protein levels parallels proteinuria in a general sense and can be manipulated by antihypertensive therapy with RAS blockade and also by inhibition of advanced glycation. However, a large proportion of filtered protein is degraded in the renal tubules through lysosomal processing. It follows that changes in albuminuria reflect not only glomerular but also tubular mechanisms.

REFERENCES

1. Wartiovaara J, Ofverstedt LG, Khoshnoodi J, et al. Nephrin strands contribute to a porous slit diaphragm scaffold as revealed by electron tomography. J Clin Invest 2004;114:1475–1483.
2. Patrakka J, Kestila M, Wartiovaara J, et al. Congenital nephrotic syndrome (NPHS1): features resulting from different mutations in Finnish patients. Kidney Int 2000;58:972–980.
3. Boute N, Gribouval O, Roselli S, et al. NPHS2, encoding the glomerular protein podocin, is mutated in autosomal recessive steroid-resistant nephrotic syndrome. Nat Genet 2000;24:349–354.
4. Shih NY, Li J, Karpitskii V, et al. Congenital nephrotic syndrome in mice lacking CD2-associated protein. Science 1999;286:312–315.
5. Deen WM. What determines glomerular capillary permeability? J Clin Invest 2004;114:1412–1414.

6. Rossi M, Morita H, Sormunen R, et al. Heparan sulfate chains of perlecan are indispensable in the lens capsule but not in the kidney. EMBO J 2003;22:236–245.
7. Haraldsson B, Sorensson J. Why do we not all have proteinuria? An update of our current understanding of the glomerular barrier. News Physiol Sci 2004;19:7–10.
8. Osterby R, Hartmann A, Nyengaard JR, Bangstad HJ. Development of renal structural lesions in type-1 diabetic patients with microalbuminuria. Observations by light microscopy in 8-year follow-up biopsies. Virchows Arch 2002;440:94–101.
9. Rudberg S, Osterby R, Dahlquist G, Nyberg G, Persson B. Predictors of renal morphological changes in the early stage of microalbuminuria in adolescents with IDDM. Diabetes Care 1997;20:265–271.
10. Caramori ML, Kim Y, Huang C, et al. Cellular basis of diabetic nephropathy: 1. Study design and renal structural-functional relationships in patients with long-standing type 1 diabetes. Diabetes 2002;51:506–513.
11. Fioretto P, Steffes MW, Mauer M. Glomerular structure in nonproteinuric IDDM patients with various levels of albuminuria. Diabetes 1994;43:1358–1364.
12. Ellis EN, Warady BA, Wood EG, et al. Renal structural-functional relationships in early diabetes mellitus. Pediatr Nephrol 1997;11:584–591.
13. Ellis EN, Steffes MW, Chavers B, Mauer SM. Observations of glomerular epithelial cell structure in patients with type I diabetes mellitus. Kidney Int 1987;32:736–741.
14. Steffes MW, Schmidt D, McCrery R, Basgen JM. Glomerular cell number in normal subjects and in type 1 diabetic patients. Kidney Int 2001;59:2104–2113.
15. White KE, Bilous RW, Marshall SM, et al. Podocyte number in normotensive type 1 diabetic patients with albuminuria. Diabetes 2002;51:3083–3089.
16. Pagtalunan ME, Miller PL, Jumping-Eagle S, et al. Podocyte loss and progressive glomerular injury in type II diabetes. J Clin Invest 1997;99:342–348.
17. Meyer TW, Bennett PH, Nelson RG. Podocyte number predicts long-term urinary albumin excretion in Pima Indians with type II diabetes and microalbuminuria. Diabetologia 1999;42:1341–1344.
18. Dalla Vestra M, Masiero A, Roiter AM, Saller A, Crepaldi G, Fioretto P. Is podocyte injury relevant in diabetic nephropathy? Studies in patients with type 2 diabetes. Diabetes 2003;52:1031–1035.
19. White KE, Bilous RW. Structural alterations to the podocyte are related to proteinuria in type 2 diabetic patients. Nephrol Dial Transplant 2004;19:1437–1440.
20. Hirschberg R, Wang S. Proteinuria and growth factors in the development of tubulointerstitial injury and scarring in kidney disease. Curr Opin Nephrol Hypertens 2005;14:43–52.
21. Kestila M, Lenkkeri U, Mannikko M, et al. Positionally cloned gene for a novel glomerular protein—nephrin—is mutated in congenital nephrotic syndrome. Mol Cell 1998;1:575–582.
22. Forbes JM, Bonnet F, Russo LM, et al. Modulation of nephrin in the diabetic kidney: association with systemic hypertension and increasing albuminuria. J Hypertens 2002;20:985–992.
23. Bonnet F, Cooper ME, Kawachi H, Allen TJ, Boner G, Cao Z. Irbesartan normalises the deficiency in glomerular nephrin expression in a model of diabetes and hypertension. Diabetologia 2001;44:874–877.
24. Kelly DJ, Aaltonen P, Cox AJ, et al. Expression of the slit-diaphragm protein, nephrin, in experimental diabetic nephropathy: differing effects of anti-proteinuric therapies. Nephrol Dial Transplant 2002;17:1327–1332.
25. Mifsud SA, Allen TJ, Bertram JF, et al. Podocyte foot process broadening in experimental diabetic nephropathy: amelioration with renin-angiotensin blockade. Diabetologia 2001;44:878–882.
26. Langham RG, Kelly DJ, Cox AJ, et al. Proteinuria and the expression of the podocyte slit diaphragm protein, nephrin, in diabetic nephropathy: effects of angiotensin converting enzyme inhibition. Diabetologia 2002;45:1572–1576.
27. Doublier S, Salvidio G, Lupia E, et al. Nephrin expression is reduced in human diabetic nephropathy: evidence for a distinct role for glycated albumin and angiotensin II. Diabetes 2003;52:1023–1030.
28. Gloy J, Henger A, Fischer KG, et al. Angiotensin II modulates cellular functions of podocytes. Kidney Int Suppl 1998;67:S168–S170.
29. Tryggvason K. Unraveling the mechanisms of glomerular ultrafiltration: nephrin, a key component of the slit diaphragm. J Am Soc Nephrol 1999;10:2440–2445.
30. Osicka TM, Kiriazis Z, Pratt LM, Jerums G, Comper WD. Ramipril and aminoguanidine restore renal lysosomal processing in streptozotocin diabetic rats. Diabetologia 2001;44:230–236.
31. Miner JH. Renal basement membrane components. Kidney Int 1999;56:2016–2024.
32. Martin J, Steadman R, Knowlden J, Williams J, Davies M. Differential regulation of matrix metalloproteinases and their inhibitors in human glomerular epithelial cells in vitro. J Am Soc Nephrol 1998;9:1629–1637.

33. Kitsiou PV, Tzinia AK, Stetler-Stevenson WG, et al. Glucose-induced changes in integrins and matrix-related functions in cultured human glomerular epithelial cells. Am J Physiol Renal Physiol 2003;284:F671–F679.
34. McLennan SV, Fisher E, Martell SY, et al. Effects of glucose on matrix metalloproteinase and plasmin activities in mesangial cells: possible role in diabetic nephropathy. Kidney Int Suppl 2000;77:S81–S87.
35. Schena F, Gesualdo L. Pathogenetic mechanisms of diabetic nephropathy. J Am Soc Nephrol 2005;16:S30–S33.
36. Coward R, Welsh G, Holman G, et al. Human podocytes rapidly utilize glucose by both GLUT1 and GLUT4 in response to insulin; with significant differences in glucose transporter levels occurring in diabetic nephropathy. J Am Soc Nephrol 2003;14:388A.
37. Heilig CW, Liu Y, England RL, et al. d-glucose stimulates mesangial cell GLUT1 expression and basal and IGF-I-sensitive glucose uptake in rat mesangial cells: implications for diabetic nephropathy. Diabetes 1997;46:1030–1039.
38. Heilig CW, Concepcion LA, Riser BL, Freytag SO, Zhu M, Cortes P. Overexpression of glucose transporters in rat mesangial cells cultured in a normal glucose milieu mimics the diabetic phenotype. J Clin Invest 1995;96:1802–1814.
39. Mathieson PW. The cellular basis of albuminuria. Clin Sci (Lond) 2004;107:533–538.
40. Inoki K, Haneda M, Maeda S, Koya D, Kikkawa R. TGF-beta 1 stimulates glucose uptake by enhancing GLUT1 expression in mesangial cells. Kidney Int 1999;55:1704–1712.
41. Yamamoto T, Nakamura T, Noble NA, Ruoslahti E, Border WA. Expression of transforming growth factor beta is elevated in human and experimental diabetic nephropathy. Proc Natl Acad Sci USA 1993;90:1814–1818.
42. Iglesias-de la Cruz MC, Ziyadeh FN, Isono M, et al. Effects of high glucose and TGF-beta1 on the expression of collagen IV and vascular endothelial growth factor in mouse podocytes. Kidney Int 2002;62:901–913.
43. Gruden G, Zonca S, Hayward A, et al. Mechanical stretch-induced fibronectin and transforming growth factor-beta1 production in human mesangial cells is p38 mitogen-activated protein kinase-dependent. Diabetes 2000;49:655–661.
44. Riser BL, Ladson-Wofford S, Sharba A, et al. TGF-beta receptor expression and binding in rat mesangial cells: modulation by glucose and cyclic mechanical strain. Kidney Int 1999;56:428–439.
45. Ziyadeh FN, Hoffman BB, Han DC, et al. Long-term prevention of renal insufficiency, excess matrix gene expression, and glomerular mesangial matrix expansion by treatment with monoclonal anti-transforming growth factor-beta antibody in db/db diabetic mice. Proc Natl Acad Sci USA 2000;97:8015–8020.
46. de Vriese AS, Tilton RG, Elger M, Stephan CC, Kriz W, Lameire NH. Antibodies against vascular endothelial growth factor improve early renal dysfunction in experimental diabetes. J Am Soc Nephrol 2001;12:993–1000.
47. Wendt TM, Tanji N, Guo J, et al. RAGE drives the development of glomerulosclerosis and implicates podocyte activation in the pathogenesis of diabetic nephropathy. Am J Pathol 2003;162:1123–1137.
48. Khamaisi M, Schrijvers BF, De Vriese AS, Raz I, Flyvbjerg A. The emerging role of VEGF in diabetic kidney disease. Nephrol Dial Transplant 2003;18:1427–1430.
49. Ferrara N, Davis-Smyth T. The biology of vascular endothelial growth factor. Endocr Rev 1997;18:4–25.
50. Gruden G, Perin P, Camussi G. Insight on the pathogenesis of diabetic nephropathy from the study of podocyte and mesangial cell biology. Curr Diabetes Rev 2005;1:27–40.
51. Foster RR, Saleem MA, Mathieson PW, Bates DO, Harper SJ. Vascular endothelial growth factor and nephrin interact and reduce apoptosis in human podocytes. Am J Physiol Renal Physiol 2005;288:F48–F57.
52. Chen S, Kasama Y, Lee JS, Jim B, Marin M, Ziyadeh FN. Podocyte-derived vascular endothelial growth factor mediates the stimulation of alpha3(IV) collagen production by transforming growth factor-beta1 in mouse podocytes. Diabetes 2004;53:2939–2949.
53. Hayashida T, Schnaper HW. High ambient glucose enhances sensitivity to TGF-beta1 via extracellular signal—regulated kinase and protein kinase Cdelta activities in human mesangial cells. J Am Soc Nephrol 2004;15:2032–2041.
54. Cha DR, Kim NH, Yoon JW, et al. Role of vascular endothelial growth factor in diabetic nephropathy. Kidney Int Suppl 2000;77:S104–S112.
55. Shulman K, Rosen S, Tognazzi K, Manseau EJ, Brown LF. Expression of vascular permeability factor (VPF/VEGF) is altered in many glomerular diseases. J Am Soc Nephrol 1996;7:661–666.

56. Cooper ME, Vranes D, Youssef S, et al. Increased renal expression of vascular endothelial growth factor (VEGF) and its receptor VEGFR-2 in experimental diabetes. Diabetes 1999;48:2229–2239.
57. Tsuchida K, Makita Z, Yamagishi S, et al. Suppression of transforming growth factor beta and vascular endothelial growth factor in diabetic nephropathy in rats by a novel advanced glycation end product inhibitor, OPB-9195. Diabetologia 1999;42:579–588.
58. Tanji N, Markowitz GS, Fu C, et al. Expression of advanced glycation end products and their cellular receptor RAGE in diabetic nephropathy and nondiabetic renal disease. J Am Soc Nephrol 2000;11:1656–1666.
59. Anavekar NS, Gans DJ, Berl T, et al. Predictors of cardiovascular events in patients with type 2 diabetic nephropathy and hypertension: a case for albuminuria. Kidney Int Suppl 2004:S50–S55.
60. Young RJ, Hoy WE, Kincaid-Smith P, Seymour AE, Bertram JF. Glomerular size and glomerulosclerosis in Australian aborigines. Am J Kidney Dis 2000;36:481–489.
61. Kriz W, Gretz N, Lemley KV. Progression of glomerular diseases: is the podocyte the culprit? Kidney Int 1998;54:687–697.
62. Durvasula RV, Petermann AT, Hiromura K, et al. Activation of a local tissue angiotensin system in podocytes by mechanical strain. Kidney Int 2004;65:30–39.
63. Schiffer M, Bitzer M, Roberts IS, et al. Apoptosis in podocytes induced by TGF-beta and Smad7. J Clin Invest 2001;108:807–816.
64. Pavenstadt H, Kriz W, Kretzler M. Cell biology of the glomerular podocyte. Physiol Rev 2003;83: 253–307.
65. Chen HC, Chen CA, Guh JY, Chang JM, Shin SJ, Lai YH. Altering expression of alpha3beta1 integrin on podocytes of human and rats with diabetes. Life Sci 2000;67:2345–2353.
66. Krishnamurti U, Rondeau E, Sraer JD, Michael AF, Tsilibary EC. Alterations in human glomerular epithelial cells interacting with nonenzymatically glycosylated matrix. J Biol Chem 1997;272: 27,966–27,970.
67. Nakamura T, Ushiyama C, Osada S, Hara M, Shimada N, Koide H. Pioglitazone reduces urinary podocyte excretion in type 2 diabetes patients with microalbuminuria. Metabolism 2001;50:1193–1196.
68. Christensen EI, Birn H. Megalin and cubilin: multifunctional endocytic receptors. Nat Rev Mol Cell Biol 2002;3:256–266.
69. Osicka TM, Houlihan CA, Chan JG, Jerums G, Comper WD. Albuminuria in patients with type 1 diabetes is directly linked to changes in the lysosome-mediated degradation of albumin during renal passage. Diabetes 2000;49:1579–1584.
70. Tojo A, Onozato ML, Kurihara H, Sakai T, Goto A, Fujita T. Angiotensin II blockade restores albumin reabsorption in the proximal tubules of diabetic rats. Hypertens Res 2003;26:413–419.
71. Yamazaki H, Saito A, Ooi H, Kobayashi N, Mundel P, Gejyo F. Differentiation-induced cultured podocytes express endocytically active megalin, a heymann nephritis antigen. Nephron Exp Nephrol 2004;96:e52–e58.
72. Farquhar MG, Saito A, Kerjaschki D, Orlando RA. The Heymann nephritis antigenic complex: megalin (gp330) and RAP. J Am Soc Nephrol 1995;6:35–47.
73. Kerjaschki D, Exner M, Ullrich R, et al. Pathogenic antibodies inhibit the binding of apolipoproteins to megalin/gp330 in passive Heymann nephritis. J Clin Invest 1997;100:2303–2309.
74. Coward RJ, Foster RR, Patton D, et al. Nephrotic plasma alters slit diaphragm-dependent signaling and translocates nephrin, Podocin, and CD2 associated protein in cultured human podocytes. J Am Soc Nephrol 2005;16:629–637.
75. Bjorn SF, Bangstad HJ, Hanssen KF, et al. Glomerular epithelial foot processes and filtration slits in IDDM patients. Diabetologia 1995;38:1197–1204.
76. Berg UB, Torbjornsdotter TB, Jaremko G, Thalme B. Kidney morphological changes in relation to long-term renal function and metabolic control in adolescents with IDDM. Diabetologia 1998;41: 1047–1056.

I

Basic Pathophysiology and Biochemistry of Diabetic Nephropathy

D. Altered Metabolic Pathways

5 Altered Glucose Transport and Its Metabolic Effects in Glomerular Cells

Charles W. Heilig, MD

Contents

INTRODUCTION

Over many years of investigation it has been found that the mechanisms contributing to the development of diabetic nephropathy (DN) are both varied and complex *(1–8)*. A key finding, however, was that hyperglycemia plays an important role in the development of diabetic tissue complications, including nephropathy. A substantial amount of effort has been expended in identifying glucose-induced pathways in the kidney, which contribute to the production of excessive extracellular matrix (ECM), which could scar the kidneys, particularly in the form of glomerulosclerosis *(3,9–12)*, but also in the form of tubulo-interstitial fibrosis *(13–17)*. More recently, the discovery of numerous new members of the glucose transporter families, both the facilitative glucose transporter family (i.e., GLUTs; solute carrier family SLC2A) and the sodium–glucose cotransporter

From: *Contemporary Diabetes: The Diabetic Kidney*
Edited by: P. Cortes and C. E. Mogensen © Humana Press Inc., Totowa, NJ

Table 1
Changes in Renal Glucose Transporter Expression Reported With Diabetes

GLUT1	Increase in glomeruli (preliminary report) and increase in whole cortex
GLUT2	Increase in proximal tubules
GLUT3	N/A
GLUT4	Decrease in glomeruli
GLUT5	Increase in mesangial cells
GLUT8	Increase in podocytes
SGLT1	Increase in proximal tubules
SGLT2	Increase in proximal tubules
SGLT3	N/A

GLUT, facilitative glucose transporter; SGLT, sodium/glucose cotransporter; N/A, information not available.

family (i.e., SGLT, SLC5A), has allowed their investigation in the kidney and a beginning assessment of their roles in normal and diabetic kidneys. The explosion of information that is now occurring in the glucose transporter field is allowing renal researchers many new opportunities to understand how these transporters contribute to normal and altered renal glucose metabolism *(18–22)*.

GLOMERULAR GLUCOSE TRANSPORTERS

The investigation of glomerular glucose transporters followed the identification of relatively higher levels of glucose transporters in the renal tubules *(23,24)*. The first glomerular glucose transporter identified was GLUT1 *(24,25)*, previously known as the red blood cell and brain glucose transporter *(26,27)*. The term "GLUT" refers to facilitative glucose transporters, of which 12 are currently known *(18,20)*. Subsequently, the GLUT3, GLUT4, GLUT5, and GLUT8 isoforms were discovered in glomeruli *(24,28,29)*. GLUTs 3, 4, and 8 are high-affinity facilitative glucose transporters, whereas GLUT5 is predominantly a fructose transporter, with less glucose transport activity. In addition, there are reports of sodium–glucose cotransporter activity, possibly SGLT1, in glomerular mesangial cells (MCs) and podocytes *(30,31)*. These latter reports remain to be confirmed and the transporters more thoroughly characterized. A description of the glomerular glucose transporters identified to date and their responses to diabetes, are provided below and in Table 1.

GLUT1

GLUT1 has been identified in whole glomeruli, MCs, podocytes, and endothelial cells (*[24]* and Heilig unpublished data on endothelial cells) and its K_m in cultured MCs has been determined to be approx 3 m*M* *(25)*. This transporter has a relatively low capacity for glucose transport, in contrast to GLUT2, which is expressed in the proximal tubule and podocytes, with a high capacity *(31,32)*. GLUT1 is believed to be near saturation at physiological glucose concentrations *(25,33)*. It typically is expressed in plasma membranes with a smaller component in intracellular vesicles *(23,24)*. In nonrenal tissues it exhibits some response to insulin by translocating to the plasma membrane, though GLUT4 is the classic insulin-responsive glucose transporter as described in muscle and adipose tissue *(34,35)*.

GLUT2

GLUT2 is a low-affinity, high-capacity glucose transporter (K_m approx 17 m*M*) that was recently identified in cultured podocytes *(31,32)*. The presence of this transporter suggests podocytes have the potential for excessive glucose uptake at high extracellular glucose concentrations and its expression in whole glomeruli and potential changes in response to diabetes mellitus have yet to be investigated.

GLUT3

GLUT3 is a high-affinity glucose transporter with a K_m of 1.4 m*M* *(22)*. This protein is expressed in glomeruli *(24)*, although the specific cell types involved have not been identified, and its response to diabetes mellitus in glomeruli is unknown *(24)*. GLUT3 mRNA has been detected in cultured podocytes, however *(31)*, and an assessment of the protein expression is needed. Therefore, characterization of GLUT3 expression in glomerular cells remains to be fully characterized. GLUT3 is undetectable in MCs that have been passed in culture, however, which impairs its study in vitro *(36)*. This glucose transporter is expressed in plasma membranes and intracellularly, and in one report a translocation response to insulin was detected in L6 myotubes *(37)*. Similar to GLUT1, GLUT3 has been proposed to play an important role in basal cell nutrition *(38)*.

GLUT4

GLUT4 is expressed in glomerular mesangial cells and podocytes *(24)*. It is a high-affinity glucose transporter with a K_m of approx 5 m*M* *(22)*. As noted earlier, it is typically located in intracellular vesicles until stimulated to translocate to the plasma membrane in response to insulin. This response of GLUT4 to insulin has been well characterized in skeletal muscle and adipose tissue *(34,39)*, although the potential regulation of renal GLUT4 by insulin has yet to be investigated. GLUT4 is suppressed in glomeruli in response to diabetes *(40)*, and this is the opposite response from glomerular GLUT1 *(41)*. Suppression of glomerular GLUT4 could be protective against diabetes, except that glomerular GLUT1 is increased in this situation and the latter transporter is typically expressed at the plasma membrane in which it can function in the uptake of excess glucose. In addition, as opposed to GLUT1, GLUT4 tends to be lost from MCs when they are repeatedly passed in culture *(25,36)*, which makes it difficult to study this glucose transporter in these cells. The expression of GLUT4 in cultured podocytes appears to be maintained at least for the short term in vitro *(31,32)*. GLUT4 expression in afferent microvessels to the glomerulus has been reported to decrease in response to diabetes *(40)*. One proposed effect of this change is that it could promote vascular dilation by reducing adenosene triphosphate (ATP) production from glycolysis, increasing ATP-dependent K^+ channel activity and hyperpolarizing the cells. The resulting shutdown of voltage-sensitive calcium channels could then lead to arteriolar vasodilation followed by glomerular hyperfiltration *(40)*. Dilation of the afferent arteriole resulting in glomerular hyperfiltration has been implicated in the pathogenesis of diabetic glomerular damage and this might be due in part to the response of the GLUT4 glucose transporter *(40)*.

GLUT5

GLUT5 has been detected in glomerular MCs by use of immunocytochemistry *(28)*. These authors also reported an apparent increase in glomerular GLUT5 with streptozotocin (STZ) type 1 diabetes. These findings await confirmation, and the role of GLUT5 in MC glucose uptake is currently unknown. This transporter is predominantly a fructose transporter (K_m of 6 m*M* for fructose), with little transport activity for glucose *(22)*.

GLUT8

GLUT8 has a high affinity for glucose, with a K_m of approx 2 m*M* *(22)*. In embryos, it has been shown to respond to insulin *(42)*. It is important in embryonic development *(42)*, and recently was identified in glomerular podocytes *(29)*. GLUT8 in podocytes has been found to increase in response to diabetes *(29)*, and the implications of this for development of DN will require further investigation. To date, GLUT8 has not been detected in other glomerular cell types. GLUT8 is located largely inside of cells in the absence of a stimulus such as insulin *(29,42)*, therefore the contribution of this glucose transporter to basal glucose metabolism in podocytes is potentially less than that of GLUT1.

IMPLICATIONS OF HIGH GLUCOSE-INDUCED ALTERATIONS OF MESANGIAL CELL GLUCOSE TRANSPORTER EXPRESSION FOR DN

High extracellular glucose in the diabetic range has been shown to stimulate MC GLUT1 expression and glucose uptake. Although such a response is not unique to MC *(43,44)*, most other cell types outside the kidney respond to high-glucose exposure by reducing their glucose transporter expression or maintaining it constant *(34,45)*. Therefore, these nonrenal cells presumably protect themselves from excessive glucose uptake and metabolism, which is potentially harmful *(25,46,47)*. Because MCs do not protect themselves from high-glucose exposure, they take up and metabolize excessive amounts of glucose, which allows them to produce excessive ECM. In vivo this would contribute to development of glomerulosclerosis *(25)*. This response of MCs has been proposed to play a key role in the kidney's well-established susceptibility to diabetic damage *(25,36)*. In other studies, it was shown that hypertension in rats is associated with increased glomerular GLUT1 expression, and that in vitro stretch of rat MCs causes an increase in GLUT1 expression leading to enhanced glucose uptake *(48)*. This suggests that in diabetes mellitus where glomerular hypertension and MC stretch are believed to occur, these processes could contribute to the increased glomerular GLUT1 expression. Therefore, both high-glucose exposure in the diabetic range and MC stretch can increase MC glucose uptake, allowing increased glucose metabolism to stimulate ECM production.

Studies have demonstrated that GLUT1 expression is limiting for glucose uptake into cultured MCs, and that GLUT1 expression regulates MC expression of ECM proteins such as fibronectin, collagen type IV, collagen type I, and laminin *(25,33)*. A model for altered GLUT1 expression in MCs has demonstrated that isolated overexpression of GLUT1 leads to excessive ECM production (Fig. 1), even in the absence of high extracellular glucose exposure *(25)*. Furthermore, suppression of MC GLUT1 prevents high-glucose stimulation of MC GLUT1 and ECM expression *(33)*. Therefore, the response of MC GLUT1 to diabetes may play an important role in the development of diabetic glomerulosclerosis. A potential role for GLUT1 susceptibility alleles in the development of diabetic nephropathy is discussed later in this chapter. In contrast to GLUT1, the potential roles of MC GLUT4, GLUT5 and SGLT1-like activities in the development of DN remain to be elucidated.

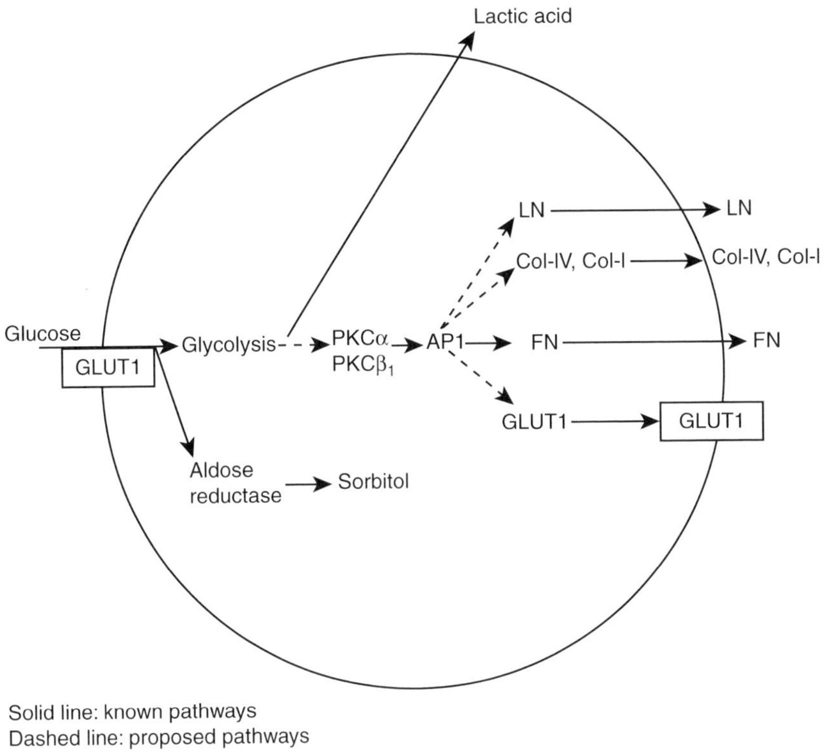

Fig. 1. Model of isolated GLUT1 overexpression in mesangial cells. (Adapted from ref. *10*)

Preliminary work in transgenic mice, which overexpress and underexpress GLUT1 in glomerular MCs indicates that reduced GLUT1 provides protection from type 2 diabetes-induced glomerulosclerosis *(41)*, whereas increased GLUT1 leads to albuminuria and glomerulosclerosis even in the absence of diabetes *(10)*. Further characterization of these models will provide information concerning the mechanisms by which isolated changes in GLUT1 affect glomerular ECM accumulation, independent of hyperglycemia. In vitro data in MCs indicates that though the effects of high extracellular glucose exposure and an isolated increase in GLUT1 expression are similar in many ways, they are not identical *(49)*. This suggests that high extracellular glucose may have effects at the plasma membrane, which are independent from the intracellular effects of glucose due to enhanced cellular uptake and metabolism. Further investigation of the transgenic mouse models should identify the resulting similarities and differences in the kidney pathology which develops with diabetes vs an isolated increased in glomerular GLUT1.

Podocytes have been shown to upregulate GLUT8 in response to diabetes mellitus *(29)*. However, the implications of this change for DN are not yet clear because GLUT8 is typically intracellular until exposed to an appropriate stimulus *(42,50)*. Glomerular podocytes also express GLUT1, GLUT4, and possibly GLUT3 *(31)*, although their responses to diabetes and high-glucose exposure in these cells remain to be clarified. SGLT1-like activity has been detected in podocytes and requires further evaluation *(31)*. Investigations underway will determine the relative roles of these transporters in podocyte glucose metabolism under normal and diabetic conditions.

Potential damage to podocytes from altered GLUT expression and the effects on ECM production by these cells have yet to be determined.

Glomerular endothelial cells express GLUT1 (Heilig, unpublished data). However, other glucose transporters have yet to be described in these cells, and the response of glomerular endothelial cell GLUT1 to diabetes has yet to be characterized. Diabetic exposure of nonrenal endothelial cells leads to different responses of GLUT1 depending on the origin of the cells, with a decrease in endothelial GLUT1 in brain and heart endothelial cells *(51)*, and no decrease in retinal endothelial cells *(51,52)*. The lack of a decrease in retinal endothelial cell GLUT1 with diabetes was suggested to make the eyes more susceptible to diabetic damage *(51,52)*. It will be of interest to find out how glomerular glucose transporters are regulated in the setting of diabetes mellitus.

In summary, much work lies ahead in order to characterize the roles of glucose transporters in glomerular glucose metabolism under both normal and diabetic conditions, though such studies should give us a much better understanding of glomerular glucose handling and the pathogenesis of diabetic nephropathy.

GLOMERULAR GLUCOSE METABOLISM

As noted, glomerular glucose transporters were initially difficult to detect, presumably owing to low expression *(23,24)*. GLUT1 was the first glucose transporter to be characterized in the glomerulus *(24,25)*, and this transporter is believed to be important for maintaining basal cell nutrition in many different cell types *(19,38)*. Partial suppression of MC GLUT1 has been shown to slow the growth rate of the cells *(33)*, an indication that GLUT1 is vital to them. Glomeruli have a relatively low level of oxygen consumption, and low levels of glycolytic and tricarboxylic acid (TCA) cycle enzymes when compared with renal tubules *(53)*, consistent with their relatively low level of glucose transporter expression *(23,24)*. The renal cortex in general tends to use fatty acids and ketones as energy substrates, with a lesser reliance on glucose *(53)*.

As noted earlier, MC glucose utilization is limited by glucose transport into the cells, and excessive glucose metabolism in MC is associated with adverse consequences in terms of excess polyol, lactic acid, and ECM production *(10)*. A role for glucose transporters in MC apoptosis has not yet been investigated but will be important to pursue, considering that GLUTs play a role in the apoptosis of other cell types *(54–56)*. In summary, the low baseline metabolism of glucose in MCs could be protective in that ECM production is controlled, whereas a diabetes-induced increase in MC GLUT1 has the potential to enhance ECM production, a process key to the development of glomerulosclerosis in vivo.

MESANGIAL CELL-SIGNALING PATHWAYS FROM GLUCOSE TRANSPORTERS TO EXTRACELLULAR MATRIX PRODUCTION

An isolated increase in MC glucose transporter expression (i.e., GLUT1) leads to persistent increases and activation of PKCα and PKCβ, even in the absence of high extracellular glucose concentrations *(57)*. A persistently elevated glucose uptake rate, polyol pathway activation with sorbitol accumulation, enhanced glycolysis, excessive glucose utilization, and excessive ECM production are also features of this model *(25,57)*. Increased PKC activity is known to stimulate assembly of the transcriptional activator protein AP-1 from cfos and cjun *(4)*, leading to increased AP-1 as described in GLUT1-overexpressing MC *(49)*. The AP-1 can then bind to TPA-responsive elements (i.e., TREs) in regulatory regions of target genes such as fibronectin and GLUT1 to increase their expression *(49)*. AP-1 is persistently increased in mesangial cells over-expressing GLUT1 *(49)*. Although acute increases in transforming growth factor (TGF)-β_1, mitogen-activated protein kinase (MAPK) and reactive oxygen species (ROS) in response to high extracellular glucose exposure have been implicated in excessive MC ECM production *(5,58)*, these processes are not necessary for maintenance of excess MC ECM production in response to an isolated increase in GLUT1 expression *(49)*. Preliminary work in which PKC was inhibited with Calphostin-C treatment and chronic PMA suppression indicated a role for PKC in GLUT1-induced GLUT1 gene transcription *(59)*.

Therefore, in the long term there appears to be an important role for the PKC pathway in maintenance of glucose-induced ECM production. It is not yet known whether chronic, intermittent high-glucose exposure would cause recurrent increases in TGF-β_1, MAPK, and ROS to stimulate MC ECM production, and this needs to be investigated. Potential roles for intracellular advanced glycosylation endproducts (AGE) and receptor for AGE (RAGE) expression also need to be examined with respect to MC glucose transporters and ECM expression, because AGE have been implicated in DN. Studies of serine/threonine Akt kinase signaling in nonrenal cell types have identified a role for this mediator in stimulating GLUT1 gene expression and translocation to the plasma membrane *(60,61)*. Investigation of Akt signaling may therefore be of value in determining mechanisms by which glomerular GLUT1 is increased in diabetes.

As noted earlier, investigations are underway to identify GLUT1-responsive genes in MC and mechanisms by which they are induced. Finally, the USF transcription factors (i.e., upstream stimulatory factors) are being investigated to determine their roles in glucose- and GLUT1-induced gene expression in MCs, as a preliminary report suggests USF2 is regulated by glucose and glucose transporters in these cells *(62)*.

RENAL TUBULAR GLUCOSE TRANSPORTERS

The renal tubules appear to have much higher expression of glucose transporters than the glomeruli. This may be due in part to the substantial energy requirement for solute reabsorption *(53)*. The renal tubules express both facilitative GLUTs and sodium–glucose cotransporters (Fig. 2). The GLUTs identified in the tubules to date include GLUT1–5 and –8. The sodium-linked glucose transporters reported in the tubules to date include SGLT1–3, and "NaGLT1" *(63,64)*. SGLT1 is a high-affinity, low-capacity glucose transporter located in the proximal tubule S3 segment in the apical membranes of the epithelial cells *(64)*. SGLT2 is a low-affinity, high-capacity glucose transporter localized to the apical membranes of proximal tubule S1 segment cells in which it is believed to play a major role in glucose reabsorption from the glomerular filtrate *(64)*. SGLT3 is not yet fully characterized, but may be expressed in the apical membranes of proximal tubule S1 segment cells *(64)*. SGLT2 in the S1 segment is associated with the high-capacity GLUT2 glucose transporter in the basolateral membrane, which would help transport glucose from the proximal tubule cells toward the blood in peritubular capillaries *(64)*. In contrast, SGLT1 in the S3 segment is associated with basolateral expression of GLUT1, which is a high-affinity, low-capacity glucose transporter. Therefore, the glucose transporters of the proximal tubule S1 segment appear better suited for large-scale reabsorption of glucose. In diabetes mellitus, SGLT2 and SGLT1 are both increased in the renal tubules, as is GLUT2 (S1 segment) and transiently

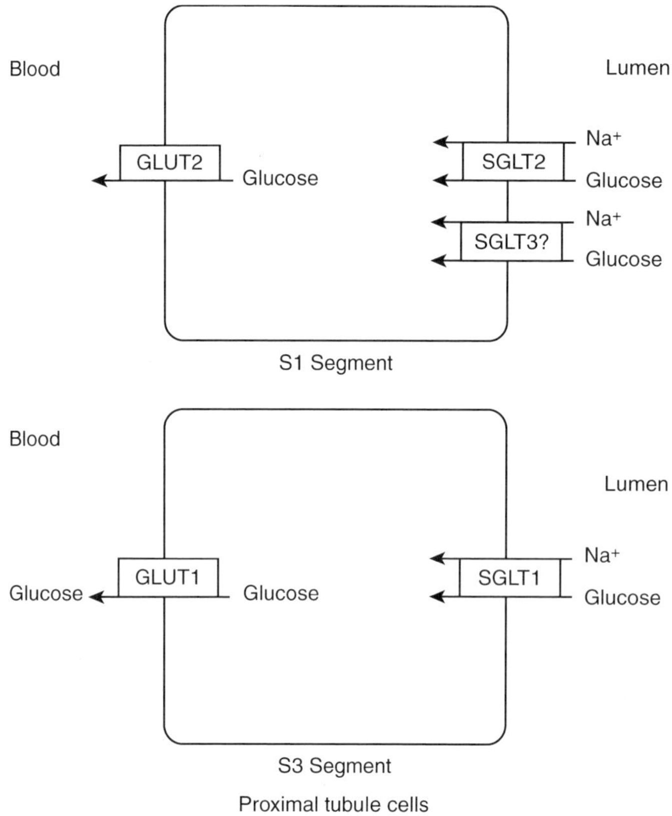

Fig. 2. Proximal tubule cells. (Reprinted by permission from Heilig et al., 2004.)

GLUT1 (distal nephron). The increases in SGLT2 and GLUT2 in the S1 segment of the proximal tubule may be particularly important for increased reabsorption of the excess filtered glucose. Therefore, there may be adaptive increases in glucose transporters to prevent excess glucose spillage into the urine. Whether or not the increases in renal tubular glucose transporters and cellular glucose uptake contribute to excessive ECM production leading to interstitial fibrosis is not yet known. This will be an important topic for future studies.

The axial distribution of facilitative GLUTs along the renal tubules differs for the individual isoforms expressed. GLUT1 appears to be most highly expressed in the thick ascending limbs (TAL) of Henle and inner medullary collecting duct (IMCD) cells *(24)*, with lower levels of expression in the cortical collecting ducts and S3 segment of proximal tubules. GLUT1 has a basolateral localization in renal tubule segments *(23,24)*. GLUT2 is expressed solely in the S1 segment of the proximal tubules, in which it has a basolateral distribution *(23)*. GLUT3 is expressed in the TAL and IMCD cells *(24)*, and is expressed both inside the cells and at the plasma membrane. GLUT4, also known as the insulin-responsive glucose transporter of adipose and muscle tissue, is expressed largely in the TAL in which it exhibits an intracellular location *(24)*. GLUT5 exhibits glucose transport activity, although it is better suited as a fructose transporter, and is expressed in the brush border membranes of S3 segment proximal tubule cells *(65)*. GLUT8 is typically intracellular, and is expressed in the TAL and collecting ducts *(29)*. GLUT1 expression in IMCD cells is positioned to provide nutrition and glucose-derived osmotically active solutes in a location of the kidney in which the oxygen tension is relatively low, and extracellular osmolality is high. GLUT1 expression tends to be high in tissues where a need for anerobic glycolysis exists *(23,24)*. GLUT3 is expressed predominantly in the TAL and IMCD cells, and like GLUT1 may supply maintenance nutrition for the cells *(19,37,38)*. GLUT4 in the TAL cells appears predominantly intracellular, and its participation in cell nutrition or the development of DN presumably depends on its translocation to the plasma membrane. However, it is not yet known which stimuli may translocate GLUT4 in renal cells. GLUT8 is expressed in the TAL and also appears to be expressed predominantly inside the cells *(29)*. Similar to the situation for GLUT4, it is not yet known if GLUT8 in the kidney responds to insulin, though GLUT8 is known to be insulin responsive in embryos *(42)*.

GENETIC STUDIES OF GLUT1 ALLELES AND THE RISK FOR DN

There are now multiple studies that have reported on the investigation of GLUT1 alleles and their potential relationship to the development of DN *(66–72)*. The initial focus of research was on the XbaI polymorphic site in intron 2 of the human GLUT1 gene. This single-nucleotide polymorphism (SNP) was associated with increased risk for development of DN in studies from China *(69)*, the United Kingdom *(67)*, and Poland *(71)*. In contrast, studies from Denmark *(70)* and Spain *(66)* did not document an increased risk. Subsequently, Ng et al. *(73)*, in the United States, identified an association between the GLUT1 XbaI (–) allele and development of DN in type 1 diabetic patients. Furthermore, a subsequent meta-analysis of the GLUT1 XbaI allele studies indicated an increased risk for DN associated with the XbaI SNP site *(74)*. Potentially more important than the XbaI data, was the finding by Ng et al. *(73)* at the Joslin Diabetes Center, that the Enhancer 2, SNP1 site in an E-box in intron 2 of the human GLUT1 gene was associated with an approximate twofold increased risk for DN (Fig. 3). The XbaI site was in tight linkage dysequilibrium with the nearby Enhancer-2, SNP 1 site, such that 100% of the patients homozygous for the Enhancer-2, SNP 1 A allele (susceptibility allele) also were homozygous for the XbaI–allele *(73)*. The authors proposed that the Enhancer-2, SNP 1 site could be the site of the disease allele. The AA genotype at this site is associated with increased risk for the nephropathy, and the linkage disequilibrium with the nearby XbaI site could explain why the XbaI site has been associated with an increased risk for DN in some of the previous reports *(73)*. A diagram depicting GLUT1 SNP sites and susceptibility alleles is shown in Fig. 3. Finally, a recent report from Hodgkinson et al. *(68)* has identified a new polymorphic site (A-2841T) in the human GLUT1 promoter that is strongly associated with an increased risk for DN (Fig. 3).

The SNP in Enhancer-2, SNP1 is an E-box, a type of motif that is potentially glucose responsive (i.e., a glucose-response element) and potentially stimulated by USF transcription factors. Because USF2 is upregulated by glucose in mesangial cells *(75)*, it has the potential to interact with the Enhancer-2, SNP1 site to affect GLUT1 transcription. If the Enhancer-2, SNP1 susceptibility allele (i.e., the A allele) were found to be associated with upregulation of GLUT1 expression, this could help explain the increased susceptibility to DN. Some evidence that this might occur comes from preliminary work in cultured mesangial cells. A segment identical to the human GLUT1 Enhancer-2, SNP1 site is found in the promoter of the mouse GLUT1 gene *(62)*. When

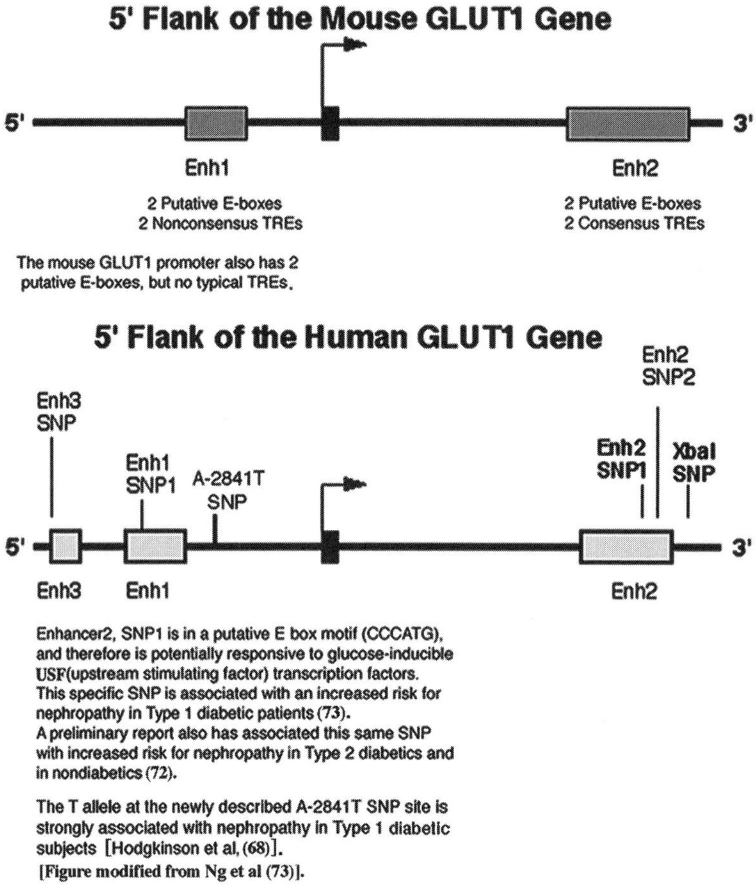

Fig. 3. Enhancer 2, SNP1 is in putative E-box motif (CCCATG), and therefore is potentially responsive to glucose-inducible USF transcription factors. This specific SNP is associated with an increased risk for nephropathy in type 1 diabetic patients *(73)*. A preliminary report also has associated this same SNP with increased risk for nephropathy in type 2 diabetics and in nondiabetics *(72)*. (Adapted from ref. *73*.)

this site was altered by site-directed mutagenesis, GLUT1 gene transcription increased in response to USF2, a glucose-inducible transcription factor in mesangial cells *(62)*. Further work is necessary to determine precisely the mechanism by which the Enhancer-2, SNP1 "A" allele predisposes to DN in humans.

EFFECTS OF ANTIDIABETIC DRUGS ON MESANGIAL CELL GLUCOSE TRANSPORTERS

Sulfonylureas

The sulfonylurea medications have been in use for decades to manage hyperglycemia in type 2 diabetic patients, however, even patients with well-controlled blood glucose levels may develop DN. It is of interest, therefore, that studies of the sulfonylurea derivative tolazemide have demonstrated that it increases MC glucose uptake *(76)*, despite its beneficial effect to improve glycemia in diabetics by increasing peripheral glucose disposal. The increase in glucose uptake into MCs appears to be via GLUT1, and may increase extracellular matrix production in vitro *(76)*. Other sulfonylureas have been shown to increase GLUT1-mediated glucose transport in nonrenal tissues *(77–80)*. However, recent work in type 1 diabetic rats suggests sulfonylurea treatment can actually protect against the development of glomerulosclerosis rather than exacerbate it *(81)*. In the same study, a similar protective effect was not observed in type 2 diabetic mice.

Thiazolidinediones

More recently, effects of the thiazolidinedione antidiabetic medications on MC glucose transport and glucose metabolism have been examined in vitro *(82,83)*. These drugs appear to suppress GLUT1 in cultured MCs, leading to improved MC glucose metabolism *(82)*. They have been used to control peripheral blood glucose levels in type 2 diabetics; therefore a beneficial effect in the kidney MC would be welcome. Again, as for the sulfonylurea effects on glucose transport, further investigations are needed to determine whether the in vitro findings translate to significant effects in vivo.

Insulin

Historically, the kidney has not been considered to be an insulin-responsive organ. Although insulin stimulates glucose uptake into skeletal muscle and adipose tissue via GLUT4, and to a lesser extent via GLUT1, it has little effect to stimulate glucose uptake into cultured MC *(84)*. More recent discoveries of GLUT4 and GLUT8 in glomeruli and renal tubules suggest the insulin responsiveness of renal cells in vivo might differ from their responsiveness in vitro. For example, the loss of GLUT4 from MCs in culture *(36)* could limit their responsiveness to insulin. A minimal response of MC glucose transporters to insulin presumably would provide some protection against excessive glucose uptake, glucose metabolism, and ECM production *(10)*, while at the same time glycemia is improving from the treatment. It would be valuable as well to know how TAL cells respond to insulin, as the TAL appears to be a major site in renal tubules in which GLUT4 and GLUT8 are expressed *(24,29)*. The TAL is a major site for solute reabsorption in which substantial energy is expended *(53)*, and additional capacity for glucose uptake could be beneficial for ATP production. Basal GLUT1 expression also appears to be relatively high in the TAL *(24)*, and for the same reasons may be beneficial to solute transport in this segment.

INHIBITORS OF GLUT1

Research to identify and characterize glucose transport inhibitors that may protect against the development of DN is in its infancy. Certainly, many different drugs and food constituents have the potential to regulate glucose transporter expression, and some examples are mentioned here with references for more in-depth reading.

Captopril has been shown to inhibit a high-glucose-induced increase in GLUT1-mediated glucose transport in retinal endothelial cells *(85)*. A role for Captopril inhibition of MC glucose transport will need to be investigated because this could identify a new and important nonhemodynamic protective effect of an angiotensin-converting enzyme (ACE) inhibitor on the kidney. The mechanism by which Captopril achieves this effect in retinal endothelial cells is not yet known, although it does not appear to result from a change in overall GLUT1 expression *(85)*.

The flavanoids and isoflavones (e.g., genestein, quercetin, and others) are tyrosine kinase inhibitors known to inhibit glucose transport via their effects on GLUT1 *(86)*. At least part of the affect results from their binding to an ATP-binding site in GLUT1, thereby impairing its transport capacity *(86)*. One article has been published in which the isoflavone quercetin was given to diabetic rats and prevented the development of DN *(87)*. Although the beneficial effect of quercetin was attributed to inhibition of ROS, the effect of this compound to inhibit glucose uptake into the mesangial cells and glomeruli was not assessed. Certainly, future studies should address the effectiveness of chemical inhibition of glucose transporters to prevent DN, because suppression of MC GLUT1 has provided protection against ECM production in vitro *(33)*, and preliminary data indicates that transgenic suppression of MC GLUT1 in vivo is protective against the development of diabetic glomerulosclerosis in mice *(41)*. Methylxanthines as well have been shown in nonrenal cells to inhibit glucose transport via GLUT1, and their avoidance has been recommended in patients with the GLUT1 deficiency syndrome in which a congenital deficiency of GLUT1 leads to hypoglycorrhachia, seizure activity, and motor abnormalities *(88–90)*. The latter example also indicates that excessive systemic inhibition of GLUT1 could have adverse consequences. Therefore, a more selective inhibition of glucose transporters in the kidney would be desirable in screening for drugs with the potential to inhibit glomerular ECM production by interfering with GLUT1-mediated glucose uptake.

The drug, rhein, an anthraquinone derived from rhubarb, which historically was used as an herbal remedy for various ailments in China, has also been effective in blocking $TGF\beta_1$-induced GLUT1 and glucose transport in cultured MCs *(91)*. The inhibitory effect of rhein on glucose transport has been known for many years in nonrenal tumor cells *(92)*. The effectiveness of rhein to prevent DN is currently under investigation.

Finally, pentobarbital is a known suppressant of GLUT1 in nonrenal tissues such as the brain *(26)*, however its potential to suppress GLUT1 in the kidney has not yet been investigated.

CONCLUSIONS

The roles of glucose transporters in renal glucose metabolism and DN have been little investigated, in part as a result of the recent discovery of numerous new glucose transporter isoforms over the last 10 yr. Renal glucose transporters continue to be identified and characterized. Information on the GLUT1 isoform suggests it could play an important role in the development of diabetic nephropathy. Studies in humans also indicate there are GLUT1 susceptibility alleles that increase the risk for nephropathy in diabetic patients. Data suggesting a role for glucose transporters in nondiabetic renal disease is more preliminary, although potentially very important as it could broaden the role of glucose transporters in the pathogenesis of renal disease. Future investigations of the more recently discovered renal glucose transporters will enhance our understanding of their roles in DN. Finally, future investigations of glucose transport inhibitors hold potential promise for new therapies to prevent and treat diabetic, and possibly even some nondiabetic kidney diseases.

REFERENCES

1. Ziyadeh FN. Mediators of diabetic renal disease: the case for TGF-beta as the major mediator. J Am Soc Nephrol 2004;15(1):S55–S57.
2. Ziyadeh FN, Han DC, Cohen JA, et al. Glycated albumin stimulates fibronectin gene expression in glomerular mesangial cells: involvement of the transforming growth factor-beta system. Kidney Int 1998;53(3):631–638.

3. Kreisberg JI, Garoni JA, Radnik R, et al. High glucose and TGF beta 1 stimulate fibronectin gene expression through a cAMP response element. Kidney Int 1994;46(4):1019–1024.
4. Kreisberg JI, Radnik RA, Ayo SH, et al. High glucose elevates c-fos and c-jun transcripts and proteins in mesangial cell cultures. Kidney Int 1994;46(1):105–112.
5. Haneda M, Araki S, Togawa M, et al. Mitogen-activated protein kinase cascade is activated in glomeruli of diabetic rats and glomerular mesangial cells cultured under high glucose conditions. Diabetes 1997;46(5):847–853.
6. Hudson BI, Schmidt AM. RAGE: a novel target for drug intervention in diabetic vascular disease. Pharm Res 2004;21(7):1079–1086.
7. Neuringer JR, Brenner BM. Glomerular hypertension: cause and consequence of renal injury. J Hypertens Suppl 1992;10(7):S91–S97.
8. Remuzzi G, Ruggenenti P, Perna A, et al. Continuum of renoprotection with losartan at all stages of type 2 diabetic nephropathy: a post hoc analysis of the RENAAL trial results. J Am Soc Nephrol 2004;15(12):3117–3125.
9. Ziyadeh FN, Hoffman BB, Han DC, et al. Long-term prevention of renal insufficiency, excess matrix gene expression, and glomerular mesangial matrix expansion by treatment with monoclonal anti-transforming growth factor-beta antibody in db/db diabetic mice. Proc Natl Acad Sci USA 2000; 97(14):8015–8020.
10. Heilig K, Chen S, Xiang M, Brosius F, Heilig C. Overexpression of GLUT1 in glomeruli produces features of diabetic nephropathy (DN) in mice. (abstract). JASN 2004;15:263A.
11. Thallas-Bonke V, Lindschau C, Rizkalla B, et al. Attenuation of extracellular matrix accumulation in diabetic nephropathy by the advanced glycation end product cross-link breaker ALT-711 via a protein kinase C-alpha-dependent pathway. Diabetes 2004;53(11):2921–2930.
12. Haneda M, Kikkawa R, Horide N, et al. Glucose-induced overproduction of type IV collagen in cultured glomerular mesangial cells. J Diabet Complications 1991;5(2,3):199, 200.
13. Hong SW, Isono M, Chen S, et al. Increased glomerular and tubular expression of transforming growth factor-beta1, its type II receptor, and activation of the Smad signaling pathway in the db/db mouse. Am J Pathol 2001;158(5):1653–1663.
14. Wolf G, Ziyadeh FN, Stahl RA. Angiotensin II stimulates expression of transforming growth factor beta receptor type II in cultured mouse proximal tubular cells. J Mol Med 1999;77(7): 556–564.
15. Bleyer AJ, Fumo P, Snipes ER, et al. Polyol pathway mediates high glucose-induced collagen synthesis in proximal tubule. Kidney Int 1994;45(3):659–666.
16. Rocco MV, Chen Y, Goldfarb S, et al. Elevated glucose stimulates TGF-beta gene expression and bioactivity in proximal tubule. Kidney Int 1992;41(1):107–114.
17. Ziyadeh FN, Simmons DA, Snipes ER, et al. Effect of myo-inositol on cell proliferation and collagen transcription and secretion in proximal tubule cells cultured in elevated glucose. J Am Soc Nephrol 1991;1(11):1220–1229.
18. Joost HG, Bell GI, Best JD, et al. Nomenclature of the GLUT/SLC2A family of sugar/polyol transport facilitators. Am J Physiol Endocrinol Metab 2002;282(4):E974–E976.
19. Joost HG, Thorens B. The extended GLUT-family of sugar/polyol transport facilitators: nomenclature, sequence characteristics, and potential function of its novel members (review). Mol Membr Biol 2001;18(4):247–256.
20. Wood IS, Trayhurn P. Glucose transporters (GLUT and SGLT): expanded families of sugar transport proteins. Br J Nutr 2003;89(1):3–9.
21. Scheepers A, Joost HG, Schurmann A. The glucose transporter families SGLT and GLUT: molecular basis of normal and aberrant function. JPEN J Parenter Enteral Nutr 2004;28(5):364–371.
22. Uldry M, Thorens B. The SLC2 family of facilitated hexose and polyol transporters. Pflugers Arch 2004;447(5):480–489.
23. Thorens B, Lodish HF, Brown D. Differential localization of two glucose transporter isoforms in rat kidney. Am J Physiol 1990;259(6 Part 1):C286–C294.
24. Heilig C, Zaloga C, Lee M, et al. Immunogold localization of high-affinity glucose transporter isoforms in normal rat kidney. Lab Invest 1995;73(5):674–684.
25. Heilig CW, Concepcion LA, Riser BL, et al. Overexpression of glucose transporters in rat mesangial cells cultured in a normal glucose milieu mimics the diabetic phenotype. J Clin Invest 1995;96(4): 1802–1814.
26. Haspel HC, Stephenson KN, Davies-Hill T, et al. Effects of barbiturates on facilitative glucose transporters are pharmacologically specific and isoform selective. J Membr Biol 1999;169(1): 45–53.

27. Baldwin SA, Baldwin JM, Lienhard GE. Monosaccharide transporter of the human erythrocyte. Characterization of an improved preparation. Biochemistry 1982;21(16):3836–3842.
28. Asada T, Ogawa T, Iwai M, et al. Recombinant insulin-like growth factor I normalizes expression of renal glucose transporters in diabetic rats. Am J Physiol 1997;273(1 Part 2):F27–F37.
29. Schiffer M, Susztak K, Ranalletta M, et al. Localization of the GLUT8 glucose transporter in murine kidney and regulation in vivo in non-diabetic and diabetic conditions. Am J Physiol Renal Physiol 2005;289(1):F186–F193.
30. Wakisaka M, He Q, Spiro MJ, et al. Glucose entry into rat mesangial cells is mediated by both Na(+)-coupled and facilitative transporters. Diabetologia 1995;38(3):291–297.
31. Lewko B, Bryl E, Witkowski JM, et al. Characterization of glucose uptake by cultured rat podocytes. Kidney Blood Press Res 2005;28(1):1–7.
32. Lewko B, Bryl E, Witkowski JM, et al. Mechanical stress and glucose concentration modulate glucose transport in cultured rat podocytes. Nephrol Dial Transplant 2005;20(2):306–311.
33. Heilig CW, Kreisberg JI, Freytag S, et al. Antisense GLUT-1 protects mesangial cells from glucose induction of GLUT-1 and fibronectin expression. Am J Physiol Renal Physiol 2001;280(4):F657–F666.
34. Dimitrakoudis D, Vranic M, Klip A. Effects of hyperglycemia on glucose transporters of the muscle: use of the renal glucose reabsorption inhibitor phlorizin to control glycemia. J Am Soc Nephrol 1992;3(5):1078–1091.
35. Deems RO, Deacon RW, Ramlal T, et al. Insulin action on whole body glucose utilization and on muscle glucose transporter translocation in mice. Biochem Biophys Res Commun 1994;199(2):662–670.
36. Heilig CW, Liu Y, England RL, et al. D-glucose stimulates mesangial cell GLUT1 expression and basal and IGF-I-sensitive glucose uptake in rat mesangial cells: implications for diabetic nephropathy. Diabetes 1997;46(6):1030–1039.
37. Bilan PJ, Mitsumoto Y, Maher F, et al. Detection of the GLUT3 facilitative glucose transporter in rat L6 muscle cells: regulation by cellular differentiation, insulin and insulin-like growth factor-I. Biochem Biophys Res Commun 1992;186(2):1129–1137.
38. Haber RS, Weinstein SP, O'Boyle E, et al. Tissue distribution of the human GLUT3 glucose transporter. Endocrinology 1993;132(6):2538–2543.
39. Chiang SH, Baumann CA, Kanzaki M, et al. Insulin-stimulated GLUT4 translocation requires the CAP-dependent activation of TC10. Nature 2001;410(6831):944–948.
40. Marcus RG, England R, Nguyen K, et al. Altered renal expression of the insulin-responsive glucose transporter GLUT4 in experimental diabetes mellitus. Am J Physiol 1994;267(5 Part 2):F816–F824.
41. Chen S, Heilig K, Brosius III F, Heilig C. Diabetes increases glomerular GLUT1, and antisense-GLUT1 protects against diabetic glomerulosclerosis. JASN 2003;14:14A.
42. Carayannopoulos MO, Chi MM, Cui Y, et al. GLUT8 is a glucose transporter responsible for insulin-stimulated glucose uptake in the blastocyst. Proc Natl Acad Sci USA 2000;97(13):7313–7318.
43. Harik SI, Behmand RA, Arafah BM. Chronic hyperglycemia increases the density of glucose transporters in human erythrocyte membranes. J Clin Endocrinol Metab 1991;72(4):814–818.
44. Miele C, Formisano P, Condorelli G, et al. Abnormal glucose transport and GLUT1 cell-surface content in fibroblasts and skeletal muscle from NIDDM and obese subjects. Diabetologia 1997;40(4):421–429.
45. Miura T, Suzuki W, Ishihara E, et al. Impairment of insulin-stimulated GLUT4 translocation in skeletal muscle and adipose tissue in the Tsumura Suzuki obese diabetic mouse: a new genetic animal model of type 2 diabetes. Eur J Endocrinol 2001;145(6):785–790.
46. Kreisberg JI, Ayo SH. The glomerular mesangium in diabetes mellitus. Kidney Int 1993;43(1):109–113.
47. Craven PA, Davidson CM, DeRubertis FR. Increase in diacylglycerol mass in isolated glomeruli by glucose from de novo synthesis of glycerolipids. Diabetes 1990;39(6):667–674.
48. Gnudi L, Viberti G, Raij L, et al. GLUT-1 overexpression: Link between hemodynamic and metabolic factors in glomerular injury? Hypertension 2003;42(1):19–24.
49. Weigert C, Brodbeck K, Brosius FC III, et al. Evidence for a novel TGF-beta1-independent mechanism of fibronectin production in mesangial cells overexpressing glucose transporters. Diabetes 2003;52(2):527–535.
50. Pinto AB, Carayannopoulos MO, Hoehn A, et al. Glucose transporter 8 expression and translocation are critical for murine blastocyst survival. Biol Reprod 2002;66(6):1729–1733.
51. Rajah TT, Olson AL, Grammas P. Differential glucose uptake in retina- and brain-derived endothelial cells. Microvasc Res 2001;62(3):236–242.

52. Fernandes R, Suzuki K, Kumagai AK. Inner blood–retinal barrier GLUT1 in long-term diabetic rats: an immunogold electron microscopic study. Invest Ophthalmol Vis Sci 2003;44(7):3150–3154.
53. Gullans S, Hebert S. The Kidney, 5th edition. W. B. Saunders, Philadelphia, 1996.
54. Chi MM, Pingsterhaus J, Carayannopoulos M, et al. Decreased glucose transporter expression triggers BAX-dependent apoptosis in the murine blastocyst. J Biol Chem 2000;275(51):40,252–40,257.
55. Heilig CW, Saunders T, Brosius FC III, et al. Glucose transporter-1-deficient mice exhibit impaired development and deformities that are similar to diabetic embryopathy. Proc Natl Acad Sci USA 2003;100(26):15,613–15,618.
56. Heilig C, Brosius F, Siu B, et al. Implications of glucose transporter protein type 1 (GLUT1)-haplodeficiency in embryonic stem cells for their survival in response to hypoxic stress. Am J Pathol 2003;163(5):1873–1885.
57. Henry DN, Busik JV, Brosius FC III, et al. Glucose transporters control gene expression of aldose reductase, PKCalpha, and GLUT1 in mesangial cells in vitro. Am J Physiol 1999;277(1 Part 2):F97–F104.
58. Ziyadeh FN, Sharma K, Ericksen M, et al. Stimulation of collagen gene expression and protein synthesis in murine mesangial cells by high glucose is mediated by autocrine activation of transforming growth factor-beta. J Clin Invest 1994;93(2):536–542.
59. Heilig C, Jin Y, Heilig K, Wu G. Regulation of GLUT1 gene transcription in mesangial cells. (abstract). JASN 2002;13:23A.
60. von der Crone S, Deppe C, Barthel A, et al. Glucose deprivation induces Akt-dependent synthesis and incorporation of GLUT1, but not of GLUT4, into the plasma membrane of 3T3-L1 adipocytes. Eur J Cell Biol 2000;79(12):943–949.
61. Rathmell JC, Fox CJ, Plas DR, et al. Akt-directed glucose metabolism can prevent Bax conformation change and promote growth factor-independent survival. Mol Cell Biol 2003;23(20):7315–7328.
62. Xiang M, Heilig C. Upstream Stimulatory Factor (USF) involvement in mesangial cell gene regulation: implications for diabetic nephropathy. (abstract). JASN 2003;14:598A.
63. Horiba N, Masuda S, Takeuchi A, et al. Cloning and characterization of a novel Na+-dependent glucose transporter (NaGLT1) in rat kidney. J Biol Chem 2003;278(17):14,669–14,676.
64. Wright EM. Renal Na(+)-glucose cotransporters. Am J Physiol Renal Physiol 2001;280(1):F10–F18.
65. Sugawara-Yokoo M, Suzuki T, Matsuzaki T, et al. Presence of fructose transporter GLUT5 in the S3 proximal tubules in the rat kidney. Kidney Int 1999;56(3):1022–1028.
66. Gutierrez C, Vendrell J, Pastor R, et al. GLUT1 gene polymorphism in non-insulin-dependent diabetes mellitus: genetic susceptibility relationship with cardiovascular risk factors and microangiopathic complications in a Mediterranean population. Diabetes Res Clin Pract 1998;41(2):113–120.
67. Hodgkinson AD, Millward BA, Demaine AG. Polymorphisms of the glucose transporter (GLUT1) gene are associated with diabetic nephropathy. Kidney Int 2001;59(3):985–989.
68. Hodgkinson AD, Page T, Millward BA, et al. A novel polymorphism in the 5′ flanking region of the glucose transporter (GLUT1) gene is strongly associated with diabetic nephropathy in patients with Type 1 diabetes mellitus. J Diabet Complications 2005;19(2):65–69.
69. Liu ZH, Guan TJ, Chen ZH, et al. Glucose transporter (GLUT1) allele (XbaI-) associated with nephropathy in non-insulin-dependent diabetes mellitus. Kidney Int 1999;55(5):1843–1848.
70. Tarnow L, Grarup N, Hansen T, et al. Diabetic microvascular complications are not associated with two polymorphisms in the GLUT-1 and PC-1 genes regulating glucose metabolism in Caucasian type 1 diabetic patients. Nephrol Dial Transplant 2001;16(8):1653–1656.
71. Grzeszczak W, Moczulski DK, Zychma M, et al. Role of GLUT1 gene in susceptibility to diabetic nephropathy in type 2 diabetes. Kidney Int 59(2):2001;631–636.
72. Hsu C, Kao W, Steffes M, et al. Genetic Variation of Glucose Transporter 1 (GLUT1) and Nephropathy in the Atherosclerosis Risk in Communities (ARIC) Study (abstract). Diabetes 2004.
73. Ng DP, Canani L, Araki S, et al. Minor effect of GLUT1 polymorphisms on susceptibility to diabetic nephropathy in type 1 diabetes. Diabetes 2002;51(7):2264–2269.
74. Zintzaras E, Stefanidis I. Association between the GLUT1 gene polymorphism and the risk of diabetic nephropathy: a meta-analysis. J Hum Genet 2005;50(2):84–91.
75. Heilig C, Elana Y, Raymondjean M, et al. Identification of potential transcription factors (TFs) for mediation of GLUT1 positive feedback in mesangial cells. (abstract). JASN 1998;9:632A.
76. Cortes P, Riser BL, Asano K, et al. Effects of oral antihyperglycemic agents on extracellular matrix synthesis by mesangial cells. Kidney Int 1998;54(6):1985–1998.
77. Smoak IW. Tolbutamide alters glucose transport and metabolism in the embryonic mouse heart. Teratology 2002;65(1):19–25.

78. Tsiani E, Ramlal T, Leiter LA, et al. Stimulation of glucose uptake and increased plasma membrane content of glucose transporters in L6 skeletal muscle cells by the sulfonylureas gliclazide and glyburide. Endocrinology 1995;136(6):2505–2512.
79. Imamur H, Morimoto I, Tanaka Y, et al. Regulation of glucose transporter 1 expression by gliclazide in rat L6 myoblasts. Diabetes Nutr Metab 2001;14(6):308–314.
80. Eckel J. Direct effects of glimepiride on protein expression of cardiac glucose transporters. Horm Metab Res 1996;28(9):508–511.
81. Biederman JI, Vera E, Rankhaniya R, et al. Effects of sulfonylureas, alpha-endosulfine counterparts, on glomerulosclerosis in type 1 and type 2 models of diabetes. Kidney Int 2005;67(2):554–565.
82. Asano T, Wakisaka M, Yoshinari M, et al. Troglitazone enhances glycolysis and improves intracellular glucose metabolism in rat mesangial cells. Metabolism 2000;49(3):308–313.
83. Isshiki K, Haneda M, Koya D, et al. Thiazolidinedione compounds ameliorate glomerular dysfunction independent of their insulin-sensitizing action in diabetic rats. Diabetes 2000;49(6):1022–1032.
84. Togawa M, Kikkawa R, Haneda M, et al. Insulin-like growth factor I (IGF-I) stimulates glucose and amino acid uptake in cultured glomerular mesangial cells. J Diabet Complications 1991;5(2-3):184, 185.
85. Zhang JZ, Gao L, Widness M, et al. Captopril inhibits glucose accumulation in retinal cells in diabetes. Invest Ophthalmol Vis Sci 2003;44(9):4001–4005.
86. Vera JC, Reyes AM, Velasquez FV, et al. Direct inhibition of the hexose transporter GLUT1 by tyrosine kinase inhibitors. Biochemistry 2001;40(3):777–790.
87. Anjaneyulu M, Chopra K. Quercetin, an anti-oxidant bioflavonoid, attenuates diabetic nephropathy in rats. Clin Exp Pharmacol Physiol 2004;31(4):244–248.
88. Ho YY, Yang H, Klepper J, et al. Glucose transporter type 1 deficiency syndrome (Glut1DS): methylxanthines potentiate GLUT1 haploinsufficiency in vitro. Pediatr Res 2001;50(2):254–260.
89. De Vivo DC, Leary L, Wang D. Glucose transporter 1 deficiency syndrome and other glycolytic defects. J Child Neurol 2002;17(3):3S15–3S23; discussion 3S24, 3S25.
90. Wang D, Pascual JM, Yang H, et al. Glut-1 deficiency syndrome: clinical, genetic, and therapeutic aspects. Ann Neurol 2005;57(1):111–118.
91. Liu ZH, Li YJ, Chen ZH, et al. Glucose transporter in human glomerular mesangial cells modulated by transforming growth factor-beta and rhein. Acta Pharmacol Sin 2001;22(2):169–175.
92. Castiglione S, Fanciulli M, Bruno T, et al. Rhein inhibits glucose uptake in Ehrlich ascites tumor cells by alteration of membrane-associated functions. Anticancer Drugs 1993;4(3):407–414.

6 mRNA Translation in Diabetic Nephropathy

Balakuntalam S. Kasinath, MD,
Myung Ja Lee, PhD, *Denis Feliers*, PhD,
and Nahum Sonenberg, PhD

Contents

INTRODUCTION

With the decoding of the human genome, there is an urgent need for greater understanding of how proteins are synthesized and how they function. This notion is predicated on the importance of proteins as ultimate arbiters of cell function. Studies restricted to investigation of changes in mRNA levels do not address changes in proteins and their function. A strict linear correlation between mRNA levels and proteins does not always exist *(1,2)*. Therefore, it is imperative that protein metabolism be studied directly.

The life history of a protein begins with the synthesis of its mRNA by transcription of its gene. Factors affecting transcription and mRNA stability regulate the ambient level of mRNA. Following its synthesis, mRNA is transported out of the nucleus and peptide chain synthesis is initiated on the ribosome. The process of synthesis of a peptide from the genetic information present in the mRNA is called translation. Following translation, the peptide commonly undergoes posttranslational modification and gets sorted to the appropriate compartment of the cell or secreted to serve discrete function after which it is degraded. Each of these stages is highly regulated by a large number of factors. The steady-state concentration of a protein is the result of transcription, mRNA stability, translation, and protein degradation. Although the processes of transcriptional and degradational control have received much attention, regulation of translation has not been as

From: *Contemporary Diabetes: The Diabetic Kidney*
Edited by: P. Cortes and C. E. Mogensen © Humana Press Inc., Totowa, NJ

thoroughly explored. Recent evidence has shown that translation is an important site of regulation of protein metabolism, cell growth, apoptosis, development, carcinogenesis, and response to cellular stress. Investigation of translational processes has provided important insights into pathogenesis of type 2 diabetes and insulin resistance syndromes *(3)*. As mRNA translation involves energy expenditure, consuming approx 20–25% of total cell energy *(4)*, it is logical to expect a derangement in its regulation in diabetes, which is characterized by significant changes in energy metabolism. In renal science, however, translation has not been investigated in detail as an independent site of regulation of protein metabolism. In this review, our aim is to focus on regulation of mRNA translation as it relates to diabetic kidney disease.

mRNA TRANSLATION

mRNA translation is thought to occur in three stages, initiation, elongation, and termination. The initiation phase is the rate-limiting step in mRNA translation *(5)*, and also the most frequently regulated phase *(6)*. Translation initiation entails the recruitment of the ribosome to the mRNA, a process that is facilitated by eukaryotic initiation factors (eIFs). During the elongation phase, amino acids are added to the nascent peptide as dictated by the codons in the mRNA by the participation of respective aminoacyl transfer RNAs (tRNAs). Eukaryotic elongation factors (eEFs) control this step in translation. In the termination phase, the polypeptide chain is released from the ribosomal complex under the direction of eukaryotic release factors. Abnormalities in any of the three phases can result in aberrant protein synthesis.

Translational Machinery: Structural Considerations

Structures within the mRNA play a critical role in translation. They include the methylated guanosine triphosphate, m^7GpppX (G for guanosine, X is any base) at the 5′ end of the mRNA (the cap), the stretch of bases from the cap to the initiator methionine AUG codon at which translation begins called the 5′ untranslated region (UTR), the stretch of bases of mRNA extending from the stop codon to the polyA stretch, called the 3′ UTR, and the polyA tail at the 3′ end (Fig. 1A). The cap, the polyA tail and the UTRs contain binding sites for a variety of proteins, for example, eIF4E, polyA binding protein. Interaction between these proteins and the mRNA results in circularization of the mRNA that is believed to improve the efficiency of translation *(7,8)*. As circularization requires intact 3′ UTR of the mRNA it may be one way to ensure that nicked or incomplete mRNAs are not translated into nonfunctional proteins.

Ribosomes consist of the 40*S* subunit made of 18*S* RNA and several proteins, the 60*S* subunit consisting of 28*S*, 5.8*S*, 5*S* RNA, and proteins, and the 80*S* ribosome formed by the association of 40*S* and 60*S* subunits (Fig. 1B). An active mRNA, which is engaged in translation, is bound to several ribosomes, resulting in a polyribosome or polysome (Fig. 1C). mRNAs for proteins that are destined for secretion or cell surface expression are sorted to ribosomes bound to endoplasmic reticulum membrane, whereas cytosolic proteins are synthesized by the free ribosomes.

Translation of mRNAs Can Occur by Two Methods

Translation of mRNAs can occur by two major mechanisms, cap-dependent or cap-independent. In the former, eIFs bind to the cap at the 5′ end of the mRNA, mediating binding of the ribosome to the mRNA. This method appears to apply to the vast majority of eukaryotic mRNAs *(9)*.

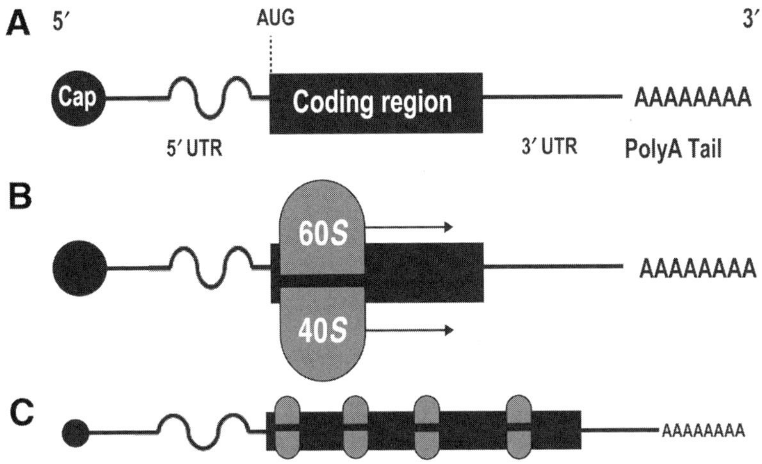

Fig. 1. mRNA and ribosome, essential components involved in mRNA translation. **(A)** Organization of mRNA showing the cap at 5′ end, 5′ and 3′ UTRs, coding region and the polyA tail. **(B)** 80S ribosome consisting of 40*S* and 60*S* subunits, bound to mRNA. **(C)** Polyribosome or polysome consists of several ribosomes bound to an mRNA transcript.

Internal Ribosomal Entry Site-Driven Translation

Translation of cellular mRNAs can continue even when the cap-dependent translation mechanism is inhibited. It is estimated that up to 10% of cellular mRNAs may be regulated in this fashion *(10–12)*. In translation of such mRNAs, the ribosome directly binds to mRNA in regions originally termed ribosome landing pads *(13)* and now called the internal ribosomal entry sites (IRES). IRES-driven translation occurs without the participation of mRNA cap at the 5′ end of the mRNA or its binding protein, eIF4E; however, other eIFs are usually used *(14)*. IRES-regulated mRNAs are generally involved in differentiation, cell cycle events and stress response, and include immunoglobulin heavy chain binding protein *(15)*, vascular endothelial growth factor (VEGF) *(16)*, fibroblast growth factor (FGF)2 *(17)*, ornithine decarboxylase *(18)*, and platelet-derived growth factor *(19)*. Recently, many non-eIF proteins that regulate ribosomal binding to IRES called IRES-transacting factors have been described and include heterogeneous nuclear RNA-binding proteins *(9,12)*. IRES-transacting factors may help bring the ribosome and the mRNA together or stabilize the active conformation of IRES and promote translation initiation. IRES-driven mRNAs do not have distinct consensus sites for ribosomal binding but are characterized by extensive secondary structures and multiple AUG sites. It is possible that secondary and tertiary structure of the 5′ UTR is important in ribosomal binding to the IRES-regulated mRNA. Translation of some capped mRNAs can occur by either cap-dependent or IRES-driven mechanisms. In some of these mRNAs, the IRES may be located within the coding region. Translation of such mRNAs can result in different lengths of peptides (isoforms) depending on initiation site, the IRES-driven peptide being smaller than cap-regulated translation product, for example, PITSLRE protein kinase, a cyclin-dependent kinase, *(20)* and FGF2 *(17,21)*. Such proteins isoforms are differentially synthesized depending on cell needs, and subserve distinct functions.

Cap-Dependent Translation: The Initiation Phase

A consensus model of initiation phase is provided here (Fig. 2). The initiation phase begins with dissociation of the 80*S* ribosome into 40*S* and 60*S* subunits, a process that

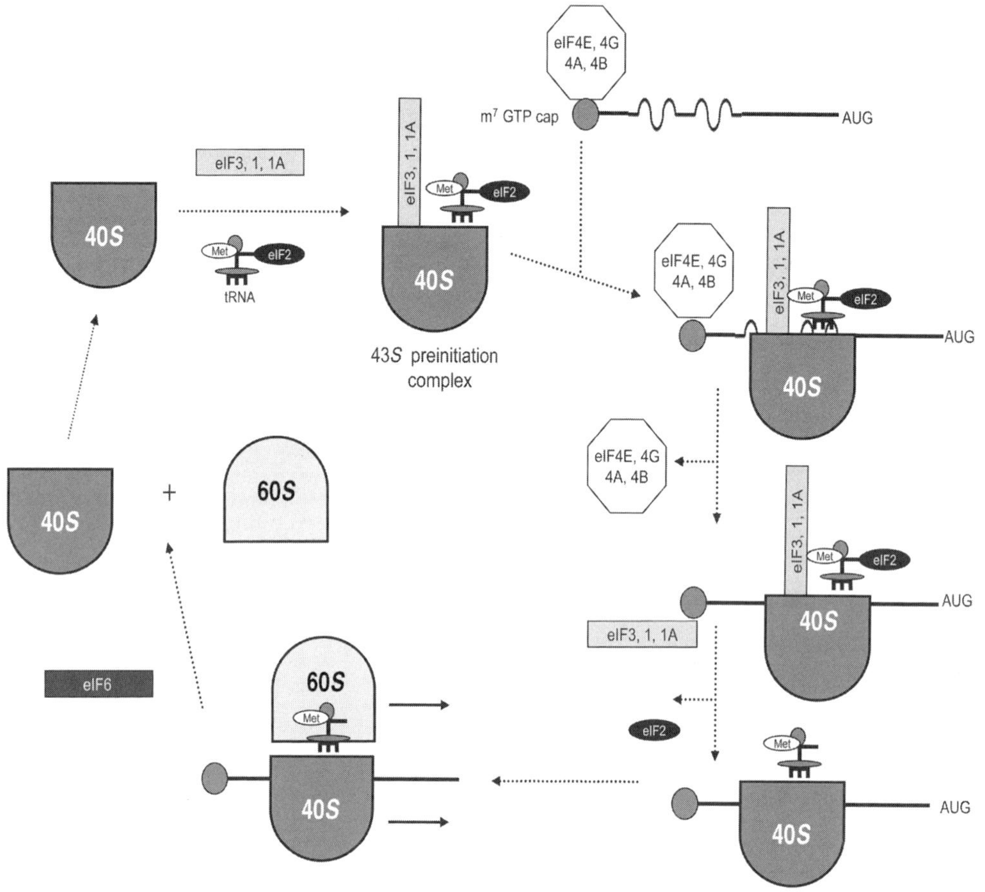

Fig. 2. Scanning model of initiation phase in cap-dependent mRNA translation.

involves regulation by eIF6. The 40*S* ribosomal subunit binds to eIF3, eIF1, eIF1A, and the initiator methionyl tRNA bound to eIF2; the resulting complex is called the 43*S* preinitiation complex. In the resting cell, the cap-binding protein, eIF4E is held inactive by its repressor-binding proteins. There are two types of repressors of eIF4E. One type is represented by proteins that are in physical association with select mRNAs and regulate their translation by binding to eIF4E although still being tethered to the mRNA, for example, maskin and cup *(6)*. The other group of proteins is not mRNA-specific and includes the eIF4E-binding proteins (4E-BPs). There are three 4E-BPs that are products of distinct genes. Of these, 4E-BP1 (also called PHAS-I) is the most commonly studied. On stimulation of protein synthesis, the eIF4E/4E-BP1 dimeric complex dissolves following phosphorylation of 4E-BP1 allowing free eIF4E to associate with eIF4G (Fig. 3). The binding sites for eIF4E on 4E-BP1 and eIF4G share the same consensus sequence (YXXXXLϕ, in which Y is tyrosine, L is leucine, X any amino acid, and ϕ is a hydrophobic amino acid) and the two proteins compete with each other for binding to eIF4E *(22)*. eIF4E and eIF4A bind to eIF4G to form the eIF4F complex. Additionally, eIF4G has binding sites for other proteins including eIF3, polyA binding protein and mitogen-activated protein (MAP) kinase-integrating kinase (Mnk-1), a kinase for eIF4E. The ability of eIF4G to bind eIF3, which interacts with 40*S* ribosomal complex enables it to function as a bridge between the mRNA and the ribosome *(14)*. The

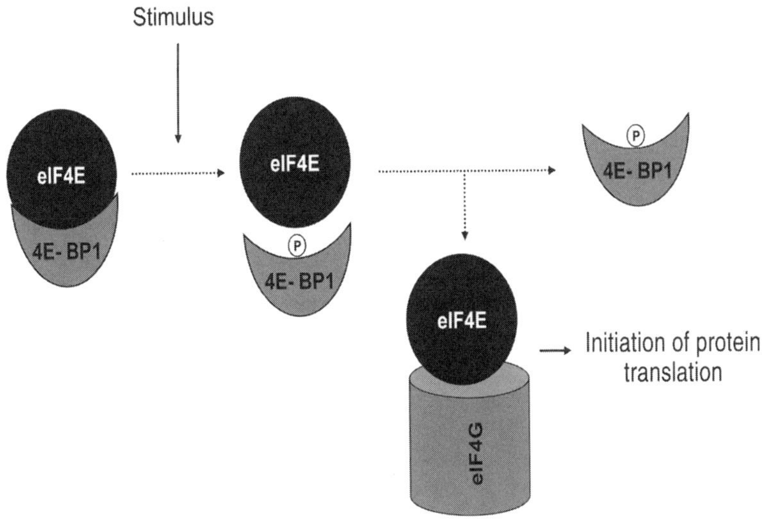

Fig. 3. Interaction between eIF4E and its binding protein, 4E-BP1. In the resting cell, eIF4E is held inactive in a dimeric complex by its binding protein, 4E-BP1. On application of a stimulus for protein synthesis, 4E-BP1 is phosphorylated with dissolution of the dimeric complex. eIF4E is now free to associate with eIF4G and facilitate initiation of mRNA translation.

eIF4F complex binds to the cap via eIF4E. The 43*S* preinitiation complex traverses the 5′ UTR of the mRNA to reach the AUG initiation codon. The 5′ UTR secondary structure is melted by the helicase activity of eIF4A, facilitating the 43*S* preinitiation complex to reach the AUG initiation codon. At this point, the initiation factors dissociate from the mRNA with assistance from eIF5, a GTPase-activating protein that promotes GTP hydrolysis by eIF2. The 60*S* ribosomal subunit now joins the 43*S* subunit, forming the 80*S* initiation complex. With the positioning of the 80*S* ribosome with the initiator methionyl tRNA on the initiator AUG codon at the translation initiation site, the initiation phase comes to an end. Activities of individual eIFs are governed by binding proteins and phosphorylation. More detailed accounts of the initiation phase have been recently published *(6,14,23)*.

Regulation of the Initiation Phase

The bulk of regulation of the initiation phase occurs by phosphorylation/dephosphorylation reactions governed by distinct kinases and phosphatases. An extensive network of signaling pathways is recruited by nutrients and growth factors to regulate translation initiation and requires a detailed examination.

Receptor Tyrosine Kinases. Recent work from our laboratory has shown that insulin, insulin-like growth factor (IGF)-I, angiotensin II and VEGF promote synthesis of both structural and matrix proteins by regulating key steps in translation in renal proximal tubular and glomerular epithelial cells in culture *(24–29)*. On exposure to insulin and VEGF, there is a rapid induction of tyrosine phosphorylation of several proteins including the respective receptors, which function as tyrosine kinases *(24,29)*. Following exposure to insulin, IGF-1 and VEGF, insulin receptor substrate 1 (IRS-1), the docking protein, binds to the respective receptor and undergoes phosphorylation; this binding serves to amplify the effects of agonist activation of its receptor (Fig. 4). In VEGF-treated cells reduction in IRS-1 expression by antisense strategy decreased both

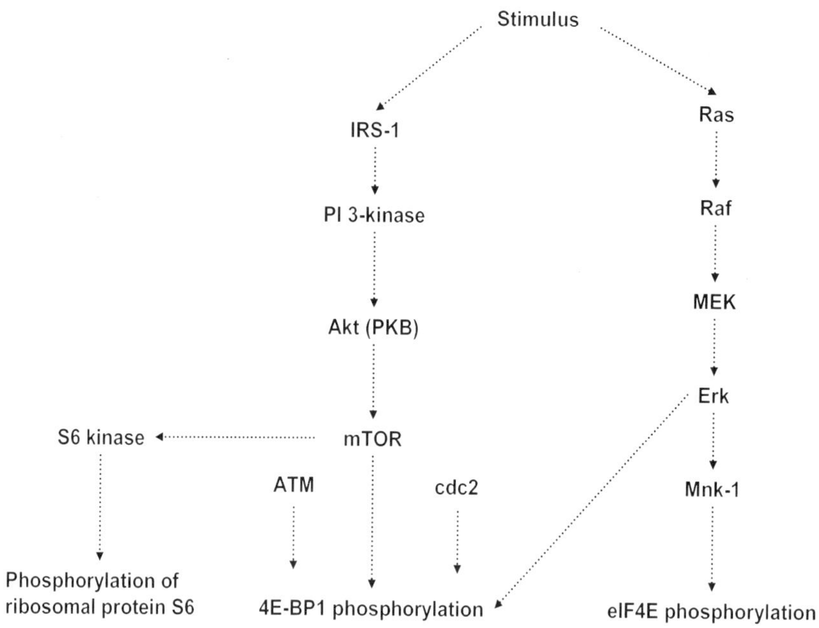

Fig. 4. Signaling pathways involved in regulation of phosphorylation of 4E-BP1 and eIF4E.

phosphatidylinositol 3 kinase (PI 3 kinase) activation and increase in protein synthesis, suggesting IRS-1 participates in the VEGF receptor signaling pathway leading to protein synthesis *(29)*.

PI 3 Kinase and Akt. In cells stimulated with growth factors, following tyrosine phosphorylation of IRS-1, the catalytic subunit of PI 3 kinase binds to the IRS protein via its 85 kDa regulatory subunit, stimulating its lipid kinase activity and generating inositol 3,4,5 triphosphate (Fig. 4). Overexpression of the 110 kDa catalytic subunit of the kinase in the absence of growth factors promotes 4E-BP1 phosphorylation, demonstrating its importance *(30)*. A phosphatase called PTEN (phosphatase and tensin homolog on chromosome 10) that dephosphorylates inositol 3,4,5 triphosphate has been identified; its role in inhibiting PI 3 kinase regulation of translation remains to be elucidated. The PI 3 kinase product, inositol 3,4,5 triphosphate translocates Akt (protein kinase B) to the cell membrane in which it is duly phosphorylated on Thr308 and Ser473. Phosphoinositide-dependent kinase 1 phosphorylates Thr308 on Akt *(31,32)*. The identity of the kinase that phosphorylates Ser473 is controversial and may include the integrin-linked kinase *(33)* or a kinase that belongs to PI 3 kinase-related kinase family called ataxia telengiectasia mutated (ATM) *(34)*. Recent reports have shown that mammalian target of rapamycin (mTOR) in a complex with a protein called rictor directly phosphorylates Ser473 on Akt *(35)*. Akt activity has been shown to be critical for phosphorylation of 4E-BP1 *(30)*. Akt activation leads to mammalian target of rapamycin (mTOR) phosphorylation, although whether Akt is a direct kinase for mTOR is controversial.

TSC-1, TSC-2 and Rheb. Because mTOR occupies a central role in mRNA translation by controlling phosphorylation of 4E-BP1 and S6 kinase that phosphorylates ribosomal proteins, its regulation merits a detailed examination (Fig. 5). It is important to note that mTOR functions as a nutrient-sensor, responding to changes in amino acid and glucose availability. The nutrient-sensing property of mTOR has obvious implications for diabetes-related complications including renal disease. Recent investigations have

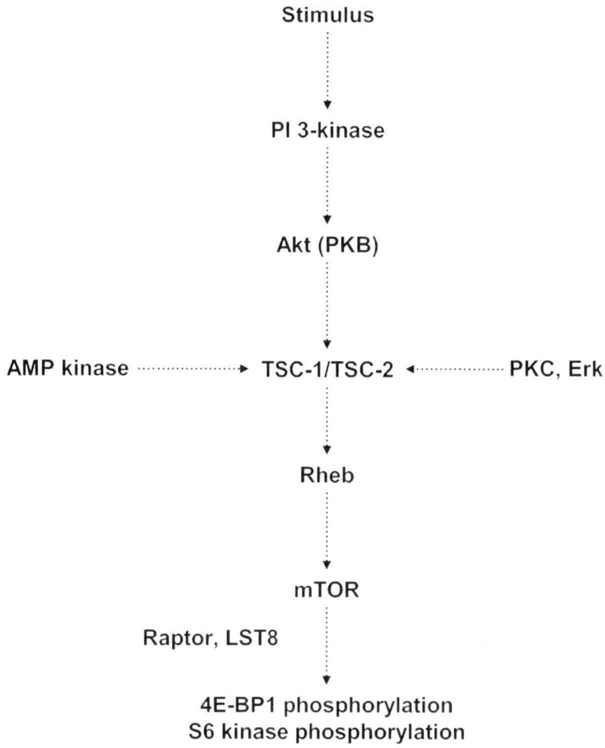

Fig. 5. Regulation of mTOR activity.

unraveled a complex series of regulatory steps involved in Akt regulation of mTOR activity. Two tuberous sclerosis complex proteins TSC-1 and TSC-2, also called hamartin and tuberin, respectively, have been found to be important mTOR regulators. Mutations in these proteins lead to tuberous sclerosis disease that is characterized by hypertrophy and growth of tumors, hamartomas, in several tissues including the kidney *(36)*. The association of cell hypertrophy with mutations in TSC genes suggests that TSC-1 and TSC-2 normally inhibit protein synthesis. TSC-1 and TSC-2 form a heterodimer that slows cell growth *(37,38)*, and inhibits mTOR activity *(39)*. Phosphorylation of TSC-2 by Akt results in its inactivation and leads to increase in mTOR activity *(40,41)*. Other kinases for TSC-2 include protein kinase C and Erk 1/2 type MAP kinase *(42)*. Nutrient supply also regulates TSC-2 phosphorylation. In states of adenosine triphosphate (ATP) deficiency, adenosine monophosphate (AMP)/ATP ratio increases, which stimulates activity of AMP-activated protein kinase (AMPK), which has been shown to promote phosphorylation of TSC-2 and increase its activity *(4)*, thereby linking nutrient sensing to an upstream regulator of mTOR activation. The control exerted by TSC-1/ TSC-2 dimer on mTOR phosphorylation is indirect and involves Rheb (Ras homolog-enriched in brain). TSC-2 acts as a GTPase-activating protein for Rheb *(43,44)*. Agonists that stimulate protein synthesis increase GTP-bound form of Rheb. In contrast, increase in TSC-1/TSC-2 dimer reduces Rheb present in GTP-bound form and increases the proportion of the GDP-bound form, thus decreasing Rheb's activity *(43,45)*. Additionally, Rheb overexpresion augments and Rheb depletion inhibits mTOR activity, respectively *(43,46,47)*. These observations show that Rheb in its GTP-bound form is a positive modulator of mTOR activity. The precise mechanism by which Rheb regulates mTOR activity remains to be elucidated.

Mammalian Target of Rapamycin. mTOR is a large modular protein (289 kDa) with a kinase domain near its carboxy terminus. It belongs to the family of PI 3 kinase-related kinases that include PI 3 kinase and ATM *(48)*. It has two important substrates relevant to translation, i.e., 4E-BP1 and S6 kinase; as such, increase in phosphorylation of these substrates is employed as a readout of mTOR activity. Rapamycin, an inhibitor of mTOR, binds a site toward N-terminus from the mTOR kinase domain. Activation of mTOR involves autophosphorylation site at Ser2481 and phosphorylation of Ser2448 regulated by the PI 3 kinase-Akt axis *(49,50)*. Increase in nutrient amino acid supply augments mTOR activity. Preliminary observations from our group suggest that increase in glucose availability also increases mTOR phosphorylation and activity in proximal tubular epithelial and glomerular epithelial cells *(50a)*. The precise mechanism by which mTOR detects changes in nutrient supply is not known; changes in the association of mTOR with its cofactors has been suggested as a possible mechanism *(51,52)*. mTOR regulation of 4E-BP1 and p70S6 kinase activity seems to depend on association with cofactors (Fig. 5). One such factor is raptor (regulatory associated protein of TOR), a 150 kDa protein that assists mTOR binding to TOR signaling motifs (TOS domains) in its substrates 4E-BP1 and S6 kinase *(53,54)*. The second cofactor for mTOR is LST8 also known as GβL (G protein β subunit-like protein), a 36 kDa protein *(52)*. LST8/GβL binds to the kinase domain of mTOR and positively modulates its activity *(52)*. The third mTOR-associated factor is called rictor. Whereas the mTOR-LST8-raptor complex is rapamycin-sensitive, another protein complex consisting of mTOR-LST8-rictor is thought to be resistant to rapamycin *(55)*. As mentioned earlier the latter complex has been implicated in the phosphorylation of Ser473 of Akt *(35)*. In summary, mTOR, a central player in regulation of initiation phase in translation, is regulated upstream by a complex network PI 3 kinase-Akt-TSC-1/TSC-2-Rheb axis and by such downstream cofactors such as raptor, rictor, and LST8/GβL. Existence of such an extensive network of regulatory factors emphasizes the critical importance of mTOR in regulation of protein synthesis.

4E Binding Protein. In the resting cell, the mRNA cap binding protein, eIF4E, is bound to 4E-BP1 that keeps eIF4E in an inactive state. An early event in the initiation phase of mRNA translation is release of eIF4E by phosphorylation of 4E-BP1, which is directly under the control of mTOR *(56,57)*. There are several serine or threonine sites for phosphorylation on 4E-BP1 *(58)*. Depending on the intensity of phosphorylation, three isoforms of 4E-BP1 with distinct migration patterns on a fractionating gel may be identified, α being the least, γ the most phosphorylated, with intensity of phosphorylation of β being intermediate between the two others. On agonist stimulation, the proportion of intensely phosphorylated isoforms increases resulting in dissolution of eIF4E complexation with 4E-BP1 (Fig. 3). The role of individual phosphorylation sites on 4E-BP1 in dissolution of its complex with eIF4E is controversial. There may be a hierarchy among the phosphorylation sites in promoting eIF4E-4E-BP1 dissociation. Thr37, 46 phosphorylation is thought to be the priming event *(58)* followed by phosphorylation at Thr70 and Ser65; phosphorylation at these four sites may be sufficient to release eIF4E *(48)*. Phosphorylated sites on 4E-BP1 seem to lie close to acidic amino acids on eIF4E *(59)*. Dissociation of the eIF4E/4E-BP1 complex following phosphorylation of the latter may be due to electrostatic repulsion of the negative charges on the two proteins. Distinct kinases may mediate phosphorylation of individual phosphorylation sites on 4E-BP1. Thus, Akt and mTOR regulate phosphorylation at Thr37, Thr46, Ser65 and Thr70. ATM, a kinase belonging to the PI 3 kinase family, and cdc42 may regulate phosphorylation at other sites *(60,61)*. The role of Erk in 4E-BP1 phosphorylation may be cell-specific and is discussed later.

Eukaryotic Initiation Factor 4E. Ser209 in eIF4E undergoes phosphorylation during initiation phase and has been identified as the physiologically important site *(62)*. Erk 1/2 MAP kinase regulates Ser209 phosphorylation, although it is not the direct kinase as eIF4E lacks proline residues around Ser209. Mnk-1 is the direct kinase for eIF4E *(63–65)*. The scaffolding protein eIF4G has binding sites for Mnk-1 and eIF4E and facilitates phosphorylation of eIF4E by Mnk-1 *(63)*. Mnk1 has a nuclear transport signal in its N terminus *(66)*, although the significance of shift from cytoplasm to nucleus is unclear. The biological implication of eIF4E phosphorylation is unsettled. In vitro studies and investigations in Drosophila suggested that phosphorylation of eIF4E promoted cell growth *(67,68)*. However, this view has been challenged recently and phosphorylation of eIF4E has been suggested to inhibit binding to mRNA cap by electrostatic repulsion between negatively charged phosphate residues on mRNA cap and eIF4E *(69,70)*.

Elongation Phase and Termination Phase

During the elongation phase, peptide propagation occurs by systematic addition of amino acids in accordance with codon sequence in the mRNA. Elongation phase is regulated by eukaryotic elongation factors (eEFs) 1 and 2; eEF2 is active when it is dephosphorylated. Detailed surveys of elongation phase have been recently published *(23,71,72)*. Termination phase begins with the arrival of the 80*S* ribosome at the termination codon on the mRNA. The release of the peptide is facilitated by the participation of ribosomal release factor, which has structural similarity to tRNA *(73,74)*. The 80*S* ribosome is split into the 40*S* and 60*S* subunits with the assistance of eIF6 and eIF3; the 40*S* ribosomal unit is recycled for another round of peptide synthesis.

mRNA TRANSLATION IN DIABETIC NEPHROPATHY

Control of mRNA translation is now receiving attention in the investigation of diabetic renal disease. A brief summary of ongoing work is provided.

Regulation of mRNA Translation by Glucose and Insulin

We have recently explored the role of hyperglycemia and hyperinsulinemia in general protein synthesis/hypertrophy and in synthesis of extracellular matrix protein, laminin, in renal cells. Whereas hyperglycemia is a pathogenic factor common to both types of diabetes, hyperinsulinemia is of relevance to type 2 diabetes. Hyperinsulinemia precedes clinical expression of diabetes during the phase of insulin resistance. Fasting plasma insulin levels and insulin levels between meals remain higher than normal in type 2 diabetes although the response of insulin to glucose loads is suboptimal *(75,76)*. This results in exposure of the individual with type 2 diabetes to considerable periods of hyperinsulinemia in a 24-h period. Mice with type 2 diabetes (db/db mice) manifest significant hyperinsulinemia during the initial phase of hyperglycemia; thus, renal abnormalities in the early phase of type 2 diabetes can be potentially due to hyperglycemia and/or hyperinsulinemia.

Translation Regulation of Glucose-Induced Hypertrophy

The first structural change in the kidney in diabetes is enlargement. Most of the kidney enlargement is accounted for by increase in size of individual renal cells from augmented protein and RNA content per cell (i.e., hypertrophy) rather than in their number *(77,78)*. Renal hypertrophy occurs rapidly with significant increase in kidney weight being evident within days of onset of type 1 or type 2 diabetes *(27)*. The importance of hypertrophy lies in the possibility that it may predispose to long-term complications of diabetes *(77)*. Glomerular visceral epithelial cells (GECs, podocytes) have recently attracted much attention for their role in diabetic renal disease. Podocyte deficiency caused by either reduced number or reduced density relative to length of the glomerular basement membrane, has been suggested as a determinant of proteinuria and progression in diabetic nephropathy *(79–81)*. The mechanism underlying podocyte loss is not well understood. In cardiac myocytes, maladaptive hypertrophy has been linked to eventual cardiac failure *(82)*; in a similar manner, podocyte loss may be linked to hypertrophy. Investigations are underway to elucidate pathways by which high glucose promotes podocyte hypertrophy. Transforming growth factor-β has been studied extensively as a mediator of glucose-induced hypertrophy in renal cells *(83)*. Other factors are likely to be involved in high-glucose-induced hypertrophy, including changes in the energy status of the cell, which has not been examined. As glucose is an important metabolic fuel for the cells, high glucose alters the energy status of the cells. The cells detect changes in the energy status by means of sensors such as the AMPK *(84)* and mTOR. However, the potential role of AMP kinase in glucose-regulated cell processes including protein synthesis has not been examined. AMPK is a trimeric protein made of the catalytic α-unit, which requires Thr172 phosphorylation for its activity, and two regulatory subunits, β and γ. AMPK activity is stimulated by increase in cellular AMP to ATP ratio. Activity of AMPK is directed at increasing ATP generation by fatty acid oxidation and inhibiting energy consuming processes *(85)*. The role played by AMPK in high glucose-induced changes in renal cell metabolism was examined in the GEC *(85a)*. High glucose stimulated significant increase in protein synthesis and induced hypertrophy in the GEC following incubation for 3 d. These changes were dependent on activation of PI 3 kinase and mTOR and were associated with increase in phosphorylation of 4E-BP1 and dephosphorylation of eEF2, respectively *(85a)*. As reviewed earlier, stimulation of initiation and elongation phases of translation requires phosphorylation of 4E-BP1 and dephosphorylation of eEF2. Under conditions of high-glucose-induced hypertrophy in the GEC, Thr172 phosphroylation of AMPK was reduced suggesting a decrease in AMPK activity. Stimulation of AMPK activity by metformin or 5-aminoimidazole-4-carboxamide 1-β-ribofuranoside prevented high-glucose-induced changes in phosphorylation status of 4E-BP1 and eEF2 and induction of hypertrophy. These data suggest that AMPK is an important regulator of initiation and elongation phases of translation in response to high glucose. The status of AMPK phosphorylation in renal tissue undergoing hypertrophy was examined in rats with streptozotocin-induced type 1 diabetes *(85a)*. There was a significant reduction in phosphorylation of AMPK in renal cortex and in isolated glomeruli in diabetic rats that coincided with hypertrophy. These in vitro and in vivo observations suggest that AMPK normally inhibits protein synthesis in renal cells. Inhibition of its activity appears to facilitate renal growth in diabetes. Availability of pharmacological agents that modulate AMPK activity, for example, metformin, makes it an attractive target for therapies aimed at ameliorating diabetic kidney disease.

Translation Regulation of Laminin Synthesis by Glucose and Insulin

Laminin is a heterotrimeric protein with distinct subunit composition in matrix compartments of the kidney. It is composed of α5, β2, γ1 chains (laminin-11) in the glomerular basement membrane and α1, β1, γ1 chains (laminin 1) or α5, β1, γ1 chains (laminin 10) in the tubular basement membrane *(86)*. Laminin is involved in cell anchorage and supramolecular assembly of extracellular matrix *(87)*. Laminin contributes to regulation of glomerular capillary permeability as mice lacking laminin β2 chain develop massive proteinuria even as other components of the glomerular basement membrane are normally expressed *(88)*. Recently, congenital nephrotic syndrome associated with ocular abnormalities owing to mutation in laminin β2 gene has been reported *(89)*. Accumulation of laminin contributes to accumulation of matrix in glomerulus as well as the tubulointerstitium in diabetic kidney *(90–93)*. We examined the molecular regulation of laminin in the kidney cortex of db/db mice with type 2 diabetes in both early (within 4 wk of onset of diabetes) and established stages of diabetes (3 mo). Accumulation of laminin chains was associated with reduced mRNA levels in the renal cortical lysates *(94)*, suggesting that nontranscriptional mechanisms were involved. Thus, decreased degradation and/or increased efficiency of laminin chain mRNA translation could account for increase in renal parenchymal laminin. The role of translation was further examined, as it has not been addressed in contrast to extensive studies on regulation of matrix degradation in diabetic renal disease. As the laminin accumulation was evident in early stages of type 2 diabetes associated with elevations not only in plasma glucose but also in plasma insulin *(95)*, the role of high glucose and high insulin in regulation of laminin synthesis were examined in renal proximal tubular epithelial cells. We employed these cells in our studies as they form the bulk of renal cortex on which in vivo studies were conducted, and laminin changes were also evident in tubular matrix in addition to that of the glomerulus *(94)*. High glucose alone (30 m*M*), high insulin alone (1 n*M*), and both together rapidly stimulated laminin β1 chain synthesis and secretion into the medium within 5 min and the effect lasted for up to 60 min; the effect of high glucose could not be explained by osmotic effect *(50a)*. Analysis of mRNA levels showed no change and laminin β1 protein increment could not be blocked by transcription inhibitors. Together these data suggested that increase in laminin β1 chain synthesis was likely owing to augmented mRNA translation. High glucose and high insulin did not increase laminin β1 chain synthesis in cells expressing mutant of 4E-BP1 in which Thr37, 46 are changed to alanine. As reviewed earlier, phosphorylation of these two "priming" sites is required for dissociation of the eIF4E/4E-BP1 complex. These data suggest that high glucose and insulin regulate laminin β1 chain synthesis at the level of initiation phase of its cap-dependent translation. Both 4E-BP1 phosphorylation and laminin synthesis induced by high glucose and high insulin could be abolished by expression of dominant negative constructs of PI 3 kinase and mTOR, demonstrating both high glucose and high insulin recruit PI 3 kinase-mTOR pathway in augmenting 4E-BP1 phosphorylation. Increase in laminin β1 chain synthesis was also associated with increase in eIF4E phosphorylation that was dependent on Erk activation. PD098059, an inhibitor of MAP kinase kinase (MEK), the upstream kinase of Erk, could abolish laminin synthesis indicating a role for Erk in laminin synthesis stimulated by high glucose and high insulin. Whether Erk regulates 4E-BP1 phosphorylation in addition to that of eIF4E remains to be studied. Computer analysis of laminin β1 chain mRNA revealed a complex 5′ UTR with extensive secondary structures; translation of such mRNAs requires assistance of cap-dependent process *(96)*. These data show that translation can be a site of regulation of matrix protein synthesis in diabetes.

An unexpected observation in these investigations was the rapidity with which high glucose and high insulin stimulated laminin synthesis. Others have noted that a 2-h exposure to high glucose commits renal fibroblasts to increase synthesis of collagen and fibronectin *(97)*. There may be a clinical correlate for these findings. Recently, postprandial peaks of plasma glucose, which tend to be short lived, have been found to be an independent risk factor for cardiovascular complications of diabetes *(98)*. Taken together, the experimental and clinical data suggest that even transient elevations of glucose may be injurious to target tissues in diabetes.

Furthermore, our data implicate hyperinsulinemia in pathogenesis of diabetic renal disease. Evaluation of insulin signaling pathway in diabetic mice has provided support for this notion. Analysis of insulin receptor activation was performed in renal cortex of mice in the early stages of type 2 diabetes in db/db mice *(99)*. In comparison with non-diabetic littermates, tyrosine phosphorylation of the insulin receptor β chain, kinase activity of the insulin receptor, and PI 3 kinase activity associated with insulin receptor were all increased several fold in the renal cortex of db/db mice. In contrast, activity of insulin receptor was unchanged in the liver of db/db mice. These data demonstrate that in contrast to the liver, an acknowledged site of insulin resistance, the renal cortex is insulin-sensitive in type 2 diabetes. The timing of insulin receptor activation suggests it may contribute to pathological changes in the kidney seen in early stages of type 2 diabetes including hypertrophy and matrix accumulation *(99)*. Insulin stimulates protein synthesis in proximal tubular epithelial cells by stimulating 4E-BP1 phosphorylation in a PI 3 kinase-Akt-mTOR-dependent manner *(24)*. Abrass et al. *(100)* have shown that insulin administration promotes appearance of type III collagen in the kidney of rodents. They have also reported that insulin promotes the synthesis of laminin in mesangial cells *(101)*. Additionally, in proximal tubular epithelial cells, insulin has been shown to promote synthesis of transforming growth factor (TGF)-β by regulating its translation and not transcription *(102)*. These data suggest that insulin may have an injurious role in kidney disease in type 2 diabetes. There is precedent implicating hyperinsulinemia in complications of diabetes, for example, vascular disease *(103)*. It should be noted that insulin effects are suboptimal in type 2 diabetes only regarding glucose transport. The compensatory hyperinsulinemia that occurs may be sufficient to amplify other properties of insulin including protein and DNA synthesis. There is probably no resistance to the non-glucose-transporting properties of insulin. Although our data suggest a pathogenic role for insulin in renal disease pathogenesis in type 2 diabetes, definitive evidence needs to be provided. It is probable that there are distinct metabolic factors in type 2 diabetes *(104)* that may operate differently from type 1 diabetes that promote a pathogenic role for insulin in the renal tissue in the hyperinsulinemic phase of type 2 diabetes. This may explain the salutary effects of insulin in management of renal disease in type 1 diabetes in contrast to its potential injurious effect in early stages of type 2 diabetes.

Other Growth Factors and Regulation of mRNA Translation

Vascular Endothelial Growth Factor (VEGF)

VEGF is an angiogenic factor with an established role in ocular complications of diabetes *(105)*; however, its involvement in diabetic kidney disease has not been well understood. In the kidney, VEGF is expressed by the podocyte *(106)* and the proximal tubular epithelial cells *(25)*. VEGF exerts its effects via VEGF receptors (VEGFRs), which function as tyrosine kinases. VEGFR1 and VEGFR2 are expressed in the glomerular endothelial cells and in vitro in the proximal tubular epithelial cells *(27)*. VEGF expression is increased several fold within a few days of onset of type 1 or type 2 diabetes in mice, coinciding with hypertrophy of the kidney *(27)*, suggesting VEGF may regulate protein synthesis. Observations in proximal tubular epithelial cells showed that VEGF stimulates protein synthesis and induces hypertrophy by recruiting PI 3 kinase-Akt-mTOR pathway to augment phosphorylation of 4E-BP1. These data provide a mechanistic explanation for the observation that administration of neutralizing antibodies to VEGF ameliorates renal hypertrophy in mice with type 1 or type 2 diabetes *(107,108)*.

The mechanism by which diabetic kidney increases VEGF expression is beginning to be addressed with focus on angiotensin II, a principal agent of renal injury in diabetes *(109)*. Administration of angiotensin II for several days resulted in elevation of VEGF synthesis by increasing its mRNA levels *(110)*. In addition to delayed phase regulation that involves transcription, recent work from our laboratory has shown that the rapid phase of VEGF synthesis induced by angiotensin II involves a different mechanism *(25)*. In proximal tubular epithelial cells, angiotensin II stimulated VEGF synthesis within 5 min that lasted for nearly 30 min. The increment in VEGF synthesis was not owing to changes in either mRNA level or stability of the mRNA, and could not be blocked by transcription inhibitors. Polysomal analysis showed that it was owing to increase in the efficiency of VEGF mRNA translation *(25)*. Angiotensin II failed to stimulate VEGF synthesis in cells expressing a phosphorylation mutant of 4E-BP1 demonstrating that the rapid phase synthesis of VEGF induced by angiotensin II is dependent on regulation of the initiation phase. Investigation of signaling mechanisms revealed that angiotensin II recruited PI 3 kinase and Akt signaling pathway to phosphorylate 4E-BP1.

The rapidity of angiotensin II regulation of VEGF synthesis suggested involvement of a mediator that is recruited almost immediately on exposure to angiotensin II. In this context, the role of reactive oxygen species (ROS) was examined. Angiotensin II has been shown to stimulate Akt by activation of ROS in mesangial cells *(111,112)*. Angiotensin II-induced VEGF synthesis was completely inhibited by antioxidants *N*-acetyl cysteine and diphenyleneiodonium. Further investigation showed that ROS were upstream of PI 3 kinase-Akt-4E BP1 pathway in angiotensin II-treated cells *(112a)*. The source of ROS that results in injury to target tissues in diabetes has attracted attention. A unifying scheme in which ROS originate in the mitochondria has been proposed as the underlying mechanism of target cell injury in diabetes *(113)*. However, amelioration of angiotensin II effect on VEGF synthesis by diphenyleneiodonium suggested involvement of flavin-containing NAD(P)H oxidase as a possible source of ROS. Preliminary studies suggest that deactivation of mitochondria does not prevent angiotensin II induction of VEGF synthesis, suggesting NAD(P)H oxidase as the potential source of ROS *(112a)*. Further studies are needed to clarify the individual roles of mitochondrial and membrane derived ROS in angiotensin II-mediated injury to the kidney.

Insulin-Like Growth Factor-I

The part played by growth factors in renal injury induced by diabetes has been reviewed recently *(114)*. We will focus on regulation of mRNA translation by growth factors as it relates to diabetic kidney disease. IGF-I has been studied for regulation of renal growth in diabetes as it is known to stimulate protein synthesis *(115)* and mice transgenic for IGF-I manifest renal hypertrophy *(116)*. Renal cells synthesize IGF-I *(117)* and may serve as the source of IGF-I in the kidney in diabetes *(118)* as systemic levels of the growth factor is reduced in diabetes *(119)*. An increase in renal parenchymal IGF-I concentration precedes rapid increase in renal weight in diabetes *(119–121)*. As proximal tubular epithelial cells express receptors for IGF-I *(122)* and constitute the bulk of cells undergoing growth in diabetes-induced renal hypertrophy, IGF-I regulation of protein synthesis at the level of translation has been studied *(26)*. IGF-I stimulated *de novo* protein synthesis by regulation of initiation phase of translation. Phosphorylation of 4E-BP1 was found to be essential for IGF-I stimulation of protein synthesis, which was dependent on stimulation of the IRS-1-PI 3 kinase-Akt signaling pathway. Interestingly, IGF-I also stimulated Erk 1/2 MAP kinase activity and blocking this kinase also inhibited both 4E-BP1 phosphorylation and protein synthesis. Further studies showed that Erk activation by IGF-I was dependent on activation of PI 3-kinase. Thus, the site of regulation of protein synthesis by IGF-I appears to be at the level of 4E-BP1 phosphorylation, a key step in the initiation phase of protein synthesis. Similar involvement of Erk in 4E-BP1 phosphorylation has also been reported in proximal tubular epithelial cells treated with insulin, with Erk activation being dependent on PI 3 kinase *(24)*. The precise site in the Erk regulatory cascade in which PI 3 kinase exerts control is not clear. Protein kinase ζ has been reported as a mediator of cross-talk between PI 3 kinase and Erk pathways in myeloid cells *(123)*. Erk involvement in regulation of 4E-BP1 phosphorylation appears to be cell-specific as it is reported to occur in smooth muscle cells *(124)*, kidney cells recovering from osmotic stress *(125)* but not in other cells *(126)*.

Platelet-Derived Growth Factor

TGF-β has been shown to be a major mediator of renal injury in diabetes *(127)*. The mechanism by which high glucose promotes TGF-β synthesis has been studied. TGF-β mRNA levels were increased by high glucose in proximal tubular epithelial cells. However, it was found that a permissive role of platelet-derived growth factor (PDGF) was needed for the accumulated mRNA to be processed into TGF-β protein *(128)*. These data suggest regulation of transcription and translation of TGF-β by distinct factors in proximal tubular epithelial cells.

CONCLUSION

Proteins are the executors of cell function. Recent advances have provided abundant evidence that mRNA translation is an important target for regulation of protein synthesis. Translational control plays an important role in such diverse cell events as development, differentiation, apoptosis, and response to environmental or endogenous stress. However, investigation of renal injury in diabetes has not adequately addressed the potential role of mRNA translation. This review has provided a brief introduction to the process and regulation of mRNA translation and summarized recent findings on its dysregulation in diabetic nephropathy.

There is a need for changing our strategy in study of proteins. We need to consider translational control of synthesis of individual proteins, in addition to their regulation at the levels of transcription, mRNA stability, posttranslational modification, and degradation. Drawing conclusions from measurement of changes in mRNA levels is hazardous as mRNA levels do not always correlate with either protein levels or protein function. It is useful to consider regulation of mRNA translation when there is lack of correlation between the mRNA concentration and that of the corresponding protein. mRNAs with complexities in the 5′ UTRs are particularly regulated by translation. Translation of mRNA is regulated predominantly by phosphorylation/dephosphorylation reactions under the control of signaling pathways. Thus, translational responses can be rapid in comparison with transcriptional regulation. It is estimated that mRNA translation can proceed at the rate of 20 amino acids per second *(72)*. Studies on mRNA translation are likely to yield important insights into cellular pathogenesis of diabetic kidney disease as its dysregulation is involved in such diverse cell events as abnormal protein synthesis, cell cycle regulation, apoptosis, differentiation, and stress response.

ACKNOWLEDGMENTS

We thank the postdoctoral trainees in our laboratory for their effort and contributions and Dr. G. Ghosh Choudhury for critical reading of the manuscript. BSK was supported by grants from the NIH (O'Brien Kidney Center Grant), American Diabetes Association, Veterans Administration, and the National Kidney Foundation of South and Central Texas.

ABBREVIATIONS

4E-BP	4E binding protein
AICAR	5-aminoimidazole-4-carboxamide 1-β-ribofuranoside
AMPK	AMP-activated protein kinase
ATM	ataxia telengiectasia mutated
BiP	immunoglobulin heavy chain-binding protein
eEF	eukaryotic elongation factor
eIF	eukaryotic initiation factor
eRF	eukaryotic release factor
FGF	fibrobalst growth factor
GβL	G protein β-subunit-like protein
GEC	glomerular epithelial cells
IRES	internal ribosomal entry site
IRS	insulin receptor substrate
ITAF	IRES-transacting factor
IGF	insulin-like growth factor
Mnk	MAP kinase-integrating kinase
mTOR	mammalian target of rapamycin
PDGF	platelet-derived growth factor
PDK	phosphoinositide-dependent kinase
PTEN	phosphatase and tensin homolog on chromosome ten
Raptor	regulatory associated protein of TOR
Rheb	Ras homolog enriched in brain
TSC	tuberous sclerosis complex
TOS	TOR signaling domain
UTR	untranslated region
VEGF	vascular endothelial growth factor
VEGFR	vascular endothelial growth factor receptor

REFERENCES

1. Gygi SP, Rochon Y, Franza BR, Aebersold R. Correlation between protein and mRNA abundance in yeast. Mol Cell Biol 1999;19:1720–1730.
2. Tew KD, Monks A, Barone L, et al. Glutathione-associated enzymes in the human cell lines of the National Cancer Institute Drug Screening Program. Mol Pharmacol 1996;50:149–159.
3. Shi Y, Taylor SI, Tan SL, Sonenberg N. When translation meets metabolism: multiple links to diabetes. Endocr Rev 2003;24:91–101.

4. Inoki K, Zhu T, Guan KL. TSC2 mediates cellular energy response to control cell growth and survival. Cell 2003;115:577–590.
5. Miron M, Sonenberg N. Regulation of translation via TOR signaling: insights from Drosophila melanogaster. J Nutr 2001;131:2988S–29893S.
6. Richter JD, Sonenberg N. Regulation of cap-dependent translation by eIF4E inhibitory proteins. Nature 2005;433:477–480.
7. Kahvejian A, Roy G, Sonenberg N. The mRNA closed-loop model: the function of PABP and PABP-interacting proteins in mRNA translation. Cold Spring Harb Symp Quant Biol 2001;66:293–300.
8. von der Haar T, Gross JD, Wagner G, McCarthy JE. The mRNA cap-binding protein eIF4E in post-transcriptional gene expression. Nat Struct Mol Biol 2004;11:503–511.
9. Komar A, Hatzoglou AM. Internal ribosome entry sites in cellular mRNAs: the mystery of their existence. J Biol Chem 2005;R400041200.
10. Bonnal S, Boutonnet C, Prado-Lourenco L, Vagner S. IRESdb: the Internal Ribosome Entry Site database. Nucleic Acids Res 2003;31:427, 428.
11. Johannes G, Carter MS, Eisen MB, Brown PO, Sarnow P. Identification of eukaryotic mRNAs that are translated at reduced cap binding complex eIF4F concentrations using a cDNA microarray. Proc Natl Acad Sci USA 1999;96:13,118–13,123.
12. Stoneley M, Willis AE. Cellular internal ribosome entry segments: structures, trans-acting factors and regulation of gene expression. Oncogene 2004;23:3200–3207.
13. Pelletier J, Sonenberg N. Internal initiation of translation of eukaryotic mRNA directed by a sequence derived from poliovirus RNA. Nature 1988;334:320–325.
14. Gingras AC, Raught B, Sonenberg N. eIF4 initiation factors: effectors of mRNA recruitment to ribosomes and regulators of translation. Annu Rev Biochem 1999;68:913–963.
15. Macejak D, Sarnow GP. Internal initiation of translation mediated by the 5' leader of a cellular mRNA. Nature 1991;353:90–94.
16. Gerlitz G, Jagus R, Elroy-Stein O. Phosphorylation of initiation factor-2 alpha is required for activation of internal translation initiation during cell differentiation. Eur J Biochem 2002;269:2810–2819.
17. Bonnal S, Schaeffer C, Creancier L, et al. A single internal ribosome entry site containing a G quartet RNA structure drives fibroblast growth factor 2 gene expression at four alternative translation initiation codons. J Biol Chem 2003;278:39,330–39,336.
18. Pyronnet S, Pradayrol L, Sonenberg N. A cell cycle-dependent internal ribosome entry site. Mol Cell 2000;5:607–616.
19. Bernstein J, Sella O, Le SY, Elroy-Stein O. PDGF2/c-sis mRNA leader contains a differentiation-linked internal ribosomal entry site (D-IRES). J Biol Chem 1997;272:9356–9362.
20. Cornelis S, Bruynooghe Y, Denecker G, Van Huffel S, Tinton S, Beyaert R. Identification and characterization of a novel cell cycle-regulated internal ribosome entry site. Mol Cell 2000;5:597–605.
21. Bonnal S, Pileur F, Orsini C, et al. Heterogeneous nuclear ribonucleoprotein A1 is a novel internal ribosome entry site trans-acting factor that modulates alternative initiation of translation of the fibroblast growth factor 2 mRNA. J Biol Chem 2005;280:4144–4153.
22. Mader S, Lee H, Pause A, Sonenberg N. The translation initiation factor eIF-4E binds to a common motif shared by the translation factor eIF-4 gamma and the translational repressors 4E-binding proteins. Mol Cell Biol 1995;15:4990–4997.
23. Thornton S, Anand N, Purcell D, Lee J. Not just for housekeeping: protein initiation and elongation factors in cell growth and tumorigenesis. J Mol Med 2003;81:536–548.
24. Bhandari BK, Feliers D, Duraisamy S, et al. Insulin regulation of protein translation repressor 4E-BP1, an eIF4E-binding protein, in renal epithelial cells. Kidney Int 2001;59:866–875.
25. Feliers D, Duraisamy S, Barnes JL, Ghosh-Choudhury G, Kasinath BS. Translational regulation of vascular endothelial growth factor expression in renal epithelial cells by angiotensin II. Am J Physiol Renal Physiol 2005;288:F521–F529.
26. Senthil D, Ghosh-Choudhury G, Abboud HE, Sonenberg N, Kasinath BS. Regulation of protein synthesis by IGF-I in proximal tubular epithelial cells. Am J Physiol Renal Physiol 2002;283: F1226–F1236.
27. Senthil D, Ghosh-Choudhury G, McLaurin C, Kasinath BS. Vascular endothelial growth factor induces protein synthesis in renal epithelial cells: a potential role in diabetic nephropathy. Kidney Int 2003;64:468–479.
28. Senthil D, Faulkner JL, Ghosh-Choudhury G, Abboud HE, Kasinath BS. Angiotensin II inhibits insulin-stimulated phosphorylation of eukaryotic initiation factor 4E-binding protein-1 in proximal tubular epithelial cells. Biochem J 2001;360:87–95.

29. Senthil D, Ghosh-Choudhury G, Bhandari BK, Kasinath BS. The type 2 vascular endothelial growth factor receptor recruits insulin receptor substrate-1 in its signalling pathway. Biochem J 2002;368: 49–56.
30. Gingras AC, Kennedy SG, O'Leary MA, Sonenberg N, Hay N. 4E-BP1, a repressor of mRNA translation, is phosphorylated and inactivated by the Akt(PKB) signaling pathway. Genes Dev 1998;12: 502–513.
31. Alessi DR, James SR, Downes CP, et al. Characterization of a 3-phosphoinositide-dependent protein kinase which phosphorylates and activates protein kinase Balpha. Curr Biol 1997;7:261–269.
32. Stephens L, Anderson K, Stokoe D, et al. Protein kinase B kinases that mediate phosphatidylinositol 3,4,5-trisphosphate-dependent activation of protein kinase B. Science 1998;279:710–714.
33. Delcommenne M, Tan C, Gray V, Rue L, Woodgett J, Dedhar S. Phosphoinositide-3-OH kinase-dependent regulation of glycogen synthase kinase 3 and protein kinase B/AKT by the integrin-linked kinase. Proc Natl Acad Sci USA 1998;95:11,211–11,216.
34. Viniegra JG, Martinez N, Modirassari P, et al. Full activation of PKB/Akt in response to insulin or ionizing radiation is mediated through ATM. J Biol Chem 2005;280:4029–4036.
35. Sarbassov DD, Guertin DA, Ali SM, Sabatini DM. Phosphorylation and regulation of Akt/PKB by the rictor-mTOR complex. Science 2005;307:1098–1101.
36. Cheadle JP, Reeve MP, Sampson JR, Kwiatkowski DJ. Molecular genetic advances in tuberous sclerosis. Hum Genet 2000;107:97–114.
37. Gao X, Pan D. TSC1 and TSC2 tumor suppressors antagonize insulin signaling in cell growth. Genes Dev 2001;15:1383–1392.
38. Potter CJ, Huang H, Xu T. Drosophila Tsc1 functions with Tsc2 to antagonize insulin signaling in regulating cell growth, cell proliferation, and organ size. Cell 2001;105:357–368.
39. Goncharova EA, Goncharov DA, Eszterhas A, et al. Tuberin regulates p70 S6 kinase activation and ribosomal protein S6 phosphorylation. A role for the TSC2 tumor suppressor gene in pulmonary lymphangioleiomyomatosis (LAM). J Biol Chem 2002;277:30,958–30,967.
40. Inoki K, Li Y, Zhu T, Wu J, Guan KL. TSC2 is phosphorylated and inhibited by Akt and suppresses mTOR signalling. Nat Cell Biol 2002;4:648–657.
41. Manning BD, Tee AR, Logsdon MN, Blenis J, Cantley LC. Identification of the tuberous sclerosis complex-2 tumor suppressor gene product tuberin as a target of the phosphoinositide 3-kinase/akt pathway. Mol Cell 2002;10:151–162.
42. Tee AR, Anjum R, Blenis J. Inactivation of the tuberous sclerosis complex-1 and -2 gene products occurs by phosphoinositide 3-kinase/Akt-dependent and -independent phosphorylation of tuberin. J Biol Chem 2003;278:37,288–37,296.
43. Castro AF, Rebhun JF, Clark GJ, Quilliam LA. Rheb binds tuberous sclerosis complex 2 (TSC2) and promotes S6 kinase activation in a rapamycin- and farnesylation-dependent manner. J Biol Chem 2003;278:32,493–32,496.
44. Inoki K, Li Y, Xu T, Guan KL. Rheb GTPase is a direct target of TSC2 GAP activity and regulates mTOR signaling. Genes Dev 2003;17:1829–1834.
45. Garami A, Zwartkruis FJ, Nobukuni T, et al. Insulin activation of Rheb, a mediator of mTOR/S6K/ 4E-BP signaling, is inhibited by TSC1 and 2. Mol Cell 2003;11:1457–1466.
46. Tee AR, Manning BD, Roux PP, Cantley LC, Blenis J. Tuberous sclerosis complex gene products, Tuberin and Hamartin, control mTOR signaling by acting as a GTPase-activating protein complex toward Rheb. Curr Biol 2003;13:1259–1268.
47. Zhang Y, Gao X, Saucedo LJ, Ru B, Edgar BA, Pan D. Rheb is a direct target of the tuberous sclerosis tumour suppressor proteins. Nat Cell Biol 2003;5:578–581.
48. Hay N, Sonenberg N. Upstream and downstream of mTOR. Genes Dev 2004;18:1926–1945.
49. Nave BT, Ouwens M, Withers DJ, Alessi DR, Shepherd PR. Mammalian target of rapamycin is a direct target for protein kinase B: identification of a convergence point for opposing effects of insulin and amino-acid deficiency on protein translation. Biochem J 1999;344(Part 2):427–431.
50. Peterson RT, Beal PA, Comb MJ, Schreiber SL. FKBP12-rapamycin-associated protein (FRAP) autophosphorylates at serine 2481 under translationally repressive conditions. J Biol Chem 2000;275:7416–7423.
50a. Mariappan MM, Ghosh Choudhury G, Kasinath BS. Rapid stimulation of laminin beta1 synthesis by high glucose, high insulin and their combination is regulated by mRNA translation in proximal tubular epithelial cells. J Am Soc Nephrol 2005;16:401A.
51. Kim DH, Sarbassov DD, Ali SM, et al. mTOR interacts with raptor to form a nutrient-sensitive complex that signals to the cell growth machinery. Cell 2002;110:163–175.

52. Kim DH, Sarbassov DD, Ali SM, et al. GbetaL, a positive regulator of the rapamycin-sensitive pathway required for the nutrient-sensitive interaction between raptor and mTOR. Mol Cell 2003;11:895–904.
53. Hara K, Maruki Y, Long X, et al. Raptor, a binding partner of target of rapamycin (TOR), mediates TOR action. Cell 2002;110:177–189.
54. Nojima H, Tokunaga C, Eguchi S, et al. The mammalian target of rapamycin (mTOR) partner, raptor, binds the mTOR substrates p70 S6 kinase and 4E-BP1 through their TOR signaling (TOS) motif. J Biol Chem 2003;278:15,461–15,464.
55. Sarbassov DD, Ali SM, Kim DH, et al. Rictor, a novel binding partner of mTOR, defines a rapamycin-insensitive and raptor-independent pathway that regulates the cytoskeleton. Curr Biol 2004;14: 1296–1302.
56. Brunn GJ, Hudson CC, Sekulic A, et al. Phosphorylation of the translational repressor PHAS-I by the mammalian target of rapamycin. Science 1997;277:99–101.
57. Burnett PE, Barrow RK, Cohen NA, Snyder SH, Sabatini DM. RAFT1 phosphorylation of the translational regulators p70 S6 kinase and 4E-BP1. Proc Natl Acad Sci USA 1998;95:1432–1437.
58. Gingras AC, Gygi SP, Raught B, et al. Regulation of 4E-BP1 phosphorylation: a novel two-step mechanism. Genes Dev 1999;13:1422–1437.
59. Gross JD, Moerke NJ, von der Haar T, et al. Ribosome loading onto the mRNA cap is driven by conformational coupling between eIF4G and eIF4E. Cell 2003;115:739–750.
60. Heesom KJ, Gampel A, Mellor H, Denton RM. Cell cycle-dependent phosphorylation of the translational repressor eIF-4E binding protein-1 (4E-BP1). Curr Biol 2001;11:1374–1379.
61. Yang DQ, Kastan MB. Participation of ATM in insulin signalling through phosphorylation of eIF-4E-binding protein 1. Nat Cell Biol 2000;2:893–398.
62. Flynn A, Proud CG. Serine 209, not serine 53, is the major site of phosphorylation in initiation factor eIF-4E in serum-treated Chinese hamster ovary cells. J Biol Chem 1995;270:21,684–21,688.
63. Pyronnet S, Imataka H, Gingras AC, Fukunaga R, Hunter T, Sonenberg N. Human eukaryotic translation initiation factor 4G (eIF4G) recruits mnk1 to phosphorylate eIF4E. EMBO J 1999;18:270–279.
64. Waskiewicz AJ, Flynn A, Proud CG, Cooper JA. Mitogen-activated protein kinases activate the serine/threonine kinases Mnk1 and Mnk2. EMBO J 1997;16:1909–1920.
65. Waskiewicz AJ, Johnson JC, Penn B, Mahalingam M, Kimball SR, Cooper JA. Phosphorylation of the cap-binding protein eukaryotic translation initiation factor 4E by protein kinase Mnk1 in vivo. Mol Cell Biol 1999;19:1871–1880.
66. Parra-Palau JL, Scheper GC, Wilson ML, Proud CG. Features in the N and C termini of the MAPK-interacting kinase Mnk1 mediate its nucleocytoplasmic shuttling. J Biol Chem 2003;278:44,197–44,204.
67. Lachance PE, Miron M, Raught B, Sonenberg N, Lasko P. Phosphorylation of eukaryotic translation initiation factor 4E is critical for growth. Mol Cell Biol 2002;22:1656–1663.
68. Minich WB, Balasta ML, Goss DJ, Rhoads RE. Chromatographic resolution of in vivo phosphorylated and nonphosphorylated eukaryotic translation initiation factor eIF-4E: increased cap affinity of the phosphorylated form. Proc Natl Acad Sci USA 1994;91:7668–7672.
69. Scheper GC, Proud CG. Does phosphorylation of the cap-binding protein eIF4E play a role in translation initiation? Eur J Biochem 2002;269:5350–5359.
70. Zuberek J, Wyslouch-Cieszynska A, Niedzwiecka A, et al. Phosphorylation of eIF4E attenuates its interaction with mRNA 5' cap analogs by electrostatic repulsion: intein-mediated protein ligation strategy to obtain phosphorylated protein. Rna 2003;9:52–61.
71. Browne GJ, Proud CG. Regulation of peptide-chain elongation in mammalian cells. Eur J Biochem 2002;269:5360–5368.
72. Frank J. Toward an understanding of the structural basis of translation. Genome Biol 2003;4:237.
73. Hirokawa G, Kiel MC, Muto A, et al. Binding of ribosome recycling factor to ribosomes, comparison with tRNA. J Biol Chem 2002;277:35,847–35,852.
74. Selmer M, Al-Karadaghi S, Hirokawa G, Kaji A, Liljas A. Crystal structure of Thermotoga maritima ribosome recycling factor: a tRNA mimic. Science 1999;286:2349–2352.
75. Hamsten A. The hemostatic system and coronary heart disease. Thromb Res 1993;70:1–38.
76. Nordt TK, Sawa H, Fujii S, Sobel BE. Induction of plasminogen activator inhibitor type-1 (PAI-1) by proinsulin and insulin in vivo. Circulation 1995;91:764–770.
77. Hostetter TH. Progression of renal disease and renal hypertrophy. Annu Rev Physiol 1995;57: 263–278.
78. Preisig PA, Franch HA. Renal epithelial cell hyperplasia and hypertrophy. Semin Nephrol 1995;15:327–340.
79. Dalla Vestra M, Masiero A, Roiter AM, Saller A, Crepaldi G, Fioretto P. Is podocyte injury relevant in diabetic nephropathy? Studies in patients with type 2 diabetes. Diabetes 2003;52:1031–1035.

80. Meyer TW, Bennett PH, Nelson RG. Podocyte number predicts long-term urinary albumin excretion in Pima Indians with Type II diabetes and microalbuminuria. Diabetologia 1999;42:1341–1344.
81. Pagtalunan ME, Miller PL, Jumping-Eagle S, et al. Podocyte loss and progressive glomerular injury in type II diabetes. J Clin Invest 1997;99:342–348.
82. Dorn GW 2nd, Force T. Protein kinase cascades in the regulation of cardiac hypertrophy. J Clin Invest 2005;115:527–537.
83. Shankland SJ, Wolf G. Cell cycle regulatory proteins in renal disease: role in hypertrophy, proliferation, and apoptosis. Am J Physiol Renal Physiol 2000;278:F515–F529.
84. Hardie DG. The AMP-activated protein kinase pathway—new players upstream and downstream. J Cell Sci 2004;117:5479–5487.
85. Viollet B, Andreelli F, Jorgensen SB, et al. Physiological role of AMP-activated protein kinase (AMPK): insights from knockout mouse models. Biochem Soc Trans 2003;31:216–219.
85a. Lee MJ, Feliers D, Mariappan MM, et al. AMP Kinase—a new regulator of renal hypertrophy in diabetes. J Am Soc Nephrol 2005;16:196A.
86. Miner JH, Patton BL, Lentz SI, et al. The laminin alpha chains: expression, developmental transitions, and chromosomal locations of alpha1-5, identification of heterotrimeric laminins 8–11, and cloning of a novel alpha 3 isoform. J Cell Biol 1997;137:685–701.
87. Miner JH, Yurchenco PD. Laminin functions in tissue morphogenesis. Annu Rev Cell Dev Biol 2004;20:255–284.
88. Noakes PG, Miner JH, Gautam M, Cunningham JM, Sanes JR, Merlie JP. The renal glomerulus of mice lacking s-laminin/laminin beta 2: nephrosis despite molecular compensation by laminin beta 1. Nat Genet 1995;10:400–406.
89. Zenker M, Aigner T, Wendler O, et al. Human laminin beta 2 deficiency causes congenital nephrosis with mesangial sclerosis and distinct eye abnormalities. Hum Mol Genet 2004;13:2625–2632.
90. Fukui M, Nakamura T, Ebihara I, Shirato I, Tomino Y, Koide H. ECM gene expression and its modulation by insulin in diabetic rats. Diabetes 1992;41:1520–1527.
91. Vleming LJ, Baelde JJ, Westendorp RG, Daha MR, van Es LA, Bruijn JA. Progression of chronic renal disease in humans is associated with the deposition of basement membrane components and decorin in the interstitial extracellular matrix. Clin Nephrol 1995;44:211–219.
92. Yang CW, Hattori M, Vlassara H, et al. Overexpression of transforming growth factor-beta 1 mRNA is associated with up-regulation of glomerular tenascin and laminin gene expression in nonobese diabetic mice. J Am Soc Nephrol 1995;5:1610–16,107.
93. Ziyadeh FN. Significance of tubulointerstitial changes in diabetic renal disease. Kidney Int Suppl 1996;54:S10–S13.
94. Ha TS, Barnes JL, Stewart JL, et al. Regulation of renal laminin in mice with type II diabetes. J Am Soc Nephrol 1999;10:1931–1939.
95. Coleman DL, Hummel KP. Hyperinsulinemia in pre-weaning diabetes (db) mice. Diabetologia 1974;10(Suppl):607–610.
96. Kozak M. Influences of mRNA secondary structure on initiation by eukaryotic ribosomes. Proc Natl Acad Sci USA 1986;83:2850–2854.
97. Polhill TS, Saad S, Poronnik P, Fulcher GR, Pollock CA. Short-term peaks in glucose promote renal fibrogenesis independently of total glucose exposure. Am J Physiol Renal Physiol 2004;287: F268–F273.
98. Ceriello A. Postprandial hyperglycemia and diabetes complications: is it time to treat? Diabetes 2005;54:1–7.
99. Feliers D, Duraisamy S, Faulkner JL, et al. Activation of renal signaling pathways in db/db mice with type-2 diabetes. Kidney Int 2001;60:495–504.
100. Abrass CK, Peterson CV, Raugi GJ. Phenotypic expression of collagen types in mesangial matrix of diabetic and nondiabetic rats. Diabetes 1988;37:1695–1702.
101. Abrass CK, Spicer D, Raugi GJ. Insulin induces a change in extracellular matrix glycoproteins synthesized by rat mesangial cells in culture. Kidney Int 1994;46:613–620.
102. Morrisey K, Evans RA, Wakefield L, Phillips AO. Translational regulation of renal proximal tubular epithelial cell transforming growth factor-beta1 generation by insulin. Am J Pathol 2001;159:1905–1915.
103. Wang CC, Goalstone ML, Draznin B. Molecular mechanisms of insulin resistance that impact cardiovascular biology. Diabetes 2004;53:2735–2740.
104. Virkamaki A, Ueki K, Kahn CR. Protein-protein interaction in insulin signaling and the molecular mechanisms of insulin resistance. J Clin Invest 1999;103:931–943.
105. Aiello LP, Avery RL, Arrigg PG, et al. Vascular endothelial growth factor in ocular fluid of patients with diabetic retinopathy and other retinal disorders. N Engl J Med 1994;331:1480–1487.

106. Simon M, Grone HJ, Johren O, et al. Expression of vascular endothelial growth factor and its receptors in human renal ontogenesis and in adult kidney. Am J Physiol 1995;268:F240–F250.
107. de Vriese AS, Tilton RG, Elger M, Stephan CC, Kriz W, Lameire NH. Antibodies against vascular endothelial growth factor improve early renal dysfunction in experimental diabetes. J Am Soc Nephrol 2001;12:993–1000.
108. Flyvbjerg A, Dagnaes-Hansen F, De Vriese AS, Schrijvers BF, Tilton RG, Rasch R. Amelioration of long-term renal changes in obese type-2 diabetic mice by a neutralizing vascular endothelial growth factor antibody. Diabetes 2002;51:3090–3099.
109. Rincon-Choles H, Kasinath BS, Gorin Y, Abboud HE. Angiotensin II and growth factors in the pathogenesis of diabetic nephropathy. Kidney Int Suppl 2002;8–11.
110. Rizkalla B, Forbes JM, Cooper ME, Cao Z. Increased renal vascular endothelial growth factor and angiopoietins by angiotensin II infusion is mediated by both AT1 and AT2 receptors. J Am Soc Nephrol 2003;14:3061–3071.
111. Gorin Y, Kim NH, Feliers D, Bhandari B, Ghosh-Choudhury G, Abboud HE. Angiotensin II activates Akt/protein kinase B by an arachidonic acid/redox-dependent pathway and independent of phosphoinositide 3-kinase. FASEB J 2001;15:1909–1920.
112. Gorin Y, Ricono JM, Kim NH, Bhandari B, Ghosh-Choudhury G, Abboud HE. Nox4 mediates angiotensin II-induced activation of Akt/protein kinase B in mesangial cells. Am J Physiol Renal Physiol 2003;285:F219–F229.
112a. Feliers D, Gorin Y, Ghosh Choudhury G, Abboud H, Kasinath BS. Angiotensin II stimulation of VEGF mRNA translation requires production of reactive oxygen species. Am J Physiology Renal, in press.
113. Brownlee M. Biochemistry and molecular cell biology of diabetic complications. Nature 2001;414:813–820.
114. Schrijvers BF, De Vriese AS, Flyvbjerg A. From hyperglycemia to diabetic kidney disease: the role of metabolic, hemodynamic, intracellular factors and growth factors/cytokines. Endocr Rev 2004;25:971–1010.
115. Canalis E. Effect of insulinlike growth factor I on DNA and protein synthesis in cultured rat calvaria. J Clin Invest 1980;66:709–719.
116. Quaife CJ, Mathews LS, Pinkert CA, Hammer RE, Brinster RL, Palmiter RD. Histopathology associated with elevated levels of growth hormone and insulin-like growth factor I in transgenic mice. Endocrinology 1989;124:40–48.
117. Abboud HE. Growth factors and diabetic nephrology: an overview. Kidney Int Suppl 1997;60: S3–S6.
118. Flyvbjerg A. Putative pathophysiological role of growth factors and cytokines in experimental diabetic kidney disease. Diabetologia 2000;43:1205–1223.
119. Flyvbjerg A, Bennett WF, Rasch R, Kopchick JJ, Scarlett JA. Inhibitory effect of a growth hormone receptor antagonist (G120K-PEG) on renal enlargement, glomerular hypertrophy, and urinary albumin excretion in experimental diabetes in mice. Diabetes 1999;48:377–382.
120. Bach L, Jerums AG. Effect of puberty on initial kidney growth and rise in kidney IGF-I in diabetic rats. Diabetes 1990;39:557–562.
121. Flyvbjerg A, Bornfeldt KE, Marshall SM, Arnqvist HJ, Orskov H. Kidney IGF-I mRNA in initial renal hypertrophy in experimental diabetes in rats. Diabetologia 1990;33:334–338.
122. Pillion DJ, Haskell JF, Meezan E. Distinct receptors for insulin-like growth factor I in rat renal glomeruli and tubules. Am J Physiol 1988;255:E504–E512.
123. Mendez R, Kollmorgen G, White MF, Rhoads RE. Requirement of protein kinase C zeta for stimulation of protein synthesis by insulin. Mol Cell Biol 1997;17:5184–5192.
124. Rao GN, Madamanchi NR, Lele M, et al. A potential role for extracellular signal-regulated kinases in prostaglandin F2alpha-induced protein synthesis in smooth muscle cells. J Biol Chem 1999;274:12,925–12,932.
125. Naegele S, Morley SJ. Molecular cross-talk between MEK1/2 and mTOR signaling during recovery of 293 cells from hypertonic stress. J Biol Chem 2004;279:46,023–46,034.
126. von Manteuffel SR, Gingras AC, Ming XF, Sonenberg N, Thomas G. 4E-BP1 phosphorylation is mediated by the FRAP-p70s6k pathway and is independent of mitogen-activated protein kinase. Proc Natl Acad Sci USA 1996;93:4076–4080.
127. Ziyadeh FN. Mediators of diabetic renal disease: the case for tgf-Beta as the major mediator. J Am Soc Nephrol 2004;15 Suppl 1:S55–S57.
128. Fraser D, Brunskill N, Ito T, Phillips A. Long-term exposure of proximal tubular epithelial cells to glucose induces transforming growth factor-beta 1 synthesis via an autocrine PDGF loop. Am J Pathol 2003;163:2565–2574.

7 The Hexosamine Biosynthesis Pathway

Contribution to the Pathogenesis of Diabetic Nephropathy

I. George Fantus, MDCM,
Howard J. Goldberg, MD,
Catharine. I. Whiteside, MD, PhD,
and Delilah Topic, MD

CONTENTS

INTRODUCTION

Prolonged hyperglycemia is the critical etiological factor in the development of the microvascular complications of diabetes including diabetic nephropathy *(1–3)*. The tissues subject to these complications appear to be susceptible by virtue of abundant expression of cell surface facilitative glucose transporters resulting in the transport of glucose down its concentration gradient. The fact that increased glucose uptake and metabolism promotes the pathological changes leading to tissue damage has led to great interest in the pathways of disposition of glucose metabolites and their regulation. There are at least five pathways of glucose metabolism that, either directly or indirectly, appear to contribute to the complications of diabetes. This current concept, reviewed by Brownlee *(4)*, is supported by a number of studies. The increased cellular entry of glucose results first in augmented glycolytic flux and glucose oxidation. A byproduct of

From: *Contemporary Diabetes: The Diabetic Kidney*
Edited by: P. Cortes and C. E. Mogensen © Humana Press Inc., Totowa, NJ

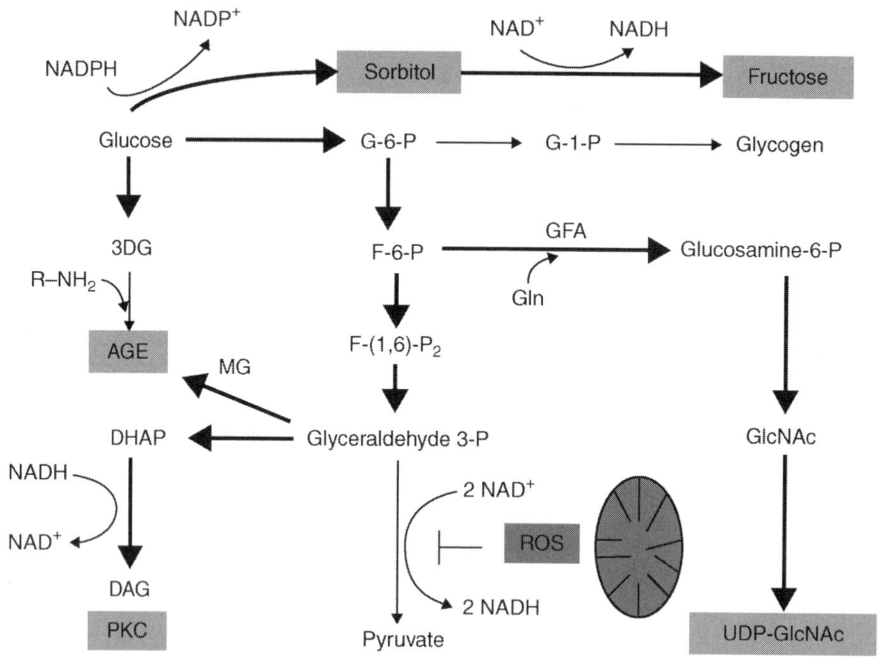

Fig. 1. Glucose metabolic pathways contributing to the microvascular complications of diabetes. Under hyperglycemic conditions, increased cellular glucose uptake and oxidative metabolism results in elevated generation of ROS and subsequent inhibition of GAPDH. Four pathways of glucose metabolism that arise at or upstream of glyceraldehyde-3-P are activated: (1) the aldose reductase/ polyol pathway, (2) formation of AGEs from 3-deoxyglucosone (3DG) and methylglyoxal (MG), (3) synthesis of DAG and activation of PKC, and (4) flux through the HBP to increase UDP-GlcNAc. (Reviewed in ref. *4*.)

mitochondrial substrate metabolism, i.e., electron transport and oxidative phosphorylation, is superoxide, O_2^-. The increased reactive oxygen species (ROS) production by mitochondria produces oxidative stress, a state in which the formation of ROS exceeds the capacity of cellular endogenous antioxidant removal systems. The excess ROS results in inhibition of the redox-sensitive glycolytic enzyme glyceraldehyde-3-phosphate dehydrogenase (GAPDH), possibly via activation of poly-ADP-ribose polymerase *(5)*. Poly-ADP-ribose polymerase activation is thought to be owing to ROS-induced DNA damage. The result of GAPDH inhibition is the increased flux of glucose metabolites through four other metabolic pathways, all of which emanate from glycolytic intermediates upstream of GAPDH. These include the following:

1. the aldose reductase or polyol pathway *(6)*,
2. the formation of advanced glycation endproducts (AGEs) *(7)*,
3. the formation of diacylglycerol (DAG), resulting in protein kinase C (PKC) activation *(8)*,
4. increased flux via the hexosamine biosynthesis pathway (HBP) and generation of the end product uridine diphosphate *N*-acetyl-glucosamine (UDP-GlcNAc), a substrate used for protein glycosylation (Fig. 1).

Other chapters review oxidative stress and the polyol, AGE formation, and PKC activation pathways in detail. In this chapter, the role of the HBP is discussed.

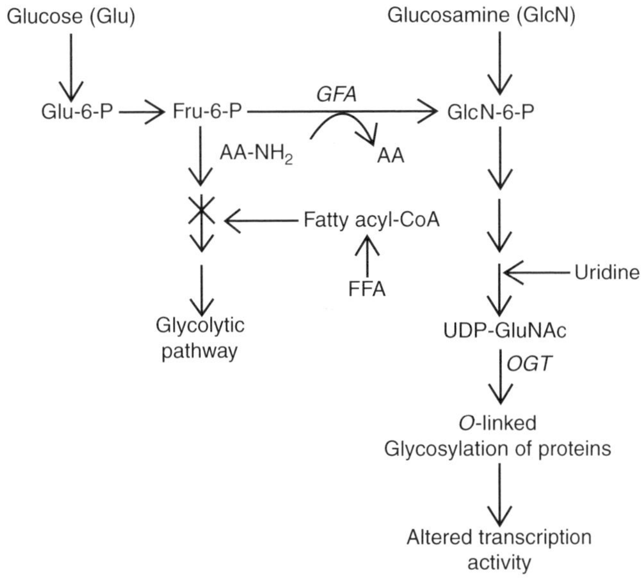

Fig. 2. The HBP. Fructose-6-P and the amino group donor, glutamine, are converted to Glc-6-P by GFA, subsequently *N*-acetylated and linked to UDP to generate UDP-GlcNAc utilized for protein glycosylation. Free fatty acid (FFA) metabolism will increase HBP flux by inhibition of glucose metabolism. Uridine availability will also enhance flux. Most commonly used in experimental systems is Glc, which bypasses the rate-limiting enzyme, GFA, and is a potent stimulator of HBP flux.

THE HEXOSAMINE BIOSYNTHETIC PATHWAY

The HBP is a glucose metabolic pathway, usually accounting for only 2–5% of total glucose metabolism that has been associated with posttranslational protein modification by glycosylation and the synthesis of glycolipids, proteoglycans, and glycosylphosphatidylinositol anchors *(9–11)*. Classical *N*- and *O*-protein glycosylation targets secreted proteins and the extracellular domains of transmembrane proteins and takes place largely in the Golgi apparatus. More recently appreciated is the process of *O*-glycosylation of intracellular proteins on Ser/Thr residues, which is a reversible, dynamic, covalent modification analogous to phosphorylation *(9–11)*. Because this intracellular *O*-glycosylation appears to be driven to a significant extent by the available concentration of UDP-GlcNAc (*see* "Protein *O*-Glycosylation and Gene Expression" section), which in turn is regulated by HBP flux, current research in the area of diabetes complications is focused largely on this phenomenon.

Interest in the relationship among glucose metabolism, diabetes, and the HBP was initiated by the discovery of its potential role in the pathogenesis of insulin resistance *(12,13)*. Although high glucose, free fatty acids, and glucosamine (Glc) can all induce insulin resistance, several studies have suggested that the HBP contributes in each case *(12–15)*. Furthermore, it has recently been proposed that the HBP functions in adipocytes, muscle cells, and pancreatic β-cells, as a "nutrient-sensing" pathway mediating responses to nutrient availability. For example, the adipocyte-derived hormone leptin is synthesized and secreted in response to increased HBP flux *(16)*. Because it is beyond the scope of this chapter to review this aspect of HBP function, the reader is referred to refs. *12–16*.

GLUTAMINE FRUCTOSE 6-PHOSPHATE AMIDOTRANSFERASE: THE RATE-LIMITING ENZYME AND DIABETES COMPLICATIONS

The HBP begins with the conversion of fructose-6-phosphate (F-6-P) and glutamine to Glc-6-P by the rate-limiting enzyme of this pathway glutamine:fructose-6-P amidotransferase (GFA; also abbreviated as GFAT or GFPT) (Fig. 2). A number of subsequent enzymatic steps result in the formation of UDP-GlcNAc. There are two isoforms of GFA encoded by separate genes *(17)*. GFA1 is ubiquitously expressed, whereas GFA2 is highly expressed in the central nervous system (CNS) as well as detected in heart, skeletal muscle, lung, and placenta. The regulation of GFA is not completely understood. Much of its activity appears to be determined by its rate of expression because it has a short half-life of 1 h. The acute effects of cAMP via protein kinase A (PKA) phosphorylation are opposite on GFA1 and GFA2. Thus, phosphorylation of Ser205 of GFA1 results in inhibition *(18)*, whereas that of Ser202 of GFA2 results in activation *(19)*. This differential regulation would allow for tissue-specific responses of HBP pathway flux depending on the relative expression of the two isoforms in each tissue. There is also allosteric feedback inhibition by the endproduct, UDP-GlcNAc *(19,20)*.

The importance of GFA as a rate-limiting step of the HBP and the data supporting its role in insulin resistance and diabetes complications have led to several studies of genetic associations. One report suggests an association of a polymorphism in the 5′ flanking region in humans (–913 G/A) with body mass index, percent body fat, and intramyocellular lipid content (–913 G associated with higher values) *(21)*. In another study, flanking sequence variations of GFA (GFPT1) showed a marginal association with diabetes in Caucasians *(22)*. In the case of diabetic nephropathy, one small study showed an association with 2/7 flanking sequence variations with diabetic nephropathy in African Americans in GFPT1 and a 60% increase in GFA1 mRNA in Caucasians with nephropathy compared with diabetic subjects without nephropathy *(22)*. In one biopsy study, immunohistochemistry revealed GFA upregulation in diabetic subjects with nephropathy *(23)*. In contrast, a larger study of type 1 diabetes mellitus (T1DM) and type 2 diabetes mellitus (T2DM) subjects with and without nephropathy revealed no association with different single-nucleotide polymorphisms (SNPs) in the 60-kb GFPT1 locus *(24)*. Recently, an amino acid substitution in GFA2, I471V, was reported to be associated with T2DM in Caucasians and a trend for an association with nephropathy in African Americans. In the same study, other variants in the 3′ UTR also showed similar associations, namely, T2DM in Caucasian and diabetic nephropathy in African Americans *(25)*. Interestingly, African Americans appeared to have a higher GFA2 mRNA in general than Caucasians. It should be noted that all these genetic association studies are small and the significance of the amino acid substitutions and the flanking region variations remain to be firmly established.

EVIDENCE FOR A ROLE OF THE HBP IN THE PATHOGENESIS OF NEPHROPATHY

Diabetic nephropathy is characterized pathologically by glomerular changes including basement membrane thickening, mesangial expansion consisting of extracellular matrix (ECM) protein accumulation, occasionally the classical Kimmelstiel-Wilson nodules, and, in advanced disease, glomerular sclerosis with obliteration of capillaries *(26–28)*. It has been proposed that the critical event leading to progressive renal failure is the unrelenting accumulation of ECM proteins such as fibronectin, laminin, and collagen.

Thus, mechanisms that increase the synthesis and/or decrease degradation of the ECM have been proposed to play important pathogenic roles. One such key effector is transforming growth factor (TGF)-β, an autocrine/paracrine growth factor that is upregulated by high glucose and stimulates ECM protein gene expression *(29,30)*. One of the first studies implicating the HBP in the pathogenesis of diabetic nephropathy showed that in cultured porcine glomerular mesangial cells, Glc could mimic high glucose to increase expression of fibronectin and TGF-β *(31)*. Glc is taken up by cells via glucose transporters and converted directly to Glc-6-P, thereby bypassing the rate-limiting enzyme GFA (Fig. 2). In this way, the HBP is very strongly activated and therefore, Glc has often been used as a probe of the effects of the HBP. Importantly, in that study the effect of high glucose on TGF-β and fibronectin was inhibited by azaserine, a glutamine analog and inhibitor of GFA, as well as by markedly decreasing GFA protein content using antisense oligonucleotides. Although Glc mimics high glucose, it likely has other effects, so that these additional approaches to modulate HBP flux in the presence of high glucose provided critical supportive data. Taken together, the evidence suggested that enhanced HBP flux increased TGF-β_1 gene expression and consequently ECM protein expression. It is noted that earlier studies had already implicated HBP activation in the stimulation of gene expression, in that case, of TGF-α and basic fibroblast growth factor in vascular smooth muscle cells *(32)*.

Another protein upregulated in diabetic nephropathy, which inhibits ECM protein degradation, is plasminogen activator inhibitor (PAI)-1. PAI-1 mRNA is also induced by high glucose via the HBP, but is independent of TGF-β_1 *(33)*. Similarly, inhibition of GFA by 6-diazo-5-oxo-1-norleucine (DON) blocked the effect of high glucose to increase PAI-1 *(33)*. Apart from using Glc, another method for driving the HBP is to overexpress GFA. This experimental maneuver can increase HBP flux even in the presence of normal glucose. Experiments in cells and transgenic mice overexpressing GFA confirm the increased expression of various proteins, for example, TGF-β1 *(34,35)*, TGF-β type 1 and type 2 receptors *(35)*, PAI-1 *(35)*, and fibronectin *(36)* in mesangial cells, angiotensinogen in renal proximal tubular cells *(37)*, and in adipose tissue, leptin *(38)*.

POTENTIAL MECHANISMS OF ALTERED GENE EXPRESSION BY HBP FLUX

Although flux through the HBP has now been well documented to influence gene expression, a number of questions have been raised about the mechanism. One is whether these effects on gene expression are dependent on the formation of the endproduct, or on some other HBP intermediate.

Oxidative Stress

In this context, it has been noted that Glc-6-P, the immediate product of GFA, can inhibit glucose-6-P-dehydrogenase, the enzyme that promotes glucose metabolism via the pentose phosphate pathway (PPP) *(39)*. One important function of the PPP is the generation of NADPH, necessary for the regeneration of reduced glutathione (GSH), a critical and major cellular antioxidant. Thus, in the presence of elevated Glc-6-P and consequent PPP inhibition caused by exposure to Glc, there occurs an associated oxidative stress. Indeed, oxidative stress has been implicated in the effects of Glc to induce pancreatic β-cell dysfunction *(40)* as well as teratogenesis *(41)*. In β-cells, both high glucose and Glc increased expression of *c*-myc, whereas in the day 7.5 mouse embryo, both glucose and Glc depleted GSH and inhibited expression of Pax-3, resulting in neural tube defects. The protection against these changes by administration of GSH ethyl ester or *N*-acetylcysteine (NAC), to maintain endogenous GSH concentrations, supports the notion that oxidative stress may be, in some cases, a key trigger of Glc action. This is important for several reasons. First, many studies that support the HBP as a mediator of hyperglycemia-induced cellular perturbations have utilized Glc. The conclusion that any of these effects are owing to increased *O*-glycosylation resulting from increased HBP flux may be erroneous. Second, both glucose and Glc may cause oxidative stress. However, they appear to act differently. Thus, Glc will inhibit the PPP, whereas glucose enhances mitochondrial oxidative metabolism and ROS generation (*see* Introduction and Fig. 1). Marshall *(42)* recently demonstrated that, at least in adipocytes, high glucose does not increase Glc-6-P concentrations, whereas exposure to 2 m*M* Glc (commonly used in in vitro experiments) results in a marked elevation. Similarly, Glc results in much higher levels of UDP-GlcNAc (about three- to fourfold) than high glucose.

In order to determine the contribution of the HBP to the pathophysiology of diabetic complications, a number of different approaches will be necessary to dissociate those consequences of increased HBP flux that are not relevant to hyperglycemia.

Protein O*-Glycosylation and Gene Expression*

Because the major function of the HBP appears to be the generation of UDP-GlcNAc used for glycosylation, increasing numbers of studies have focused on this process. Whereas more complex glycosylation of secreted and extracellular domains of proteins appears to be regulated by enzymes localized to the endoplasmic reticulum and Golgi apparatus, the addition of a single *O*-GlcNAc moiety to protein Ser/Thr residues is catalyzed by uridine diphospho-*N*-acetyl-Glc:polypeptide β-*N*-acetylglucosaminyltransferase (OGT) (EC 2.4.1.94). OGT is encoded by a single gene and resides largely in the nucleus. An alternatively spliced variant is localized to the mitochondria *(43,44)*. Although the regulation of OGT is not completely understood, Hart has proposed that the intracellular levels of UDP-GlcNAc are limiting for intracellular protein *O*-glycosylation *(9,11)*. For this reason, glucose concentration and activity of GFA are important determinants of overall levels of protein *O*-glycosylation. OGT targeting via protein–protein interactions likely imposes some substrate specificity under certain conditions *(45)*. There is also one enzyme, *O*-GlcNAcase (*O*-β-*N*-acetylglucosaminidase EC 3.2.1.52 [hexosaminidase C]) which removes the *O*-GlcNAc moiety *(46,47)*. This results in reversible alterations of protein function.

The protein targets of *O*-glycosylation are those primarily involved in transcriptional regulation, for example, RNA polymerase-associated proteins, transcription factors, and coactivators and corepressors *(9–11)*. Several functional consequences of *O*-glycosylation have been documented such as increased DNA-binding *(48)*, altered protein–protein binding *(49,50)*, and decreased protein degradation *(51)*. Depending on the cellular context, activation or repression of gene expression has been documented *(52–55)*.

In the context of diabetic nephropathy, as outlined above, the expression of several genes; TGF-β_1, laminin, fibronectin, and PAI-1 were stimulated by high glucose, Glc, and overexpression of GFA. Furthermore, inhibition of GFA blocked the effect of high glucose but not Glc (Fig. 3). These data support increased *O*-glycosylation secondary to HBP flux as playing a role.

Transcription Factor Regulation by the HBP

In the case of PAI-1, our laboratory has examined the role of the transcription factor Spl. Although the PAI-1 promoter can be stimulated by TGF-β_1 via a Smad-binding

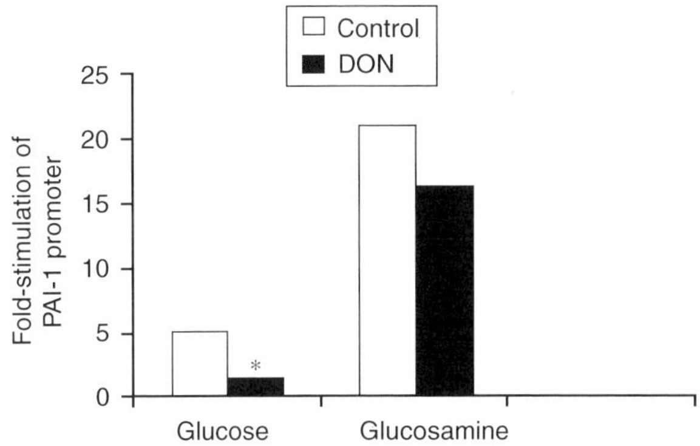

Fig. 3. Inhibition of GFA by DON blocks high glucose but not Glc stimulation of the PAI-1 promoter. Rat mesangial cells were transfected with a PAI-1 promoter (nucleotides from –740 to +44) fused to the luciferase reporter gene and then exposed to 20 m*M*, high glucose (glucose) or 2 m*M* Glc, in the presence and absence of DON to inhibit GFA. Cells were harvested and luciferase activity determined. Values are expressed relative to basal glucose defined as 1.0. (Adapted from ref. *33*.)

site, we found that HBP flux could increase gene expression independent of TGF-β_1 *(33)*. Other PAI-1 promoter sequences had been identified, which bound the transcription factor specificity protein 1 (Sp1), a known target of *O*-glycosylation *(56)*. We were able to demonstrate that a PAI-1 promoter luciferase reporter gene was activated by Glc and mutation of the Spl-binding sites abolished this stimulation (Fig. 4). In keeping with at least one function of *O*-glycosylation, *O*-glycosylated Sp1 showed enhanced DNA binding *(33)*. It was also shown that under hyperglycemic conditions, there is increased glycosylation and reciprocally decreased overall phosphorylation of Sp1 *(34)*. It has been proposed that one mechanism by which protein *O*-glycosylation alters function is by competition with phosphorylation which may occur on the same or adjacent sites *(9)* (Fig. 5). It is important to note, however, that in the case of Spl, with at least nine potential *O*-glycosylation sites, it is possible that specific sites may regulate different or even opposing functions.

Although we noted that the enhanced DNA binding was relatively modest (~30%), there was a marked stimulation of the promoter *(33)*. Thus, the transactivation function of Sp1 was examined by fusing the entire transcription factor (holo Sp1) or only the transactivation domain (TAD) with the yeast GAL4 DNA-binding domain. This chimeric, fused Sp1 GAL4 was cotransfected into mesangial cells with an expression vector encoding a luciferse reporter gene driven by a GAL4-binding promoter (GAL4-Luc). Both Glc and high glucose strongly stimulated luciferase gene expression and the glucose effect was blocked by DON, a GFA enzyme inhibitor *(57)* (Fig. 6). Thus, it appeared that increased flux through the HBP could alter gene expression by modulating transcription factor function in at least two ways, namely, DNA binding and transactivation. The mechanism of altered transactivation could be direct, i.e., mediated by Sp1 *O*-glycosylation, or indirect, for example, glycosylation-independent and mediated by an upstream HBP product such as Glc-6-P, and/or *O*-glycosylation of other targets that regulate Sp1 function such as signaling proteins or transcriptional coactivators/corepressors. To test whether “upstream” HBP metabolites were involved, we took advantage of cells derived from embryos of EMeg32 knockout mice *(58)*. Glc-6-P *N*-acetyltransferase (EMeg32) catalyzes the acetylation of Glc-6-P. The targeted deletion of EMeg32 is embryonic lethal but embryonic fibroblasts could be generated. These cells have

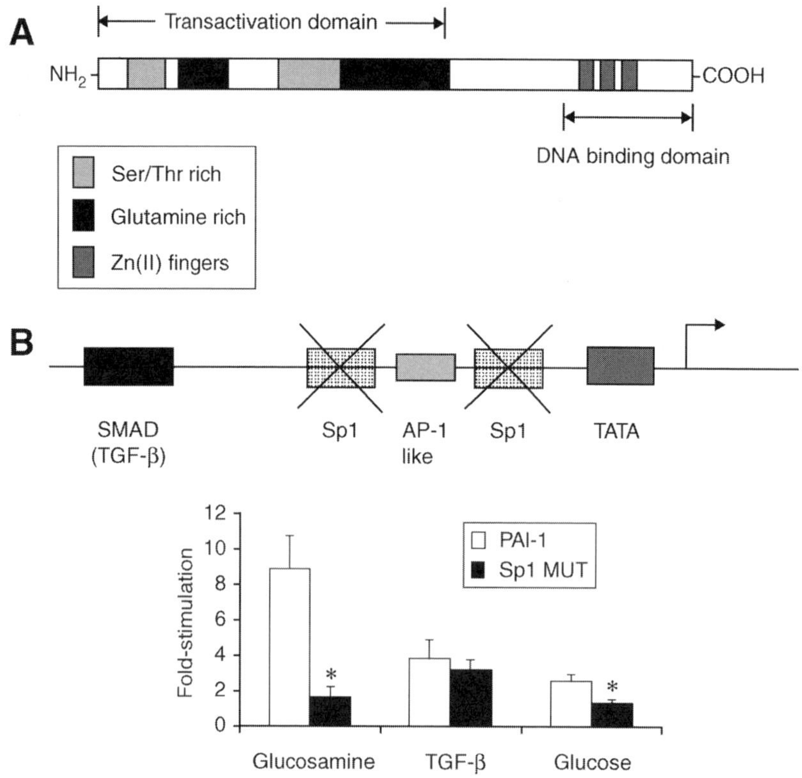

Fig. 4. Activation of the PAI-1 promoter by high glucose and Glc is dependent on Sp1 binding sites. **(A)** Schematic representation of the transcription factor Sp1, which contains nine potential sites of *O*-glycosylation on Ser/Thr residues. Note the Ser/Thr rich regions in the TAD. **(B)** A portion of the PAI-1 promoter (nucleotides from –740 to +44) fused to a luciferase reporter (PAI-1, open bars) or the PAI-1 promoter –Luc with the Sp1 sites mutated (Sp1 mut, filled bars) was transfected into rat mesangial cells which were subsequently exposed to 2 m*M* Glc, 20 ng/mL TGF-β, or 20 m*M* glucose. Cells were harvested and luciferase activity measured. Although Glc and high glucose stimulated the wild-type PAI-1 promoter, mutation of the Sp1 sites abolished this effect. However, TGF-β_1 was able to stimulate both wild type and mutant promoters, presumably via the intact smad, transcription factor, binding site. $*p < 0.05$ vs stimulation of wild-type promoter. (Adapted from ref. *33*.)

extremely low levels of UDP-GlcNAc that do not rise on exposure to elevated glucose. When transfected with the PAI-1 promoter luciferase-expressing cDNA, basal levels of expression were low and did not increase in response to glucose or Glc (Fig. 7). However, addition of serum did lead to an increase demonstrating the specificity of a lack of the HBP end product to high glucose-induced gene expression (not shown).

Altered Cell Signaling

Another effect of increased HBP flux that we considered was altered cell signaling. There were a number of suggestions that Glc could activate PKC enzymes *(59,60)*. It had been well documented that high glucose results in PKC activation, which appears to be a key event in the pathogenesis of the complications of diabetes *(8)*. Furthermore, PKC signaling had been noted to activate Sp1-mediated gene expression

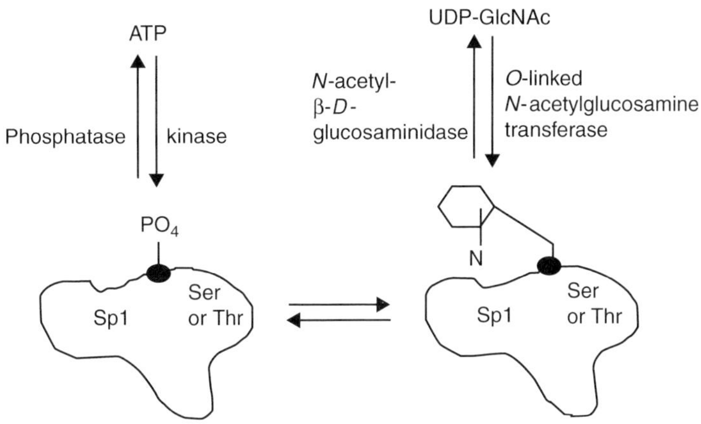

Fig. 5. Reciprocal phosphorylation and *O*-glycosylation. A number of transcription factors, including Sp1, are subject to both phosphorylation and *O*-glycosylation which may occur at the same site and modulate protein function. Such alternating covalent modification may serve as an additional level of control to that exerted by activation and inhibition of kinases, phosphatases, OGT, and *O*-GlcNAcase. (Reviewed in ref. *9*.)

(61). We found that both high glucose and Glc-activated PKC-β and -δ in cultured mesangial cells, and that specifically inhibiting each isoform by transfection of dominant negative (DN) PKCs was able to block PAI-1 promoter-driven luciferase expression. Moreover, the DN PKC-β_1 (but not DN PKC-δ) and a PKC-β specific pharmacological inhibitor, LY379196, were able to block the transactivation function of the Sp1-GAL4 chimeric transcription factor (Fig. 8) *(57)*. These data implicated PKC activation, and specifically PKC-β, as part of the mechanism. Although high glucose is known to activate cPKCs (conventional PKCs) such as PKC-β by stimulating *de novo* DAG synthesis, blocking the HBP flux with DON, surprisingly, also decreased PKC activation (Fig. 8). The precise contribution of the HBP to PKC activation remains unclear; however, *O*-glycosylation of PKCs was not detected (not shown).

Requirement of O*-Glycosylation: OGT*

The evidence thus far strongly suggested, but did not directly prove the requirement of *O*-glycosylation for the stimulation of PAI-1 gene expression and Sp1 activation by high glucose. To demonstrate this we have recently employed genetic and pharmacological approaches to specifically modulate *O*-glycosylation. Thus, transfection of a DN-OGT (lacking the catalytic domain) blocked the high glucose-induced increase in expression of the endogenous PAI-1 mRNA and the PAI-1 promoter-driven luciferase reporter gene. Similar results were obtained with transfection of an OGT siRNA that depleted OGT by 60–80%. Third, overexpression of *O*-GlcNAcase, to rapidly remove the *O*-GlcNAc from proteins, also inhibited the effect of high glucose. This was demonstrated for endogenous PAI-1 mRNA, as well as reporter gene expression driven by either the PAI-1 promoter or the GAL4 promoter (in the presence of the fused Spl-GAL4 transcription factor), indicating that the stimulation of the transactivation function of Spl was *O*-glycosylation-dependent. Finally, inhibition of *O*-GlcNAcase with PUGNAc, in the presence of normal physiological glucose concentrations, increased protein *O*-glycosylation and mimicked high glucose to

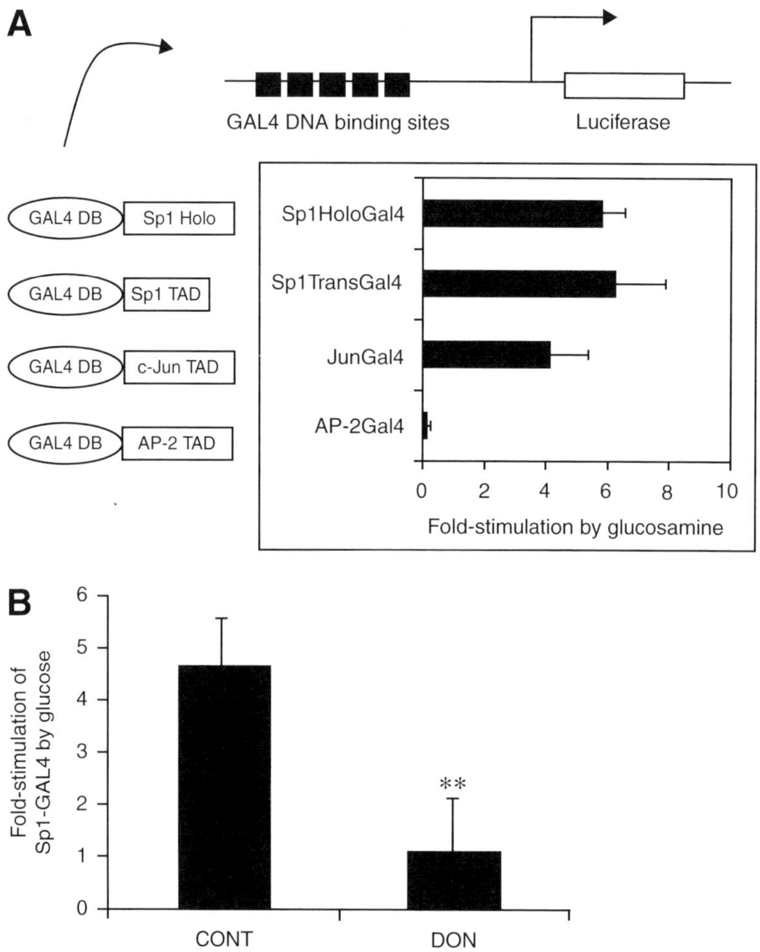

Fig. 6. High glucose and Glc stimulate the transactivation function of Sp1 via the HBP. **(A)** A cDNA coding for the entire transcription factor Sp1 (Sp1 Holo) or its TAD (Sp1 Trans), or the *c*-Jun TAD (Jun), or a portion of the AP-2 TAD was fused to the yeast GAL4 DNA binding domain (GAL4). These cDNAs were cotransfected into mesangial cells with an expression vector for the luciferase reporter gene driven by a promoter containing GAL4 DNA binding sites and exposed to Glc. Glc strongly stimulated the transactivation of Sp1, as well as Jun (likely via the AP-1 like site in the promoter, *see* Fig. 4B), but not AP-2. **(B)** Rat mesangial cells were cotransfected as in **A** with plasmids expressing the Spl GAL4 "chimeric" transcription factor and the GAL4-Luc reporter and exposed to 20 m*M* glucose in the presence and absence of 20 μ*M* DON to inhibit GFA. Inhibition of GFA completely blocked the stimulation of Sp1 transactivation function by high glucose. (Adapted from ref. *57*.)

stimulate PAI-1 mRNA and luciferase expression *(62)*. These results formally prove that the effects of HBP flux on gene expression, at least in the case of PAI-1, and likely for many other genes, is mediated by increased *O*-glycosylation. It should be emphasized that, although correlating with Sp1 glycosylation, the relevant target protein(s) of OGT, which enhance gene expression remain unknown. In the case of Sp1, for example, glycosylation of at least one amino acid, Ser484, has been associated with decreased transcriptional activity *(53)*. In the case of enhanced TGF-β_1 expression by high glucose and the HBP, the transcription factor USF (upstream stimulatory factor) has been implicated, but increased glycosylation of USF was not detected *(63)*. Furthermore, cAMP response element-binding protein (CREBP) phosphorylation

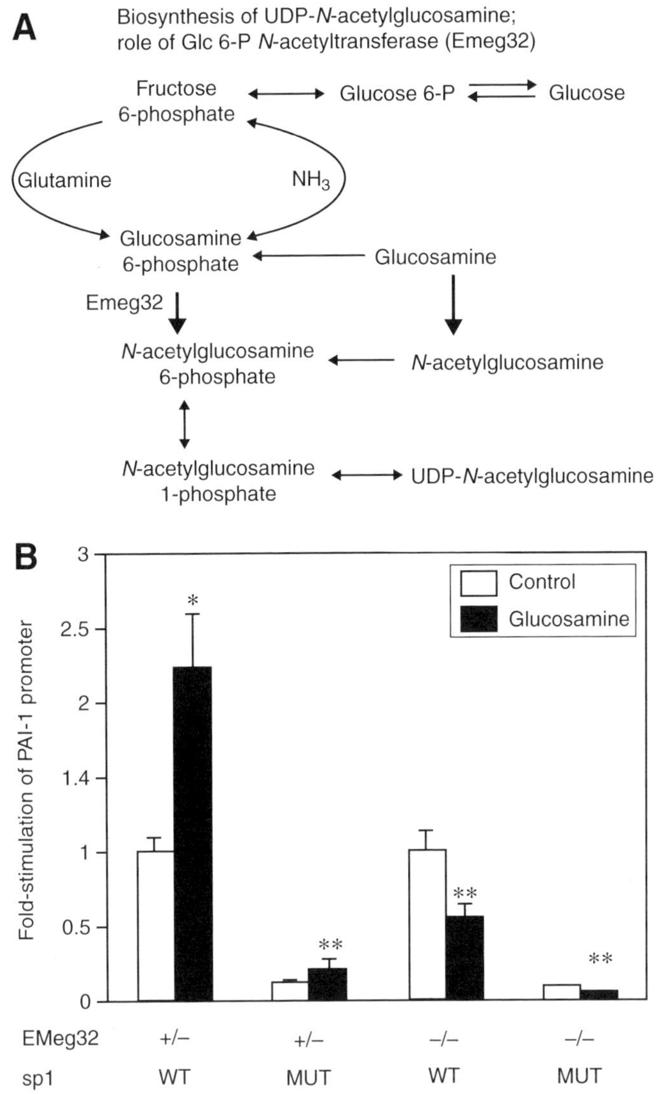

Fig. 7. EMeg32$^{-/-}$ cells with an impaired HBP do not respond to Glc. **(A)** The HBP includes the enzyme, Glc-6-P *N*-acetyltransferase (EMeg 32), which is necessary for the generation of the end product, UDP-GlcNAc. **(B)** EMeg32$^{+/-}$ (heterozygote) and EMeg32$^{-/-}$ (knockout) embryonic fibroblasts were cultured and transfected with the wild-type PAI-1 promoter or the PAI-1 promoter with the Spl sites mutated fused to the luciferase reporter as in Fig. 4. The cells were exposed or not to 2 m*M* Glc. The EMeg32$^{+/-}$ cells containing the wild-type promoter responded to Glc whereas the mutation of the Sp1 sites blocked this effect. In contrast, in the EMeg32$^{-/-}$ cells, there was no stimulation of the wild-type PAI-1 promoter by Glc. UDP-GlcNAc concentrations were very low in the EMeg32$^{-/-}$ cells and not altered by Glc. *$p < 0.05$ compared with control. **$p < 0.01$ compared with Glc in EMeg32$^{+/-}$ with wild-type promoter.

and activation has also been associated with enhanced HBP flux *(64)*. Thus, in addition to transcription factors, proteins which alter cell signaling (e.g., kinases, phosphatases *[65,66]*), or coactivator/corepressor proteins resulting in altered protein–protein interactions with transcription factors, may be equally or more important targets of *O*-glycosylation depending on the cellular context and specific gene being studied.

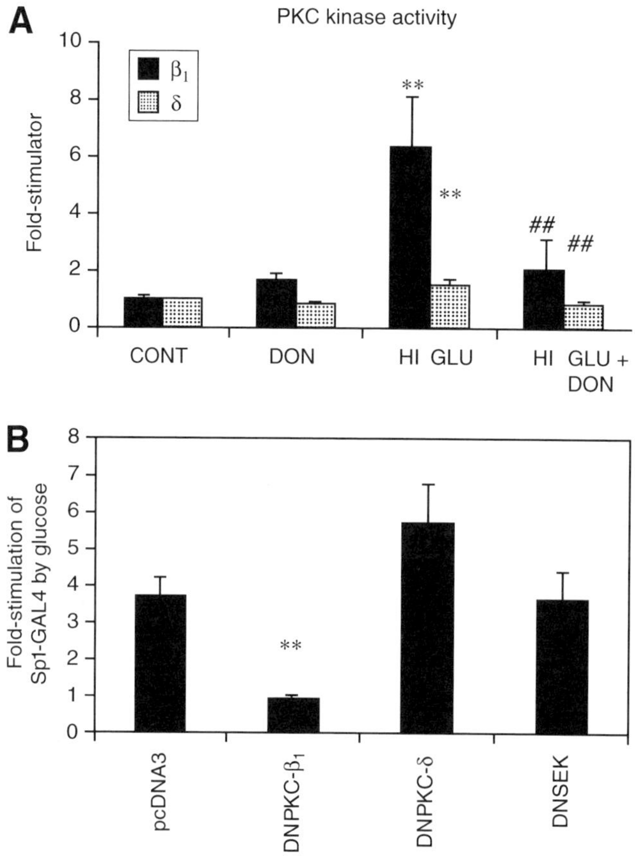

Fig. 8. High glucose activates PKC-β and -δ and PKC-β is required to stimulate Sp1 transactivation. **(A)** Cultured rat mesangial cells were exposed to 20 m*M* glucose (HI GLU) for 4 d and with or without 20 μ*M* DON for the final 2 d. Cells were homogenized and PKCs immunoprecipitated with isoform-specific antibodies and subjected to in vitro kinase assays. High glucose activated PKC-β_1 and PKC-δ, which were both inhibited in the presence of the GFA inhibitor, DON. $^{**}p < 0.01$ vs PKC activity in basal glucose. $^{\#\#}p < 0.01$ vs HI GLU in the absence of DON. **(B)** Mesangial cells were cotransfected with the expression vectors for Sp1-GAL4 and GAL4-Luc as in Fig. 6, along with an empty vector or DN mutants of PKC-β_1, PKC-δ, or stress-activated protein kinase/extracellular signal activated protein kinase kinase. Only DN-PKC-β_1 blocked the transactivation function of Sp1. $^{**}p < 0.01$ vs empty vector pcDNA3. (Adapted from ref. *57.*)

CONCLUSIONS

The HBP begins with conversion of the glycolytic intermediate F-6-P, in combination with glutamine, to Glc-6-P. Subsequent steps yield the endproduct, UDP-GlcNAc, utilized in glycosylation reactions. Flux through the HBP, usually comprising only 2–5% of glucose metabolism, is elevated in diabetes by hyperglycemia. This is due not only to increased cellular glucose uptake but also to an oxidative stress induced block of glycolysis, downstream of F-6-P, at the level of GAPDH. The augmented synthesis of UDP-GlcNAc drives intracellular protein *O*-glycosylation, a posttranslational, dynamic, and reversible modification of Ser/Thr residues analogous to phosphorylation. Many of the targets of *O*-glycosylation, namely, nuclear proteins, for example, transcription factors, cofactors, and signaling molecules, for example, eNOS, regulate

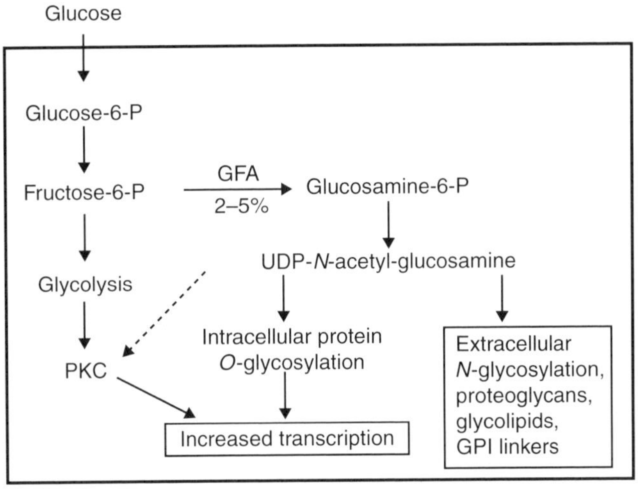

Fig. 9. Proposed mechanism of the contribution of the HBP to the pathogenesis of diabetic nephropathy. Increased flux through the HBP results in elevated UDP-GlcNAc levels that drive intracellular protein *O*-glycosylation. This posttranslational modification of nuclear proteins, for example, transcription factors, cofactors and potentially of signaling molecules, leads to altered gene expression. Increased expression of such prosclerotic proteins as TGF-β_1, fibronectin, laminin, collagen, and PAI-1, which are documented to contribute to diabetic nephropathy are mediated, at least in part, by the HBP. The most relevant protein targets of *O*-glycosylation that play a role in the pathogenesis of nephropathy and altered gene expression remain to be identified.

gene expression. Indeed, expression of prosclerotic proteins, for example, TGF-β_1, fibronectin, laminin, collagen, and PAI-1, has been found to be stimulated in the kidney via enhanced HBP flux. These proteins are critical components of the development and progression of diabetic nephropathy, involved in basement membrane thickening, extracellular mesangial matrix accumulation, and glomerulosclerosis. Thus the HBP, along with other glucose metabolic pathways, appears to be a significant contributor to the altered tissue structure and function observed in diabetes caused by hyperglycemia. A goal of future research is to test whether inhibition of the increased *O*-glycosylation in vivo is a feasible and effective approach to prevent and treat diabetic nephropathy.

In conclusion, the HBP is implicated as a major contributor to the microvascular complications of diabetes, along with the polyol pathway, PKC activation, and AGE formation. It has been associated not only with diabetic nephropathy, but also more recently with diabetic embryopathy *(41)*, cardiomyopathy *(67)*, and cataract formation *(68)*. This pathway has been shown to be a contributor to insulin resistance, particularly in the context of high glucose, and to β-cell dysfunction. Taken together, the data support augmented intracellular *O*-glycosylation as one of the major mediators of "glucose toxicity." In this chapter and in the context of diabetic nephropathy, we have focused on altered gene expression as the major consequence of increased HBP flux (Fig. 9). However, proteins other than transcriptional regulators are known to be modified by *O*-glycosylation, which results in functional consequences. Important examples are the Rpt2 ATPase subunit of the 26S proteasome, which results in inhibition of protein degradation *(51)*, and endothelial nitric oxide synthase (eNOS) which is *O*-glycosylated on Ser1146, the amino acid target of phosphorylation by Akt/PKB *(66)*. This results in resistance of eNOS activation by insulin and other Akt/PKB activators in endothelial cells. Such dysregulation may contribute to atherosclerosis, a process that begins with endothelial dysfunction.

We are just beginning to discover the multiple targets and functional consequences of reversible, intracellular protein *O*-glycosylation *(11)*. The HBP and this posttranslational modification appear to play a critical role in the physiology and pathophysiology of diseases associated with abnormal glucose metabolism. Further in vivo work is required to explore these relationships and determine if, and under what circumstances, inhibition of the HBP and/or protein *O*-glycosylation may be a feasible and effective therapeutic strategy to limit the vascular complications of diabetes.

ACKNOWLEDGMENTS

This work was supported by grants from the Canadian Institutes for Health Research and the Juvenile Diabetes Research Foundation International. The authors would like to thank Dr. G. Boehmelt and J. Dennis for the EMeg32$^{-/-}$ cells and G. Hart for helpful discussion. D. Topic was supported by summer studentships from the Banting and Best Diabetes Centre, University of Toronto, and the Samuel Lunenfeld Research Institute, Mount Sinai Hospital.

REFERENCES

1. Nathan DM. Long-term complications of diabetes mellitus. N Engl J Med 1993;328:1676–1685.
2. The Diabetes Control and Complications Trial Research Group. The effect of intensive treatment of diabetes on the development and progression of long-term complications in insulin-dependent diabetes mellitus. N Engl J Med 1993;329:977–986.
3. UK Prospective Diabetes Study (UKPDS) Group. Intensive blood-glucose control with sulphonylureas or insulin compared with conventional treatment and risk of complications in patients with type 2 diabetes (UKPDS 33). Lancet 1998;352:837–853.
4. Brownlee M. Biochemistry and molecular cell biology of diabetic complications. Nature 2001;415: 813–820.
5. Du X, Matsumura T, Edelstein D, et al. Inhibition of GAPDH activity by poly (ADP-ribose) polymerase activates three major pathways of hyperglycemic damage in endothelial cells. J Clin Invest 2003;112:1049–1057.
6. Greene D, Latimer SA, Sima AAF. Sorbitol, phosphoinositides, and sodium potassium-ATPase in the pathogenesis of diabetic complications. N Engl J Med 1987;316:599–606.
7. Brownlee M. Advanced protein glycosylation in diabetes and aging. Annu Rev Med 1995;46: 223–234.
8. Koya D, King GL. Protein kinase C activation and the development of diabetic complications. Diabetes 1998;47:859–866.
9. Wells L, Vosseller K, Hart GW. Glycosylation of nucleocytoplasmic proteins: Signal transduction and *O*-GlcNAc. Science 2001;291:2376–2378.
10. Vosseller K, Sakabe K, Wells L, Hart CW. Diverse regulation of protein function by *O*-GlcNAc a nuclear and cytoplasmic carbohydrate post-translational modification. Curr Opin Chem Biol 2002;6: 851–857.
11. Zachara NE, Hart GW. *O*-GlcNAc a sensor of cellular state: the role of nucleocytoplasmic glycosylation in modulating cellular function in response to mutation and stress. Biochem Biophys Acta 2004; 1673:13–28.
12. Marshall S, Garvey WT, Traxinger RR. New insights into the metabolic regulation of insulin action and insulin resistance: role of glucose and amino acids. FASEB J 1991;5:3032–3036.
13. Rossetti L, Hawkins M, Chen W, Gividi J, Barzilai N. In vivo glucosamine infusion induces insulin resistance in normoglycemic but not in hyperglycemic conscious rats. J Clin Invest 1995;96:132–140.
14. Hawkins M, Barzilai N, Liu R, Hu M, Chen W, Rossetti L. Role of the glucosamine pathway in fat-induced insulin resistance. J Clin Invest 1997;99:2173–2181.
15. McClain DA, Crook ED. Hexosamines and insulin resistance. Diabetes 1996;45:1003–1009.

16. Wang J, Liu R, Hawkins M, Barzilai N, Rossetti L. A nutrient-sensing pathway regulates leptin gene expression in muscle and fat. Nature 1998;393:684–688.
17. Oki T, Yamazaki K, Kuromitsu J, Okada M, Tanaka I. cDNA cloning and mapping of a novel subtype of glutamine:fructose-6-phosphate amidotransferase (GFAT2) in human and mouse. Genomics 1999;57:227–234.
18. Chang Q, Su K, Baker JR, Yang X, Paterson AJ, Kudlow JE. Phosphorylation of human glutamine: fructose-6-phosphate amidotransferase by cAMP-dependent protein kinase at serine 205 blocks the enzyme activity. J Biol Chem 2000;275:21,981–21,987.
19. Hu Y, Riesland L, Paterson AJ, Kudlow JE. Phosphorylation of mouse glutamine-fructose-6-phosphate amidotransferase 2 (GFAT2) by cAMP-dependent protein kinase increases the enzyme activity. J Biol Chem 2004;279:29,988–29,993.
20. Broschat KO, Gorka C, Page JD, et al. Kinetic characterization of human glutamine-fructose-6-phosphate amidotransferase I: potent feedback inhibition by glucosamine 6-phosphate. J Biol Chem 2002;277: 14,764–14,770.
21. Weigert C, Thamer C, Brodbeck K, et al. The -913 G/A glutamine:fructose-6-phosphate aminotransferase gene polymorphism is associated with measures of obesity and intramyocellular lipid content in nondiabetic subjects. J Clin Endocrinol Metab 2005;90:1639–1643.
22. Elbein SC, Zheng H, Jia Y, Chu W, Cooper JJ, Hale T, Zhang Z. Molecular screening of the human glutamine-fructose-6-phosphate amidotransferase 1 (GFPT1) gene and association studies with diabetes and diabetic nephropathy. Mol Genet Metab 2004;82:321–328.
23. Nerlich AG, Sauer U, Kolm-Litty V, Wagner E, Koch M, Schleicher ED. Expression of glutamine: fructose-6-phosphate amidotransferase in human tissues. Diabetes 1998;47:170–178.
24. Ng DP, Walker WH, Chia KS, Choo S, Warram JH, Krolewski AS. Scrutiny of the glutamine-fructose-6-phosphate transaminase 1 (GFPT1) locus reveals conserved haplotype block structure not associated with diabetic nephropathy. Diabetes 2004;53:865–869.
25. Zhang H, Jia Y, Cooper JJ, Hale T, Zhang Z, Elbein SC. Common variants in glutamine:fructose-6-phosphate amidotransferase 2 (GFPT2) gene are associated with Type 2 diabetes, diabetic nephropathy, and increased GFPT2 mRNA levels. J Clin Endocrinol Metab 2004;89:748–755.
26. Steffes MW, Bilous RW, Sutherland DER, Mauer SM. Cell and matrix components of the glomerular mesangium in type 1 diabetes. Diabetes 1992;41:679–684.
27. Kreisberg JI, Ayo S. The glomerular mesangium in diabetes mellitus. Kidney Int 1993;43:109–113.
28. Sharma K, Ziyadeh F. Biochemical events and cytokine interactions linking glucose metabolism to the development of diabetic nephropathy. Semin Nephrol 1997;17:80–92.
29. Yamamoto T, Noble NA, Cohen AH, et al. Expression of transforming growth factor-β isoforms in human glomerular diseases. Kidney Int 1996;49:461–469.
30. Ziyadeh FN, Sharma K, Eriksen M, Wolf G. Stimulation of collagen gene expression and protein synthesis in murine mesangial cells by high glucose is mediated by autocrine activation of transforming growth factor-β. J Clin Invest 1994;93:536–542.
31. Kolm-Litty V, Sauer U, Nerlich A, Lehmann F, Schleicher ED. High glucose-induced transforming growth factor β1 production is mediated by the hexosamine pathway in porcine glomerular mesangial cells. J Clin Invest 1998;101:160–169.
32. McClain DA, Paterson AJ, Roos MD, Wei X, Kudlow JE. Glucose and glucosamine regulate growth factor gene expression in vascular smooth muscle cells. Proc Natl Acad Sci USA 1992;89: 8150–8154.
33. Goldberg HJ, Scholey J, Fantus IG. Glucosamine activates the plasminogen activator inhibitor 1 gene promoter through Spl DNA binding sites in glomerular mesangial cells. Diabetes 2000;49: 863–871.
34. Schleicher ED, Weigert C. Role of the hexosamine biosynthetic pathway in diabetic nephropathy. Kidney Int 2000;58(77):S13–S18.
35. James LR, Fantus IG, Goldberg H, Ly H, Scholey JW. Overexpression of GFAT activates PAI-1 promoter in mesangial cells. Am J Physiol Renal Physiol 2000;279:F718–F727.
36. Singh LP, Alexander M, Greene K, Crook ED. Overexpression of the complementary DNA for human glutamine:fructose-6-phosphate amidotransferase in mesangial cells enhances glucose-induced fibronectin synthesis and transcription factor cyclic adenosine monophosphate-responsive element binding phosphorylation. J Invest Med 2003;51:32–41.
37. Hsieh T-J, Fustier P, Zhang S-L, et al. High glucose stimulates angiotensinogen gene expression and cell hypertrophy via activation of the hexosamine biosynthesis pathway in rat kidney proximal tubular cells. Endocrinology 2003;144:4338–4349.

38. Hazel M, Cooksey RC, Jones D, et al. Activation of the hexosamine signaling pathway in adipose tissue results in decreased serum adiponectin and skeletal muscle insulin resistance. Endocrinology 2004;145:2118–2128.
39. Wu G, Haynes TE, Li H, Yan W, Meininger CJ. Glutamine metabolism to glucosamine is necessary for glutamine inhibition of endothelial nitric oxide synthesis. Biochem J 2001;353:245–252.
40. Kaneto H, Xu G, Song K-H, et al. Activation of the hexosamine pathway leads to deterioration of pancreatic β-cell function through the induction of oxidative stress. J Biol Chem 2001;276:31,099–31,104.
41. Horal M, Zhang Z, Stanton R, Virkamaki A, Loeken MR. Activation of the hexosamine pathway causes oxidative stress and abnormal embryo gene expression: Involvement in diabetic teratogenesis. Birth Defects Res (Part A) Clin Mol Teratol 2004;70:519–527.
42. Marshall S, Nadeau O, Yamasaki K. Dynamic actions of glucose and glucosamine on hexosamine biosynthesis in isolated adipocytes: Differential effects on glucosamine 6-phosphate, UDP-*N*-acetylglucosamine and ATP levels. J Biol Chem 2004;279:35,313–35,319.
43. Kreppel LK, Blomberg MA, Hart GW. Dynamic glycosylation of nuclear and cytosolic proteins. J Biol Chem 1997;272:9308–9315.
44. Love DC, Kochran J, Cathey RL, Shin S-H, Hanover JA. Mitochondrial and nucleocytoplasmic targeting of *O*-linked GlcNAc transferase. J Cell Sci 2002;116:647–654.
45. Iyer SPN, Hart GW. Roles of the tetratricopeptide repeat domain in *O*-GlcNAc transferase targeting and protein substrate specificity. J Biol Chem 2003;278:24,608–24,616.
46. Gao Y, Wells L, Comer FI, Parker GJ, Hart GW. Dynamic *O*-glycosylation of nuclear and cytosolic proteins: cloning and characterization of a neutral, cytosolic β-*N*-acetylglucosaminidase from human brain. J Biol Chem 2001;276:9838–9845.
47. Hanover JA. Glycan-dependent signaling: *O*-linked *N*-acetylglucosamine. FASEB J 2001;15:1865–1876.
48. Gao Y, Miyazaki J, Hart GW. The transcription factor PDX-1 is post-translationally modified by *O*-linked *N*-acetylglucosamine and this modification is correlated with its DNA binding activity and insulin secretion in Min 6 beta cells. Arch Biochem Biophys 2003;415:155–163.
49. Roos MD, Su K, Baker JR, Kudlow JE. *O*-glycosylation of an Spl-derived peptide blocks known Spl protein interactions. Mol Cell Biol 1997;17:6472–6480.
50. Gewinner C, Hart GW, Zachara N, Cole R, Beisanherz-Huss C, Groner B. The coactivator of transcription CREB binding protein interacts preferentially with the glycosylated form of Stat5. J Biol Chem 2003;279:3563–3572.
51. Zhang F, Su K, Yang X, Bowe OB, Paterson AJ, Kudlow JE. *O*-GlcNAc modification is an endogenous inhibitor of the proteasome. Cell 2003;115:715–725.
52. Du XL, Edelstein D, Rossetti L, et al. Hyperglycemia-induced mitochondrial superoxide overproduction activates the hexosamine pathway and induces plasminogen activator inhibitor-1 expression by increasing Spl glycosylation. Proc Natl Acad Sci USA 2000;97:12,222–12,226.
53. Yang X, Su K, Roos MD, Chang Q, Paterson AJ, Kudlow JE. *O*-linkage of *N*-acetylglucosamine to Sp1 activation domain inhibits its transcriptional capability. Proc Natl Acad Sci USA 2001;98: 6611–6616.
54. Brasse-Lagnel C, Fairand A, Lavoinne A, Husson A. Glutamine stimulates argininosuccinate synthetase gene expression through cytosolic *O*-glycosylation of Sp1 in Caco-2 cells. J Biol Chem 2003;278:52,504–52,510.
55. Yang X, Zhang F, Kudlow JE. Recruitment of *O*-GlcNAc transferase to promoters by corepressor mSin3A: coupling protein *O*-GlcNAcylation to transcriptional repression. Cell 2002;110:69–80.
56. Jackson SP, Tjian R. *O*-glycosylation of eukaryotic transcription factors: implications for mechanisms of transcriptional regulation. Cell 1988;55:125–133.
57. Goldberg HJ, Whiteside CI, Fantus IG. The hexosamine pathway regulates the plasminogen activator inhibitor-1 gene promoter and Spl transcriptional activation through protein kinase C-βI and -δ. J Biol Chem 2002;277:33,833–33,841.
58. Boehmelt G, Wakeham A, Elia A, et al. Decreased UDP-GlcNAc levels abrogate proliferation control in EMeg32-deficient cells. EMBO J 2000;19:5092–5104.
59. Filippis A, Clark S, Proetto J. Increased flux through the hexosamine biosynthesis pathway inhibits glucose transport acutely by activating protein kinase C. Biochem J 1997;324:981–985.
60. Singh LP, Crook ED. Hexosamine regulation of glucose-mediated laminin synthesis in mesangial cells involves protein kinases A and C. Am J Physiol 2000;279:F646–F654.
61. Biggs JR, Kraft AS. The role of the smad3 protein in phorbol ester-induced promoter expression. J Biol Chem 1999;274:36,987–36,994.

62. Goldberg HJ, Whiteside CI, Hart GW, Fantus IG. Posttranslational, reversible *O*-glycosylation is stimulated by high glucose and mediates plasminogen activator inhibitor-1 (PAI-1) gene expression and Sp1 transcriptional activity in glomerular mesangial cells. Endocrinology 2005 (e-pub ahead of print).
63. Weigert C, Brodbeck K, Sawadogo M, Haring HU, Schleicher ED. Upstream stimulatory factor (USF) proteins induce human TGF-beta1 gene activation via the glucose-response element-1013/-1002 in mesangial cells: up-regulation of USF activity by the hexosamine biosynthetic pathway. J Biol Chem 2004;279:15,908–15,915.
64. Singh LP, Green K, Alexander M, Basely S, Crook ED. Hexosamines and TGF-β1 use similar signaling pathways to mediate matrix protein synthesis in mesangial cells. Am J Physiol Renal Physiol 2004; 286:F409–F416.
65. Wells L, Kreppel LK, Corner FI, Wadzinski BE, Hart GW. *O*-GlcNaAc transferase is in a functional complex with protein phosphatase 1 catalytic subunits. J Biol Chem 2004;279:38,466–38,470.
66. Du XL, Edelstein D, Dimmeler S, Ju Q, Sui C, Brownlee M. Hyperglycemia inhibits endothelial nitric oxide synthase activity by posttranslational modification at the Akt site. J Clin Invest 2001; 108:1341–1348.
67. Clark RJ, McDonough PM, Swanson E, et al. Diabetes and the accompanying hyperglycemia impairs cardiomyocyte calcium cycling through increased nuclear *O*-GlcNAcylation. J Biol Chem 2003; 278:44,230–44,237.
68. Akimoto Y, Kawakami H, Yamamoto K, Munetomo E, Hida T, Hirano H. Elevated expression of *O*-GlcNAc-modified proteins and *O*-GlcNAc transferase in corneas of diabetic Goto-Kakizaki rats. Invest Ophthalmol Vis Sci 2003;44:3802–3809.

I

Basic Pathophysiology and Biochemistry of Diabetic Nephropathy

E. Non-Enzymatic Glycosylation

8 Glycation

Receptor for Advanced Glycation Endproducts and Diabetic Nephropathy

Vivette D'Agati, MD
and Ann Marie Schmidt, MD

CONTENTS

INTRODUCTION

The products of nonenzymatic glycation and oxidation of proteins and lipids are enriched in diabetic tissues. Driven by hyperglycemia and oxidative stress, the production and accumulation of these species result in multiple perturbations in the diabetic kidney. One of these, a "gain-of-function" outcome results from the interaction of advanced glycation endproducts (AGEs) with their signal transduction receptor, RAGE (receptor for AGE). Multiple epidemiological studies support the contention that AGEs are increased in diabetic nephropathy (DN) and may be a biomarker of disease activity. Studies in animal models support the premise that blockade of AGE or RAGE pathways results in significant suppression of diabetes-associated nephropathic changes, including decreases in albuminuria, expansion of the mesangial matrix, and production of prosclerotic cytokines and growth factors. First, studies in human clinical trials targeting the AGE axis provide support for the contribution of AGEs to the pathogenesis of DN. Trials to assess the role of RAGE antagonism are on the horizon.

From: *Contemporary Diabetes: The Diabetic Kidney*
Edited by: P. Cortes and C. E. Mogensen © Humana Press Inc., Totowa, NJ

GLYCATION AND RAGE

AGEs and Diabetic Kidney Disease

A number of key consequences ensue from elevated levels of glucose; one of these, the generation of AGEs, is linked to the development of diabetic complications *(1,2)*. AGEs are a heterogeneous class of compounds formed by a number of mechanisms in the tissues, including nonenzymatic glycation and oxidation of proteins and lipids. Examples of AGEs that have been found in diabetic tissues, including in the diabetic kidney, include pentosidine, carboxymethyl lysine (CML) AGEs, and pyrallines *(3–10)*. In addition to measurement of tissue AGEs in the kidney, many researchers have reported the utility of measurement of serum/plasma AGEs as markers of the presence and/or degree of DN *(11–16)*. Certainly, examination of peripheral blood provides a more readily available source of material for initial determination of AGEs, particularly for serial assessments. It is important to note that confounding factors in at least some of these studies are the following. First, these studies support the premise that as renal function declines, levels of AGEs rise in parallel with reduced clearance of these species. Thus, beyond a certain degree of renal insufficiency, AGE levels may not solely reflect the degree of microvascular complications, but, in addition, the general severity of impending renal failure. Second, it is well established that AGEs are a heterogeneous class of molecules. Thus, although some types of AGEs are increased in renal consequences of diabetes, it is likely that some of these species reflect markers of disease. In other cases, such elevated AGEs may not only be biomarkers of disease, but, also, contributing pathogenetic factors in the development of nephropathy. More study is needed in the AGE field to better establish the precise role(s) of distinct AGE species in microvascular disease in the kidney. Despite these caveats, however, such studies underscore the concept that at least certain classes of AGEs likely play a role in the pathogenesis of nephropathy.

One of the principal AGEs found in vivo are the CML-AGE species *(6,7)*. CML-AGEs are not members of the crosslinking family of AGEs. Evidence indicates that CML adducts interact with the signal transduction receptor, RAGE. The interaction of CML-AGE with RAGE is linked to the pathogenesis of diabetic complications in both the macro- and microvasculature *(17)*.

RAGE is Expressed in Diabetic Kidney

Multiple different types of receptor or binding molecules have been reported for AGEs, such as scavenger receptor type A, CD36, galectin-3, and others *(18–21)*. Our work has focused on RAGE as a receptor for AGEs *(22,23)*. There is no evidence that RAGE serves as a scavenger receptor for AGEs *(22)*. Rather, as RAGE is a member of the immunoglobulin superfamily of cell-surface molecules, extensive evidence suggests that RAGE transduces the effects of AGEs in the tissue by virtue of its ability to activate a range of signal transduction pathways inside the cell *(23)*. The predicted hydropathy plot indicates that RAGE is composed of an extracellular domain, itself containing three immunoglobulin (Ig)-like domains (one V-type Ig domain followed by two C-type domains). This portion of the molecule is followed by a single transmembrane spanning domain and, lastly, a short intracellular cytoplasmic domain that is essential for RAGE-mediated modulation of cellular function *(23)*.

Multiple studies have indicated that RAGE is expressed at low levels in homeostasis but at enhanced degrees in kidney tissues affected by chronic types 1 or 2 diabetes

(24–27). Studies by our group showed for the first time that the principal site of RAGE expression in diabetic kidney is the glomerular visceral epithelial cell, or podocyte *(27)*.

Studies have now indicated clearly that RAGE is not solely a receptor for AGEs. Rather, RAGE also transduces the effects of distinct ligands that accumulate not only in diabetic kidney, but also in euglycemic foci characterized by chronic inflammatory injury, cellular transformation, or degenerative processes. Specifically, RAGE interacts with S100/calgranulins *(28)*. S100/calgranulins are a family of molecules with multiple potential functions. These molecules may have roles inside the cell, in which they have been demonstrated to bind calcium *(29–31)*. Outside the cell, S100/calgranulins are not merely markers of inflammatory disease or malignancy. Rather, the demonstration that RAGE is a signaling receptor for S100/calgranulins supports the premise that interaction of these ligands with RAGE may augment inflammatory mechanisms. In this context, blockade of RAGE has been shown to suppress various inflammatory pathways in euglycemic animals, such as delayed-type hypersensitivity, collagen-induced arthritis, inflammatory colitis, and experimental autoimmune encephalitis *(28,32,33)*. Furthermore, in euglycemic animals predisposed to the development of type 1 diabetes, by virtue of injection of diabetogenic splenocytes, RAGE blockade significantly prolongs the time to development of hyperglycemia vs vehicle-treated mice *(34)*.

In addition to S100/calgranulins, recent work has suggested that the RAGE ligand amphoterin, or high-mobility group box 1 (HMGB1) protein, is also linked to amplification of inflammatory mechanisms *(35–37)*. HMGB1 is a nuclear protein, however, a plethora of evidence suggests that this molecule may exist on the surface of cells, especially at the leading edges, and outside the cell, and may interact with RAGE. The relationship between RAGE, HMGB1, and inflammation is complex, however, as it has been demonstrated that HMGB1 also interacts with toll like receptors 2 and 4 *(38)*.

Additional studies indicate that RAGE interacts with amyloid-β peptide and other β-sheet fibrils *(39–41)*. Such studies suggest roles for RAGE in Alzheimer's disease as well as in amyloidoses. Lastly, it has been recently shown that RAGE is a receptor for Mac-1, thereby further implicating RAGE in inflammatory mechanisms *(42)*. To date, it has been shown that at least two ligand families of RAGE are upregulated in human DN, AGEs and S100/calgranulins *(27)*. The challenge of linking these phenomena with the pathogenesis of nephropathy has been approached by the use of pharmacological blockade of RAGE as well as genetic modification.

RAGE IS LINKED TO THE PATHOGENESIS OF DIABETIC NEPHROPATHY

Pharmacological Blockade of RAGE and Its Impact in Diabetic Nephropathy

Studies demonstrating the enhanced expression of RAGE in the diabetic kidney did not shed light on whether this observation was linked mechanistically to the pathogenesis of nephropathy. To approach this question, pharmacological approaches have been taken to test the role of the RAGE axis in diabetes-associated nephropathy. In the first experiments, we employed the soluble form of the receptor. Soluble RAGE (sRAGE) was produced and purified from a baculovirus expression system and administered to animals once daily based on the pharmacokinetic profile of distribution and elimination *(43)*.

In diabetes, it has been speculated that vascular leakiness, a surrogate marker of endothelial dysfunction, is a harbinger of diabetic vascular complications *(44,45)*.

To test the potential role of RAGE in this setting, we modeled endothelial dysfunction by measurement of "vascular permeability," using the tissue blood isotope ratio (TBIR). Diabetes was induced using streptozotocin (STZ) in rats. By 11 wk after induction of hyperglycemia, diabetic animals displayed increased vascular leakage as measured by TBIR. Increased vascular permeability in diabetic rats was most evident in intestine, skin, and kidney, in which albumin leakage was increased approx 2.8-, 3- and 2.8-fold, respectively, compared with nondiabetic controls. The ligand decoy, sRAGE was administered to the rats by once daily intraperitoneal administration, at two different doses, 2.25 mg/kg or 5.15 mg/kg. sRAGE was administered immediately before sacrifice of the animals. Administration of sRAGE at the lower dose completely blocked vascular leakage in the intestine and skin, and largely prevented vascular leakage in the kidney (approx 60%). In the presence of the higher dose of sRAGE, hyperpermeability was completely suppressed in both intestine and skin, and by approx 90% in the kidney *(43)*. These studies suggested that key features of endothelial function were strikingly impaired in diabetes, and that this dysfunction could be reversed by blockade of RAGE.

To extend these studies to a chronic model in which early changes of nephropathy of diabetes develop, we employed db/db mice, a murine model of insulin resistance and type 2 diabetes. Mice were treated once daily with sRAGE or vehicle, phosphate-buffered saline from age 8 wk. db/db Mice displayed increased expression of RAGE and S100/calgranulins in the kidney, particularly in podocytes and in infiltrating inflammatory cells, respectively *(46)*. Mice, 8 wk of age, were chosen for those studies as, at that time, all of the mice displayed marked insulin resistance and hyperglycemia. After an extended period of treatment, mice were sacrificed *(46)*. Multiple studies revealed significant protection from the adverse impact of diabetes on the kidney in these animals. Specifically, albuminuria was significantly less in sRAGE-treated diabetic mice compared with that observed in vehicle-treated db/db animals. Mesangial expansion and thickening of the glomerular basement membrane were significantly lower in mice treated with sRAGE *(46)*. At the molecular level, transcripts for TGF-β and α-1,4 collagen were decreased in the renal cortices of sRAGE-treated mice *(46)*. Furthermore, antigen levels of vascular endothelial growth factor (VEGF) were also decreased by sRAGE in the diabetic mice, particularly in podocytes *(46)*. Because previous studies linked VEGF expression selectively to podocytes in the diabetic kidney *(47)*, these studies suggested that generation of this factor was, at least in part, under control of RAGE. It may be speculated that VEGF might function to enhance permeability or recruit mononuclear cells to the perturbed glomerulus *(46)*. Other potential functions of VEGF in this setting include roles in fibrosis *(48)*. Consistent with pathogenic roles for VEGF in early nephropathy, administration of antibodies against VEGF improved early renal dysfunction in STZ-treated diabetic rats *(49)*.

Flyvbjerg and colleagues *(50)* addressed the impact of direct antagonism of RAGE in db/db mice by means of long-term administration of a neutralizing antibody against the receptor. Animals were treated for 2 mo with anti-RAGE antibody vs an irrelevant IgG. Compared with mice receiving irrelevant IgG, anti-RAGE IgG-treated mice displayed reduced increases in kidney weight, glomerular volume, mesangial volume, and urinary albumin excretion rate. Full normalization of creatinine clearance and basement membrane thickness was affected by administration of anti-RAGE IgG in these animals.

Taken together, these studies were the first to demonstrate that blockade of the ligand–RAGE axis, using either sRAGE or neutralizing antibody to RAGE blocked key elements of the DN phenotype in diabetic mice.

An additional pharmacological approach to the blockade of RAGE targeting production of type IV collagen was demonstrated by the studies of Tsuji and colleagues *(51)*. A stable mouse mesangial cell (MC) line producing the RAGE-specific ribozymes was generated in which RAGE mRNA and protein were effectively diminished vs control cells. Exposure to AGEs in the RAGE-ribozyme-expressing cells resulted in significantly decreased production of type IV collagen mRNA *(51)*. Although these studies were limited to the in vitro setting, they nevertheless underscored the relevance of the RAGE axis to mechanisms linked to DN.

Genetic Models of RAGE Modification and Diabetic Nephropathy

In order to definitively address the role of RAGE in the pathogenesis of DN, genetic models have been employed in experimental systems. In the first studies, Yamamoto and colleagues *(52)* generated transgenic mice that overexpress RAGE in vascular cells (and to some degree on mononuclear phagocytes) and cross-bred these mice with animals that develop insulin-dependent diabetes shortly after birth. The double-transgenic diabetic mice displayed increased enlargement of the kidney, glomerular hypertrophy, increased albuminuria, mesangial expansion, advanced glomerulosclerosis, and increased serum creatinine compared with the diabetic littermates that lacked the RAGE transgene. In those studies, consistent with roles for advanced glycation in amplifying RAGE-mediated perturbation in this setting, these authors found that administration of OPB-9195, an inhibitor of AGEs, prevented the nephropathy phenotype in the double-transgenic mice *(52)*.

In other studies, to test the impact of genetic deletion of RAGE, homozygous RAGE null mice and their RAGE-expressing littermates were rendered diabetic with STZ. After 3 mo of established hyperglycemia, diabetic RAGE null and wild-type mice were sacrificed for analyses. Compared with RAGE-expressing diabetic mice, diabetic RAGE null mice displayed decreased kidney weight/body weight ratio and decreased renal cortex expression of VEGF antigen and transcripts for TGF-β *(46)*. Together with studies in RAGE-overexpressing mice, these experiments in mice devoid of RAGE highlighted the central role of RAGE in the pathogenesis of the DN phenotype.

RAGE SIGNALING AND IMPLICATIONS FOR DIABETIC NEPHROPATHY

The signaling cascades activated on ligand-engagement of RAGE are diverse and reflect the cell type and duration of stimulation by ligand. We and others have shown that RAGE signaling triggers recruitment of p21ras, erk1/2 (p44/p42) MAP kinases, p38 and SAPK/JNK MAP kinases, rho GTPases, phosphoinositol-3 kinase, and the JAK/STAT pathway. Key downstream consequences such as activation of the key transcription factors nuclear factor (NF)-κB and CREB have also been reported *(28,36,53–61)*.

Recent studies have linked RAGE signaling to TGF-β-Smad signaling pathways, and, further, have suggested key links between AGE–RAGE pathways and angiotensin (Ang) II. In cultured rat MCs, incubation with AGEs resulted in RAGE-dependent generation of reactive oxygen species in parallel with production of Ang II *(62)*. AGE-induced TGF-β overproduction was blocked by the Ang II type 1 receptor blocker candesartan. AGE-induced phosphorylation of Smad 2 and TGF-β inducible promoter activity were reduced by candesartan and antibody to TGF-β. In these MCs, AGEs inhibited

DNA synthesis and stimulated protein synthesis and fibronectin production, in parallel with upregulation of p27, processes blocked by candesartan or antibody to TGF-β *(62)*. These studies linked for the first time AGE–RAGE signaling to TGF-β and Smad signaling in MCs.

Other studies demonstrated that AGEs and TGF-β induced p21waf expression and collagen production in cultured MCs. Signaling via STAT5 was required for the effects on AGE adducts and TGF-β on p21 waf expression and growth arrest, but not required for the impact on collagen production. These studies were confirmed in fibroblasts retrieved from p21waf null mice *(63)*.

A potential effect of RAGE signaling in the progression of tubulo-interstitial disease has been suggested by the effects of AGEs on epithelial–myofibroblast transdifferentiation. AGE exposure to cultured rat proximal tubule cells resulted in epithelial–myofibroblast transdifferentiation determined by *de novo* α-smooth muscle actin expression and loss of epithelial E-cadherin staining, effects blocked by antibodies to either RAGE or to TGF-β *(64)*. These effects were prevented by incubation with ALT-711, an AGE crosslink breaker. Li and colleagues *(65)* extended these findings to show that these effects were consequent to signaling through MEK1-ERK 1/2 MAP kinases and were independent of TGF-β.

Our studies indicated that RAGE signaling exerted effects on VEGF expression in cultured podocytes. When immortalized cultured murine podocytes were incubated with the prototypic RAGE ligand, S100b, increased VEGF antigen was demonstrated by Western blotting. Consistent with an important role for RAGE, pretreatment of the podocytes with anti-RAGE IgG or sRAGE significantly attenuated S100b-mediated upregulation of VEGF *(46)*.

Although the implications of these findings to the in vivo setting in long-term diabetic kidney remain to be elucidated in human studies, they nevertheless suggest that AGE–RAGE pathways may exert diverse effects in cells susceptible to the long-term adverse effects of hyperglycemia in the kidney.

TARGETING AGE–RAGE PATHWAYS: PERSPECTIVES FOR CLINICAL TRIALS

AGEs as Therapeutic Targets

Substantial evidence supporting the AGE hypothesis in the pathogenesis of DN is now accruing in both experimental systems and human clinical trials.

Initial studies employed aminoguanidine, an inhibitor of AGE formation, antiantioxidant, and inhibitor of iNOS in animal models of diabetic complications, including nephropathy. Aminoguanidine displayed preclinical benefit in reduction of albuminuria and mesangial expansion when administered to such animals as STZ-treated diabetic rats, Otsuka Long-Evans Tokushima Fatty rats, and STZ-treated diabetic apolipoprotein E (apo-E) null mice *(66–68)*. In-depth studies using aminoguanidine implicated roles for protein kinase C in the pathogenesis of nephropathy *(69)*. Furthermore, in aminoguanidine-treated diabetic Sprague-Dawley rats, significantly decreased expression of TGF-β, PDGF-B, and type IV collagen was noted in the renal cortex tissue *(70)*.

These promising findings led to clinical trials in which pimagedine (aminoguanidine) was tested in human subjects with type 1 diabetes in a randomized clinical trial. The primary endpoint of the trial was the time of doubling of serum creatinine; the secondary endpoints included evaluation of proteinuria, kidney function, and retinopathy. Serum creatinine doubled in 26% of the placebo-treated subjects and in 20% of those receiving pimagedine ($p = 0.099$) *(71)*. The estimated glomerular filtration rate decreased more slowly in the subjects treated with pimagedine over 36 mo ($p = 0.05$) and pimagedine significantly reduced the 24-h protein excretion ($p < 0.001$). However, three patients receiving the high-dose pimagedine in this trial developed glomerulonephritis *(71)*. Despite the fact that the trial failed to show efficacy based on the primary endpoint, in their entirety, these studies provided strong support for the AGE hypothesis in the pathogenesis of DN.

More recently, the AGE crosslink breaker, ALT-711 has been tested for efficacy in animal models of DN. Promising findings have been reported in STZ-induced diabetic rats and diabetic apo-E null mice *(72,73)*. Although not yet tested in human trials in nephropathy, administration of ALT-711 to the elderly resulted in improved arterial compliance in aged humans with vascular stiffening when administered over a 56-d period *(74)*.

Other experimental agents that target AGEs, such as pyridoxamine and LR-90, have also been tested in preclinical models of nephropathy and have demonstrated promising results *(75,76)*. Pyridoxamine targets both AGEs and advanced lipoxidation endproducts, thereby implicating lipid peroxidation products as well in the pathogenesis of nephropathy *(75)*.

RAGE as a Therapeutic Target

Although RAGE antagonism has yet to be tested in clinical trials, preclinical studies using sRAGE, anti-RAGE IgG, or ribozymes directed against RAGE in nephropathy models support the relevance of this axis to the pathogenesis of injury in the diabetic kidney *(46,50–51)*. Importantly, in each of these cases, there was no evidence that blockade of RAGE (using sRAGE, anti-RAGE IgG or in RAGE-null mice) altered levels of glucose, insulin, or lipids in the animals. These studies suggest strongly that RAGE is a downstream effector pathway in hyperglycemic injury, and not the cause of initial perturbation. In this context, it is likely that complementary therapies targeting this axis, as well as other established targets, might exert additive benefit in the kidney. Additional strategies to antagonize RAGE, including small-molecule antagonists and siRNA are also possible means to break the cycle of AGE–RAGE perturbation in the diabetic kidney.

Combination Therapies in Diabetic Nephropathy

The finding that RAGE antagonism in diabetic animals does not impact on levels of glucose or lipids strongly supports that optimal strategies to attenuate the course of nephropathy will include agents targeting multiple key axes. For example, Davis and colleagues have shown superior protective effects of combination therapy with ACE inhibitors (perindopril) and aminoguanidine in STZ-induced spontaneously hypertensive rats *(77)*. Interestingly, other studies have suggested that there is interplay between ACE and AGE pathways. Administration of ACE inhibition (ramipril) or aminoguanidine attenuated AGE formation in the kidney of STZ diabetic animals to the same degree, thereby suggesting that accumulation of AGEs in experimental DN may be linked through oxidative stress *(77)*. Other studies confirmed this relationship; STZ-treated diabetic rats receiving the AT1 receptor antagonist valsartan displayed reduction of tissue and plasma CML-AGEs *(78)*.

Thus, it would not be surprising that combination therapies may exert synergistic benefit in nephropathy. Such experimental findings set the stage for optimal design of renoprotective regimens in chronic diabetes. If and how RAGE antagonism might be included in these treatment regimens remains to be determined.

CONCLUSIONS

Evidence is accruing that the AGE–RAGE pathway plays critical roles in the pathogenesis of DN. We hypothesize that AGEs, via RAGE, impact on multiple distinct cell types implicated in nephropathy. Experimental evidence supports the premise in vitro and in vivo that AGE–RAGE interaction in podocytes results in upregulation of VEGF, and, thereby, a mechanism to attract inflammatory cells and release of pro-inflammatory RAGE ligands, such as S100/calgranulins and HMGB1. In addition, ligand–RAGE interaction activates MCs, thereby providing a mechanism to augment generation of prosclerotic growth factors and cytokines such as TGF-β. RAGE is also expressed by endothelial cells, thus, interaction of RAGE ligands with RAGE in the endothelium may directly amplify vascular perturbation in the glomerulus. A key consequence of such injury is the development of albuminuria. Future studies must dissect the potential impact of inflammatory RAGE signaling in the pathogenesis of nephropathy.

Although studies in proximal tubular cells suggest roles for AGE–RAGE signaling in epithelial myofibroblast transdifferentiation, such concepts have yet to be explored in vivo and thus represent solely theoretical considerations at this time.

We conclude that future clinical trials should include studies focused on combination therapy strategies to target the AGE–RAGE axis. Importantly, the critical impact of stringent control of hyperglycemia is the foremost goal. Studies in the Diabetes Control and Complications (DCCT) research group clearly indicated that rigorous control of hyperglycemia was associated with decreased microvascular complications, including nephropathy *(79)*. Recently, fascinating findings published by the Epidemiology of Diabetes Interventions and Complications (EDIC) study suggested that subjects in the original intensively treated DCCT group continued to display renoprotection (decreased albuminuria, hypertension, and rise in serum creatinine level) vs subjects originally in the conventional treatment group *(80)*. This extended benefit occurred despite the fact that levels of glycosylated hemoglobin in the originally intensively treated subjects gradually became indistinguishable between the two groups. Such considerations suggest that earlier and substantive reduction in hyperglycemia in the original intensively treated group left an indelible mark in the vasculature of these diabetic subjects, and support the hypothesis that high levels of glucose may be linked to long-term "memory" in vascular targets in diabetes. It is plausible that AGE–RAGE interaction is one of the mechanisms underlying glycemic memory, thereby further supporting the targeting of this axis in chronic nephropathy.

ACKNOWLEDGMENTS

This work was supported, in part, by grants from the US Public Health Service and the Juvenile Diabetes Research Foundation International. AMS is a recipient of a Burroughs Wellcome Fund Clinical Scientist Award in translational research.

REFERENCES

1. Brownlee M, Cerami A, Vlassara H. Advanced glycoslyation endproducts in tissue and the biochemical basis of diabetic complications. N Engl J Med 1988;318:1315–1321.
2. Brownlee M. Advanced glycosylation in diabetes and aging. Ann Rev Med 1995;46:223–234.

3. Dyer D, Blackledge S, Thorpe SR, Baynes JW. Formation of pentosidine during nonenzymatic browning of protein by glucose: identification of glucose and other carbohydrates as possible precursors of pentosidine in vivo. J Biol Chem 1991;266:11,654–11,660.
4. Grandhee S, Monnier VM. Mechanisms of formation of the Maillard protein crosslink pentosidine: ribose, glucose, fructose and ascorbate as pentosidine precursors. J Biol Chem 1991;266: 11,649–11,653.
5. Beisswenger P, Moore L, Brinck-Johnsen T, Curphey TJ. Increased collagen-linked pentosidine levels and AGEs in early diabetic nephropathy. J Clin Invest 1993;92:212–217.
6. Ikeda K, Higashi T, Sano H, et al. Carboxymethyllysine protein adduct is a major immunological epitope in proteins modified with AGEs of the Maillard reaction. Biochem 1996;35:8075–8083.
7. Reddy S, Bichler J, Wells-Knecht K, Thorpe SR, Baynes JW. Carboxymethyllysine is a dominant AGE antigen in tissue proteins. Biochem 1995;34:10,872–10,878.
8. Anderson MM, Requena JR, Crowley JR, Thorpe SR, Heinecke JW. The myeloperoxidase system of human phagocytes generates Nepsilon-(carboxymethyl)lysine on proteins: a mechanism for producing advanced glycation endproducts at sites of inflammation. J Clin Invest 1999;104:103–113.
9. Schleicher ED, Wagner E, Nerlich AG. Increased accumulation of the glycoxidation product N(epsilon)-(carboxymethyl)lysine in human tissues in diabetes and aging. J Clin Invest 1997;99: 457–468.
10. Horie K, Miyata T, Maeda K, et al. Immunohistochemical colocalization of glycoxidation products and lipid peroxidation products in diabetic renal glomerular lesions. Implication for glycoxidative stress in the pathogenesis of diabetic nephropathy. J Clin Invest 1997;100:2995–3004.
11. Sebekova K, Podracka L, Heidland A, Schinzel R. Enhanced plasma levels of advanced glycation end products (AGE) and pro-inflammatory cytokines in children/adolescents with chronic renal insufficiency and after renal replacement therapy by dialysis and transplantation—are they inter-related? Clin Nephrol 2001;56:S21–S26.
12. Shimoike T, Inoguchi T, Umeda F, Nawata H, Kawano K, Ochi H. The meaning of serum levels of advanced glycosylation end products in diabetic nephropathy. Metab 2000;49:1030–1035.
13. Aso Y, Inukai T, Tayama K, Takemura Y. Serum concentrations of advanced glycation endproducts are associated with the development of atherosclerosis as well as diabetic microangiopathy in patients with type 2 diabetes. Acta Diabetol 2000;37:87–92.
14. Miura J, Yamagishi S, Uchigata Y, et al. Serum levels of non-carboxymethyllysine advanced glycation endproducts are correlated to severity of microvascular complications in patients with type 1 diabetes. J Diabet Complications 2003;17:16–21.
15. Wagner Z, Wittmann I, Mazak I, et al. N(epsilon)-(carboxymethyl)lysine levels in patients with type 2 diabetes: role of renal function. Am J Kidney Dis 2001;38:785–791.
16. Kanauchi M, Nishioka H, Dohi K. Serum levels of advanced glycosylation end products in diabetic nephropathy. Nephron 2001;89:228–230.
17. Kislinger T, Fu C, Huber B, et al. Ne (carboxymethyl)lysine modifications of proteins are ligands for RAGE that activate cell signaling pathways and modulate gene expression. J Biol Chem 1999;274: 31,740–31,749.
18. El Khoury J, Thomas CA, Loike JD, Hickman SE, Cao L, Silverstein SC. Macrophages adhere to glucose-modified basement membrane collagen IV via their scavenger receptors. J Biol Chem 1994;269:10,197–10,200.
19. Vlassara H, Li YM, Imani F, et al. Identification of galectin-3 as a high-affinity binding protein for advanced glycation end products (AGE): a new member of the AGE-receptor complex. Mol Med 1995;1:634–646.
20. Li YM, Mitsuhashi T, Wojciechowicz D, et al. Advanced glycation end products induce glomerular sclerosis and albuminuria in normal rats. Proc Natl Acad Sci 1996;93:11,047–11,052.
21. Ohgami N, Nagai R, Ikemoto M, et al. CD36 serves as a receptor for advanced glycation endproducts (AGE). J Diabet Complications 2002;16:56–59.
22. Schmidt AM, Vianna M, Gerlach M, et al. Isolation and characterization of two binding proteins for advanced glycosylation end products from bovine lung which are present on the endothelial cell surface. J Biol Chem 1992;267:14,987–14,997.
23. Neeper M, Schmidt AM, Brett J, et al. Cloning and expression of a cell surface receptor for advanced glycosylation end products of proteins. J Biol Chem 1992;267:14,998–15,004.
24. Brett J, Schmidt AM, Zou YS, et al. Tissue distribution of the receptor for advanced glycation endproducts (RAGE): expression in smooth muscle, cardiac myocytes, and neural tissue in addition to vasculature. Am J Pathol 1993;143:1699–1712.

25. Ritthaler U, Deng Y, Zhang Y, et al. Expression of RAGE in peripheral occlusive vascular disease. Am J Pathol 1995;146:688–694.
26. Hou FF, Ren H, Owen WF Jr, et al. Enhanced expression of receptor for advanced glycation end products in chronic kidney disease. J Am Soc Nephrol 2004;15:1889–1896.
27. Tanji N, Markowitz GS, Fu C, et al. The expression of advanced glycation endproducts and their cellular receptor RAGE in diabetic nephropathy and non-diabetic renal disease. J Am Soc Nephrol 2000;11:1656–1666.
28. Hofmann MA, Drury S, Fu C, et al. RAGE mediates a novel proinflammatory axis: a central cell surface receptor for S100/calgranulin polypeptides. Cell 1999;97:889–901.
29. Schafer BW, Heinzmann CW. The S100 family of EF-hand calcium-binding proteins: functions and pathology. TIBS 1996;21:134–140.
30. Zimmer DB, Cornwall EH, Landar A, Song W. The S100 protein family: history, function, and expression. Brain Res Bull 1995;37:417–429.
31. Donato R. S100: a multigenic family of calcium-modulated proteins of the EF-hand type with intracellular and extracellular functional roles. Intl J Biochem Cell Biol 2001;33:637–668.
32. Hofmann MA, Drury S, Hudson BI, et al. RAGE and arthritis: The G82S polymorphism amplifies the inflammatory response. Genes Immun 2002;3:123–135.
33. Yan SS, Wu ZY, Zhang HP, et al. Suppression of experimental autoimmune encephalomyelitis by selective blockade of encephalitogenic T-cell infiltration of the central nervous system. Nat Med 2003;9:287–293.
34. Chen Y, Yan SS, Colgan J, et al. Blockade of the late stagtes of autoimmune diabetes by inhibition of the receptor for advanced glycation end products. J Immunol 2004;173:1399–1405.
35. Hori O, Brett J, Slattery T, et al. RAGE is a cellular binding site for amphoterin: mediation of neurite outgrowth and co-expression of RAGE and amphoterin in the developing nervous system. J Biol Chem 1995;270:25,752–25,761.
36. Taguchi A, Blood DC, del Toro G, et al. Blockade of amphoterin/RAGE signaling suppresses tumor growth and metastases. Nature 2000;405:354–336.
37. Wang H, Bloom O, Zhang M, et al. HMG-1 as a late mediator of endotoxin lethality in mice. Science 1999;285:248–251.
38. Park JS, Svetkauskaite D, He Q, et al. Involvement of toll-like receptors 2 and 4 in cellular activation by high mobility group box 1 protein. J Biol Chem 2004;279:7370–7377.
39. Yan SD, Chen X, Chen M, et al. RAGE and amyloid-β peptide neurotoxicity in Alzheimer's disease. Nature 1996;382:685–691.
40. Yan SD, Zhu H, Fu J, et al. Amyloid beta peptide-receptor for advanced glycation endproduct interaction elicits neuronal expression of macrophage-colony stimulating factor: a proinflammatory pathway in Alzheimer disease. Proc Natl Acad Sci USA 1997;94:5296–5301.
41. Yan SD, Zhu H, Zhu A, et al. Receptor-dependent cell stress and amyloid accumulation in systemic amyloidosis. Nat Med 2000;6:643–651.
42. Chavakis T, Bierhaus A, Al-Fakhri N, et al. The pattern recognition receptor (RAGE) is a counter-receptor for leukocyte integrins: a novel pathway for inflammatory cell recruitment. J Exp Med 2003; 198:1507–1515.
43. Wautier JL, Zoukourian C, Chappey O, et al. Receptor-mediated endothelial cell dysfunction in diabetic vasculopathy: soluble RAGE blocks hyperpermeability. J Clin Invest 1996;97:238–243.
44. Mattock M, Morrish N, Viberti G, Keen H, Fitzgerald AP, Jackson G. Prospective study of microalbuminuria as predictor of mortality in NIDDM. Diabetes 1992;41:736–741.
45. Johnstone MT, Creager SJ, Scales KM, Cusco JA, Lee BK, Creager MA. Impaired endothelium-dependent vasodilation in patients with insulin-dependent diabetes mellitus. Circulation 1993;88:2510–2516.
46. Wendt TM, Tanji N, Guo J, et al. RAGE drives the development of glomerulosclerosis and implicates podocyte activation in the pathogenesis of diabetic nephropathy. Am J Pathol 2003;162:1123–1137.
47. Cooper ME, Vranes D, Youssef S, et al. Increased renal expression of vascular endothelial growth factor (VEGF) and its receptor VEGFR-2 in experimental diabetes. Diabetes 1999;48:2229–2239.
48. Kang DH, Johnson RJ. Vascular endothelial growth factor: a new player in the pathogenesis of renal fibrosis. Curr Opin Nephrol Hypertens 2003;12:43–49.
49. de Vriese AS, Tilton RG, Elger M, Stephan CC, Kriz W, Lameire NH. Antibodies against vascular endothelial growth factor improve early renal dysfunction in experimental diabetes. J Am Soc Nephrol 2001;12:993–1000.
50. Flyvbjerg A, Denner L, Schrijvers BF, et al. Long-term renal effects of a neutralizing RAGE antibody in obese type 2 diabetic mice. Diabetes 2004;53:166–172.

51. Tsuji H, Iehara N, Masegi T, et al. Ribozyme targeting of receptor for advanced glycation endproducts in mouse mesangial cells. Biochem Biophys Res Commun 1998;245:583–588.
52. Yamomoto Y, Kato I, Doi T, et al. Development and prevention of advanced diabetic nephropathy in RAGE-overexpressing mice. J Clin Invset 2001;108:261–268.
53. Yan SD, Schmidt AM, Anderson GM, et al. Enhanced cellular oxidant stress by the interaction of advanced glycation endproducts with their receptors/binding proteins. J Biol Chem 1994;269: 9889–9897.
54. Lander HL, Tauras JM, Ogiste JS, Moss RA, Schmidt AM. Activation of the Receptor for Advanced Glycation Endproducts triggers a MAP Kinase pathway regulated by oxidant stress. J Biol Chem 1997;272:17,810–17,814.
55. Wautier MP, Chappey O, Corda S, Stern DM, Schmidt AM, Wautier JL. Activation of NADPH oxidase by AGE links oxidant stress to altered gene expression via RAGE. Am J Physiol Endocrinol Metab 2001;280:E685–E694.
56. Deora AA, Win T, Vanhaesebroeck B, Lander HM. A redox-triggered ras-effector interaction. Recruitment of phosphatidylinositol 3'-kinase to ras by redox stress. J Biol Chem 1998;273:29,923–29,928.
57. Huang JS, Guh JY, Chen HC, Hung WC, Lai HY, Chuang LY. Role of receptor for advanced glycation end-product (RAGE) and the JAK/STAT-signaling pathway in AGE-induced collagen production in NRK-49F cells. J Cell Biochem 2001;81:102–113.
58. Huttunen HJ, Fages C, Rauvala H. Receptor for Advanced Glycation Endproducts (RAGE)-mediated neurite outgrowth and activation of NF-kB require the cytoplasmic domain of the receptor but different downstream signaling pathways. J Biol Chem 1999;294:19,919–19,924.
59. Huttunen HJ, Kuja-Panula J, Rauvala H. RAGE signaling induces CREB dependent chromogranin expression during neuronal differentiation. J Biol Chem 2002;277:38,635–38,646.
60. Yeh C-H, Sturgis L, Haidacher J, et al. Requirement for p38 and p44/42 Mitogen-activated protein kinases in RAGE-mediated Nuclear Factor Kappa B transcriptional activation and cytokine secretion. Diabetes 2001;50:1495–1504.
61. Sakaguchi T, Yan SF, Yan SD, et al. Central role of RAGE-dependent neointimal expansion in arterial restenosis. J Clin Invest 2003;111:959–972.
62. Fukami K, Ueda S, Yamagishi S, et al. AGEs activate mesangial TGF-beta-SMAD signaling via an angiotensin II type 1 receptor interaction. Kidney Int 2004;66:2137–2147.
63. Brizzi MF, Dentelli P, Rosso A, et al. RAGE- and TGF-beta receptor-, mediated signals converge on STAT5 and p21waf to control cell cycle progression of mesangial cells: a possible role in the development and progression of diabetic nephropathy. FASEB J 2004;18:1249–1251.
64. Oldfield MD, Bach LA, Forbes JM, et al. Advanced glycation endproducts cause epithelial-myofibroblast transdifferentiation via the receptor for advanced glycation endproducts (RAGE). J Clin Invest 2001;108:1853–1863.
65. Li JH, Wang W, Huang XR, et al. Advanced glycation endproducts induce tubular epithelial-myofibroblast transition through the RAGE ERK 1/2 MAP kinase signaling pathway. Am J Pathol 2004;164:1389–1397.
66. Soulis-Liparota T, Cooper M, Papazoglou D, Clarke B, Jerums G. Retardation by aminoguanidine of development of albuminuria, mesangial expansion, and tissue fluorescence in streptozotocin-induced diabetic rats. Diabetes 1991;40:1328–1334.
67. Yamauchi A, Takei I, Makita Z, et al. Effects of aminoguanidine on serum advanced glycation endproducts, urinary albumin excretion, mesangial expansion, and glomerular basement membrane thickening in Otsuka Long-Evans Tokushima fatty rats. Diabetes Res Clin Pract 1997;34:127–133.
68. Lassila M, Seah KK, Allen TJ, et al. Accelerated nephropathy in diabetic apolipoprotein E knockout mouse: role of advanced glycation end products. J Am Soc Nephrol 2004;15:2125–2138.
69. Osicka TM, Yu Y, Panagiotopoulos S, et al. Prevention of albuminuria by aminoguanidine or ramipril in streptozotocin-induced diabetic rats is associated with the normalization of glomerular protein kinase C. Diabetes 2000;49:87–93.
70. Kelly DJ, Gilbert RE, Cox AJ, Soulis T, Jerums G, Cooper ME. Aminoguanidine ameliorates overexpression of prosclerotic growth factors and collagen deposition in experimental diabetic nephropathy. J Am Soc Nephrol 2001;12:2098–2107.
71. Bolton WK, Cattran DC, Williams ME, et al. Randomized trial of an inhibitor of formation of advanced glycation endproducts in diabetic nephropathy. ACTION I Investigator Group. Am J Nephrol 2004;24:32–40.
72. Forbes JM, Thallas V, Thomas MC, et al. The breakdown of preexisting advanced glycation endproducts is associated with reduced renal fibrosis in experimental diabetes. FASEB J 2003;17:1762–1764.

73. Thallas-Bonke V, Lindschau C, Riskalla B, et al. Attenuation of extracellular matrix accumulation in diabetic nephropathy by the advanced glycation end product cross link breaker ALT 711 via a protein kinase C alpha dependent pathway. Diabetes 2004;53:2921–2930.
74. Kass DA, Shapiro EP, Kawaguchi M, et al. Improved arterial compliance by a novel advanced glycation endproduct cross link breaker. Circulation 2001;104:1464–1470.
75. Alderson NL, Chachich ME, Frizzell N, et al. Effect of antioxidants and ACE inhibition on chemical modifications of proteins and progression of nephropathy in the streptozotocin diabetic rat. Diabetologia 2004;47:1385–1395.
76. Figarola JL, Scott S, Loera S, et al. LR-90, a new advanced glycation endproduct inhibitor prevents progression of diabetic nephropathy in streptozotocin-diabetic rats. Diabetologia 2003;46:1140–1152.
77. Davis BJ, Forbes JM, Thomas MC, et al. Superior renoprotective effects of combination therapy with ACE and AGE inhibition in the diabetic spontaneously hypertensive rat. Diabetologia 2004;47:89–97.
78. Forbes JM, Thomas MC, Thorpe SR, Alderson NL, Cooper ME. The effects of valsartan on the accumulation of circulating and renal advanced glycation endproducts in experimental diabetes. Kidney Int Suppl 2004;92:S105–S107.
79. The Diabetes Control and Complications Research Group. The effect of intensive treatment of diabetes on the development and progression of long-term complications in insulin-dependent diabetes mellitus. N Engl J Med 1993;318:977–986.
80. Writing Team for the Diabetes Control and Complications Trial/Epidemiology of Diabetes Interventions and complications Research Group. Sustained effect of intensive treatment of type 1 diabetes mellitus on development and progression of diabetic nephropathy: the Epidemiology of Diabetes Interventions and Complications (EDIC). JAMA 2003;290:2159–2167.

I

Basic Pathophysiology and Biochemistry of Diabetic Nephropathy

F. Oxidative Stress

9 Oxidative and Glycooxidative Stress in Diabetic Nephropathy

Frederick R. DeRubertis, MD
and Patricia A. Craven, PhD

CONTENTS

INTRODUCTION

Diabetic nephropathy (DN) is currently the leading cause of end-stage renal disease (ESRD) in the United States and most other developed nations. Approximately 40% of new patients who entered ESRD programs in the United States in 2003 had DN; the overall rate of ESRD resulting from diabetes in the United States has risen 68% since 1992 *(1)*. Moreover, even the earliest clinically detected stage of renal injury in diabetes (microalbuminuria) is associated with an increased prevalence of macrovascular disease *(2–5)*. Thus, the mortality, morbidity, and costs associated with DN extend far beyond those directly attributable to ESRD *per se*. They include costs associated with the increased burden of macrovascular disease seen at earlier stages of DN *(2–5)*. Common pathogenic mechanisms operative in both microvascular and macrovascular injury in diabetes may account at least in part for this association *(6,7)*.

Over the past several decades, much progress has been made in our understanding of the pathogenesis of DN. Genetic *(8–11)*, hemodynamic *(12–14)*, and metabolic risk factors *(15)* have all been implicated. The independent and interactive benefits of glycemic and blood pressure control in the suppression of the development of

From: *Contemporary Diabetes: The Diabetic Kidney*
Edited by: P. Cortes and C. E. Mogensen © Humana Press Inc., Totowa, NJ

microalbuminuria and its progression to overt nephropathy *(13,16–20)*, and the powerful effect of blood pressure control to retard the progression of overt nephropathy *(19,20)* have been clearly demonstrated in both types 1 and 2 diabetes. The added beneficial effects of angiotensin-converting enzyme inhibitors (ACEIs) and/or angiotensin receptor blockers (ARBs) on the development and the progression of DN beyond those attributable to blood pressure reduction alone are also now well established in both types 1 and 2 diabetes *(21–26)*. Dyslipidemia has been similarly implicated as a risk factor for renal injury in diabetes but this association requires further examination *(27)*. Unfortunately, none of the interventions currently available has been shown to completely prevent the development or arrest the progression of DN. Accordingly, there is a need to develop additional strategies for intervention based on a more complete understanding of the pathogenesis of renal injury in diabetes.

In this regard, there is accumulating evidence to support a role for oxidative and glycooxidative (carbonyl) stress in the pathogenesis of DN, as well as in other diabetic complications *(28–30)*. The formation of increased quantities of labile intermediate dicarbonyls and advanced glycosylation endproducts (AGEs) in diabetes is well recognized *(31,32)*. These products arise via nonenzymatic extracellular protein glycation or from intracellular pathways of glucose metabolism, which result in generation of reactive dicarbonyl precursors *(31,32)*. Formation of some of these products involves redox reactions, including glucose autooxidation (glycooxidative stress) *(31,32)*. Once formed, extracellular AGE also contributes to oxidative stress by increasing cellular generation of reactive oxygen species (ROS) through receptor-mediated pathways *(33)*. Other multiple metabolic processes in diabetes may lead to enhanced levels of ROS. Thus, nonphysiological and potentially cytotoxic levels of ROS may develop in kidney and other tissues as direct or indirect consequences of hyperglycemia, elevated free fatty acids, other intermediary metabolites, and/or due to compromised antioxidant defense mechanisms in diabetes *(28,34,35)*. In experimental diabetes, evidence for increased renal oxidative stress includes accumulation of malondialdehyde (MDA) in renal cortex (a marker of increased lipid peroxidation), increased content of 8-hydroxy 2′-deoxyguanosine in glomeruli (an index of enhanced oxidation of nucleic acid), depletion of reduced glutathione in renal cortex, and increased production of ROS, NADPH oxidase, and heme-oxygenase-1 activities in glomeruli *(35–38)*. These renal changes are all suppressed by treatment of diabetic animals with antioxidants *(35–38)*. However, the conventional concept that ROS act predominantly as cellular toxins via pathological interactions with lipids, proteins, and nucleic acids has been revised. Recent studies have supported a physiological role for ROS in normal cell signal transduction, including cell signaling by angiotensin (Ang) II whose participation in renal injury in diabetes, similar to that of hyperglycemia, is firmly established *(28,39–41)*. Thus, interventions targeted at modification of key redox reactions in diabetes might alter not only ROS generated pathophysiologically, such as that occurs in response to hyperglycemia or AGE, but also those formed as part of otherwise physiological cell signaling pathways which are overexpressed in diabetes.

In this chapter, the major mechanisms that may mediate increased oxidative and glycooxidative stress in diabetes, the pathways through which redox and/or glycooxidative reactions may participate in the pathogenesis of renal injury, and evidence for involvement of redox and/or glycooxidative mechanisms in the development of DN in vivo will be reviewed.

Table 1
Pathways Implicated in Increased ROS or Dicarbonyl Generation in Diabetes

- Increased mitochondrial electron transport activity induced by hyperglycemia and fatty acids *(42,43)*.
- Altered activity of endothelial nitric oxide synthase (eNOS) *(44,45)*.
- Activation of nonphagocytic cell NADH/NADPH oxidase *(46)*.
- Increased glucose autooxidation *(47,48)*.
- Activation of RAGE receptors by AGE *(33)*.
- Increased cyclooxygenase and/or lipoxgenase activity *(28)*.
- Increased xanthine oxidase activity *(49)*.
- Increased cytochrome P-450 activity *(50)*.

MECHANISMS OF INCREASED OXIDATIVE AND GLYCOOXIDATIVE STRESS IN DIABETES

Multiple pathways may contribute to enhanced oxidative and glycooxidative stress in diabetes via increased generation of reactive oxygen species (ROS) and dicarbonyls (Table 1). The relative importance of various metabolic pathways as sources of these labile moieties in diabetes may differ significantly as a function of the cell type in question. The major pathways implicated are reviewed below.

Increased Mitochondrial Electron Transport

In many cell types under physiological conditions, mitochondria are the major intracellular source of ROS production *(39)*. In an elegant series of studies conducted predominantly in cultured bovine aortic endothelial cells, Brownlee and coworkers *(34)* implicated overproduction of superoxide by the mitochondrial electron transport chain, induced by hyperglycemia and/or fatty acids, as a potential major source of ROS generation in diabetes. Overproduction of superoxide by mitochondria, in turn, may be a key mechanism by which hyperglycemia increases activity of the polyol and hexosamine pathways, the formation of AGE and activation of protein kinase C (PKC), all of which have been implicated in the pathogenesis of vascular and renal injury in diabetes *(34)*. This proposed common pathogenetic mechanism for expression of multiple cellular actions of high ambient concentrations of glucose has previously been reviewed in detail by Brownlee et al. *(34)*. Briefly, in cells in which glucose uptake is not regulated by insulin, including endothelial and glomerular mesangial cells (MCs) *(42,51)*, a high extracellular concentration of glucose leads to an elevated intracellular glucose level. Metabolism of glucose via glycolysis and the tricarboxylic acid (TCA) cycle results in reduction in the coenzymes NAD^+ and FADH with generation of CO_2. The NADH and $FADH_2$ formed donate electrons to the electron transport chain located in the inner mitochondrial membrane and are thus reoxidized. Electron transport through the chain generates a proton gradient across the inner mitochondrial membrane *(52–54)*. The latter drives oxidative phosphorylation with production of adenosine triphosphate (ATP). When the proton gradient across the membrane is enhanced via metabolism of excess glucose, there is evidence that electron transport at complex III (ubiquinol: cytochrome-*c* oxidoreductase) of the chain is suppressed, and that electrons carried by coenzyme Q (ubiquinone) reduce O_2 to superoxide rather than being passed to complex III *(52–54)*.

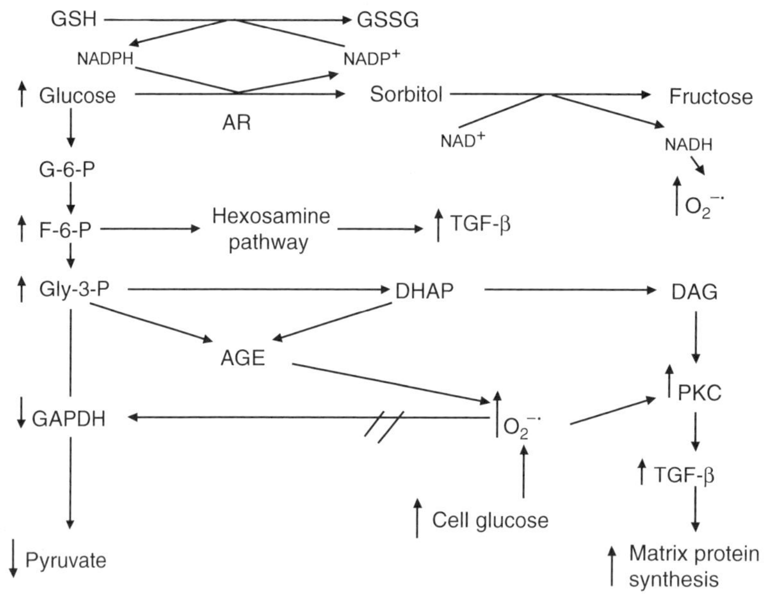

Fig. 1. Effects of glucose-induced increases in superoxide ($O^{2-\cdot}$) production on pathways of glucose-mediated cell injury. GSH, reduced glutathione; GSSG, oxidized glutathione; G-6-P, glucose 6-phosphate; F-6-P, fructose 6-phosphate; Gly-3-P, glyceraldehyde-3-phosphate; GAPDH, glyceraldehyde-3-phosphate dehydrogenase; TGF-β, transforming growth factor-β; DHAP, dihydroxyacetone phosphate; DAG, diacylglycerol; AGE, advanced glycosylation endproducts; PKC, protein kinase C; AR, aldose reductase. (For description, *see* text.)

The increase in mitochondrial superoxide production that results from high intracellular glucose has in turn been linked to suppression of glyceraldehyde-3-phosphate dehydrogenase (GAPDH), and generation of increased levels of intermediary metabolites of glucose (Fig. 1). It has been proposed that this sequence may lead to (a) an increase in diacylglycerol from the glycolytic intermediate dihydroxyacetone phosphate (DHAP) with consequent activation of PKC; (b) an increase in fructose 3-phosphate formation which enhances the activity of the hexosamine pathway; the latter promotes glycosylation and increased activity of several transcription factors through formation of UDP-*N*-acetylglucosamine. These include specificity factor 1 and transforming growth factor (TGF)-β_1, a central mediator of progressive glomerular mesangial expansion in DN *(55,56)*; (c) an increase in formation of AGE from dicarbonyl metabolites (glyoxal and methylglyoxal), which in turn are derived from high glucose (HG) and the glycolytic intermediates DHAP and glyceraldehyde-3-phosphate; and (d) activation of the polyol pathway by HG *per se*, in which aldose reductase uses NADPH as a cofactor to convert glucose to sorbitol (Fig. 1). The conversion of $NADP^+$ back to NADPH consumes reduced glutathione and thus may impair cellular antioxidant defenses *(34)*. In addition, during the subsequent oxidation of sorbitol to fructose by sorbitol dehydrogenase, NAD^+ is reduced to NADH (Fig. 1). In a hyperglycemic environment, NAD^+ is also consumed by activated poly-ADP-ribose polymerase, an effect of glucose that has been linked to increased mitochondrial superoxide production *(34,57)*. The resultant increase in the cytosolic ratio of $NADH/NAD^+$ impairs the activity of GAPDH, which as noted above, fosters generation of intermediate glucose metabolites (Fig. 1).

In support of a key role for mitochondrial electron transport in the increase in superoxide induced by HG in cultured endothelial cells, this increase is suppressed by (a) inhibitors of mitochondrial metabolism, (b) overexpression of manganese superoxide dismutase (Mn^{+2} SOD), the mitochondrial form of SOD, or (c) overexpression of uncoupling protein 1, which collapses the protein gradient across the inner mitochondrial membrane *(42)*. Recent studies have similarly supported a role for enhanced mitochondrial metabolism in the increases in superoxide induced by HG in cultured human MCs *(58)*. Other studies have suggested mitochondria as a major source of the increases in superoxide induced in cultured endothelial cells by high levels of fatty acids *(43)*.

Altered Endothelial NO Synthase

NO derived from eNOS plays a critical physiological role in normal vascular function and structure *(7,59,60)*. Reduced bioavailability of NO in diabetes has been linked to impaired endothelium-dependent vasodilation, an altered vascular redox state, abnormal vascular smooth muscle cell (VSMC) growth, and prothrombotic properties of the vessel wall *(7,59,60)*. The rapid interaction of NO with superoxide may be an important determinant of the redox state of some cells, including endothelial cells *(7,61,62)*. Of note, there is evidence to support eNOS *per se* as a significant source of superoxide in diabetes *(7,63)*. Under conditions of reduced access of eNOS to either substrate (arginine) or the cofactor tetrahydrobiopterin, conditions which may pertain in diabetes *(7,63,64)*, the enzyme preferentially transfers electrons to molecular oxygen and produces increased quantities of superoxide relative to NO. This altered synthetic capacity has been referred to as "uncoupled" eNOS. The eNOS production of superoxide is enhanced in vitro in endothelial cells exposed to HG *(65)*, whereas inhibition of eNOS in vivo has been shown to suppress aortic endothelial superoxide levels in diabetic animals *(66)*. Notably, eNOS mRNA and protein are increased in the aorta of diabetic animals *(64,65,67)*. Thus, an increased vascular content of eNOS and the propensity of the enzyme to generate more superoxide relative to NO under diabetic conditions may both contribute to increased oxidative stress *(64,67)*. Similar changes in eNOS activity and eNOS superoxide production have been reported in diabetic rat renal cortex *(68)*. In rats with early proteinuric DN, expression of both glomerular eNOS and NADPH oxidase are increased, in association with indexes of enhanced renal-oxidative and nitrosative stress *(69)*. These and other data support altered NO bioavailability in glomeruli of diabetic animals, which is at least in part attributable to enhanced NO interaction with superoxide *(70)*. Uncoupled eNOS *per se* thus may be a source of both superoxide and NO in the glomeruli of diabetics.

Nonphagocytic Cell NADH/NADPH Oxidase

Endothelial cell (EC), VSMC, glomerular MC, renal tubular cells, and fibroblasts contain oxidases that use NADH and/or NADPH as substrates for electron transfer to molecular oxygen *(46)*. These oxidases are structurally similar but functionally different from the plasma membrane-associated NADPH oxidase first characterized in neutrophils *(71,72)*. The latter enzyme complex releases millimolar amounts of superoxide extracellularly during phagocytosis *(71)*. The oxidases identified in nonphagocytic cells are similar to neutrophil NADPH oxidase, a membrane-associated cytochrome-*b*558 complex, in that they possess both flavin and heme-binding regions likely involved in electron transfer *(71,72)*. They also share at least one protein subunit, P22 phox (phox stands for phagocyte oxidase). However, several differences have been noted between the NADPH oxidase systems of neutrophils and those of nonphagocytic cells. These include the following: (1) the neutrophil enzyme system preferentially uses NADPH as substrate, whereas nonphagocytic cells use either NADH or NADPH; (2) the nonphagocytic systems seem to constitutively generate consistently low levels of superoxide which can be upregulated by stimuli, but not to the high levels produced in bursts by activated neutrophils; and (3) a significant fraction of superoxide generated by the NADPH oxidase of nonphagocytic cells seems to occur intracellularly, whereas that of neutrophils is released extracellularly *(46,71–74)*. The latter difference may in turn be linked to the subcellular distribution of NADPH oxidase in neutrophils vs nonphagocytic cells *(75–77)*. In resting neutrophils, regulatory subunits of NADPH oxidase (p47 phox, p67 phox, and others) are in the cytosol. They translocate to the plasma membrane and associate with the membrane-bound cytochrome catalytic components gp 91 phox and p22 phox during neutrophil activation. By contrast, in nonphagocytic cells NADPH oxidase subunit may be preassembled in the cytosol and associated with the intracellular cytoskeleton *(46,75–77)*.

Studies in kidney from normal rats have indicated that NADH/NADPH oxidase is the major source of superoxide production in renal cortex and outer medulla, exceeding that derived from mitochondria in this region of the kidney *(78)*. Of note, VSMC and/or MC NADH/NADPH oxidase is activated by Ang II, AGE, HG, fatty acids, and platelet-derived growth factor *(46,72,79–81)*, whereas NADPH oxidase of EC is activated by TNF-α, thrombin, and other moieties *(46,82)*. In diabetes, upregulation of NADPH oxidases by these and other agonists in cells may contribute to oxidative stress *(33,46,78,83)*. However, superoxide derived from NADH/NADPH oxidase has also been implicated as an important step in the cell signaling cascade of several extracellular messengers implicated in diabetic renal injury (*see* Fig. 3, p.159), and most notably in expression of the cellular actions of Ang II *(79,84)*. Thus, a number of the cellular actions of Ang II are blocked by inhibitors of NADPH oxidase and in NADPH-oxidase knockout mouse models *(72,79,85,86)*.

As noted above, NADPH oxidase is upregulated in glomeruli of diabetic rats with proteinuria, as assessed by immunostaining of the p47 phox cytosolic component *(69)*. Treatment of the diabetic rats with either an ACEI or an angiotensin subtype-1 ARB suppressed the increases in immunoreactive NADPH oxidase and eNOS, as well as the increases in urinary protein excretion and indexes of oxidative and nitrosative stress *(69)*. Enhanced superoxide production via activation of NADPH oxidase in kidney in diabetes has also been postulated to have several consequences which contribute to the pathogenesis of DN. They include suppression of the bioavailability of NO *(66)*, increases in glomerular TGF-β_1 and matrix protein accumulation, and decreased expression of renal matrix metalloproteinases *(87)*.

Glucose Auto-Oxidation and Formation of AGE

AGE, predominantly NG-(carboxymethyl) lysine (CML), pentosidine, and pyrraline, can arise in excess in diabetes from sequential glycation and oxidation reactions termed glycooxidation or auto-oxidative glycosylation *(30,34,47,48,88,89)*. Formation of CML and pentosidine in particular depend on oxidative processes *(31)*.

Glucose and other reducing sugars can be auto-oxidized by metal-catalyzed oxidative processes that generate ROS and the reactive intermediate dicarbonyl, glyoxal (Fig. 2). The latter reacts with amino groups on protein to form CML *(90)*.

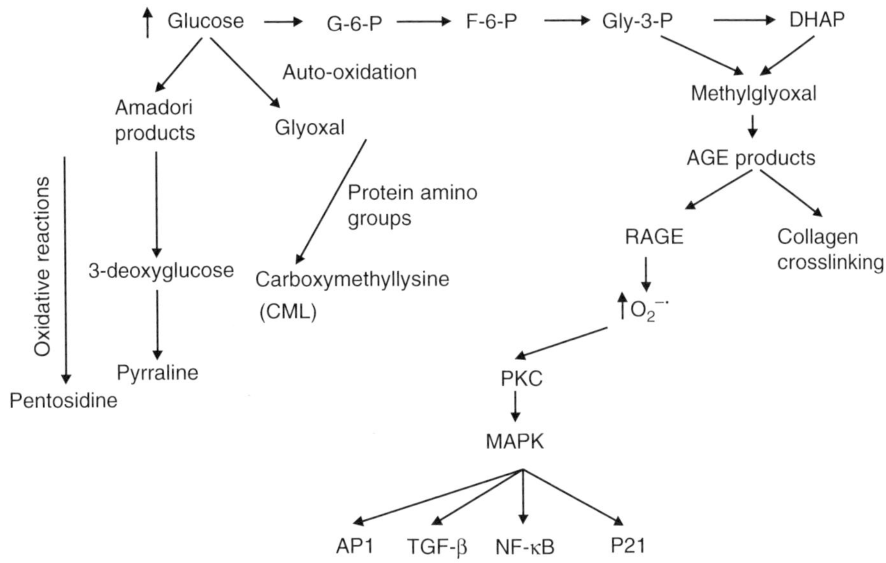

Fig. 2. Metabolic pathways in the formation of AGE. (For description, *see* text.) RAGE, receptor for AGE; MAPK, mitogen-activated protein kinase; AP1, activator protein 1; NF-κB, nuclear factor-κB. (For other abbreviations, *see* Fig. 1.)

Pentosidine is also formed from the Amadori product (glucose-derived 1-amino-1-deoxyfructose lysine adducts) by oxidative reactions *(31,91)*. The Amadori product may decompose to 3-deoxyglucosone, which reacts with amino groups of proteins to form pyrraline *(47)*. The reactive diacarbonyl intermediate methylglyoxal, which also participates in formation of AGE adducts, is generated from glyceraldehydes 3-phosphate and DHAP *(34)*. In renal biopsies obtained from humans with DN *(31)*, the glycooxidation products CML and pentosidine were colocalized by immunohistochemical staining with the lipid peroxidation product MDA (a marker of oxidative stress). These products were colocalized in the expanded glomerular mesangium and in thickened glomerular capillaries in early DN and in nodular glomerular accumulation of matrix and renal arteriolar walls in advanced DN *(31)*. By contrast, pyrraline did not colocalize with MDA in these areas. The findings suggest that accumulation, and presumably increased formation of at least some AGE reflects local oxidative stress *(31)*.

Formation of reactive AGE precursors may result in renal and other cell injury by a variety of mechanisms (Fig. 2) involving direct alterations of protein function and/or structure *(34,91,92)*. In DN, these include alterations in matrix proteins such as intermolecular crosslinking of collagen *(34,83,91,92)*. However, in addition to these effects, extracellular AGE-modified proteins also interact with several cell surface receptors *(33,34,93,94)*, including the receptor for AGE (RAGE), a multiligand member of the immunoglobulin superfamily of cell surface molecules *(33)*. Activation of RAGE increases ROS generation in EC and MC *(32,83,95)*. This increase (Fig. 2), which may be mediated via RAGE stimulation of NADPH oxidase, is part of a cell signaling cascade by which extracellular AGE activates PKC, mitogen-activated protein kinase, TGF-β and the pleiotropic gene transcription factors, nuclear factor (NF)-κB, activator protein 1, and p21 *(32–34,87)*.

Depletion of Endogenous Antioxidants and Altered Activity of Antioxidant Enzymes

Depletion of endogenous antioxidants and free radical scavengers may occur in diabetes *(28,96–101)*. In plasma or serum, lower levels of vitamins C, E, and A, lycopene, and lipoic acid have been reported in human diabetics compared with nondiabetic controls *(28,96–99,102–104)*. Similarly, impaired total serum antioxidant capacity and reduced antioxidant properties of serum albumin and high-density lipoprotein have been described in human diabetics *(102,105–109)*. In experimental diabetes, depletion of reduced glutathione occurs in kidney and other tissues *(36,49,70)*. Depletion of endogenous antioxidants and radical scavengers in diabetes may be a consequence rather than a cause of oxidative stress.

Depending on the tissue examined and the duration and severity of diabetes, activities of some antioxidant enzymes are reduced, whereas those of others are increased or unchanged *(14,38,110–117)*. Thus, activities of both cytosolic Cu^{2+}/Zn^{2+} SOD (SOD1) and mitochondrial Mn^{2+} SOD (SOD2) of neutrophils from diabetic human subjects are lower than corresponding values in nondiabetics *(111)*. In the kidney of streptozotocin (STZ) diabetic rats, the changes described in antioxidant enzyme activities have not been consistent. In one study *(113)*, renal activities of SOD1 and glutathione peroxidase increased, whereas SOD2 did not change 1–6 wk after induction of diabetes. Catalase activity in kidney from diabetic rats showed a biphasic response with an early increase at 1 wk and later decline to levels below that of control kidney *(113)*. In another report, increased mRNA levels for SOD1 and catalase were found in kidney from STZ diabetic rats, but enzyme activities were not examined *(38)*. In STZ diabetic and db/db mice with diabetes for 2–5 mo duration, renal cortical, SOD1, SOD2, and catalase activities did not differ from corresponding values of renal cortex from nondiabetics *(14,70)*. By contrast, after several months of diabetes, glutathione peroxidase activity of renal cortex from the diabetic mice was higher than the corresponding values from age-matched control mice. The potential roles of specific antioxidant enzymes in the pathogenesis of renal injury in diabetes, or in renoprotection, are at present incompletely understood. However, there is now evidence that genetic enhancement of SOD1 activity may be renoprotective in experimental diabetes *(14,70)*.

REDOX AND GLYCOOXIDATIVE REACTIONS IN THE PATHOGENESIS OF DIABETIC RENAL INJURY

Redox-Regulated Signaling Pathways

A characteristic feature of early and advanced DN is expansion of the glomerular mesangium, owing predominantly to deposition of extracellular matrix *(118)*. Indeed, in human DN, the severity of this histological change correlates best with loss of glomerular filtration rate *(118,119)*. Studies in cultured glomerular MCs have demonstrated that high ambient concentrations of glucose, Ang II, extracellular AGE proteins, and a thromboxane analog—all increase synthesis and reduce degradation of extracellular matrix proteins (ECMs) *(81,120–123)*. These same factors also have been implicated in the pathogenesis of glomerular mesangial expansion in vivo in experimental diabetes *(16,22,34,124–126)*. A central common mediator of the cellular actions of these agonists in MC matrix protein deposition is TGF-β_1 *(127–129)*. Redox reactions have been implicated in cell signaling pathways leading to increased production and release

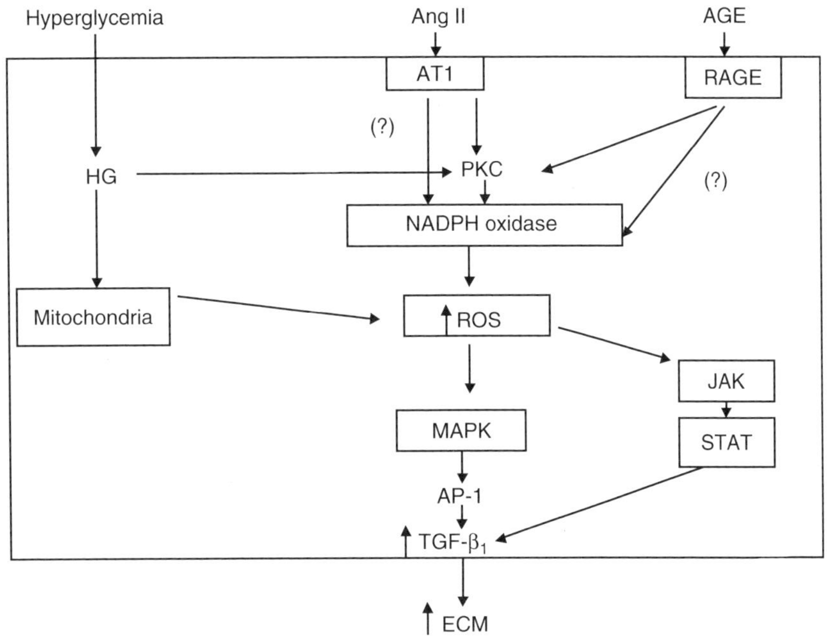

Fig. 3. Redox-regulated signaling of increased accumulation of extracellular matrix (ECM) in diabetes in response to high intracellular levels of glucose (HG), angiotensin II (Ang II), and AGE (for description, *see* text); AT1, angiotensin receptor type 1; ROS, reactive oxygen species; JAK, Janus family of protein kinases; STAT, signal transducers and activators of transcription. (For other abbreviations, *see* Fig. 2.)

of TGF-β_1 *(95,130–133)* and in the expression of at least some of the actions of TGF-β_1 *per se* in kidney *(41)*.

As summarized in Fig. 3, the expression of the actions of HG, Ang II, and AGE to signal increases in TGF-β_1 in matrix protein synthesis in MC involves ROS generation. There is evidence that the latter may be derived at least in part from activation of NADPH oxidase *(40,41,81,94,134,135)* in response to HG, Ang II, and AGE, and in the case of HG also from mitochondria *(41,42)*. Activation of NADPH oxidase by HG, Ang II, and AGE in MC may in turn be mediated via activation of PKC *(37,41,81,134)*. In support of this possibility, adenovirus-mediated overexpression of PKC-β_2 in cultured MC increases ROS *(37)*. However, studies suggest the converse is also true, namely, that activation of NADPH oxidase and the consequent increase in ROS leads to activation of PKC *(95,135)*. Accordingly, the interrelations of these two early steps in the signaling pathway are complex and may differ as a function of cell type.

In MC, evidence to support a key role for redox reactions in the increases in ECM induced by HG, Ang II, and AGE include (a) demonstration of increases in ROS generation in cultured MC in response to these agonists *(40–42,81,94,134,135)*; (b) suppression of increases in TGF-β_1 and ECM by inhibitors of NADPH oxidase *(41,81,134)*, and/or in the case of HG also by inhibitors mitochondrial electron transport *(41)*; and (c) suppression of increases in PKC activity, TGF-β_1, and/or ECM in cultured MC by a variety of exogenous antioxidants, or by overexpression of either SOD1 or SOD2 *(14,95,131,136,137)*. The actions of HG, Ang II, AGE, TXA_2 to activate NF-κB and specificity factor 1, and to increase monocyte chemoattractant protein-1 or PAI-1 in MC also involve redox mechanisms, as reflected by inhibition of these responses by antioxidants *(87)*. TGF-β_1 *per se* has been shown to enhance the transition of renal tubular epithelial cells to mesenchymal cells, a process implicated in the development of interstitial fibrosis in diabetes *(138)*. There is evidence that expression of this effect of TGF-β involves enhanced generation of ROS as part of the pathway which signals cell transition *(138)*.

In EC, as noted above, increased mitochondrial production of ROS in response to HG has been linked to activation of metabolic pathways that may mediate vascular injury in diabetes *(34,42)*. In this cascade (Fig. 1), superoxide suppresses GAPDH with diversion of upstream glycolytic metabolites into pathways which may mediate hyperglycemic damage, including activation of PKC and an increase in AGE formation *(34)*. In cultured bovine EC, benfotiamine, a lipid-soluble thiamine derivative, has recently been reported to suppress the actions of HG to activate PKC, the hexosamine pathway, and NF-κB, and to inhibit AGE formation *(139)*. Benfotiamine activates the pentose phosphate pathway enzyme transketolase, which converts the glycolytic intermediates glyceraldehydes 3-phosphate and fructose 6-phosphate to pentose 5-phosphates and other sugars. By this action, benfotiamine may reduce the availability of the glycolytic intermediates to activate PKC and several other pathways leading to hyperglycemic damage. Benfotiamine also suppressed the development of early retinopathy when administered to STZ diabetic rats *(139)*, but its effect on DN has not been examined.

Thus, multiple, redox-regulated signaling pathways may participate in the pathogenesis of renal cell injury in diabetes. Targeted interruption of one or more of these pathways may be protective against renal injury and other vascular complications of diabetes.

Interactions Between ROS and NO

Alterations in NO signaling in diabetes have been linked to hemodynamic and structural changes in the kidney. As recently reviewed in detail, the contribution of altered NO signaling to renal hemodynamic changes in diabetes is quite complex, incompletely understood, and may vary with the duration of the disease and other factors *(64)*. There is evidence that renal generation of both NO and superoxide are enhanced in diabetes *(14,28,39,70,140–143)*. An imbalance between renal NO and superoxide production in diabetes might lead to altered renal hemodynamic through several pathways (Fig. 4): (1) inactivation of NO via its reaction with superoxide may lead to vasoconstriction owing to loss of the vasodilator action of NO *(62)*; (2) excess superoxide production *per se*, independent of its inactivation of NO, may mediate renal vasoconstriction *(40)*; and (3) increased renal production of superoxide and its subsequent conversion to H_2O_2 by SOD may result in vasodilation mediated by H_2O_2 *(144)*. In vitro studies indicate that the relative kinetics of the two potential metabolic fates of superoxide above (i.e., inactivation by NO or conversion to H_2O_2 by SOD) favor the former pathway *(145)*. Nevertheless, the net renal hemodynamic impact of increased production of both NO and superoxide in diabetes cannot be readily predicted. At least early in experimental diabetes, enhanced renal NO production by neuronal NOS in the macula densa, eNOS or both may result in increased NO bioavailability, which contributes to renal vasodilation and glomerular hyperfiltration *(140,141)*. However, not all data support this conclusion *(62)*. Studies of Ang II-induced vasoconstriction of afferent arteriole isolated from diabetic rats illustrate the complexity of factors which may govern vasomotor responses in diabetes in addition to altered production rates and interactions between

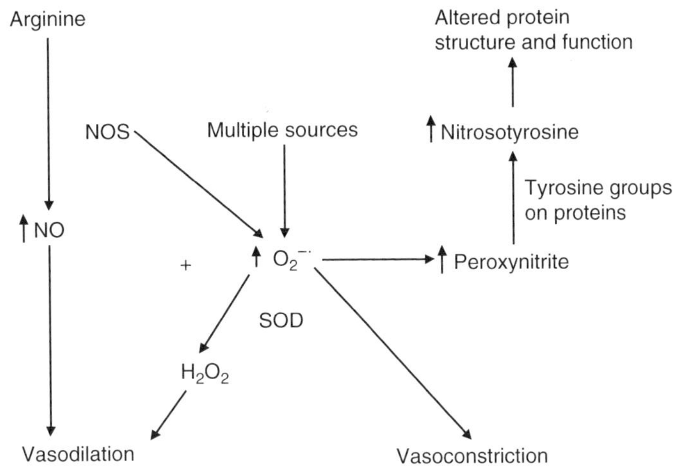

Fig. 4. Potential hemodynamic and cytotoxic effects of nitric oxide (NO)-superoxide interaction in diabetes. For description, *see* text. NOS, nitric oxide synthase; H_2O_2, hydrogen peroxide; SOD, superoxide dismutase.

NO and superoxide *(62)*. The results indicated that increased superoxide production in response to Ang II in afferent arterioles from diabetic rats attenuated the vasodilatory influence of endogenously produced NO *(62)*. Nevertheless, afferent arterioles from diabetic rats remained vasodilated after exposure to Ang II, presumably owing to a concurrent defect in expression of the action of Ang II to depolarize the cell membrane and open voltage-gated Ca^{2+} channels, a step essential to the vasoconstrictor response *(62)*. Clearly, the net effects of reactions between NO and superoxide on renal hemodynamics are highly complex and require further study.

NO also modulates the proliferation of MC and production of ECM in response to HG, Ang II, and other stimuli *(146–149)*. Thus, altered NO signaling may also participate in the expansion of glomerular mesangium characteristic of DN. In general, evidence in cultured MC and VSMC supports antiproliferative actions of NO and NO suppression of ECM protein production by MC *(146–152)*. Studies in cultured MC have shown that increases in endogenous NO production or NO donors can suppress several steps in the signaling cascade by which HG, Ang II, and TXA_2 increase ECM production, including activation of PKC and increases in TGF-β *(146,148,149)*. As noted above, some of these same agonists increase ROS generation in MC *(81,131,135)*. Thus, expression of the action of HG and Ang II to increase MC matrix protein may be owing, in part, to quenching of NO by ROS. This conclusion is supported by the action of antioxidants to potentiate NO suppression of MC synthesis of ECM in response to HG *(148)*. Observations in glomeruli isolated from rats or mice with either STZ or genetic (db/db mice) diabetes have demonstrated that NO-dependent increases in cGMP, induced by either cholinergic stimuli or exogenous NO donors, are suppressed compared with corresponding responses in glomeruli from nondiabetic rats *(70,153)*. Overexpression of SOD1 in glomeruli from db/db mice restores NO-dependent cGMP responses to levels seen in the glomeruli from nondiabetic mice *(70)*. Thus, the attenuated cGMP responses to NO observed in glomeruli from wild-type diabetic mice may be owing to quenching of NO by superoxide.

The reaction between NO and superoxide leads to the formation of peroxynitrite (Fig. 4), a reactive intermediate which nitrosylates tyrosine moieties of protein *(154)*.

The latter process may alter protein structure and function, and thus represents an additional pathway for cell injury under conditions in which both the generation of NO and superoxide are increased *(154)*. Enhanced accumulation of nitrotyrosine in tissues in diabetes is thus at least in part an index of increased peroxynitrite generation, which in turn may reflect increased generation of NO, superoxide, or both *(154)*. Nitrotyrosine accumulates in the kidney of rodents with STZ or genetic diabetes *(68,70,142,143)*, consistent with enhanced renal production of NO and/or superoxide *(154)*. Genetic overexpression of SOD1 in diabetic mice suppresses accumulation of nitrotyrosine in glomeruli to levels observed in nondiabetic, wild-type mice, and also attenuates renal injury in the diabetics. Thus, a reduction in the availability of superoxide to react with NO may be renoprotective in diabetes, in part by reducing formation of the toxic-reactive intermediate peroxynitrite *(70)*.

INVOLVEMENT OF REDOX AND GLYCO-OXIDATIVE MECHANISMS IN THE PATHOGENESIS OF DN IN VIVO

Evidence to support a role for oxidative and/or glycooxidative stress in the pathogenesis of DN in vivo has come largely from studies of the effects of inhibitors of AGE formation and those of conventional exogenous antioxidants on renal function and structure in experimental diabetes. There are only limited data on the effects of these same interventions on renal injury in human diabetes, and on the impact of genetically induced alterations in antioxidant enzymes on renal injury in diabetic animals. However, there is increasing recognition that the renoprotective actions of interventions of proven efficacy in human DN, notably those of ACEIs and ARBs, may involve or at least are associated with, reductions in oxidative stress and AGE formation *(142,143)*. Similarly, though not yet assessed with respect to DN, vascular protection afforded by statins in diabetics may be linked to antioxidant and anti-inflammatory, as well as lipid-lowering actions of these agents *(155)*. Thus, at least two classes of agents with established benefits in reducing vascular injury in diabetes, although not previously thought of as antioxidants, may in fact have antioxidant actions.

Inhibitors of AGE Formation and RAGE Blockade

In STZ diabetic rats, two structurally different inhibitors of AGE formation have been reported to ameliorate renal injury *(124,156–158)*. Aminoguanidine, the most extensively studied inhibitor of AGE formation, has been reported to prevent the development of albuminuria and mesangial matrix expansion, as well as renal accumulation of AGE *(124)*. Similarly, this agent has been reported to prevent retinal and neural injury in experimental diabetes *(34,159)*. In addition to its antioxidant properties, aminoguanidine also inhibits the activity of inducible NOS *(124,150, 157)*. However, a recent study suggests that its renoprotective actions in diabetes are owing largely to its antioxidant properties *(124)*. Clinical trials with aminoguanidine in human diabetics with nephropathy have found a reduction in proteinuria and retardation of loss of renal function *(34)*, but drug toxicity has complicated interpretation of these benefits *(6)*. Consistent with the possibility that extracellular AGE moieties may also mediate cellular injury in diabetes via cell surface receptors, administration of a soluble blocker of RAGE has been reported to attenuate renal and vascular injury in experimental diabetes *(160,161)*. Additional studies of this interventional approach are needed.

Antioxidant Therapy

The effects of dietary supplementation with exogenous antioxidants on renal injury in experimental diabetes have been extensively examined *(36,162–165)*. Agents studied include vitamins E and C, lipoic acid, and taurine *(36,162–165)*. Most studies have found renoprotective effects associated with evidence of reduced oxidative stress, including reduction in indices of renal lipid peroxidation and restoration of renal cortical levels of reduced glutathione *(36,162–165)*. Lipoic acid, in particular, has been shown not only to suppress albumin excretion, glomerular volume, and glomerular content of TGF-β and collagen (α_1) IV, but also to attenuate subsequent increases in mesangial matrix volume and glomerulosclerosis *(36,165)*. However, not all studies have found that conventional antioxidants ameliorate DN in experimental models *(163)*. The dose of antioxidants employed may be critical, perhaps because agents such as vitamin E may have either pro- or antioxidant effects in vivo *(164)*. Thus, potentiation of renal injury in diabetes has been reported with vitamin E in one study *(163)*. In another study, administration of antioxidants have been shown to improve some indices of end-organ injury in diabetes but worsen others *(166)*. In general, results of clinical trials employing conventional antioxidants for secondary prevention of macrovascular diseases in either diabetics or nondiabetic subjects, have shown no significant benefits *(167–171)*. Few clinical studies have specifically examined the effects of antioxidants on DN. These trials included small study groups and were relatively brief in duration. Thus, although antioxidant attenuation of proteinuria has been reported in short-term trials with diabetic subjects given either lipoic acid or a combination of vitamins C and E *(172,173)*, definitive data to support sustained benefits of these agents on the progression of DN are lacking.

Clinical trials with antioxidants in the secondary prevention of vascular disease have been disappointing. However, this does not necessarily negate a key role for redox mechanisms in the mediation of vascular injury in diabetes. Both the complexity of the cellular pathways involved and of the actions of the antioxidants tested should temper extrapolation of these negative outcomes to the conclusion that redox reactions do not participate in vascular injury in diabetes.

Genetic Alterations of SOD

The role of superoxide in the mediation of renal injury in diabetes in vivo has been assessed in transgenic mice which overexpress SOD1 *(14,70)*. SOD1-transgenic mice with either STZ-induced or genetic (db/db) diabetes were examined and alterations in renal function and structure compared with those in corresponding age-matched, wild-type diabetic mice. In these experimental mouse models of types 1 and 2 diabetes, overexpression of SOD-1 suppressed increases in urinary albumin excretion, glomerular volume, glomerular content of collagen IV, TGF-β and mesangial matrix volume compared with the corresponding values in diabetic wild-type mice. Overexpression of SOD-1 in the diabetic mice was associated with decreases in renal cortical accumulation of MDA and/or higher GSH levels, indices of reduced renal oxidative stress *(14,70)*. Overall, these findings support a role for superoxide in the pathogenesis of renal injury in vivo in diabetes. Conversely, in STZ diabetic mice with reduced expression of SOD1 (homozygous SOD1 knockouts) renal injury is accelerated compared with the wild-type diabetic counterparts (unpublished), further supporting a role for superoxide in the pathogenesis of DN. Of note, the GFR of diabetic mice which overexpressed SOD-1 was higher that that of the diabetic wild-type mice before, but not after, treatment with a NOS inhibitor; the latter reduced GFR in the transgenic but not the wild-type diabetics. These findings implied that the higher GFR in the diabetic mice overexpressing SOD1 was at least in part dependent on NO *(70)*. Ex vivo studies of glomeruli from the wild-type db/db mice demonstrated impaired cGMP responses to both endogenously generated NO and to exogenous NO donors compared with corresponding responses of glomeruli from nondiabetic mice *(70)*. By contrast, cGMP responses to endogenous and exogenous NO of glomeruli from db/db mice which overexpress SOD1 did not differ from those of glomeruli from nondiabetic mice *(70)*. The renoprotection observed in the db/db mice which overexpressed SOD-1 was thus associated with evidence of increased NO action on GFR in vivo and enhanced bioavailability of glomerular NO ex vivo, possibly owing to reduced quenching of NO by superoxide. The latter possibility was supported by the finding that the nitrotyrosine content of glomeruli from diabetic mice which overexpress SOD1 was significantly lower than that of the nontransgenic db/db mice, an index of reduced glomerular peroxynitrite formation in the SOD1 overexpressors *(70)*. An interaction between NO and superoxide in the regulation of systemic blood pressure and GFR in STZ diabetic rats has also been described *(174)*. Thus, chronic administration of the NOS inhibitor L-NAME induces systemic hypertension and reduces GFR in the diabetic rats. These changes are reversed by chronic treatment with the SOD mimetic tempol *(174)*.

CONCLUSIONS

DN is the leading cause of end-stage renal disease in most developed nations. Mounting evidence supports a role for oxidative and glyco-oxidative stress in the pathogenesis of DN and other diabetic complications. Multiple metabolic processes participate in the increased generation of ROS, reactive dicarbyonyl species, or both in diabetes. Sources include (a) increased mitochondrial electron transport activity induced by hyperglycemia and fatty acids, (b) increased production of superoxide relative to nitric oxide (NO) by "uncoupled" eNOS; (c) activation of nonphagocytic cell NADH/NADPH oxidase by hyperglycemia and Ang II; (d) increased glucose auto-oxidation, and several others. Moreover, interactions among different sources of ROS have been described, which may further amplify cellular production of ROS in diabetes *(175,176)*. An example is oxidative degradation of the eNOS cofactor tetrahydobiopterin by ROS derived from several sources *(176)*. This in turn leads to uncoupling of eNOS and consequent enhanced superoxide generation by the enzyme *(176)*. Increased production of ROS in diabetes may result in renal injury and other complications by direct cytotoxic actions or via overexpression of physiological redox regulated signaling pathways, such as Ang II activation of NADPH oxidase.

Among the consequences of increased superoxide production by glomerular cells in diabetes are inactivation of NO and enhanced formation of the highly reactive radical peroxynitrite. In addition to direct renal cytotoxic actions of peroxynitrite, reduced availability of NO as a consequence of its reaction with superoxide may contribute to renal hemodynamic changes, and to increases in matrix production by MCs which results in the expansion of the glomerular mesangium, characteristic of DN. Therapeutic interventions targeted at interruption of redox-mediated signaling pathways, ROS-mediated cytotoxicity, and/or the interaction of superoxide with NO have shown renoprotective effects in experimental DN. These include exogenous antioxidants such as lipoic acid and genetic overexpression of superoxide dismutase. However, the clinical efficacy and safety of antioxidant interventions in the prevention or treatment of human DN remain to be demonstrated.

REFERENCES

1. U.S. Renal Data System, USRDS 2003 Annual Data Report: Atlas of End-Stage Renal Disease in the United States, National Institutes of Health, National Institute of Diabetes and Digestive and Kidney Diseases, Bethesda, MD, 2004.
2. Valmadrid CT, Klein R, Moss SE, Klein BEK. The risk of cardiovascular disease mortality associated with microalbuminuria and gross proteinuria in persons with older onset diabetes mellitus. Arch Intern Méd 2000;160:1093–1100.
3. Gerstein HC, Mann JFE, Yi Q, et al. Albuminuria and risk of cardiovascular events, death, and heart failure in diabetic and nondiabetic individuals. The HOPE Study Investigators. JAMA 2001;286: 421–426.
4. Ritz E, McClellan WM. Overview: increased cardiovascular risk in patients with minor renal dysfunction: an emerging issue with far-reaching consequences. J Am Soc Nephrol 2004;15:513–516.
5. Collins AJ, Li S, Gilbertson DT, Liu J, Chen SC, Herzog CA. Chronic kidney disease and cardiovascular disease in the medical population. Kidney Int 2003;87:S24–S31.
6. Sheetz MJ, King GL. Molecular understanding of hyperglycemia's adverse effects for diabetic complications. JAMA 2002;288:2579–2588.
7. Harrison DG. Cellular and molecular mechanisms of endothelial cell dysfunction. J Clin Invest 1997;100:2153–2157.
8. Sequist ER, Goetz FC, Rich S, Barbosa J. Familial clustering of diabetic kidney disease. Evidence for genetic susceptibility to diabetic nephropathy. N Engl J Med 1989;320:1161–1165.
9. Viberti G. Why do we invoke genetic susceptibility for diabetic nephropathy? Kidney Int 1999;55:2526–2527.
10. Vardarli I, Baier LJ, Hanson RL, et al. Gene for susceptibility to diabetic nephropathy in type 2 diabetes maps to 18q22.3–33. Kidney Int 2002;62:2176–2183.
11. Neuberger S, Baba T, Wantanabe T. Association of nitric oxide synthase gene polymorphism with an increased risk for progression to diabetic nephropathy in type 2 diabetes. Diabetes 2000;49: 500–503.
12. O'Bryan GT, Hostetter TH. The renal hemodynamic basis of diabetic nephropathy. Semin Nephrol 1997;17:93–100.
13. Cortes P, Zhao X, Riser BL, Narins RG. Role of glomerular mechanical strain in the pathogenesis of diabetic nephropathy. Kidney Int 1997;51:57–68.
14. Craven PA, Melhem MF, Phillips SL, DeRubertis FR. Overexpression of Cu^{2+}/Zn^{2+} superoxide dismutase protects against early diabetic glomerular injury in transgenic mice. Diabetes 2001;50: 2114–2125.
15. Vats A, DeRubertis F. The kidney: diabetic nephropathy: contemporary endocrinology: type 1 diabetes: etiology and treatment. In: Sperling, MA, ed. Humana, Totowa, NJ, 2003, pp. 409–436.
16. DCCT Research Group. The effect of intensive treatment of diabetes on the development and progression of long-term complications in insulin-dependent diabetes mellitus. N Engl J Med 1993;329:977–986.
17. United Kingdom Prospective Diabetes Study (UKPDS). Intensive blood-glucose control with sulphonylurea or insulin compared to conventional treatment and risk of complications in patients with type 2 diabetes (UKPDS 33). Lancet 1998;38:516–523.
18. Mauer SM, Goetz FC, McHugh CE. Long term studies of normal kidneys transplanted into patients with type 1 diabetes. Diabetes 1989;38:516–523.
19. Kasiske BL, Kalil RS, Ma JZ, Liao M, Keane WF. Effect of antihypertensive therapy on the kidney in patients with diabetes: a meta-regression analysis. Ann Intern Med 1993;118:129–138.
20. UK Prospective Diabetes Study Group. Efficacy of atenolol and captopril in reducing the risk of macrovascular complications in type 2 diabetes (UKPDS 39). Br Med J 1998;317:713–720.
21. Ravid M, Lang R, Rachmani R, Lishner M. Long-term renoprotective effect of angiotensin-converting enzyme inhibition in non-insulin-dependent diabetes mellitus: a 7-year follow-up study. Arch Intern Med 1996;156:286–289.

22. Lewis EJ, Hunsicker LG, Bain RP, Rohde RD, Collaborative Study Group. The effect of angiotensin-converting-enzyme inhibition on diabetic nephropathy. N Engl J Med 1993;118:129–138.
23. Parving HH, Rossing P, Hommel E, Smidt UM. Angiotensin-converting enzyme inhibition in diabetic nephropathy: ten years' experience. Am J Kidney Dis 1995;26:99–107.
24. Laffel LMB, McGill JB, Gans DJ, North American Microalbuminuria Study Group. The beneficial effect of angiotensin-converting enzyme inhibition with captopril on diabetic nephropathy in normotensive IDDM patients with microalbuminuria. Am J Med 1995;99:497–504.
25. Brenner BM, Cooper ME, de Zeeuw D, et al. Effects of losartan on renal and cardiovascular outcomes in patients with type 2 diabetes and nephropathy. N Eng J Med 2001;345:861–869.
26. Parving HH, Lehnert H, Brochner-Mortensen J, Gomis R, Andersen S, Arner P. The effect of irbesartan on the development of diabetic nephropathy in patients with type 2 diabetes. N Engl J Med 2001;345:870–878.
27. Fried LF, Orchard TJ, Kasiske BL. Effect of lipid reduction on the progression of renal disease: a meta-analysis. Kidney Int 2001;59:260–269.
28. Evans JL, Goldfine D, Maddux BA, Grodsky GM. Oxidative stress and stress-activated signaling pathways: a unifying hypothesis of type 2 diabetes. Endocr Rev 2002;23(5):599–622.
29. Baynes JW, Thorpe SR. The role of oxidative stress in diabetic complications. Curr Opin Endocrinol 1996;3:277–284.
30. Baynes JW, Thorpe SR. Role of oxidative stress in diabetic complications: a new perspective on an old paradigm. Diabetes 1999;48:1–9.
31. Horie K, Miyata T, Maeda, K, Miyata S, et al. Immunohistochemical colocalization of glycooxidation products and lipid peroxidation products in diabetic renal glomerular lesions. J Clin Invest 1997;12:2995–3004.
32. Wendt T, Tanji N, Guo J, et al. Glucose, glycation, and RAGE: implications for amplification of cellular dysfunction in diabetic nephropathy. J Am Soc Nephrol 2003;14:1383–1395.
33. Wautier M-P, Chappey O, Corda S, Stern DM, Schmidt AM, Wautier JL. Activation of NADPH oxidase by AGE links oxidant stress to altered gene expression via RAGE. Am J Physiol Endocrinol Metab 2001;280:E685–E694.
34. Brownlee M. Biochemistry and molecular cell biology of diabetic complications. Nature 2001;414:813–820.
35. Dickinson PJ, Carrington AL, Frost GS, Boulton AJM. Neurovascular disease, antioxidants and glycation in diabetes. Diabetes Metab Res Rev 2002;18:260–272.
36. Melhem MF, Craven PA, Liachenko J, DeRubertis FR. α-Lipoic acid attenuates hyperglycemia and prevents glomerular mesangial matrix expansion in diabetes. J Am Soc Nephrol 2002;13: 108–116.
37. Kitada M, Koya D, Sugimoto T, et al. Translocation of glomerular p47phox and p67phox by protein kinase C-β activation is required for oxidative stress in diabetic nephropathy. Diabetes 2003;52: 2603–2614.
38. Koya D, Hayashi K, Munehiro K, Kashiwagi A, Kikkawa R, Haneda M. Effects of antioxidants in diabetes-induced oxidative stress in the glomeruli of diabetic rats. J Am Soc Nephrol 2003;14: S250–S253.
39. Finkel T, Holbrook N. Oxidants, oxidative stress and the biology of ageing. Nature 2000;408: 239–247.
40. Schnackenberg CG. Physiological and pathophysiological roles of oxygen radicals in the renal microvasculature. Am J Physiol Regul Integrat Comp Physiol 2002;282:R335–R342.
41. Lee HB, Yu M-R, Yang Y, Jiang Z, Ha H. Reactive oxygen species-regulated signaling pathways in diabetic nephropathy. J Am Soc Nephrol 2003;14:S241–S245.
42. Nishikawa T, Edelstein D, Du XL, et al. Normalizing mitochondrial superoxide production blocks three pathways of hyperglycaemic damage. Nature 2000;404:787–790.
43. Yamagishi S-I, Guzman M, Brownlee M. Leptin induces mitochondrial superoxide production and monocyte chemoattractant protein-1 expression in aortic endothelial cells by increasing fatty acid oxidation via protein kinase A. J Biol Chem 2001;276(27):25,096–25,100.
44. Vasquez-Vivar J, Kalyanaraman B, Martasek P, et al. Superoxide generation by endothelial nitric oxide synthase: the influence of cofactors. Proc Natl Acad Sci USA 1998;95:9220–9225.
45. Zia Y, Tsai AL, Berka V, Zweier JL. Superoxide generation from endothelial nitric-oxide synthase. A Ca^{2+}/calmodulin-dependent and tetrahydrobiopterin regulatory process. J Biol Chem 1998;273: 25,804–25,808.
46. Li J-M, Shah AM. ROS generation by nonphagocytic NADPH oxidase: potential relevance in diabetic nephropathy. J Am Soc Nephrol 2003;14:S221–S226.

47. Wolff SP, Dean RT. Glucose autooxidation and protein modification. The potential role of autoxidative glycosylation in diabetes. Biochem J 1987;245:205–212.
48. Hunt JV, Dean RT, Wolff SP. Hydroxyl radical production and autoxidative glycosylation: glucose autooxidation as the cause of protein damage in the experimental glycation model of diabetes mellitus and aging. Biochem J 1988;256:9889–9897.
49. Desco MC, Asensi M, Marquez R, et al. Xanthine oxidase is involved in free radical production in type 1 diabetes: protection by allopurinol. Diabetes 2002;51:1118–1124.
50. Hannon-Fletcher MP, O'Kane MJ, Moles KW, Barnett YA, Barnett CR. Lymphocyte cytochrome P450-CYP2E1 expression in human IDDM subjects. Food Chem Toxicol 2001;39:125–132.
51. Haneda M, Koya D, Isono M, Kikkawa R. Overview of glucose signaling in mesangial cells in diabetic nephropathy. J Am Soc Nephrol 2003;14:1374–1382.
52. Wallace DC. Diseases of the mitochondrial DNA. Annu Rev Biochem 1992;61:1175–1212.
53. Trumpower BL. The protonmotive Q cycle. J Biol Chem 1990;265:11,409–11,412.
54. Korshunov SS, Sikulachev VP, Starkov AA. High protonic potential actuates a mechanism of production of reactive oxygen species in mitochondria. FEBS Lett 1997;416:15–18.
55. Sharma K, Ziyadeh FN. Hyperglycemia and diabetic kidney disease: the case for transforming growth factor-(beta) as a key mediator. Diabetes 1995;44:1139–1146.
56. Kolm-Litty V, Sauer U, Nerlich A, Lehmann R, Schleicher ED. High glucose-induced transforming growth factor beta1 production is mediated by the hexosamine pathway in porcine glomerular mesangial cells. J Clin Invest 1998;101:160–169.
57. Garcia Soriano F, Virag L, Jagtap P, et al. Diabetic endothelial dysfunction: the role of poly(ADP-ribose) polymerase activation. Nat Med 2001;7:108–113.
58. Kiritoshi S, Nishikawa T, Sonda K, et al. Reactive oxygen species from mitochondria induce cyclooxygenase-2 gene expression in human mesangial cells. Potential role in diabetic nephropathy. Diabetes 2003;52:2570–2577.
59. Raij L, Baylis C. Glomerular actions of nitric oxide. Kidney Int 1995;48:20–32.
60. Moncada S, Palmer RM, Higgs EA. Nitric oxide: Physiology, pathophysiology, and pharmacology. Pharmacol Rev 1991;43:109–142.
61. Rabelink TJ, Bakris GL. The renin-angiotensin system in diabetic nephropathy: the endothelial connection. Miner Electrolyte Metab 1998;24:381–388.
62. Schoonmaker GC, Fallet RW, Carmines PK. Superoxide anion curbs nitric oxide modulation of afferent arteriolar ANG II responsiveness in diabetes mellitus. Am J Physiol Renal Physiol 2000;278: F302–F309.
63. Pieper GM, Peltier BA. Amelioration by L-arginine of a dysfunctional arginine/nitric oxide pathway in diabetic endothelium. J Cardiovas Pharmacol 1995;25:398–403.
64. Komers R, Anderson S. Paradoxes of nitric oxide in the diabetic kidney. Am J Physiol Renal Fluid, Electrolyte Physiol 2003;284:1121–1137.
65. Cosentino F, Hishikawa K, Katusic ZS, Luscher TF. High glucose increases nitric oxide synthase expression and superoxide anion generation in human aortic endothelial cells. Circulation 1997;96:25–28.
66. Hink U, Li H, Mollnau H, et al. Mechanisms underlying endothelial dysfunction in diabetes mellitus. Circ Res 2001;88:E14–E22.
67. Piper GM. Review of alterations in endothelial nitric oxide production in diabetes: protective role of arginine on endothelial dysfunction. Hypertension 1998;31:1047–1060.
68. Ishii N, Patel KP, Lane PH, et al. Nitric oxide synthesis and oxidative stress in the renal cortex of rats with diabetes mellitus. J Am Soc Nephrol 2001;12:1630–1639.
69. Onozato ML, Tojo A, Goto A, Wilcox CS. Oxidative stress and nitric oxide synthase in rat diabetic nephropathy. Effects of ACEI and ARB. Kidney Int 2002;61:186–194.
70. DeRubertis FR, Craven PA, Melhem MF, Salah EM. Attenuation of renal injury in db/db mice overexpressing superoxide dismutase: evidence for reduced superoxide-nitric oxide interaction. Diabetes 2004;53:762–768.
71. Babior BM, Lambeth JD, Nauseef W. The neutrophil NADPH oxidase. Arch Biochem Biophys 2002;397:342–344.
72. Griendling KK, Sorescu D, Ushio-Fukkai M. NAD(P)H oxidase: Role in cardiovascular biology and disease. Circ Res 2000;86:494–501.
73. Jones SA, Hancock JT, Jones OT, Neubauer A, Topley N. The expression of NADPH oxidase components in human glomerular mesangial cells: detection of protein and mRNA for p47phox, p67phox and p22phox. J Am Soc Nephrol 1995;5:1483–1491.

74. Hattori M, Sakaki Y, Suminmoto H. A novel superoxide-producing NAD(P)H oxidase in kidney. J Biol Chem 2001;276:1417–1423.
75. Geiszt M, Kopp JB, Varnai P, Leto TL. Identification of renox, an NAD(P)H oxidase in kidney. Proc Natl Acad Sci USA 2000;97:8010–8014.
76. Li J-M, Shah AM. Intracellular localization and pre-assembly of the NADPH oxidase complex in cultured endothelial cells. J Biol Chem 2002;277:19,952–19,960.
77. Baraktutan U, Blayney L, Shah AM. Molecular characterization and localization of the NAD(P)H oxidase components gp91-phox and p22-phox in endothelial cells. Arterioscler Thromb Vasc Biol 2000;1903–1911.
78. Zou A-P, Ningjun L, Cowley AW. Production and actions of superoxide in the renal medulla. Hypertension 2001;37:547–553.
79. Griendling KK, Ushio-Fukai M. Reactive oxygen species as mediators of angiotensin II signaling. Cardiovasc Res 2000;91:21–27.
80. Berry C, Hamilton CA, Brosnan MJ, et al. Investigation into the sources of superoxide in human blood vessels. Circulation 2000;101:2206–2212.
81. Jaimes EA, Galceran JM, Raij L. Angiotensin II induced superoxide anion production by mesangial cells. Kidney Int 1998;54:775–784.
82. Li J-M, Mullen AM, Yun S, et al. Essential role of the NADPH oxidase subunit p47 Phox in endothelial cell superoxide production in response to phorbol ester and tumor necrosis factor-α. Circ Res 2002;90:143–150.
83. Forbes JM, Cooper ME, Oldfield MD, Thomas MC. Role of advanced glycation end products in diabetic Nephropathy. J Am Soc Nephrol 2003;14:5254–5258.
84. Mollnau H, Wendt M, Szocs K, et al. Effect of angiotensin II infusion on the expression and function of NAD(P)H oxidase and components of nitric oxide/cGMP signaling. Circ Res 2002;90:E58–E65.
85. Kappert K, Schmidt G, Doerr G, Wollert-Wulf B, Fleck E, Graf K. Angiotensin II and PDGF-BB stimulate β1-integrin-mediated adhesion and spreading in human VSMCs. Hypertension 2000;35:255–261.
86. Bendall JK, Cave AC, Heymes C, Gall N, Shah AM. Pivotal role of pg91-phox-containing NADPH oxidase in angiotentin II-induced cardiac hypertrophy in mice. Circulation 2002;105:293–296.
87. Lee HB, Yu M, Yang Y, Jiang Z, Ha H. Reactive oxygen species-regulated signaling pathways in diabetic nephropathy. J Am Soc Nephrol 2003;14:S241–S245.
88. Wells-Knecht KJ, Zyzak DV, Litchfield SR, Thorpe SR, Baynes JW. Mechanism of autoxidative glycosylation: identification of proteins by glucose. Biochemistry 1995;34:3702–3709.
89. Glomb MA, Monnier VM. Mechanism of protein modification by glyoxal and glycoaldehyde reactive intermediates of the Maillard reaction. J Biol Chem 1995;270:10,017–10,026.
90. Baynes JW. Perspectives in diabetes: role of oxidative stress in development of complications in diabetes. Diabetes 1991;40:405–412.
91. Ahmed MU, Thorpe SR, Baynes JW. Identification of N-carboxymethyllysine as a degradation product of fructoselysine in glycated protein. J Biol Chem 1986;261:4889–4894.
92. Monnier VAM, Sell DR, Nagaraj RH, et al. Maillard reaction-mediated molecular damage to extracellular matrix and other tissue proteins in diabetes, aging, and uremia. Diabetes 1992;41:36–41.
93. Neeper M, Schmidt AM, Brett J, et al. Cloning and expression of a cell surface receptor for advanced glycosylation end products of proteins. J Biol Chem 1992;267:14,998–15,004.
94. Skolnick EY, Zang Z, Makita Z, Radoff S, Kirstein M, Vlassara H. Human and rat mesangial cell receptors for glucose-modified proteins: potential role in kidney tissue remodeling and diabetic nephropathy. J Exp Med 1991;174:931–939.
95. Lal MA, Brismar H, Eklof A-C, Aperia A. Role of oxidative stress in advanced glycation end product-induced mesangial cell activation. Kidney Int 2002;61:2006–2014.
96. Maxwell SRJ, Thomason H, Sandler D, et al. Antioxidant status in patients with uncomplicated insulin-dependent and non-insulin-dependent diabetes mellitus. Eur J Clin Invest 1997;27:484–490.
97. Salonen JT, Nyyssonen K, Tuomainen TP, et al. Increased risk of non-insulin dependent diabetes mellitus at low plasma vitamin E concentrations: a four year follow up study in men. BMJ 1995;311: 1124–1127.
98. Shigeta Y, Hiraizumi G, Wada M, Oji K, Yoshida T. Study on the serum level of thioctic acid in patients with various diseases. J Vitaminol (Kyoto) 1961;7:48–52.
99. Packer L, Witt EH, Tritschler HJ. [alpha]-Lipoic acid as a biological antioxidant. Free Radic Biol Med 1995;19:227–250.
100. Cameron NE, Cotter MA. Potential therapeutic approaches to the treatment and prevention of diabetic neuropathy: evidence from experimental studies. Diabet Med 1993;10:593–605.

101. Cameron NE, Cotter MA. Effects of antioxidants on nerve and vascular dysfunction in experimental diabetes. Diabetes Res Clin Pract 1999;45:137–146.
102. Upritchard JE, Sutherland W, Mann JL. Effect of supplementation with tomato juice, vitamin E and vitamin C on LDL oxidation and products of inflammatory activity in type 2 diabetes. Diabetes Care 2000;23:733–738.
103. Basu TK, Basuald C. Vitamin A homeostasis and diabetes mellitus. Nutrition 1997;13:804–806.
104. Ford ES, Will JC, Bowman BA, Narayan KM. Diabetes mellitus and serum carotenoids, findings from the third national health and nutrition examination survey. Am J Epidemiol 1999;149:168–176.
105. Wen Y, Sahni A, Rea C, Zhang X, Khokher MA, Singh BM. Differential antioxidant status among Indo Asians compared with Caucasians with and without diabetes. Diabetes Care 2000;22: 254–255.
106. Opara EC, Abdel-Rahman E, Soliman S, et al. Depletion of total antioxidant capacity in type 2 diabetes. Metabolism 1999;48:1414–1417.
107. Bourdon E, Loreau N, Blache D. Glucose and free radicals impair the antioxidant properties of serum albumin, FASEB J 1999;13:233–244.
108. Lyons TJ. Lipoprotein glycation and its metabolic consequences. Diabetes 1999;41(2):67–73.
109. Ren S, Shen GX. Impact of antioxidants and HDL on glycated LDL-induced generation of fibrinolytic regulators from vascular endothelial cells. Arterioscler Thromb Vasc Biol 2000;20:1688–1693.
110. Vijayalingam S, Parthiban A, Shanmugasundaram KR, Mohan V. Abnormal antioxidant status in impaired glucose tolerance and non insulin dependent diabetes mellitus. Diabet Med 1996;13: 715–719.
111. Nath N, Chari SN, Rathi AB. Superoxide dismutase in diabetic polymorphonuclear leukocytes. Diabetes 1984;33:586–589.
112. Volkovova K, Chorvathova V, Jurcovicova M, Kosezeghyova L. Antioxidative state of myocardium and kidneys in acute diabetic rats. Physiol Res 1993;42:251–255.
113. Kakkar R, Mantha SV, Radhi J, Prasad K, Kalra J. Antioxidant defense system in diabetic kidney: a time course study. Life Sci 1997;60:667–679.
114. Wohaieb S, Godin DV. Alterations in free radical tissue defense mechanisms in streptozotocin induced diabetes in rat: effects of insulin treatment. Diabetes 1987;36:1014–1018.
115. Dohi T, Kawamura K, Morita K, Okamoto H, Tsujimoto A. Alterations of the plasma selenium concentrations and the activities of tissue peroxide metabolising enzymes in streptozotocin-induced diabetic rats. Horm Metab Res 1988;20:671–675.
116. Asayama K, Hayashibe H, Dobashi K, Nitsu T, Miyao A, Kato K. Antioxidant enzyme status and lipid peroxidation in various tissues of diabetic and starved rats. Diabetes Res 1989;12:85–105.
117. Kakkar R, Kalra J, Mantha SV, Orasad K. Lipid peroxidation and activity of antioxidant enzymes in diabetic rats. Mol Cell Biochem 1995;151:113–119.
118. Caramori ML, Mauer M. Diabetes and nephropathy. Cur Opin Nephrol Hypertens 2003;12(3): 273–282.
119. Caramori ML, Fioretto P, Mauer M. Low glomerular filtration rate in normoalbuminuric type 1 diabetic patients: an indicator of more advanced glomerular lesions. Diabetes 2003;52(4):1036–1040.
120. Ziyadeh FN, Sharma K, Ericksen M, Wolf G. Stimulation of collagen gene expression and protein synthesis in murine mesangial cells by high glucose is mediated by activation of transforming growth factor-β. J Clin Invest 1994;93:536–542.
121. Wolf G, Haberstroh U, Neilson EG. Angiotensin II stimulates the proliferation and biosynthesis of Type I collagen in cultured murine mesangial cells. Am J Pathol 1992;140:95–107.
122. Kim YS, Kim BC, Song CY, Hong HK, Moon KC, Lee HS. Advanced glycosylation end products stimulate collagen mRNA synthesis in mesangial cells mediated by protein kinase C and transforming growth factor-beta. J Lab Clin Med 2001;138:59–68.
123. Studer RK, DeRubertis FR, Craven PA. Nitric oxide suppresses increases in mesangial cell protein kinase C, transforming growth factor B and fibronectin synthesis induced by thromboxane. J Am Soc Nephrol 1996;7:999–1005.
124. Soulis-Liparota T, Cooper M, Papazoglou D, Clarke B, Jerums G. Retardation by aminoguanidine of development of albuminuria, mesangial expansion and tissue fluorescence in streptozotocin induced diabetic rat. Diabetes 1999;40:1328–1334.
125. Soulis T, Cooper ME, Sastra S, et al. Relative contributions of advanced glycation and nitric oxide synthase inhibition to aminoguanidine mediated renoprotection in diabetic rats. Diabetologia 1997;40:1141–1151.
126. Craven PA, Melhem MF, DeRubertis FR. Thromboxane in the pathogenesis of glomerular injury in diabetes. Kidney Int 1992;42:937–946.

127. Sharma K, Ziyadeh FN. Biochemical events and cytokine interactions linking glucose metabolism to the development of diabetic nephropathy, Semin Nephrol 1997;17:80–92.
128. Ziyadeh FN, Hoffmann BB, Han DC, et al. Long-term prevention of renal insufficiency, excess matrix gene expression and glomerular mesangial matrix expansion by treatment with monoclonal anti-transforming growth factor-beta antibody in db/db diabetic mice. Proc Natl Acad Sci USA 2000;97: 8015–8021.
129. Border W, Yamamoto T, Noble NA. Transforming growth factor-beta in diabetic nephropathy. Diabetes Metab Rev 1996;12:309–339.
130. Nath KA, Grande J, Croatt A, Haugen J, Kim Y, Rosenberg ME. Redox regulation of renal DNA synthesis, transforming growth factor-beta1 and collagen gene expression. Kidney Int 1998;53:367–381.
131. Ha H, Lee HB. Reactive oxygen species as glucose signaling molecules in mesangial cells cultured under high glucose. Kidney Int 2000;77:S19–S25.
132. Iglesias-de la Cruz MC, Ruiz-Torres P, Alcami J, et al. Hydrogen peroxide increases extracellular matrix mRNA through TGF beta in human mesangial cells. Kidney Int 2001;59:87–95.
133. Wilmer WA, Dixon CL, Hebert C, Lu L, Rovin BH. PPAR-alpha ligands inhibit H2O2 mediated activation of transforming growth factor beta1 in human mesangial cells. Antioxidants Redox Signaling 2002;4:877–884.
134. Yoo CW, Song Cy, Kim BC, Hong HK, Lee HS. Glycated albumin induces superoxide generation in mesangial cells. Cell Physiol Biochem 2004;14:361–368.
135. Hua H, Munk S, Goldberg H, Fantus IG, Whiteside CI. High glucose-suppressed endothelin-1 Ca^{2+} signaling via NADPH oxidase and diacylglycerol-sensitive protein kinase C isozymes in mesangial cells. J Biol Chem 2003;278:33,951–33,962.
136. Craven P, Phillips S, Melhem M, Liachenko J, DeRubertis FR. Overexpression of Mn2+ superoxide dismutase suppresses increases in collagen accumulation induced by culture of mesangial cells in high media glucose. Metabolism 2001;50:1043–1048.
137. Studer RK, Craven PA, DeRubertis FR. Antioxidant inhibition of protein kinase C-signaled increases in transforming growth factor-beta in mesangial cells. Metabolism 1997;46:918–925.
138. Yang Y, Ha H, Lee HB. Role of reactive oxygen species in TGF β induced epithelial to mesenchymal transition. Nephrol Dial Transplant 2003;18(4):300.
139. Hammes HP, Du X, Edelstein D, et al. Benfotiamine blocks three major pathways of hyperglycemic damage and prevents experimental diabetic retinopathy. Nat Med 2003;9:294–299.
140. Bank N, Aynedijan HS. Role of EDRF in diabetic renal hyperfiltration. Kidney Int 1993;43: 1306–1312.
141. Komers R, Allen TJ, Cooper ME. Role of endothelium derived nitric oxide in the pathogenesis of the renal hemodynamic changes of experimental diabetes. Diabetes 1997;43:1190–1197.
142. Onozato ML, Tojo A, Goto A, Fujita T, Wilcox CS. Oxidative stress and nitric oxide synthase in rat diabetic nephropathy: effects of ACE-I and ARB. Kidney Int 2002;61:186–194.
143. Forbes JM, Cooper ME, Thallas V, et al. Reduction of the accumulation of advanced glycation end products by ACE inhibition in experimental diabetic nephropathy. Diabetes 2002;51:3 274–3282.
144. Burke TM, Wolin MS. Hydrogen peroxide elicits pulmonary arterial relaxation and guanylate cyclase activation. Am J Physiol 1987;252:H721–H732.
145. Kojda G, Harrison D. Interactions between NO and reactive oxygen species: pathophysiological importance in atherosclerosis, hypertension, diabetes and heart failure. Cardiovasc Res 1999;43: 562–571.
146. Craven PA, Studer RK, Felder J, Phillips S, DeRubertis FR. Nitric oxide inhibition of transforming growth factor-beta and collagen synthesis in mesangial cells. Diabetes 1997;46:671–681.
147. Garg UC, Hassid A. Inhibition of rat mesangial cell mitogenesis by nitric oxide generating vasodilators. Am J Physiol Renal Fluid Electrolyte Physiol 1989;257:F60–F66.
148. Studer RK, DeRubertis FR, Craven PA. Nitric oxide suppresses increases in mesangial cell protein kinase C, transforming growth factor beta, and fibronectin synthesis induced by thromboxane. J Am Soc Nephrol 1996;7:999–1005.
149. Wang S, Shiva S, Poczatek MH, Darley-Usmar V, Murphy-Ullrich JE. Nitric oxide and cGMP-dependent protein kinase regulation of glucose- mediated thrombospondin1-dependent TGF-β activation in mesangial cells. J Biol Chem 2002;277:9880–9888.
150. Von der Leyen HE, Gibbons GH, Morishita R, et al. Gene therapy inhibiting neointimal vascular lesion: in vivo transfer of endothelial cell nitric oxide synthase gene. Proc Natl Acad Sci USA 1995;92:1137–1141.

151. Janssens S, Flaherty D, Nong Z, et al. Human endothelial nitric oxide synthase gene transfer inhibits vascular smooth muscle cell proliferation and neointima formation after balloon injury in rats. Circulation 1998;97:1274–1281.
152. Tanner FC, Meier P, Greutert H, Champion C, Nabel EG, Luscher TF. Nitric oxide modulates expression of cell cycle regulatory proteins: a cytostatic strategy for inhibition of human vascular smooth muscle cell proliferation. Circulation 2000;101:1982–1989.
153. Craven PA, Studer RK, DeRubertis FR. Impaired nitric oxide dependent cyclic guanosine monophosphate generation in glomeruli from diabetic rats: evidence for protein kinase C mediated suppression of the cholinergic response. J Clin Invest 1994;93:311–320.
154. Beckman JS, Koppenol WH. Nitric oxide, superoxide and peroxynitrite, the good, the bad and the ugly. Am J Physiol 1996;271:C1424–C1437.
155. Christ M, Bauersachs J, Liebetrau C, Heck M, Gunther A, Wehling M. Glucose increases endothelial dependent superoxide formation in coronary arteries by NAD(P)H oxidase activation: attenuation by the 3-hydroxy-3-methylglutaryl coenzyme A reductase inhibitor atorvastatin. Diabetes 2002;51: 2648–2652.
156. Nakamura S, Makita Z, Ishikawa S, et al. Progression of nephropathy in spontaneous diabetic rats is prevented by OPB-9195, a novel inhibitor of advanced glycation. Diabetes 1997;46:895–899.
157. Forbes JM, Soulis T, Thallas V, et al. Renoprotective effects of a novel inhibitor of advanced glycation. Diabetologia 2001;44:108–114.
158. Wilkinson-Berka JL, Kelly DJ, Koerner SM, et al. ALT-946 and aminoguanidine, inhibitors of advanced glycation, improve severe nephropathy in the diabetic transgenic (mREN-2)27 rat. Diabetes 2002;51:3283–3289.
159. Hammes HP, Martin S, Federlin K, Geisen K, Brownlee M. Aminoguanidine treatment inhibits the development of experimental diabetic retinopathy. Proc Natl Acad Sci USA 1991;88: 11,555- 11,559.
160. Park L, Raman KG, Lee KJ, et al. Suppression of accelerated diabetic atherosclerosis by the soluble receptor for advanced glycation endproducts. Nat Med 1998;4:1025–1031.
161. Wautier JH, Zoukourian C, Chappey O, et al. Receptor mediated endothelial cell dysfunction in diabetic vasculopathy. J Clin Invest 1996;97:238–243.
162. Koya D, Lee IK, Ishi H, Kanoh H, King GL. Prevention of glomerular dysfunction in diabetic rats by treatment with d-alpha-tocopherol. J Am Soc Nephrol 1997;8:426–435.
163. Trachtman H, Futterweit S, Maesaka J, et al. Taurine ameliorates chronic streptozotocin induced diabetic nephropathy in rats. Am J Physiol 1995;269:F429–F438.
164. Craven P, DeRubertis FR, Kagan VE, Melhem MF, Studer RK. Effects of dietary supplementation with vitamin C or E on albuminuria, glomerular TGF[beta] and size in diabetes. J Am Soc Nephrol 1997;8:1405–1407.
165. Melhem MF, Craven PA, DeRubertis FR. Effects of dietary supplementation of [alpha]-lipoic acid on early glomerular injury in diabetes mellitus. J Am Soc Nephrol 2001;12:124–133.
166. Mustata GT, Rosca M, Biemel KM, et al. Paradoxical effects of green tea (*Camellia sinensis*) and antioxidant vitamins in diabetic rats: improved retinopathy and renal mitochondrial defects but deterioration of collagen matrix glycoxidation and cross-linking. Diabetes 2005;54:517–526.
167. Economides PA, Khaodhiar L, Caselli A, et al. The effect of vitamin E on endothelial function of micro-and macrocirculation and left ventricular function in type 1 and type 2 diabetic patients. Diabetes 2005;54:204–211.
168. Stephens NG, Parsons A, Schofield PM, Kelly F, Cheeseman K, Mitchinson MJ. Randomised controlled trial of vitamin E in patients with coronary disease: Cambridge Heart Antioxidant Study (CHAOS). Lancet 1996;347:781–786.
169. Heart Protection Study Collaborative Group. MRC/BHF heart protection study of antioxidant vitamin supplementation in 20 536 high-risk individuals: a randomised placebo-controlled trial. Lancet 2002;360:7–22.
170. Waters DD, Alderman EL, Hsia J, et al. Effects of hormone replacement therapy and antioxidant vitamin supplements on coronary atherosclerosis in postmenopausal women: a randomized controlled trial. JAMA 2002;288:2432–2440.
171. Lonn E, Yusuf S, Hoogwerf B, et al. HOPE study, MICRO-HOPE study: Effects of vitamin E on cardiovascular and microvascular outcomes in high-risk patients with diabetes: results of the HOPE study and MICRO-HOPE substudy. Diabetes Care 2002;25:1919–1927.
172. Morcos M, Borcea V, Isermann B, et al. Effect of alpha lipoic acid on the progression of endothelial cell damage and albuminuria in patients with diabetes mellitus: an exploratory study. Diabetes Res Clin Pract 2001;52:175–183.

173. Gaede P, Poulsen HE, Parving HH, Pedersen O. Double-blind, randomised study of the effect of combined treatment with vitamin C and E on albuminuria in type 2 diabetic patients. Diabet Med 2001;18:756–760.
174. Brands MV, Bell TD, Gibson B. Nitric oxide may prevent hypertension early in diabetes by counteracting renal actions of superoxide. Hypertension 2004;43:57–63.
175. Li M-M, Shah AM. Endothelial cell superoxide generation: regulation and relevance for cardiovascular pathophysiology. Am J Physiol Regul Integr Comp Physiol 2004;287:R1014–R1030.
176. Zorov DB, Filburn CR, Klotz LO, Zweier JL, Sollott SJ. Reactive oxygen species (ROS)-induced ROS release: a new phenomenon accompanying induction of the mitochondrial permeability transition in cardiac myocytes. J Exp Med 2000;192:1001–1014.

I

Basic Pathophysiology and Biochemistry of Diabetic Nephropathy

G. Growth Factors

10 Connective Tissue Growth Factor in the Pathogenesis of Diabetic Nephropathy

A Target for Therapeutic Intervention

Bruce L. Riser, PhD, *Alessia Fornoni,* MD, PhD, *and Sujatha Karoor,* PhD

CONTENTS

INTRODUCTION

Since its discovery in 1991, connective tissue growth factor (CCN2; formerly named CTGF), a member of the CCN family of genes, has been shown to have quite diverse biological functions. Our laboratory was among the first to provide evidence for a causal role for CCN2 in the pathogenesis of diabetic nephropathy (DN). We suggested its criticality as downstream profibrotic factor stimulated by both transforming growth factor (TGF)-β-dependent and -independent mechanisms, and as such, a novel target for therapeutic intervention. Proof is now being provided for its role in the fibrosis and sclerosis that occurs in the glomerulus, and likely in the interstitium, in DN. This chapter will focus first on the evidence for a causal role, second on the recently discovered mechanisms and factors involved in regulation of CCN2, and third on the direction we envision the research heading, including possibilities for novel therapeutics and diagnostics targeting CCN.

CCN2: DISCOVERY AND STRUCTURE

CTGF is a cysteine-rich (CR) peptide first described as a molecule capable of inducing proliferation of endothelial cells *(1)*. It is now recognized that CTGF belongs to a family

From: *Contemporary Diabetes: The Diabetic Kidney*
Edited by: P. Cortes and C. E. Mogensen © Humana Press Inc., Totowa, NJ

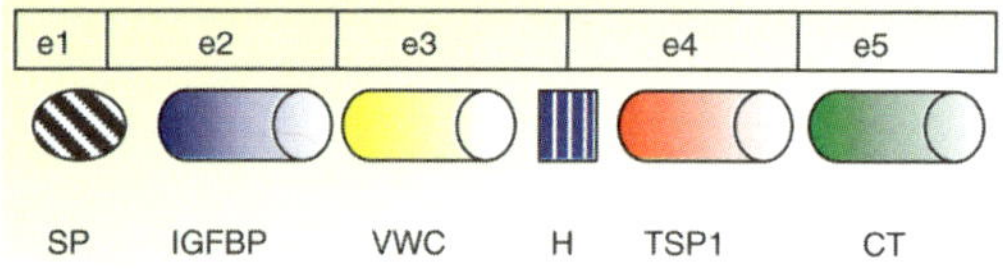

Fig. 1. Schematic representation of basic CCN2 structure. Five exons encode a signal peptide (SP), an insulin-like growth factor-binding protein domain, a VWC, a thrombospondin type-1 repeat, and a C-terminal (CT) module. At the junction between the domains II and III is a region proposed to act as a hinge. (Reprinted by permission of author, B. Perbal et al., University of Paris, from Lancet, 363, 2004.)

of at least six related genes, recently named the CCN family *(2)*. The letters, C–C–N, arise from the first letter of the first three members to be reported, CTGF, Cyr-61, and NOV. As CTGF was the second to be reported, the newly proposed name for this molecule is CCN2. All of the members share a common motif consisting of four modules:

1. an insulin-like growth factor-binding protein domain;
2. a von Willebrand factor type-C repeat (VWC);
3. a thrombospondin type-1 repeat; and
4. a C-terminal (CT) module (Fig. 1).

These members share a 40–60% sequence homology with the modules of the other members. Full-length CCN2 typically exists as approx 36- and 39-kDa molecules, the two likely representing differences in glycosylation.

CCN2: A CAUSAL FACTOR IN THE PATHOGENESIS OF DN

Ito et al. *(3)* first reported the presence of CCN2 mRNA in the adult human kidney, and suggested that increased CCN2 might be associated with renal disease. CCN2 mRNA staining in human kidney sections was faint and limited to a few areas in non-diseased tissue, but was substantially greater among those with a variety of different kidney diseases, including two cases of DN. Soon thereafter, our laboratory reported that cultured mesangial cells (MCs) produced relatively low constitutive levels of CCN2 mRNA and protein *(4)*. However, in an in vitro model of DN, exposure to either TGF-β, or elevated glucose concentrations, markedly increased both the transcript and protein levels of MC CCN2, a change accompanied by increased extracellular matrix (ECM) accumulation *(4)*. A causal role was indicated by the finding that exposure of cultured MCs to rhCCN2 resulted in an augmentation of collagen and fibronectin protein levels equal to, or greater than, those stimulated by TGF-β or high glucose levels. Furthermore, using the db/db mouse model of human type 2 diabetes and DN, we found an early and dramatic upregulation of CCN2 mRNA in the glomerulus (27-fold). This compared with a mild, but statistically significant (twofold), increase in the kidney cortex *(4)*. Overall, these findings suggested that CCN2 was a major causal factor in DN and that the primary source, at least at this stage of DN, was the glomerulus. The MC was the likely contributor. Our findings were substantiated by those from a number of other laboratories *(5,6)* and extended to implicate CCN2 in other renal fibrosis models, including the streptozotocin (STZ) model of type 1 diabetes and those with reduced renal mass, that is, in nondiabetic animals *(7–10)*.

Tubulo-interstitial fibrosis is considered a late stage and final common pathway in the progression to end-stage renal failure in numerous afflictions, including DN. Models of DN share the deficiency of a lack of progression to the advanced disease seen in humans, often without tubulo-interstitial fibrosis. We must therefore extrapolate from comparable studies. However, in a partial nephrectomy rat model, CCN2 mRNA expression is minimal in controls but increases strongly after 4–8 wk in interstitial fibroblasts, coinciding with damage, regeneration, and fibrosis *(11)*. TGF-β, but not high glucose exposure, has been reported to induce increased expression of CCN2 in cultured mouse proximal convoluted tubule cells, and rhCCN2 exposure moderately increased fibronectin in mouse proximal convoluted tubule cells, with rhCCN2 increasing collagen type I and III in cultured normal rat kidney fibroblasts (NRK-49F) *(10,12)*. This suggests then that CCN2 may also play an important role in the interstitial fibrosis that occurs in later stage DN.

In consideration of the present data supporting a casual role for CCN2 in DN, final proof is not yet available, but will come from in vivo blockade studies using CCN2-specific inhibitors. Along these lines, a recent preliminary study has described the use CCN2-specific antisense oligonucleotides (AS-ODN), administered in both STZ and db/db mouse diabetic models *(13)*. Using a prevention protocol, systemic treatment was able to substantially block the upregulation of CCN2. In the STZ model, this treatment resulted in a blockade of albuminuria development, and a significant attenuation of fibronectin and mesangial matrix expansion *(13)*. In the same report, similar results were observed in the db/db model, with a substantial reduction in the development of albuminuria, collagen gene expression, and mesangial matrix expansion. These preliminary findings are supported by two recent peer-reviewed publications also using CCN2 AS-ODN treatments to demonstrate a causal role in nondiabetic models of renal fibrosis. For example, CCN2 is upregulated in the proximal tubular epithelial cells of mice after partial (5/6) nephrectomy. This upregulation can be blocked by an intravenous administration of CCN2 AS-ODN. The increased level of TGF-β mRNA that also occurs in the model is not reduced. This paralleled a reduction in mRNA levels of matrix molecules as well as proteinase inhibitors, plasminogen activator inhibitor-1, and tissue inhibitor of metalloproteinase (TIMP)-1, suppressing renal interstitial fibrogenesis *(14)*. Furthermore, AS-ODN directed against CCN2-specific sequences, when injected into the renal artery, were able to markedly attenuate the upregulation of CCN2 that occurs in unilateral uretheral obstruction, a rapidly developing model of tubulo-interstitial fibrosis in rats *(15)*. This treatment simultaneously and markedly attenuated the upregulation of fibronectin and collagen type I, without affecting the expression of TGF-β and appeared to reduce the number of myofibroblasts, but not proliferating tubule or interstitial cells.

POSITIVE REGULATORY FACTORS FOR CCN2 IN DN

We currently envision CCN2 as a very downstream mediator of ECM overaccumulation and fibrosis/sclerosis in DN. This means that multiple factors act to drive (either directly or indirectly) CCN2 activity. The schematic in Fig. 2 provides an overview of the proposed interaction and hints to its complexity.

Altered Glucose Metabolism and CCN2

Altered metabolism of glucose, unique in diabetes as opposed to other forms of renal disease, is a critical factor contributing to increased CCN2 and DN. As described earlier, the exposure of a variety of renal cell types, including MCs, to elevated glucose levels has been shown to markedly increase CCN2 activity. This is likely to occur through at least two pathways in vivo. First, high glucose is able to increase protein kinase C, which

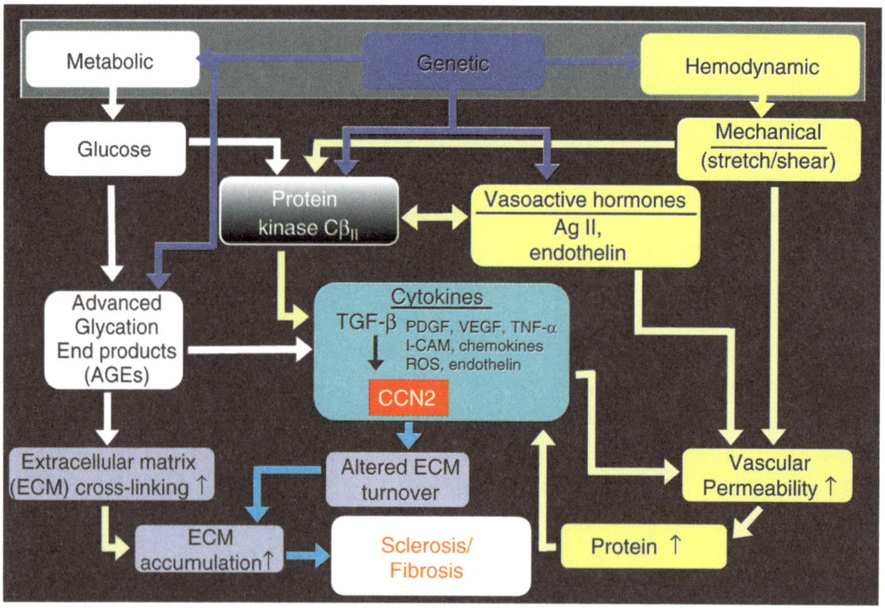

Fig. 2. Schematic diagram proposing a central role of CCN2 in the pathogenesis of diabetic nephropathy, and the interplay of contributing factors. (From ref. *52* with permission.)

then acts to upregulate TGF-β activity *(16)*. As described earlier, TGF-β activity is well established as a major stimulatory factor for CCN2 production in a variety of renal and nonrenal cells. An increase in its activity is able to then increase CCN2, via a TGF-β responsive element on the CCN2 molecule *(17)*.

A second pathway for glucose metabolism-driven CCN2 stimulation is via the generation of advanced glycation endproducts (AGE). These irreversibly formed biochemical endproducts of nonenzymatic glycosylation have been implicated as causal in the expansion of ECM that occurs in DN. AGE are present in the serum and in many tissues of diabetic patients. They have the ability to covalently crosslink and biochemically modify protein structure and function. AGE exposure upregulates, in a dose-dependent and dose-specific manner, CCN2 mRNA and protein level in dermal fibroblasts *(18)*. In a similar manner, the exposure of cultured MCs to AGE increases both CCN2 and fibronectin expression *(19)*. Further support for a role of AGE in this pathway has come from several in vivo studies using specific inhibitors of AGE formation (*see* the section on nonspecific inhibitors).

Altered Hemodynamics and CCN2

A third major pathway for the upregulation of CCN2 activity in DN likely results from increased hemodynamic stretching or sheer forces. Systemic hypertension is an established causal factor in progressive renal disease. In experimental diabetes, one early change is that of impaired normal dampening of blood pressure fluctuations at the afferent arteriole of the glomerulus. This results in the exposure of the glomerulus and its vessels to increased pressure, with pathological effects likely occurring even in the absence systemic hypertension, but likely worsened as systemic pressure increases. Our laboratory in conjunction with that of Kritz in Germany previously showed that the MC, with foot-like processes attached to the perimesangial basement membrane is subjected to mechanical stretching force as the glomerulus expands *(20,21)*. The MC response to increased cyclic stretch is an upregulation of both TGF-β and ECM accumulation *(21)*. We more recently showed that this same cyclic stretch acts to markedly upregulate CCN2 expression in MCs *(4)*, an observation supported by the findings of others *(22)*. It stands to reason that provided enough time, CCN2 activity will increase as a result of a stretch-induced TGF-β upregulation, the latter requiring 24–48 h *(23)*. However, we showed that CCN2 expression levels increase dramatically, as early as 4 h following the application of cyclic stretch and remain upregulated for a least 48 h. Collectively, this indicates that mechanical force resulting from glomerular hypertension may act to upregulate CCN2 production and activity both through TGF-β-dependent and -independent pathways. Increased stretch and sheer forces also act to increase vascular permeability, which could result in increased proteinuria and the release of vasoactive hormones. The latter, including angiotensin (Ang) II and endothelin, may increase protein kinase C and in turn TGF-β and CCN2, either directly or indirectly *(24–28)* (Fig. 2).

Inflammatory Mediators and CCN2

Recent attention has focused on inflammation and inflammatory cytokines as contributing factors in the pathogenesis of DN. Along these lines we investigated the MC response to the proinflammatory cytokine tumor necrosis factor (TNF)-α. We found that a 24-h treatment increased MC CCN2 protein to levels similar to that induced by TGF-β. When TNF-α was used in combination with TGF-β, there was an additive stimulatory effect on CCN2 protein and mRNA. This suggested that the presence of TNF-α under inflammatory conditions would result in augmentation of CCN2 activity and thus further enhance ECM deposition. Surprisingly, however, this same treatment with TNF-α failed to correspondingly increase collagen type-I protein levels, but instead decreased levels, compared with those in unstimulated cells (measured by ELISA). In a similar manner, TNF-α markedly reduced the level of collagen type-I mRNA stimulated by TGF-β (manuscript submitted). When the exposure was extended to a second treatment, i.e., over a 6 d total period, neither TGF-β nor TNF-α alone simulated CCN2 protein production, but in combination did synergistically increase CCN2 protein accumulation. These findings demonstrate the complexity of examining and interpreting the role of multiple cytokine interactions. Although such studies do not appear to have been done previously, TNF-α (in the absence of other cytokines) was reported to have no effect on constitutive CCN2 protein levels in cultured human scleroderma fibroblasts *(29)*, primary bovine aortic endothelial cells *(30)*, and murine 3T3 fibroblasts *(31)*. However, increased TGF-β and TIMP-1 in MCs occurred following treatment with TNF-α and TGF-β in combination *(32)*. Increased TGF-β would then be expected to further increase CCN2 and ECM accumulation. Our results suggest that in rat MCs, TNF-α does not act directly on CCN2 gene expression at the level of transcription but may instead have a posttranslational effect, perhaps via the modulation of levels of TIMP-1 and/or matrix metalloproteinase (MMP)-3 as described earlier (submitted for publication). The response of MCs to CCN2 then, may be greatly modified in the presence of TNF-α. Other cytokines including platelet-derived growth factor, vascular endothelial growth factor, and endothelin may also have a regulatory, or modifying, effect on CCN2 activity. Reactive oxygen species are likely to upregulate CCN2 activity. Although there does not appear to be information addressing this element in kidney cells, it has been reported that hydrogen peroxide increased CCN2 mRNA levels in a dose-dependent manner in human lens epithelial cell line B3 *(33)*. Message levels were increased as early as 2 h poststimulation, suggesting that the response was independent of TGF-β. This is supported by the additional finding that same exposure failed to stimulate either TGF-β mRNA expression or that of plasminogen activator inhibitor-1. The upregulation of CCN2 expression was blocked by AG490, an inhibitor of Janus kinase *(33)*.

Genetics and CCN2

Genetics are thought to play a role in the development and progression of DN, and may be a key factor in explaining why 30–40% of diabetic patients progress to DN, whereas the remaining live free of the disease for decades. Although implicated, the exact contribution(s) of genetics is not yet clear. As depicted in Fig. 2, it is thought that the genetic background may act at the levels of altered glucose metabolism and altered hemodynamics. We investigated the possibility that genetics might also operate at the level of CCN2 regulation, with differences in genetic background determining the level of constitutive CCN2 produced, or the potential for the cellular response to upregulation of CCN2. To test this, MCs were isolated from the glomeruli of two different mouse strains. These strains model the two outcomes described above for patients with diabetes, namely those who have a propensity (ROP; B6 mouse; Jackson Labs) or resistance (C57BL/6 mouse; Jackson Labs) for developing progressive DN *(34)*. After switching these early passage MC cultures to serum-deprived conditions, CCN2 protein and mRNA expression were determined. Interestingly, the cultures from the DN susceptible ROP strain produced CCN2 protein levels that were nearly twofold greater than those produced by the MCs from the DN-resistant C57B/6 strain. A correspondingly similar increase in CCN2 mRNA level was obtained from the DN-susceptible strain as compared with the resistant strain. These findings suggest that genetic differences at the MC level may be reflected in the baseline levels of CCN2 produced, and may therefore influence directly the potential for development of DN.

Many, if not all, of the factors outlined in Fig. 2 are likely to interact in DN to upregulate CCN2 and to drive the overaccumulation of ECM that characterizes the disease. Additionally, once upregulated, CCN2 may be able to autoinduce its own activity. We found that MCs, when exposed to rhCCN2, increased the expression of CCN2 transcripts fourfold *(4)*. In fact, the level of induction was equal to that in response to TGF-β at 2 ng/mL. We did not find the reverse to be true, that is, rhCCN2 (even at 20 ng/mL) failed to upregulate TGF-β message levels.

THERAPEUTIC INTERVENTION TARGETING CCN2

Because CCN2 appears to exert its effect in a very downstream manner, concerning injurious factors in DN, it would seem to be a potentially attractive therapeutic target. In fact, we first began our investigations into the role of CCN2 in DN seeking a new downstream element that might provide advantages over targeting molecules such as TGF-β. For example, TGF-β, an established profibrotic factor is ubiquitous, exists in multiple isoforms, and appears to play a role in a diverse array of biological functions including immune surveillance. CCN2 as a factor acting downstream of TGF-β and with the potential to also be stimulated independently of TGF-β would appear, *a priori*, to be a potentially more effective target. However, as recent evidence is solidifying its role as an important causal factor, it is also becoming increasingly clear that CCN2,

Table 1
Potential Candidates for Therapeutic Intervention of CCN2 Activity

CCN2-specific inhibitors	*CCN2-nonspecific inhibitors*	*Endogenous CCN2 inhibitors*
Antibodies	ACEI/ARBs	IFN-γ
AS-ODNs	Cyclooxygenase inhibitors	BMP-7
siRNAs	AGE inhibitors	Others ??

CCN2, connective tissue growth factor; ACE, angiotensin II-converting enzyme; ARB, angiotensin II receptor blockers; IFN, interferon; AS-ODNs, antisense oligonucleotides; BMP, bone morphogenic protein; AGE, advanced glycation endproduct.

like TGF-β, is important in a diverse array of biological functions. Furthermore, it is produced under a variety of different stimuli, and in many organs. It is also present in circulation, and is excreted in urine *(35)*. It will be important to determine the effect, if any, of chronic reduction in CCN2 on normal physiology. This may define a necessity of developing CCN2 inhibitory agents that are site specific. Current evidence suggests a number of agents, or methods, for negatively regulating CCN2 (Table 1).

Specific Inhibitors of CCN2

One method for the control, or inhibition, of CCN2 activity may be the administration of neutralizing antibodies. Antibodies directed against CCN2 have been generated in a number of different species, and to different sites on the molecule, and may therefore seem to have potential as therapeutic agents. However, very few of these antibodies have been reported to demonstrate neutralizing activity. In fact, we have observed that some anti-CCN2 antibodies not only fail to neutralize, but may actually enhance CCN2 biological activity (unpublished observation). The mechanism for this enhancement is not known. However, our observation is supported by a recent study of both polyclonal and monoclonal antibodies generated to full-length CCN2. The authors reported that most antibodies produced were directed against the VWC module, and were not neutralizing. One antibody that bound to the CT module was able to neutralize the proliferative effect of CCN2 on chrondrocytes. They also found that most of the antibodies enhanced the proteoglycan synthesis by these cells *(36)*. At least one company, however, has developed a human anti-CCN2 monoclonal antibody that is currently in an open-label, phase-I clinical trial (FibroGen public announcement, October 27, 2004) and plans to enter phase II with an indication of pulmonary fibrosis. The results of these trials should be most interesting.

Our laboratory has been interested in the development of inhibitors of CCN2 RNA regulation and utilization in the form of both AS-ODN and siRNAs. This approach has the potential advantage of highly specific targeting. Some of the greatest obstacles to this technology, however, involve delivery to the target organ and proof of limited off-target effects. These factors are often not effectively addressed in initial reports. Nevertheless, AS-ODN to CCN2 administered via the renal artery has been reported to successfully attenuate the fibrosis observed in the unilateral uretheral obstruction model, as described earlier. This ostensibly, is a reasonable model to test such agents because of the rapid development of fibrosis. However, the use of such an agent to treat chronic kidney disease will likely require a long-term stable agent and the acceptability of an oral or infrequent intravenous parenteral administration, with targeted delivery to the appropriate renal site.

Nonspecific Inhibitors of CCN2

As described earlier, Ang II is likely an important positive regulatory factor for CCN2, and may help to explain the ability of angiotension II- converting enzyme (ACE) inhibitor therapy to slow progression in at least some patients. Understanding how this effect is mediated may lead to improvement within these classes of drugs. Several studies have shown the ability of ACE inhibitors, or angiotension II receptor blockers (ARBs) to reduce CCN2 expression in vitro *(27,37)*. Another potential method for indirectly targeting CCN2 would be one directed at altered glucose metabolism. For example, a 32-wk treatment of diabetic rats with aminoguanidine, an inhibitor of AGE formation, was reported to prevent the expression of excess expression CCN2 and fibronectin *(19)*. In another study with STZ-induced diabetes in rats, similar effects were seen with both early (16-wk) and late (8-wk) treatment with aminoguanidine. Both reduced TGF-β and CCN2, as well as the albumin excretion rate, blood pressure, and renal hypertrophy. However, the glomerulosclerotic index, tubulo-interstitial area, renal collagen, and TGF-β only showed improvement with the early treatment *(38)*. Finally, another method for potential indirect targeting of CCN2 is suggested by a study reporting that chronic aspirin treatment in diabetic rats effectively suppressed CCN2 induction and fibronectin expression, and significantly attenuated mesangial expansion *(39)*. This treatment also inhibited the upregulation of TGF-β. In cultured MCs, aspirin treatment abolished high glucose-stimulated CCN2 upregulation, suggesting that modulation of the cyclooxygenase pathway may slow the progression of DN via a downregulation of multiple elements impacting on CCN2 and ultimately ECM accumulation *(39)*.

Endogenous Factors as Therapeutics

We are currently exploring the possibility of utilizing endogenous mechanisms that are part of the normal control of CCN2 expression and/or activity in the kidney. Along these lines, previous reports have suggested that the interferon (IFN)-γ may act to slow the development of pulmonary fibrosis by its ability its ability to downregulate TGF-β *(40–42)*. We examined IFN-γ as a possible negative regulatory cytokine for CCN2. However, in our hands, a 24-h exposure of MCs to IFN-γ alone (50 U/mL) had no effect on CCN2 or collagen protein expression measured at 3 d poststimulation, and failed to block the induction by TGF-β of CCN2 or collagen type I, over a dose range of 5–500 U/mL (manuscript submitted).

Certain of the bone morphogenic proteins (BMPs) may also be endogenous negative regulatory factors for CCN2 activity. For example, BMP-7 is able to repress CCN2 expression in MCs *(43)*. However, this treatment also reduces the activity of TGF-β. It has apparently not yet been determined if the effect on CCN2 can occur independent of TGF-β. These findings are particularly interesting because, the primary organ for production of this cytokine/hormone appears to be the kidney. Production and circulation of BMP-7 appears to be greatly reduced in chronic kidney disease, being most apparent in end-stage renal disease. In models of DN it has been demonstrated that the replacement of BMP-7 (i.e., treatment with rhBMP-7) is able to ameliorate progression of disease *(44,45)*. The treatment of human patients with a systemic administration of BMP-7 does not appear to have as yet been reported. As an additional note, it has been shown that CCN2 can directly bind BMP-4 and TGF-β_1 through its CR chordin-like domain (shown in Fig. 1 as VWC domain) and antagonizes BMP-4 activity *(46)*, indicating a possible coregulation by some of the members of these two different families of molecules.

A number of studies have indicated a role for hepatocyte growth factor (HGF) as a potential endogenous antifibrotic factor, although some original reports suggested the reverse effect. A human HGF (hHGF) plasmid administered by intramuscular injection over a 30-d period in rats, with early and advanced STZ-DN, upregulated endogenous HGF expression in kidney *(47)*. This gene therapy did not improve early DN but reduced albuminuria and was reported to induce a regression of mesangial expansion and glomerulosclerosis in advanced DN *(47)*. These findings were associated with suppression of renal TGF-β_1, and mesangial CCN2 upregulation, and were therefore suggested as an innovative therapeutic strategy to treat advanced DN. Endogenous administration of HGF to mice transgenic for TGF-β expression and with an added partial nephrectomy, counteracted TGF-β_1 through attenuation of CCN2 induction, and was reported to prevent renal fibrogenesis *(48)*.

PREDICTING THE ONSET AND PROGRESSION OF DN

One of the problems inherent in the treatment of DN is that of early diagnosis. More effective treatment, or prevention, might be possible if these 30–40% of patients destined to develop DN could be identified before the formation of irreversible renal damage. Microalbuminuria, often considered a predictor, is most likely an indicator of already established renal disease. We showed, for the first time, that CCN2 is present in urine of healthy individuals as well as in rodents *(35)*. Interestingly, the amount (and possibly the molecular form) of urinary CCN2 is altered early in DN. This occurred both in humans and in rodent models and suggests that the measurement of urinary CCN2 may be a predictor of those patients destined for development of disease. In support of this hypothesis, we also examined glomerular mRNA levels for CCN2 from kidney biopsy of living renal donors ($n = 10$), and patients with type 1 diabetes and normoalbuminuria ($n = 12$), microalbuminuria ($n = 5$), and overt proteinuria ($n = 6$) *(49)*. Values were established for those falling within the 95% confidence interval (CI) for the live donors and those falling within the 95% CI for those with abnormal albuminuria. After 44 mo of follow-up, one patient converted to from normoalbuminuria to microalbuminuria. This was the only patient in the study whose CCN2 mRNA levels were above the 95% CI of the living renal donors *(49)*.

In addition to urine and renal tissue, CCN2 is present in circulation. A recent study using an antibody that measures the amino-terminal fragment of CCN2, reported an elevation of the molecule in the plasma of patients with type 1 diabetes and nephropathy that correlated with proteinuria and creatinine clearance *(50)*. In another recent investigation, we studied 18 patients who were either proteinuric (0.2–4.9 g/dL) and/or who had elevated serum creatinine levels (1.2–3.8 mg/dL). Spot urine samples were collected, measured by ELISA for urinary CCN2, and the relationship to creatinine, urinary protein, and/or blood pressure studied. We found a significant and positive relationship between the level of CCN2 excretion and the levels of both proteinuria, as well as serum creatinine. Perhaps most remarkable, however, was the highly positive correlation (R2 0.878) between urinary CCN2 levels and mean arterial blood pressure. The latter results support the findings from our in vitro modeling experiments, indicating that intraglomerular hypertension and the resulting mechanical strain are critical determinants for the positive regulation of CCN2, and thus the development of renal fibrosis/sclerosis *(51)*.

CONCLUSIONS

In DN, the overall casual factors include metabolic, genetic, and hemodynamic alterations. These factors interact to drive progression. We envision CCN2 as a central, downstream mediator of the effects of these three elements. For example, pathological force (shear or stretch) resulting from intraglomerular hypertension appears to stimulate the production of cytokines including CCN2. This same force is likely to be responsible for increased vascular permeability leading to both proteinuria and an elevated production of vasoactive hormones such as Ang II and endothelin, which in turn also elevate CCN2 and further enhance the mechanical force. The abnormal accumulation of AGE that occurs with the altered metabolism of glucose present in DN may also work to directly increase ECM crosslinking and accumulation, as well as to stimulate CCN2 activity. The genetic background of the individual can influence the elements of hemodynamics and metabolism and, as a result, the pathways described. However, the genetic background may also exert its effect at a more direct cellular level, seen as a differential cellular capacity for production of, and perhaps response to, CCN2. In consideration of intervention, recent information has suggested a number of potential methods for therapeutically reducing or preventing the increase in CCN2 in DN. These include both specific as well as nonspecific targeting of CCN2. Although recent animal studies appear encouraging, most have utilized prevention, rather than treatment, protocols. Nevertheless, CCN2, as a downstream molecule in the pathway to DN, does appear to greatly influence the accumulation of ECM and fibrosis, and is upregulated both by TGF-β-dependent and -independent mechanisms, including possible autoinduction. This suggests a high potential as an effective target for therapeutic intervention. As a caveat, however, there remains much we do not know about this molecule including the role, if any, of partial CCN2 fragments, CCN2 complexed with other molecules (including other members of the CCN family of genes). Additionally, unknown is the effect of CCN2 blockade, or reduction, on normal physiology including the capacity to upregulate its activity when needed.

REFERENCES

1. Bradham DM, Igarashi A, Potter RL, Grotendorst GR. Connective tissue growth factor: a cysteine-rich mitogen secreted by human vascular endothelial cells is related to the SRC-induced immediate early gene product CEF-10. J Cell Biol 1991;114(6):1285–1294.
2. Brigstock DR, Goldschmeding R, Katsube KI, et al. Proposal for a unified CCN nomenclature. Mol Pathol 2003;56(2):127,128.
3. Ito Y, Kasuga H, Matsuo S. Connective tissue growth factor (CTGF) in renal fibrosis. Igaku no Ayumi 1999;190(1):68–73.
4. Riser BL, Denichilo M, Cortes P, et al. Regulation of connective tissue growth factor activity in cultured rat mesangial cells and its expression in experimental diabetic glomerulosclerosis. J Am Soc Nephrol 2000;11(1):25–38.
5. Murphy M, Godson C, Cannon S, et al. Suppression subtractive hybridization identifies high glucose levels as a stimulus for expression of connective tissue growth factor and other genes in human mesangial cells. J Biol Chem 1999;274(9):5830–5834.
6. Wahab NA, Yevdokimova N, Weston BS, et al. Role of connective tissue growth factor in the pathogenesis of diabetic nephropathy. Biochem J 2001;359(Part 1):77–87.
7. Tan Y, Wang B, Keum JS, Jaffa AA. Mechanisms through which bradykinin promotes glomerular injury in diabetes. Am J Physiol Renal Fluid Electrolyte Physiol 2005;288(3).
8. Liu BC, Luo DD, Sun J, Ma KL, Ruan XZ. Influence of irbesartan on renal hypertrophy and thickening of glomerular basement-membrane in streptozotocin-induced diabetic rats. Chung Hua Nei Ko Tsa Chih Chin J Internal Med 2003;42(5):320–323.

9. Forbes JM, Cooper ME, Oldfield MD, Thomas MC. Role of advanced glycation end products in diabetic nephropathy. J Am Soc Nephrol 2003;14(3):S254–S258.
10. Wang S, Denichilo M, Brubaker C, Hirschberg R. Connective tissue growth factor in tubulointerstitial injury of diabetic nephropathy. Kidney Int 2001;60(1):96–105.
11. Frazier KS, Paredes A, Dube P, Styer E. Connective tissue growth factor expression in the rat remnant kidney model and association with tubular epithelial cells undergoing transdifferentiation. Vet Pathol 2000;37(4):328–335.
12. Yokoi H, Sugawara A, Mukoyama M, et al. Role of connective tissue growth factor in profibrotic action of transforming growth factor-b: A potential target for preventing renal fibrosis. Am J Kidney Dis 2001;38(4 Suppl 1):S134–S138.
13. Guha M, Xu Z, DeFalco C, et al. Antisense Oligonucleotides (ASOs) to connective tissue growth factor (CTGF) attenuates progression of diabetic nephropathy in mouse models of type 1 and type 2 diabetes. J Am Soc Nephrol 2004;15:29A.
14. Okada H, Kikuta T, Kobayashi T, et al. Connective tissue growth factor expressed in tubular epithelium plays a pivotal role in renal fibrogenesis. J Am Soc Nephrol 2005;16(1):133–143.
15. Yokoi H, Mukoyama M, Nagae T, et al. Reduction in connective tissue growth factor by antisense treatment ameliorates renal tubulointerstitial fibrosis. J Am Soc Nephrol 2004;15(6):1430–1440.
16. Chen Y, Blom IE, Sa S, Goldschmeding R, Abraham DJ, Leask A. CTGF expression in mesangial cells: involvement of SMADs, MAP kinase, and PKC. Kidney Int 2002;62(4):1149–1159.
17. Grotendorst GR, Okochi H, Hayashi N. A novel transforming growth factor beta response element controls the expression of the connective tissue growth factor gene. Cell Growth Differentiation 1996;7(4):469–480.
18. Twigg SM, Chen MM, Joly AH, et al. Advanced glycosylation end products up-regulate connective tissue growth factor (insulin-like growth factor-binding protein-related protein 2) in human fibroblasts: a potential mechanism for expansion of extracellular matrix in diabetes mellitus. Endocrinology 2001;142(5):1760–1769.
19. Twigg SM, Cao Z, SV MC, et al. Renal connective tissue growth factor induction in experimental diabetes is prevented by aminoguanidine. Endocrinology 2002;143(12):4907–4915.
20. Kriz W, Elger M, Lemley K, Sakai T. Structure of the glomerular mesangium: a biomechanical interpretation. Kidney Int 1990;30:S2–S9.
21. Riser BL, Cortes P, Zhao X, Bernstein J, Dumler F, Narins RG. Intraglomerular pressure and mesangial stretching stimulate extracellular matrix formation in the rat. J Clin Invest 1992;90(5):1932–1943.
22. Hishikawa K, Oemar BS, Nakaki T. Static pressure regulates connective tissue growth factor expression in human mesangial cells. J Biol Chem 2001;276(20):16,797–16,803.
23. Riser BL, Cortes P, Heilig C, et al. Cyclic stretching force selectively up-regulates transforming growth factor-beta isoforms in cultured rat mesangial cells. Am J Pathol 1996;148(6):1915–1923.
24. Liu B-C, Sun J, Chen Q, Ma K-L, Ruan X-Z, Phillips AO. Role of connective tissue growth factor in mediating hypertrophy of human proximal tubular cells induced by angiotensin II. Am J Nephrol 2003;23(6):429–437.
25. Finckenberg P, Inkinen K, Ahonen J, et al. Angiotensin II induces connective tissue growth factor gene expression via calcineurin-dependent pathways. Am J Pathol 2003;163(1):355–366.
26. Iwanciw D, Rehm M, Porst M, Goppelt-Struebe M. Induction of connective tissue growth factor by angiotensin II: integration of signaling pathways. Arteriosclerosis Thromb Vascular Biol 2003; 23(10):1782–1787.
27. Ruperez M, Ruiz-Ortega M, Esteban V, et al. Angiotensin II increases connective tissue growth factor in the kidney. Am J Pathol 2003;163(5):1937–1947.
28. Wolf G, Mueller E, Stahl RA, Ziyadeh FN. Angiotensin II-induced hypertrophy of cultured murine proximal tubular cells is mediated by endogenous transforming growth factor-beta. J Clin Invest 1993;92(3):1366–1372.
29. Abraham DJ, Shiwen X, Black CM, Sa S, Xu Y, Leask A. Tumor necrosis factor alpha suppresses the induction of connective tissue growth factor by transforming growth factor-beta in normal and scleroderma fibroblasts. J Biol Chem 2000;275(20):15,220–15,225.
30. Aburatani H, Yamamoto S, inventors (NGK Insulators, Ltd., Japan) assignee. Human tissue-specific housekeeping genes identified by expression profiling. Wo patent 2004035785, 2004.
31. Dammeier J, Beer HD, Brauchle M, Werner S. Dexamethasone is a novel potent inducer of connective tissue growth factor expression. Implications for glucocorticoid therapy. J Biol Chem 1998;273(29): 18,185–18,190.

32. Pawluczyk IZ, Harris KP. Cytokine interactions promote synergistic fibronectin accumulation by mesangial cells. Kidney Int 1998;54(1):62–70.
33. Park SK, Kim J, Seomun Y, et al. Hydrogen peroxide is a novel inducer of connective tissue growth factor. Biochem Biophys Res Comm 2001:966–971, 2001 Jun 22.
34. Fornoni A, Striker LJ, Zheng F, Striker GE. Reversibility of glucose-induced changes in mesangial cell extracellular matrix depends on the genetic background. Diabetes 2002;51(2):499–505.
35. Riser BL, Cortes P, DeNichilo M, et al. Urinary CCN2 (CTGF) as a possible predictor of diabetic nephropathy: preliminary report. Kidney Int 2003;64(2):451–458.
36. Minato M, Kubota S, Kawaki H, et al. Module-specific antibodies against human connective tissue growth factor: utility for structural and functional analysis of the factor as related to chondrocytes. J Biochem 2004;135(3):347–354.
37. Huang S, Liu F, Sha Z, et al. Effect of high glucose, angiotensin II and receptor antagonist Losartan on the expression of connective tissue growth factor in cultured mesangial cells. Chin Med J (Beijing, China, English Edition) 2003;116(4):554–557.
38. Forbes JM, Thallas V, Thomas MC, et al. The breakdown of preexisting advanced glycation end products is associated with reduced renal fibrosis in experimental diabetes. FASEB J 2003;17(12): 1762–1764.
39. Makino H, Mukoyama M, Sugawara A, et al. Roles of connective tissue growth factor and prostanoids in early streptozotocin-induced diabetic rat kidney: the effect of aspirin treatment. Clin Exp Nephrol 2003;7(1):33–40.
40. Gurujeyalakshmi G, Giri SN. Molecular mechanisms of antifibrotic effect of interferon gamma in bleomycin-mouse model of lung fibrosis: downregulation of TGF-beta and procollagen I and III gene expression. Exp Lung Res 1995;21(5):791–808.
41. Eickelberg O, Pansky A, Koehler E, et al. Molecular mechanisms of TGF-(beta) antagonism by interferon (gamma) and cyclosporine A in lung fibroblasts. FASEB J 2001;15(3):797–806.
42. Ziesche R, Hofbauer E, Wittmann K, Petkov V, Block LH. A preliminary study of long-term treatment with interferon gamma-1b and low-dose prednisolone in patients with idiopathic pulmonary fibrosis. N Engl J Med 1999;341(17):1264–1269.
43. Wang S, Hirschberg R. BMP7 antagonizes TGF-b-dependent fibrogenesis in mesangial cells. Am J Physiol 2003;284(5 Part 2):F1006–F1013.
44. Gonzalez EA, Lund RJ, Martin KJ, et al. Treatment of a murine model of high-turnover renal osteodystrophy by exogenous BMP-7. Kidney Int 2002;61(4):1322–1331.
45. Wang S, Chen Q, Simon TC, et al. Bone morphogenic protein-7 (BMP-7), a novel therapy for diabetic nephropathy. Kidney Int 2003;63(6):2037–2049.
46. Abreu JG, Ketpura NI, Reversade B, De Robertis EM. Connective-tissue growth factor (CTGF) modulates cell signalling by BMP and TGF-beta. Nat Cell Biol 2002;4(8):599–604.
47. Cruzado JM, Lloberas N, Torras J, et al. Regression of advanced diabetic nephropathy by hepatocyte growth factor gene therapy in rats. Diabetes 2004;53(4):1119–1127.
48. Inoue T, Okada H, Kobayashi T, et al. Hepatocyte growth factor counteracts transforming growth factor-b1, through attenuation of connective tissue growth factor induction, and prevents renal fibrogenesis in 5/6 nephrectomized mice. FASEB J 2003;17(2):268–270, 10.1096/fj.02-0442fje.
49. Adler SG, Kang SW, Feld S, et al. Can glomerular mRNAs in human type 1 diabetes be used to predict transition from normoalbuminuria to microalbuminuria? Am J Kidney Dis 2002;40(1):184–188.
50. Roestenberg P, van Nieuwenhoven FA, Wieten L, et al. Connective tissue growth factor is increased in plasma of type 1 diabetic patients with nephropathy. Diabetes Care 2004;27(5):1164–1170.
51. Mohammed A, Frinak S, Yee J, Riser BL. Urinary CCN2 (CTGF): A new tool to stage progression of diabetic nephropathy. J Am Soc Nephrol 2002;13(Suppl):250A.
52. Riser B. In: CCN proteins: a new family of cell growth and differentiation Regulators London, UK: Imperial College Press, 2005.

11 Vascular Endothelial Growth Factor as a Determinant of Diabetic Nephropathy

Geoffrey Boner, MBBCh,
and Mark E. Cooper, MBBS, PhD

CONTENTS

INTRODUCTION

Diabetic nephropathy is the major cause of end-stage renal disease in the United States and in many other countries *(1–3)*. The development of diabetic nephropathy is thought to occur as a result of an interplay between hemodynamic and metabolic factors *(4,5)*. The various metabolic factors, such as the renal accumulation of advanced glycation end (AGE) products and activation of the polyol pathway, as well as hemodynamic changes, including changes in vasoactive hormones such as the renin–angiotensin system (RAS), act through the stimulation of various intracellular second messengers, cytokines and growth factors to induce end-organ injury *(5,6)*. Vascular endothelial growth factor (VEGF), originally known as vascular permeability factor because of its ability to stimulate vascular permeability, was later shown to have a mitogenic effect in endothelial cells *(7,8)*. Indeed, VEGF was shown to stimulate angiogenesis *(8)* and has subsequently been postulated to play a role in the pathogenesis of various complications of diabetes *(9)*. In this chapter, we will discuss the role of VEGF, as yet not fully delineated in the development of diabetic nephropathy.

From: *Contemporary Diabetes: The Diabetic Kidney*
Edited by: P. Cortes and C. E. Mogensen © Humana Press Inc., Totowa, NJ

VASCULAR ENDOTHELIAL GROWTH FACTOR

VEGF and its functions have been described in many excellent reviews *(7–10)*. It is a specific mitogen of endothelial cells and has been described as having at least five isoforms *(7,8)*. A number of receptors for VEGF have been described including two specific tyrosine-kinase receptors, VEGFR-1 (*flt-1*) and VEGFR-2 (KDR/*flk-1*) *(7,8)*. VEGF stimulates endothelial cell proliferation and differentiation, increases vascular permeability, endothelium-dependent vasodilatation via NO, and plays a central role in physiological and pathological angiogenesis as well as modulating leukocyte migration *(6,8)*. The importance of VEGF in angiogenesis is critical as deletion of the gene in mice results in major vascular defects and intrauterine death *(11)*. In fact, topical application of VEGF improves wound healing by stimulating growth factors and by mobilizing cells, which contribute to new vessel formation *(12)*. In addition, VEGF has been shown to promote tumor angiogenesis with clinical trials of agents, which block VEGF dependent pathways currently underway *(7,8)*. VEGF has also been shown to play a role in hematopoiesis and hematological malignancies *(8)*.

The importance of VEGF in the pathogenesis of proliferative diabetic retinopathy has been extensively examined. This role of VEGF has been substantiated in both animal *(13–15)* and human studies *(16,17)* and has recently been reviewed *(18)*.

VEGF AND THE KIDNEY

VEGF mRNA and protein have been localized to glomerular epithelial cells and collecting duct cells using *in situ* hybridization and immunohistochemistry *(19–22)*. In addition, using sensitive techniques to assess gene expression of VEGF, the presence of three isoforms of VEGF in fetal kidney and cortex, isolated glomeruli and medulla of human adult kidney has been demonstrated. Gene expression of the two tyrosine kinase receptors has been reported in endothelia from glomerular and peritubular capillaries in fetal and adult kidneys *(19,21,22)*. The presence of both VEGF and its receptors within the kidney suggests that this factor may play an important role in renal physiology and pathology. The importance of VEGF in development of glomerular abnormalities and disease has been investigated in genetically modified mice with specific loss or gain of VEGF function in the glomerular podocytes *(23)*. Mice, which had complete absence of VEGF in the podocytes, died at birth or within 18 h of birth, some of them being born with hydrops as seen in congenital nephrotic syndrome. The mice, which were heterozygotic for podocyte VEGF, developed endotheliosis and "bloodless" kidneys by 2.5 wk of age, which progressed to nephrotic syndrome and end-stage renal failure by 9–12 wk of age. Overexpression of VEGF led to a form of collapsing glomerulopathy *(23)*. These studies demonstrate the importance of regulation of glomerular VEGF and the development of renal disease as a result of both under- and overexpression of this growth factor. Interactions between important renal factors and the release of VEGF have also been described. For instance, angiotensin II stimulates the release of VEGF from human vascular *(24)* and mesangial cells *(25)*.

VEGF AND NONDIABETIC RENAL DISEASE

Shulman et al. *(26)* examined the expression of VEGF in renal biopsies of a series of patients with various renal diseases including diabetic nephropathy. They found a decreased number of cells expressing VEGF in areas of focal glomerular sclerosis in the setting of amyloidosis, diabetes, crescentic glomerulonephritis, and diffuse endocapillary proliferative glomerulonephritis associated with systemic lupus erythematosus *(26)*. In a previous study we have found decreased VEGF gene expression in a series of patients with minimal change disease *(27)*. These findings have been interpreted to be consistent with VEGF being important for the repair of renal tissue, as previously postulated by other investigators *(28)*.

VEGF IN EXPERIMENTAL DIABETIC KIDNEY DISEASE

The possible role of VEGF in diabetic nephropathy has been investigated in several animal models of diabetes mellitus, initially in essentially descriptive studies but more recently in experiments in which the effects of VEGF have been blocked. Cooper et al. *(21)* demonstrated an early and sustained increase in VEGF gene and protein expression in the visceral epithelial cells of the glomerulus from rats with streptozotocin-induced diabetes. On the other hand, the expression of VEGFR-2, mainly in the glomeruli was increased at the earlier 3-wk time-point but not at 32 wk, suggesting a more important role for VEGF in the earlier stages of diabetic renal disease. A similar increased expression of VEGF mRNA and protein has been reported at early time-points in the development of nephropathy in spontaneously diabetic rats. These investigators suggested that hypoxia and cAMP played a regulatory role in the expression of VEGF at the onset of diabetes *(29)*. Changes in VEGF expression have been examined in a longitudinal manner in Otsuka-Long-Evans-Tokushima-Fatty rats, a model of type-2 diabetes mellitus. These rats had increased albuminuria throughout the study *(30)*. Urinary VEGF levels were greater from 25 to 37 wk and then decreased but remained higher than observed in control rats. Urinary VEGF levels correlated with albuminuria. VEGF was found mainly in the podocytes, as had been reported in the type-1 models of diabetes. Interestingly, the increase in VEGF gene expression was observed in the early period of diabetic nephropathy and was associated with increased urinary albumin excretion. Other investigators have described similar findings in these Otsuka-Long-Evans-Tokushima-Fatty rats *(31)* as well as in Zucker Diabetic fatty rats, another model of type-2 diabetes *(32)*.

The importance of this early increase in VEGF expression in the diabetic kidney has been further investigated using a variety of different interventions. Monoclonal antibodies against VEGF were administered intraperitoneally to rats with streptozotocin diabetes. The antibodies were shown to inhibit serum VEGF levels and caused a decrease in hyperfiltration, albuminuria, and glomerular hypertrophy *(33)*. As experimental diabetes is associated with renal hypertrophy, Schrijvers et al. *(34)* used another model of glomerular hypertrophy induced by high protein intake in mice. The administration of a neutralizing antibody to VEGF prevented the glomerular hypertrophy in that model but had no effect on kidney and body weight, consistent with a specific action of VEGF on glomerular hypertrophy. Furthermore, these investigators demonstrated in a mouse model of obese type-2 diabetes the db/db mouse that the administration of a neutralizing VEGF antibody resulted in attenuation in the increases in kidney weight, glomerular volume, and basement membrane thickness, seen in untreated diabetic mice *(35)*. In addition the increase in creatinine clearance, a relatively crude marker of hyperfiltration, was prevented. These findings are consistent with the view that direct inhibition of VEGF may prevent the renal damage seen in diabetes.

Of particular interest is whether other agents, which ameliorate diabetic nephropathy, work through VEGF-dependent mechanisms. Diabetic rats were treated with either an angiotensin converting enzyme inhibitor (ACE-I) (enalapril) or an angiotensin II receptor blocker (ARB) (candesartan) *(36)*. Both treatment regimens reduced the urinary excretion of albumin, whereas only the ACE-I attenuated renal VEGF protein content, consistent with the antialbuminuric effect of ACE inhibition, which may be partly via reducing renal VEGF accumulation. Recently Satoh et al. *(37)* examined the effects of an ARB and a calcium channel blockade in hypertensive Wistar fatty rats, a model of type-2 diabetes. ARB administration reduced blood pressure and the increase in urinary albumin excretion, whereas the calcium channel blocker did not affect albuminuria despite reducing blood pressure to a similar extent. The ARB reduced renal expression of VEGF, whereas the calcium channel blocker had no effect on this growth factor. The authors concluded that in this model the concomitant systemic hypertension accelerates nephropathy through hemodynamic mechanisms involving angiotensin II's action on VEGF synthesis. Of interest is the report showing that the administration of a cyclo-oxygenase-2 inhibitor to a rat model of diabetes and hypertension resulted in the reduction of several putative mediators of renal injury including PAI-I, VEGF, and tumor growth factor (TGF)-β_1 *(38)*. This was associated with a decrease in proteinuria and mesangial sclerosis, suggesting that various mediators of renal disease in diabetes, such as VEGF may involve cyclo-oxygenase-2 dependent pathways. In a study to determine if HMG Coenzyme A reductase inhibitors influence the progression of diabetic nephropathy diabetic rats were treated with losartan (ARB), simvastatin or both *(39)*. Injury to the kidney was attenuated by losartan but not by simvastatin. Both drugs individually and in combination resulted in a similar attenuation of the increase in not only glomerular expression of TGF-β_1 but also VEGF. However, only the combination resulted in a reduction in the plasma concentrations of urea and creatinine.

In a study investigating the relationship between AGE products and the intracellular second messenger, protein kinase C (PKC) in diabetic nephropathy, diabetic rats were treated with pharmacological approaches to attenuate renal AGE accumulation, either the crosslink breaker, ALT-711 or the inhibitor of AGE formation, aminoguanidine *(40)*. Both treatments reduced the glomerular deposition of AGEs and attenuated increased expression of certain PKC isoforms. However, the increased renal expression of VEGF was attenuated only by ALT-711 and not by aminoguanidine. Further studies indicated that ALT-711, in both in vitro and in vivo experiments, inhibited phosphorylation of the PKC-α isoform suggesting a link between certain PKC isoforms and VEGF expression. The importance of the PKC-α isoform has been further suggested in experiments in which induction of diabetes in PKC-α–/– mice was associated with reduced renal VEGF expression and interestingly less albuminuria *(41)*.

In an attempt to correlate the effects of VEGF with other angiogenic growth factors, Rizkalla et al. *(42)* measured the expression not only of VEGF and the receptor VEGF-R2 but other angiogenesis related factors such as, angiopoietin (Ang)-1, Ang-2, and their cognate receptor, Tie2 in diabetic rat, kidneys. Furthermore, the investigators assessed the effects of blockade of the RAS with AT-1 and AT-2 receptor antagonists on these growth factors and their receptors. Diabetes was associated with increased gene and protein expression of VEGF, the VEGF receptor VEGFR-2, Ang-1, Ang-2, and Tie-2. Blockade of the AT-1 receptor prevented the increased expression of these cytokines and their respective receptors, whereas the AT-2 blocker had less widespread effects, reducing VEGF receptor and Ang-1 gene expression and decreasing VEGF, Ang-1, and Ang-2 protein levels.

Although not directly relevant to this chapter, further evidence linking the RAS to expression of VEGF, related proteins and receptors has been described in AII infused rodent kidneys *(43)* as well as in the diabetic retina *(44)* and in a nondiabetic model of retinal neovascularization *(45)*.

VEGF AND RENAL CELLS: IN VITRO STUDIES

VEGF signaling and production has been assessed in cultured mesangial cells, in response to high glucose concentrations. The high glucose concentration resulted in increased VEGF mRNA and protein expression. This increase was prevented by inhibition of PKC *(46,47)*. Other investigators have demonstrated VEGF production in glomerular endothelial cells, proximal and distal tubular cells as well as confirming the mesangial cell findings *(25,48,49)*. High ambient glucose concentrations have also been shown to stimulate production of VEGF in mouse podocytes *(50)*. Exogenous VEGF stimulated the production of $\alpha 3$ (IV) collagen by immortalized mouse podocytes *(51)*. SU5416, a pan-VEGF receptor inhibitor prevented the increase in VEGF-stimulated collagen production and collagen production secondary to TGF-β_1 seen in this model *(51)*. However, VEGF had no effect on $\alpha 5$ (IV) collagen. These results suggest that podocyte-derived VEGF may play an important role in collagen production in diabetic glomerulopathy and that TGF-β_1 induced matrix accumulation may work partly through this mechanism. In a subsequent study by the same group, pilot results suggest that the stimulatory effect of TGF-β_1 on $\alpha 3$ (IV) collagen is partly dependent on the podocyte's endogenous VEGF system, operating in an autocrine loop, possibly involving the receptor, VEGFR-1 and signaling through the PI3 kinase and PKC pathways *(52)*. AGE products and angiotensin II, stimuli highly relevant to the diabetic milieu, have also been reported to induce VEGF secretion in cultured human mesangial cells *(25,49,53)*. Moreover, VEGF stimulation of endothelial cells caused an increase in nuclear factor-κB and an increase in ACE further extending the relationship, probably a two way interaction, between VEGF and the renin-angiotensin system *(54,55)*.

VEGF IN DIABETIC NEPHROPATHY IN HUMANS

In spite of the large amount of experimental evidence implicating VEGF in the development of experimental diabetic nephropathy, there is a lack of convincing evidence of a pivotal role for VEGF in human diabetic nephropathy. Of interest is a patient described by Baba et al. *(56)*. This patient had a syndrome known as POEMS (polyneuropathy, organomegaly, endocrinopathy, monoclonal gammopathy, and skin changes) and type 2 diabetes for 30 yr, when he died from cardiac failure. Plasma levels of VEGF had been markedly elevated, yet before death renal function was not severely impaired and at autopsy there were only slight glomerular changes. Thus, it is possible that rather than VEGF playing a pathophysiological role in the diabetic kidney, it acts as a survival factor protecting the kidney from ongoing injury. A recent report has described various VEGF gene polymorphisms in a large group of diabetic patients with retinopathy and nephropathy *(57)*. The VEGF-460 polymorphism was associated with retinopathy, but neither this nor the other polymorphism was associated with nephropathy. This would suggest the importance of this specific VEGF gene polymorphism in retinopathy, but not nephropathy. However, most of the current evidence is not uniform in its findings with respect to VEGF and diabetic nephropathy and thus it is virtually impossible to draw definite conclusions at this stage. It needs to be noted that various methods have been used to examine the role of

VEGF in diabetic patients and thus it is difficult to compare the results among the various studies. The studies can be divided essentially into two types of clinical investigation. First, VEGF has been measured in body fluids including serum, plasma, or urine and then these levels have been linked to various biochemical markers of diabetic nephropathy. Second, investigations have assessed the expression of VEGF gene, VEGF protein, and VEGF receptors in histological specimens.

VEGF Levels in Plasma, Serum, or Urine

In a group of patients with both types of diabetes, serum VEGF concentrations were found to be increased, especially in those with proliferative retinopathy (Table 1). Furthermore, levels of VEGF were higher in patients with macroalbuminuria than in those with lesser degrees of albuminuria *(58)*. Indeed, there was a significant correlation between serum VEGF concentrations and albuminuria. Similar findings have been reported in a group of type-2 diabetic subjects with serum creatinine concentrations less than 2 mg/dL *(46)*. However, in a large group of patients with type-1 diabetes, plasma VEGF concentrations were only increased in males but not females with nephropathy (micro- or macroalbuminuria) *(59)*. Serum VEGF levels were found to be increased in preschool, prepubertal diabetic children and to be markedly increased in adolescents with microvascular complications *(60)*. In a group of type-1 diabetic children and adolescents, who were followed for 8 yr, initial VEGF levels were increased in those subjects who subsequently developed microalbuminuria *(61)*. In another study, Lenz et al. *(62)* found serum concentrations of the VEGF isoform, VEGF165 to be increased in type-1 diabetic patient, who were receiving ACE-I or ARBs. Another group reported that plasma VEGF concentrations were increased in hypertensive diabetic individuals and this measurement correlated with urinary excretion of albumin *(63)*. In a study of type-2 diabetic patients with or without cardiovascular disease, Lim et al. *(64)* observed increased serum VEGF concentrations in diabetic subjects, which correlated with serum Ang-2 concentrations. These authors also noted that HbA1c predicted the levels of VEGF. By contrast, some investigators have not been able to demonstrate an increase in serum or plasma VEGF in diabetic subjects with or without complications. Serum VEGF and basic fibroblast growth factor levels were unchanged in a group of type-1 diabetic children and adolescents without clinical complications when compared with nondiabetic children *(65)*. Furthermore, in a large group of type-1 diabetic subjects, who participated in the EUCLID study, there was no correlation between plasma VEGF concentrations at baseline and duration of diabetes or glycemic control *(66)*. As one would have predicted, there was a tendency for the plasma VEGF level to increase in those patients with proliferative retinopathy. In another study in type-2 diabetic patients, plasma VEGF concentrations were not related to the degree of nephropathy *(67)*. Another group found a nonsignificant increase in serum VEGF concentrations in type-2 diabetic, hypertensive patients, but there was no correlation between this growth factor and renal function and metabolic control *(68)*. Finally serum VEGF165 levels were not different in type-2 diabetic subjects with varying degrees of albuminuria *(69)*. At this stage, measurement of serum VEGF does not appear to contribute significantly to the understanding of the involvement of VEGF in the pathogenesis of diabetic nephropathy and other diabetic complications.

Urinary excretion of VEGF seems to be a better marker of renal involvement in diabetes. Cha et al. *(46)* showed in type-2 diabetic patients, that urinary VEGF excretion was greater in those subjects with macroalbuminuria than in those with microalbuminuria,

Table 1
Circulating and Urinary VEGF Levels in Relation to Diabetic Nephropathy

Ref no./yr	*No and description of subjects*	*Results*
58/1997	20 T1, 56 T2	Serum VEGF increased in diabetics, highest in proliferative retinopathy. Significantly higher in macro than micro.
65/1998	40 T1 No clinical complications	Serum VEGF and basic fibroblast growth factor no different from control.
46/2000	73 T2 SCr <2	Plasma VEGF–macro>micro or normo. Urine VEGF–macro>micro>normo.
59/2000	199 T1	Plasma VEGF increased in nephropathy (micro + macro), but only in males.
60/2000	196 T1	Serum VEGF significantly increased in preschool, prepubertal and pubertal diabetics, and markedly elevated in adolescents with microvascular complications. Increased VEGF with poor control and improved with glycemic control.
61/2001	101 T1	Initial plasma VEGF higher in those developing micro. 8-yr follow-up.
66/2001	299 T1 (EUCLID)	No correlation between plasma VEGF at baseline and duration of diabetes and glycemic control. Tendency to increase in proliferative retinopathy No effect of ACEI.
67/2002	71 T2	Plasma VEGF not related to degree of nephropathy.
62/2004	35 T1, 37 T2	Serum VEGF 165 increased in T1 receiving ACEI/ARB. Urine VEGF no different in diabetics to healthy subjects. Correlation between urine VEGF and albuminuria in T2.
63/2004	107 T2	Plasma VEGF increased in hypertensive diabetic, correlated with ACR. Urine VEGF increased with advancing disease and correlated with ACR.
68/2004	50 T2 + hypertension	Serum VEGF higher in diabetic than normal subjects (not significant). No correlation with renal function and metabolic control.
64/2004	94 T2 ± cardiovascular disease	VEGF increased in diabetics. VEGF correlated with increased Ang-2 and HbA1c predicted increased VEGF.
69/2005	107 T2	Serum VEGF 165, no different in varying degrees of albuminuria. Urine VEGF and soluble FLT-1 (VEGFR-1) increased and correlated with degree of albuminuria.

Abbreviations: T1, type-1 diabetic patients; T2, type-2 diabetic patients; macro, macroalbuminuria; micro, microalbuminuria; normo, normalbuminuria; ACE-I, angiotensin converting enzyme inhibitor; ARB, angiotensin receptor blocker; ACR, urine albumin/creatinine.

Table 2
Renal Expression of VEGF

Ref. no./yr	*Number, type of disease and specimen*	*Method of examination*	*Results*
26/1996	5 BX	IH, ISH	VEGF mRNA—strong in normal glomeruli, weak to absent in areas of sclerosis. VEGF protein—similar.
71/2001	12 T2 BX	RT/PCR	VEGF 121 greater expression than VEGF 165 in glomeruli and tubulo-interstitium (TI). KDR (VEGFR-2) and Flt-1 (VEGFR-1) in most specimens. In mainly TI involvement less VEGF and receptors.
72/2004	2 T2 PM 5 T2 BX	MIH, IH	Almost 100 genes were upregulated and over 500 genes were downregulated. VEGF and nephrin were downregulated. In the biopsies decreased VEGF mRNA and VEGF protein.
70/2004	17 T2 BX	RT/PCR	Glomerular VEGF mRNA inversely related to albuminuria. Mesangial expansion inversly related to VEGF 165 mRNA and directly related to VEGF 121 mRNA. VEGF and VEGFR-2 directly related.
73/2005	18 T2 BX	IH, ISH	VEGF protein in glomeruli and proximal tubule. Increased expression of VEGF in glomeruli in diabetes. Increased VEGF mRNA cells in glomeruli in diabetes. Significant correlation between VEGF mRNA and glomerular matrix index. No correlation with clinical parameters and parameters of glycemic control. Glomerular VEGF expressed early in disease.

Abbreviations: T1, type-1 diabetic patients; T2, type-2 diabetic patients; PM, autopsy specimens; BX, biopsy specimens; IH, immunohistochemistry; ISH, *in situ* hybridization; RT/PCR, reverse transcription/polymerase chain reaction; MIH, microarray hybridization.

with nonalbuminuric patients having the lowest levels of VEGF in their urine. However, Lenz et al. *(62)* found that urinary VEGF excretion was similar in diabetic subjects in comparison with healthy controls. Nevertheless, these authors showed a correlation between urinaryVEGF levels and albuminuria in type-2 diabetic patients. Two recent studies have reported increased urinary VEGF excretion in type-2 diabetic patients and correlated this finding to the degree of albuminuria *(63,64)*. Furthermore, it has been shown that these changes were associated with increased excretion of the soluble VEGF receptor *Flt-1* (VEGFR-1). Thus, overall there appears to be a correlation between the magnitude of urinary VEGF excretion and the degree of renal involvement in diabetic subjects and this has been interpreted as consistent with a local role for VEGF in the pathogenesis of kidney diseases including diabetic nephropathy.

VEGF Expression in Renal Specimens

Shulman et al. *(26)* demonstrated significant expression of VEGF mRNA and protein in relatively normal glomeruli but weak to absent expression of this growth factor in areas of sclerosis (Table 2). Bortoloso et al. *(70)* examined the changes in VEGF gene expression in glomeruli of 17 patients with type 2 diabetes. Glomerular VEGF gene expression was inversely related to urinary albumin excretion. Mesangial expansion was inversely related to the gene expression of the VEGF isoform, VEGF165 and directly related to the gene expression of the isoform, VEGF121. The same investigators also examined the expression of VEGF and its receptors in the tubulo-interstitium in renal biopsies from 12 patients with type 2 diabetes *(71)*. They demonstrated VEGF mRNA in all kidney samples, whereas the VEGF receptors, KDR, (VEGFR-2), and Flt-1 (VEGFR-1) were found in most but not all specimens. Furthermore, the expression of VEGF121 was greater than VEGF165 in glomeruli and interstitium. In the patients with mainly tubulointerstitial involvement there was a decreased expression of VEGF and its receptors. The investigators concluded that the VEGF system is crucial in maintaining the structural and functional integrity of the kidney. Baelde et al. *(72)* used a microarray strategy to profile gene expression in kidneys taken at autopsy from two patients with type 2 diabetes and specifically examined gene and protein expression of VEGF and the podocyte specific slit pore protein, nephrin in biopsy specimens from five individuals with type 2 diabetes. More genes were downregulated than were upregulated in the diabetic kidneys in comparison with the normal kidney. Specifically, VEGF and nephrin gene expression were downregulated in the microarray experiments. Furthermore, in the biopsy specimens the gene and protein expression of both nephrin and VEGF were decreased. Kanesaki et al. *(73)* have recently examined the expression of VEGF in open renal biopsies taken from 18 patients with type 2 diabetes. VEGF protein was demonstrated in the glomeruli and proximal tubule. There was increased expression of VEGF in glomeruli from the diabetic subjects. The authors also found a significant correlation between VEGF mRNA levels and glomerular extracellular matrix accumulation. There was no correlation between VEGF expression and clinical parameters of renal injury or markers of glycemic control. These investigators suggested that glomerular VEGF upregulation occurs early in the disease process consistent with previous animal findings *(21)*.

CONCLUSIONS

The role of VEGF in renal disease remains to be fully delineated, particularly in the context of diabetes. Early on in the nephropathic process, there appears to be upregulation of VEGF and/or some of its receptors and this could explain some of the features of the diabetic kidney including hyperfiltration and albuminuria. As the renal disease progresses, the pattern becomes more complex with some investigators reporting a decrease in renal VEGF expression occurring in association with increased renal structural damage including podocyte loss. The postulate that the repair functions of the VEGF became impaired with increasing duration of diabetes resulting in accelerated renal injury in progressive diabetic nepthropathy remains to be proven. Preliminary studies using various approaches to inhibit VEGF levels or action suggest a role for this growth factor in diabetic renal disease but these studies are still at a very early stage with limited approaches currently available to adequately examine this issue.

REFERENCES

1. US Renal Data System: Excerpts from the USRDS 2004 Annual Data Report. Am J Kidney Dis 2005;45(1):S57–S70.
2. US Renal Data System: Excerpts from the USRDS 2001 Annual Data Report. Am J Kidney Dis 2001;38(3):S195–S200.
3. Ritz E, Rychlik I, Locatelli F, Halimi S. End-stage renal failure in type-2 diabetes; A medical catastrophe of worldwide dimensions. Am J Kidney Dis 1999;34:795–808.
4. Cooper ME, Gilbert RE, Epstein M. Pathophysiology of Diabetic Nephropathy. Metabolism 1998;47:3–6.
5. Cooper ME. Interaction of metabolic and haemodynamic factors in mediating experimental diabetic nephropathy. Diabetologia 2001;44:1957–1972.
6. Schrijvers BF, De Vriese AS, Flyvbjerg A. From hyperglycemia to diabetic kidney disease: the role of metabolic, hemodynamic, intracellular factors and growth factors/cytokines. Endocrine Rev 2004;25:971–1010.
7. Neufeld G, Cohen T, Gengrinovitch S, Poltorak Z. Vascular endothelial growth factor (VEGF) and its receptors. FASEB J 1999;13:9–22.
8. Ferrara N, Gerber H-P. The role of vascular endothelial growth factor in angiogenesis. Acta Haematol 2001;106:148–156.
9. Khamaisi M, Schrijvers BF, De Vriese AS, Raz I, Flyvbjerg A. The emerging role of VEGF in diabetic kidney disease. Nephrol Dial Transplant 2003;18:1427–1430.
10. Schrijvers BF, Flyvbjerg A, De Vriese AS. The role of vascular endothelial growth factor (VEGF) in renal pathophysiology. Kidney Int 2004;65:2003–2017.
11. Ferrara N, Carver-Moore K, Chen H, et al. Heterozygous embryonic lethality induced by targeted inactivation of the VEGF gene. Nature 1996;380:439–442.
12. Galiano RD, Tepper OM, Pelo CR, et al. Topical vascular endothelial growth factor accelerates diabetic wound healing through increased angiogenesis and by mobilizing and recruiting bone marrow-derived cells. Am J Pathol 2004;164:1935–1947.
13. Gilbert RE, Vranes D, Berka JL, et al. Vascular endothelial growth factor and its receptors in control and diabetic rat eyes. Lab Invest 1998;78:1017–1027.
14. Zhang X, Lassila M, Cooper ME, Cao Z. Retinal expression of vascular endothelial growth factor is mediated by angiotensin type 1 and type 2 receptors. Hypertension 2004;43:276–281.
15. Cukiernik M, Hileeto D, Evans T, Mukherjee S, Downey D, Chakrabarti S. Vascular endothelial growth factor in diabetes induced early retinal abnormalities. Diabetes Res Clin Pract 2004;65: 197–208.
16. Nicoletti VG, Nicoletti R, Ferrara N, Meli G, Reibaldi M, Reibaldi A. Diabetic patients and retinal proliferation: an evaluation of the role of vascular endothelial growth factor (VEGF). Exp Clin Endocrinol Diabetes 2003;111:209–214.
17. Itakura H, Kishi S, Kotajima N, Murakami M. Persistent secretion of vascular endothelial growth factor into the vitreous cavity in proliferative diabetic retinopathy after vitrectomy. Ophthalmology 2004;111:1880–1884.
18. Caldwell RB, Bartoli M, Behzadian MA, et al. Vascular endothelial growth factor and diabetic retinopathy: pathophysiological mechanisms and treatment perspectives. Diabetes Metab Res Rev 2003;19:442–455.
19. Simon M, Grone HJ, Johren O, et al. Expression of vascular endothelial growth factor and its receptors in human renal ontogenesis and in adult kidney. Am J Physiol 1995;268:F240–F250.
20. Brown LF, Berse B, Tognazzi K, et al. Vascular permeability factor mRNA and protein expression in human kidney. Kidney Int 1992;42:1457–1461.
21. Cooper ME, Vranes D, Youssef S, et al. Increased renal expression of vascular endothelial growth factor (VEGF) and its receptor VEGFR-2 in experimental diabetes. Diabetes 1999;48:2229–2239.
22. Simon M, Rockl W, Hornig C, et al. Receptors of vascular endothelial growth factor/vascular permeability factor (VEGF/VPF) in fetal and adult human kidney: localization and [125I]VEGF binding sites. J Am Soc Nephrol 1998;9:1032–1044.
23. Eremina V, Sood M, Haigh J, et al. Glomerular-specific alterations of VEGF-A expression lead to distinct congenital and acquired renal diseases. J Clin Invest 2003;111:707–716.
24. Williams B, Baker AQ, Gallacher B, Lodwick D. Angiotensin II increases vascular permeability factor gene expression by human vascular smooth muscle cells. Hypertension 1995;25:913–917.
25. Pupilli C, Lasagni L, Romagnani P, et al. Angiotensin II stimulates the synthesis and secretion of vascular permeability factor/vascular endothelial growth factor in human mesangial cells. J Am Soc Nephrol 1999;10:245–255.

26. Shulman K, Rosen S, Tognazzi K, Manseau EJ, Brown LF. Expression of vascular permeability factor (VPF/VEGF) is altered in many glomerular diseases. J Am Soc Nephrol 1996;7:661–666.
27. Boner G, Cox AJ, Kelly DJ, et al. Does vascular endothelial growth factor (VEGF) play a role in the pathogenesis of minimal change disease? Nephrol Dial Transplant 2003;18:2293–2299.
28. Remuzzi G, Benigni A. Repairing renal lesions: will VEGF be the builder? Kidney Int 2000;58: 2594–2595.
29. Braun L, Kardon T, Reisz-Porszasz ZS, Banhegyi G, Mandl J. The regulation of the induction of vascular endothelial growth factor at the onset of diabetes in spontaneously diabetic rats. Life Sci 2001;69:2533–2542.
30. Cha DR, Kang YS, Han SY, et al. Vascular endothelial growth factor is increased during early stage of diabetic nephropathy in type II diabetic rats. J Endocrinol 2004;183:183–194.
31. Tsuchida K, Makita Z, Yamagishi S, et al. Suppression of transforming growth factor beta and vascular endothelial growth factor in diabetic nephropathy in rats by a novel advanced glycation end product inhibitor, OPB-9195. Diabetologia 1999;42:579–588.
32. Hoshi S, Shu Y, Yoshida F, et al. Podocyte injury promotes progressive nephropathy in zucker diabetic fatty rats. Lab Invest 2002;82:25–35.
33. de Vriese AS, Tilton RG, Elger M, Stephan CC, Kriz W, Lameire NH. Antibodies against vascular endothelial growth factor improve early renal dysfunction in experimental diabetes. J Am Soc Nephrol 2001;12:993–1000.
34. Schrijvers BF, Rasch R, Tilton RG, Flyvbjerg A. High protein-induced glomerular hypertrophy is vascular endothelial growth factor-dependent. Kidney Int 2002;61:1600–1604.
35. Flyvbjerg A, Dagnaes-Hansen F, De Vriese AS, Schrijvers BF, Tilton RG, Rasch R. Amelioration of long-term renal changes in obese type-2 diabetic mice by a neutralizing vascular endothelial growth factor antibody. Diabetes 2002;51:3090–3094.
36. Kakizawa H, Itoh Y, Imamura S, et al. Possible role of VEGF in the progression of kidney disease in streptozotocin (STZ)-induced diabetic rats: effects of an ACE inhibitor and an angiotensin II receptor antagonist. Horm Metab Res 2004;36:458–464.
37. Sato T, Murao M, Kumal T, et al. Hemodynamic mechanisms involved in the early stage of diabetic nephropathy in the Wistar fatty rats, a model of type-2 diabetes: Roles of renal NO metabolisms and VEGF. Abstract 2693, American Society of Nephrology, Renal Week, St Louis, October 2004.
38. Cheng HF, Wang CJ, Moeckel GW, Zhang MZ, McKanna JA, Harris RC. Cyclo-oxygenase-2 inhibitor blocks expression of mediators of renal injury in a model of diabetes and hypertension. Kidney Int 2002;62:929–939.
39. Qin J, Zhang Z, Liu J, et al. Effects of the combination of an angiotensin II antagonist with an HMG-CoA reductase inhibitor in experimental diabetes. Kidney Int 2003;64:565–571.
40. Thallas-Bonke V, Lindschau C, Rizkalla B, et al. Attenuation of extracellular matrix accumulation in diabetic nephropathy by the advanced glycation end product cross-link breaker ALT-711 via a protein kinase C-alpha-dependent pathway. Diabetes 2004;53:2921–2930.
41. Menne J, Park JK, Boehne M, et al. Diminished loss of proteoglycans and lack of albuminuria in protein kinase C-alpha-deficient diabetic mice. Diabetes 2004;53:2101–2109.
42. Rizkalla B, Forbes JM, Cao Z, Boner G, Cooper ME. Temporal renal expression of angiogenic growth factors and their receptors in experimental diabetes: role of the renin-angiotensin system. J Hypertens 2005;23:153–164.
43. Rizkalla B, Forbes JM, Cooper ME, Cao Z. Increased renal vascular endothelial growth factor and angiopoietins by angiotensin II infusion is mediated by both AT1 and AT2 receptors. J Am Soc Nephrol 2003;14:3061–3071.
44. Zhang X, Lassila M, Cooper ME, Cao Z. Retinal expression of vascular endothelial growth factor is mediated by angiotensin type 1 and type 2 receptors. Hypertension 2004;43:276–281.
45. Sarlos S, Rizkalla B, Moravski CJ, Cao Z, Cooper ME, Wilkinson-Berka JL. Retinal angiogenesis is mediated by an interaction between the angiotensin type 2 receptor, VEGF, and angiopoietin. Am J Pathol 2003;163:879–887.
46. Cha DR, Kim NH, Yoon JW, et al. Role of vascular endothelial growth factor in diabetic nephropathy. Kidney Int Suppl 2000;77:S104–S112.
47. Kim NH, Jung HH, Cha DR, Choi DS. Expression of vascular endothelial growth factor in response to high glucose in rat mesangial cells. J Endocrinol 2000;165:617–624.
48. El Awad B, Kreft B, Wolber EM, et al. Hypoxia and interleukin-1beta stimulate vascular endothelial growth factor production in human proximal tubular cells. Kidney Int 2000;58:43–50.
49. Gruden G, Thomas S, Burt D, et al. Interaction of angiotensin II and mechanical stretch on vascular endothelial growth factor production by human mesangial cells. J Am Soc Nephrol 1999;10:730–737.

50. Iglesias-de la Cruz MC, Ziyadeh FN, Isono M, et al. Effects of high glucose and TGF-beta1 on the expression of collagen IV and vascular endothelial growth factor in mouse podocytes. Kidney Int 2002;62:901–913.
51. Chen S, Kasama Y, Lee JS, Jim B, Marin M, Ziyadeh FN. Podocyte-derived vascular endothelial growth factor mediates the stimulation of alpha3(IV) collagen production by transforming growth factor-beta1 in mouse podocytes. Diabetes 2004;53:2939–2949.
52. Chen S, Lee JS, Kasama Y, Marin M, Ziyadeh FN, Sung SH. TGF-β1 stimulation of α3(IV) collagen production in mouse podocytes is partly mediated VEGF autocrine loop involving PI3K and PKC. J Am Soc Nephrol 2004;15:31A, "abstract."
53. Yamagishi S, Inagaki Y, Okamoto T, et al. Advanced glycation end product-induced apoptosis and overexpression of vascular endothelial growth factor and monocyte chemoattractant protein-1 in human-cultured mesangial cells. J Biol Chem 2002;277:20,309–20,315.
54. Marumo T, Schini-Kerth VB, Busse R. Vascular endothelial growth factor activates nuclear factor-kappaB and induces monocyte chemoattractant protein-1 in bovine retinal endothelial cells. Diabetes 1999;48:1131–1137.
55. Saijonmaa O, Nyman T, Kosonen R, Fyhrquist F. Upregulation of angiotensin-converting enzyme by vascular endothelial growth factor. Am J Physiol Heart Circ Physiol 2001;280:H885–H891.
56. Baba T, Osterby R, Neugebauer-Baba S, et al. No nephropathy in type-2 diabetic patient with POEMS syndrome with an elevated plasma VEGF. Diabet Med 2004;21:292–294.
57. Ray D, Mishra M, Ralph S, Read I, Davies R, Brenchley P.Association of the VEGF gene with proliferative diabetic retinopathy but not proteinuria in diabetes. Diabetes 2004;53:861–864.
58. Abdel Aziz MY, Ben Gharbia O, el-Sayed Mohamed K, Muchaneta-Kubara EC, el Nahas AM. VEGF and diabetic microvascular complications. Nephrol Dial Transplant 1997;12:1538.
59. Hovind P, Tarnow L, Oestergaard PB, Parving HH. Elevated vascular endothelial growth factor in type-1 diabetic patients with diabetic nephropathy. Kidney Int Suppl 2000;75:S56–S61.
60. Chiarelli F, Spagnoli A, Basciani F, et al. Vascular endothelial growth factor (VEGF) in children, adolescents and young adults with type-1 diabetes mellitus: relation to glycaemic control and microvascular complications. Diabet Med 2000;17:650–656.
61. Santilli F, Spagnoli A, Mohn A, et al. Increased vascular endothelial growth factor serum concentrations may help to identify patients with onset of type-1 diabetes during childhood at risk for developing persistent microalbuminuria. J Clin Endocrinol Metab 2001;86:3871–3876.
62. Lenz T, Haak T, Malek J, Grone HJ, Geiger H, Gossmann J. Vascular endothelial growth factor in diabetic nephropathy. J Biol Chem 2004;279:3941–3948.
63. Kim NH, Kim KB, Kim DL, et al. Plasma and urinary vascular endothelial growth factor and diabetic nephropathy in type-2 diabetes mellitus. Diabet Med 2004;21:545–551.
64. Lim HS, Blann AD, Chong AY, Freestone B, Lip GY. Plasma Vascular Endothelial Growth Factor, Angiopoietin-1, and Angiopoietin-2 in Diabetes: Implications for cardiovascular risk and effects of multifactorial intervention. Diabetes Care 2004;27:2918–2924.
65. Malamitsi-Puchner A, Sarandakou A, Tziotis J, Dafogianni C, Bartsocas CS. Serum levels of basic fibroblast growth factor and vascular endothelial growth factor in children and adolescents with type-1 diabetes mellitus. Pediatr Res 1998;44:873–875.
66. Chaturvedi N, Fuller JH, Pokras F, Rottiers R, Papazoglou N, Aiello LP. EUCLID Study Group. Circulating plasma vascular endothelial growth factor and microvascular complications of type-1 diabetes mellitus: the influence of ACE inhibition. Diabet Med 2001;18:288–294.
67. Shimada K, Baba T, Neugebauer S, et al. Plasma vascular endothelial growth factor in Japanese type-2 diabetic patients with and without nephropathy. J Diabetes Complications 2002;16:386–390.
68. Cipriani R, Sensi M, Gabriele A, et al. The impairment of renal function is not associated to altered circulating vascular endothelial growth factor in patients with type-2 diabetes and hypertension. Diabetes Nutr Metab 2004;17:90–94.
69. Kim NH, Oh JH, Seo JA, et al. Vascular endothelial growth factor (VEGF) and soluble VEGF receptor FLT-1 in diabetic nephropathy. Kidney Int 2005;67:167–177.
70. Bortoloso E, Del Prete D, Dalla Vestra M, et al. Quantitave and qualitative changes in vascular endothelial growth factor gene expression in glomeruli of patients with type-2 diabetes. Eur J Endocrinol 2004;150:799–807.
71. Bortoloso E, Del Prete D, Gambaro G, et al. Vascular endothelial growth factor (VEGF) and VEGF receptors in diabetic nephropathy: expression studies in biopsies of type-2 diabetic patients. Ren Fail 2001;23:483–493.

72. Baelde HJ, Eikmans M, Doran PP, Lappin DW, de Heer E, Bruijn JA. Gene expression profiling in glomeruli from human kidneys with diabetic nephropathy. Am J Kidney Dis 2004;43: 636–650.
73. Kanesaki Y, Suzuki D, Uehara G, et al. Vascular endothelial growth factor gene expression is correlated with glomerular neovascularization in human diabetic nephropathy. Am J Kidney Dis 2005; 45:288–294.

12 Transforming Growth Factor-β Signal Transduction in the Pathogenesis of Diabetic Nephropathy

Identifying Molecular Targets for Therapeutic Intervention

Sheldon Chen, MD *and Fuad N. Ziyadeh,* MD

Contents

INTRODUCTION

The pathogenesis of diabetic nephropathy (DN) can be broadly divided into hemodynamic and metabolic causes, but this chapter will focus on the metabolic theories. Among the numerous metabolic derangements in diabetes, the abnormality that plays a central role in the pathogenesis of diabetic renal disease is overactivity of the renal transforming growth factor (TGF)-β system. TGF-β can be thought of as a growth factor or cytokine that causes cellular hypertrophy and stimulates the production of extracellular matrix (ECM), i.e., proteins such as fibronectin, proteoglycans, and several

From: *Contemporary Diabetes: The Diabetic Kidney*
Edited by: P. Cortes and C. E. Mogensen © Humana Press Inc., Totowa, NJ

collagen isotypes. These actions are especially relevant to DN, a disease characterized by glomerular and tubular hypertrophy and ECM accumulation. The consequences of matrix buildup manifest as arteriolar hyalinosis, glomerular basement membrane thickening, mesangial matrix expansion (glomerulosclerosis), and tubulo-interstitial fibrosis. In turn, these sclerotic lesions are thought to contribute to progressive renal dysfunction by obliterating the glomerular capillary loops and by displacing or destroying the tubulo-interstitium, causing loss of nephron mass and progressive kidney dysfunction.

EVIDENCE FOR ROLE OF TGF-β IN DIABETIC NEPHROPATHY

Koch's postulates have classically been used to determine whether an agent is the cause of an infectious disease, but the paradigm can be adapted to ascertain the role of TGF-β in DN *(1)*. If TGF-β is a causative agent, then it should be found in diabetic kidneys in increased levels. TGF-β has been shown to be elevated intrarenally in human DN *(2–5)* and in experimental animal models of diabetic renal disease, at both the mRNA and protein levels, and in both the glomerular and tubulo-interstitial compartments *(6–9)*. Increased amounts of TGF-β_1 (one of the three mammalian isoforms of TGF-β) are also excreted in the urine of diabetic patients *(10–12)*. The kidney in diabetes can also be a source of TGF-β. When the TGF-β_1 mass balance was calculated across the renal vascular bed (in patients undergoing cardiac catheterization), it was estimated that nondiabetic kidneys were extracting TGF-β_1 from the circulation whereas diabetic kidneys were adding TGF-β_1 to the bloodstream *(13)*.

If TGF-β contributes to DN, the increase in renal TGF-β should be attributable to the diabetic state. High glucose, elevated angiotensin II, amadori-modified proteins, advanced glycation endproducts, thromboxane, endothelin, platelet-derived growth factor, and leptin have all been shown to stimulate TGF-β production by cultured renal cells, which include mesangial, proximal tubular, interstitial fibroblast, and glomerular endothelial cells *(14–22)*. In humans with type 2 diabetes, the degree of glycemic control correlates with the increase in glomerular expression of TGF-β_1 *(2)*. Even in the absence of diabetes, TGF-β can reproduce the deleterious effects of diabetic metabolic features on kidney cells. For example, high glucose causes mesangial cell (MC) hypertrophy *(23,24)* and stimulates collagen I and IV expression *(14)*. In normal glucose media, exogenously added TGF-β_1 also promotes MC hypertrophy and ECM production *(14,23)*. For interstitial fibroblasts in culture, high glucose caused cellular proliferation and stimulated collagen I synthesis *(25)*. Likewise, exogenous TGF-β_1 was mitogenic for the interstitial fibroblast and TGF-β_1 increased type-I collagen expression *(25)*. Finally, experiments on cultured proximal tubular cells show that high glucose and TGF-β_1 share similar actions (inhibition of proliferation, induction of cellular hyerptrophy, and stimulation of ECM production) *(15)*.

Perhaps the most important part of the modified Koch's postulates is that therapy targeted against the causative agent should ameliorate or cure the disease. In the case of DN, blocking the effects of TGF-β should prevent diabetes from causing renal pathology and dysfunction. Inhibition of the TGF-β system can be achieved with a PAN-selective, neutralizing anti-TGF-β antibody *(26)*. Treating renal cells with this antibody, effectively prevented high glucose and other mediators of diabetes from inducing cellular hypertrophy and increasing matrix protein production, proving that these pathobiological effects are mediated by the cellular TGF-β system *(14,23,27,28)*. Even more striking, the systemic treatment of diabetic animals with injected anti-TGF-β antibody prevented many of the structural and functional defects of DN, even though hyperglycemia was left untreated *(6,8)*. In fact, neutralizing the TGF-β system ameliorated renal hypertrophy, normalized the overexpression of collagen IV and fibronectin, prevented the mesangial matrix expansion, and preserved renal function *(8)*. These findings constitute the strongest evidence that the harmful effects of diabetes on the kidney are largely mediated by heightened activity of the intrarenal TGF-β system.

DETAILS ABOUT THE TGF-β SYSTEM

In mammals, the three isoforms of TGF-β, named TGF-β_1, -β_2, and -β_3, share similar actions in vitro but not in vivo *(29,30)*. This is partly owing to differences in developmental regulation and tissue-specific expression. In the adult kidney, TGF-β1 has been described in tubular epithelial cells (both proximal and distal), in interstitial cells, and to a lesser extent in glomerular mesangial, endothelial, and epithelial cells. TGF-β_3 follows a similar pattern of expression but in quantitatively lower amounts. The TGF-β_2 protein is largely restricted to the juxtaglomerular apparatus in which it may play an important role in renin metabolism *(20,31)*. It should be kept in mind that nonrenal cells like platelets, macrophages, and vascular smooth muscle cells can also contribute to the overall TGF-β activity in the kidney. Unless otherwise specified, we will focus on TGF-β_1 because it is the most highly expressed isoform in the kidney and has been most closely linked to the pathophysiology of DN *(32)*.

The active form of TGF-β_1 is a homodimer of two cysteine-rich 12.5-kDa polypeptide subunits derived from the C-terminal end of the gene product and linked by a single disulfide bond. This active form can bind to its receptor and propagate a signal *(33)*. Normally, however, TGF-β is secreted as a latent complex that exists in a soluble form or an insoluble form bound to extracellular matrix constituents *(34,35)*. The latent complex is made up of the mature TGF-β dimer linked noncovalently to a latency-associated peptide (LAP) that is also encoded by the TGF-β gene *(36)*. LAP imparts latency by blocking TGF-β binding to the signaling receptor. In certain tissues including the glomerulus, the latent complex exists in covalent association with the product of another gene, the latent TGF-β binding protein. In the kidney, tubular epithelial cells secrete the small latent complex (mature TGF-β_1 + LAP), whereas glomerular parenchymal and arteriolar cells secrete the large latent complex (mature TGF-β_1 + LAP + latent TGF-β binding protein) *(37)*. This pattern of tissue expression implies potentially important differences in activation and functional regulation of the TGF-β system between the glomerular/vascular compartment and the tubular compartment.

The activation of latent TGF-β in vivo is largely controlled by proteases (e.g., plasmin) that cleave the LAP from the bioactive TGF-β dimer *(38)*. Plasmin-mediated activation of TGF-β involves the binding of the latent form to a mannose-6-phosphate receptor on the cell surface and then the concerted action of transglutaminase and plasmin to remove LAP. A protease-independent conformational change of the latent complex can also occur when thrombospondin (TSP), derived from the α-granules of platelets, allows the active TGF-β moiety to bind to its cell-surface receptor. The TSP system may partly explain how TGF-β_1 can be activated in MCs by high-ambient glucose.

Three different receptor proteins are involved in TGF-β signaling: types I–III *(39–41)* The type-III receptor, which does not signal, appears to enhance the delivery of TGF-β to the receptors that do signal. Signaling commences when the free TGF-β homodimer binds to the type-II receptor. This ligand–receptor complex recruits the binding of a type-I receptor to form a heterotetramer. Within this complex, the type-II receptor, via its serine/threonine kinase activity, phosphorylates and activates the type-I receptor in a glycine/serine region *(42,43)*. Via its own serine/threonine kinase, the type-I receptor phosphorylates the Smad proteins, which carry the TGF-β signal intracellularly.

The Smad proteins are a family of transcription factors that, so far, are the only TGF-β receptor substrates with a demonstrated ability to propagate signals *(44)*. After phosphorylation by the type-I receptor, the receptor-regulated Smads (R-Smad), Smad2 and Smad3, associate with a common partner Smad (Co-Smad), also known as Smad4. The Smad2–Smad4 or Smad3–Smad4 complexes translocate into the nucleus in which they can bind to the promoters of multiple genes. Optimal binding is achieved with the 5-bp DNA sequence CAGAC, also known as the Smad-binding element (SBE—although technically the Smad-binding element is GTCTAGAC) *(45,46)*. In conjunction with other transcription factors, coactivators, and corepressors, the Smad complexes coordinate the expression of target genes *(44,47)* In this way, the TGF-β signal is transduced from the cell surface to the nucleus, and the cell responds by activating certain genes and repressing others.

Ultimately, the predominant effect of TGF-β is to promote matrix accumulation. The matrix-stimulating effects of TGF-β involve several key systems:

- Stimulation of gene expression of matrix molecules such as fibronectin, proteoglycans, and several collagen isotypes.
- Inhibition of matrix degradation via a dual-pronged pathway of suppressing the expression and activity of serine, thiol, and metalloproteinases (e.g., plasminogen activator, collagenase, elastase, and stromelysin) as well as stimulating tissue inhibitors of metalloproteinases and plasminogen activator inhibitor-1 *(48)*; and
- Upregulation of integrins (the cell-surface receptors for ECM), thereby enhancing the ability of cells to interact with specific matrix proteins.

Additionally, excess TGF-β activity is important in mediating fibroproliferative disorders because of its potent chemotactic properties for macrophages and fibroblasts and its ability under certain conditions to stimulate proliferation of fibroblasts (including renal interstitial cells). Finally, TGF-β has the peculiar ability to autoinduce its own expression *(49,50)*, potentially resulting in a positive feedback loop and amplifying the fibrotic response in some situations.

INTERCEPTING THE EXPRESSION OF TGF-β

Antisense Oligodeoxynucleotides

Inhibition of TGF-β expression can be achieved by antisense oligodeoxynucleotides (ODNs), which bind to the complementary sequence of TGF-β mRNA and prevent its translation *(51–55)*. This antisense strategy was used to inhibit the TGF-β system in the cultured proximal tubular cell *(51)*. This cell type was chosen because in diabetes the proximal tubule is exposed to high concentrations of TGF-β coming from the glomerular filtrate. In addition, the proximal tubule is a site that is amenable to antisense therapy because circulating antisense ODNs can be filtered and may accumulate in the tubular lumen. We found in cultured proximal tubular cells that antisense ODN significantly reduced the high glucose-induced increases in [^{3}H]-leucine incorporation (general marker of protein synthesis) and in TGF-β_1 protein production. Furthermore, antisense

ODN treatment of streptozotocin (STZ)-diabetic mice partially but significantly decreased kidney TGF-β_1 protein levels and attenuated the increase in kidney weight and the α1(IV) collagen and fibronectin mRNAs *(51)*. Therefore, therapy with antisense TGF-β_1 ODN decreases TGF-β_1 production and attenuates high glucose-induced proximal tubular cell hypertrophy in vitro and partially prevents the increase in kidney weight and extracellular matrix expression in diabetic mice. However, it must be stressed that the effect of antisense therapy was only partial.

An unexpected and perhaps novel way to inhibit TGF-β-induced matrix production by antisense therapy is to target the cyclin kinase inhibitor (CKI), $p21^{Waf1/Cip1}$, which is stimulated by TGF-β and would normally inhibit progression through the cell cycle. Using this $p21^{Waf1/Cip1}$ antisense ODN, Weiss et al. *(56)* showed in cultured vascular smooth muscle cells that the production and secretion of fibronectin and laminin were markedly reduced, despite continued stimulation by TGF-β_1.

BLOCKING THE ACTIVATION OF TGF-β

Furin

Before TGF-β is secreted as a 25-kDa homodimer attached to one or more peptides that confer latency, it must first be processed from a larger, biologically inactive precursor, pre-pro-TGF-β made up of 390 amino acids *(57)*. Cleavage then occurs to yield pro-TGF-β (amino acids 30–390) *(58)*. Final proteolytic processing to yield mature TGF-β takes place at a cluster of basic amino acids, R–H–R–R *(59)*, that immediately precedes the NH_2-terminal of the mature TGF-β peptide. Interestingly, the R–X–K/R–R is the optimal motif for cleavage by furin, a calcium-dependent serine endoprotease in the family of processing enzymes called SPCs (subtilisin-like proprotein convertases) or PCs (proprotein convertases) for short *(60,61)*. The TGF-β_1 precursor was shown to be effectively cleaved both in vitro and in vivo by human furin, releasing the mature TGF-β_1 moiety *(62)*. By Western blotting, pro-TGF-β was cleaved from its 55-kDa form down to the 44- and 12.5-kDa peptides that corresponded to the proregion and the active monomer of TGF-β *(62)*. However, other convertases in the same class as furin could conceivably cleave pro-TGF-β. Therefore, the ability to process pro-TGF-β was tested in the LoVo colon carcinoma cell line, which expresses all of the proprotein convertases except for furin because of point mutations in both *fur* alleles (which encode furin). In these cells, less than 5% of the TGF-β precursor was converted into active TGF-β. Furthermore, genetic complementation with wild-type furin significantly raised production of bioactivatable TGF-β_1 *(58)*. In a similar furin inhibition experiment, a bioengineered serpin, α_1-antitrypsin Portland (α_1-PDX), was used because it mimics the consensus sequence R–X–X–R and therefore inhibits furin with a K_i of 0.6 nmol/L *(63–66)*. The introduction of α_1-PDX into furin-positive BSC-40 cells with a vaccinia vector diminished the release of active TGF-β1 into the culture media by an average of 78% *(58)*. Not only does furin cleave pro-TGF-β, but through a mechanism involving cross-talk between the p42/p44 MAP kinase (i.e., extracellular signal-regulated kinase or ERK) and Smad (in particular, Smad2) pathways, active TGF-β also increases the expression of furin *(67–69)*. This physiological coupling between TGF-β and furin potentially sets up a system whereby TGF-β augments its own bioavailability. All of these data strongly support the contention that furin is the predominant convertase that is responsible for the processing of intracellular pro-TGF-β into active TGF-β.

Interestingly, there are no studies yet on the role of furin in renal disease. Perhaps this is related to the widespread importance of furin in the processing of many precursor proteins besides TGF-β. Other members of the TGF-β superfamily share the consensus R–X–X–R motif at the junction of the proregion and the mature polypeptide. Therefore, blocking furin may indiscriminately inhibit the processing of many TGF-β-related proteins such as the activin/inhibins, bone morphogenetic proteins, nodal, lefty-1, and lefty-2, all of which have important functions in growth, differentiation, and development *(70–72)*. It is not surprising that a loss-of-function mutation in the *fur* gene results in embryonic lethality owing to several developmental defects *(73)*. In addition, furin processes other substrates like von Willebrand factor *(74)*, nerve growth factor *(75)*, insulin-like growth factor receptor *(76)*, and the hepatocyte growth factor receptor *(77)*. A more targeted approach to inhibit just the furin-mediated conversion of TGF-β in the kidney will probably be necessary to investigate the therapeutic utility of furin in DN.

ROLE OF THROMBOSPONDIN IN ACTIVATING TGF-β

TGF-β_1 is produced as a latent complex that requires extracellular activation before it can bind to its receptor. Although there are many physiological ways of activating TGF-β, one mechanism involving the extracellular glycoprotein, thrombospondin, may be particularly important in vivo *(78)*. The TSPs are a small family of secreted, modular glycoproteins that are similar to structural proteins but mostly function by influencing cell–matrix interactions *(79)*. For this reason, they have been classified as "matricellular" proteins *(79)*. TSP was first discovered to complex strongly with TGF-β among the substances released during platelet degranulation *(80)*, and then TSP was found to possess the ability to activate latent TGF-β secreted by bovine aortic endothelial cells in culture *(81,82)*. This activation could occur in the absence of cells and without the need for proteases that normally activate TGF-β such as plasmin *(81)*. The mechanism of TSP-mediated activation of TGF-β appears to involve two discrete peptide sequences within the domain of the three type-1 repeats of TSP-1 *(83,84)*. One sequence in the first type-1 repeat (GGWSHW—amino acids 418–423, or generically the WXXW motif) binds latent TGF-β and perhaps orients it properly, whereas the other sequence between the first and second type-1 repeats (KRFK—amino acids 412–415) induces a conformational rearrangement of the latency-associated peptide (LAP) at the LSKL sequence *(85)*, thus freeing active TGF-β *(79,84,86,87)*. Synthetic peptides based on the type-1 repeat sequences could potentially have therapeutic uses in modulating TGF-β activation *(88)*. For example, the minimal GGWSHW peptide can bind to TGF-β but cannot activate it, thereby blocking TGF-β activation by TSP-1 *(84)*. In therapeutic experiments, one group was able to demonstrate that normal type-1 repeat peptides (especially the one containing RFK) could activate TGF-β and inhibit melanoma tumor growth, but that a mutant type-1 repeat peptide could not produce this effect *(89)*. More relevant to DN, MCs exposed to high glucose showed significantly suppressed levels of bioactive TGF-β and fibronectin when treated with either the LSKL or GGWSHW peptide *(90)*. In another study, the synthetic GGWSHW peptide was also able to decrease the level of biologically active TGF-β_1 in the media of cultured MCs exposed to high glucose *(87)*. This peptide treatment completely suppressed the increases in fibronectin and plasminogen activator inhibitor-1 expression. The same group confirmed their finding with antisense ODNs directed against TSP-1, highlighting another potential means of inhibiting activation of TGF-β *(87)*. Finally, it should be noted that despite the evidence presented so far, at least three studies have failed to confirm that TSP either interacts with or even activates latent TGF-β_1 *(91–93)*.

The role of TSP in diabetic nephropathy is being investigated. Type-1 diabetic patients have elevated plasma levels of TSP-1 as do platelets from patients with diabetes *(94,95)*. In vitro studies show that high glucose upregulates TSP-1 expression at both the mRNA and protein levels in MCs *(96,97)*. Also in MC culture, it is well known that high glucose increases the activity of TGF-β, but the mechanisms are incompletely understood *(87)*. One possibility is that high glucose increases the production of TSP-1, perhaps through a protein kinase C- or TGF-β-dependent mechanism *(98)*, and TSP-1 in turn activates latent TGF-β and increases the synthesis of fibronectin *(97)* and other matrix molecules. When cultured MCs in high-glucose media were treated with peptides that antagonize TSP-activation of TGF-β (but not plasmin-mediated activation of TGF-β), the glucose-dependent stimulation of fibronectin was inhibited *(90)*. These studies demonstrate that high glucose increases TGF-β and the resultant matrix production by the autocrine action of TSP to convert latent TGF-β to its biologically active form.

The extent of chronic tubulo-interstitial fibrosis is another important lesion that contributes to progressive renal failure in diabetic kidney disease. The role of TSP in the pathogenesis of tubulo-interstitial scarring has not been well studied in diabetes, but perhaps this can be inferred from studies of TSP in other sclerotic renal diseases. In one study, the temporal and spatial expression of TSP-1 was correlated with tubulo-interstitial fibrosis in several animal models of glomerulonephritis. They found that TSP-1 expression localized with and always preceded the development of tubulo-interstitial fibrosis and that the extent of TSP-1 expression correlated quantitatively with the severity of fibrosis *(99)*. Similar results were found in the rat remnant kidney model in that TSP-1 expression was frequently localized to the sites of increased TGF-β and preceded the development of glomerular and tubulo-interstitial fibrosis *(100)*.

ANTAGONIZING EXTRACELLULAR TGF-β

Decorin

Up to this point, we have discussed the gene expression, intracellular processing, and extracellular activation of TGF-β. Once TGF-β is in its active homodimer form (25 kDa) and ready to bind to its receptors, other techniques can be used to inhibit TGF-β at this stage. Decorin is a naturally occurring inhibitor of TGF-β. This is a 92.5-kDa extracellular proteoglycan with a 40-kDa leucine-rich core and a single chondroitin sulfate side chain. The decorin core scavenges and neutralizes TGF-β or possibly sequesters TGF-β in the ECM, thus antagonizing the prosclerotic effect of this cytokine *(101)*. In experimental glomerulonephritis in the rat, systemic administration of decorin or transfection of decorin cDNA (to deliver decorin into the bloodstream) improved proteinuria, decreased glomerular TGF-β, and alleviated excess matrix accumulation in the kidney *(102)*. It has been assumed that acute glomerulonephritis is characterized by a relative lack of decorin and an excess of TGF-β activity, but the pattern may be different in chronic renal diseases that do not have a significant inflammatory component. In human biopsy specimens of various chronic renal diseases, intrarenal decorin was actually enhanced and was the best predictor of the severity of interstitial fibrosis and renal failure *(103)*. In experimental hydronephrosis in the rat, renal decorin mRNA and TGF-β activity were both elevated *(104)*.

Likewise, the findings in DN show an intricate pattern of TGF-β and decorin expression. An early study showed that high glucose increased decorin mRNA and protein in human MCs *(105)*. Our more recent study showed that high glucose increased decorin mRNA in rat and mouse MCs as well as mouse proximal tubular cells *(106)*. On the contrary, neither the glomerular endothelial nor the glomerular epithelial cell showed constitutive expression of decorin or displayed increased expression in response to high glucose *(106)*. TGF-β also affects the expression of decorin, but unlike high glucose, it suppresses decorin gene transcription *(106)*. The negative TGF-β-responsive element of the decorin gene appears to be located in the proximal promoter, between –140- and –111-bp *(107)*. In the STZ diabetic mouse (C57Bl female), there was an early and sustained 2- to 2.5-fold increase in decorin mRNA in the renal cortex at up to 6 wk of diabetes *(106)*. Based on the previous in vitro experiments, this probably reflects an upregulation of decorin expression in the MCs and proximal tubule epithelial cells.

The antagonistic relationship between decorin and TGF-β raises the possibility of using decorin to treat DN. This approach would be justified if DN were characterized by a deficiency of decorin and an excess of TGF-β, but in fact DN is characterized by surpluses of both decorin and TGF-β. The increased decorin may represent a protective mechanism by which renal cells counteract the injury produced by hyperglycemia-stimulated TGF-β *(108)*. Would supplying exogenous decorin in even higher concentrations benefit diabetic kidney disease? This remains to be established. If supplementation with decorin were to be tried, some methods seem promising. One could directly supply the decorin protein. For example, recombinant decorin has been injected into knee joints *(109)* and muscle *(110)*. Unfortunately, there are no reports in the literature regarding the best way to deliver decorin protein to the kidney. However, the short half-life of exogenous peptides, in general, makes decorin administration somewhat problematic. An alternative approach that may achieve long-lasting levels of decorin is gene transfer. Some have successfully used a retroviral vector *(111)*, whereas others have used an adenoviral vector *(112)*. One group has transfected decorin cDNA (cloned in a eukaryotic expression vector) into human MCs and shown that TGF-β_1, α1(IV) collagen, and fibronectin mRNAs all decreased, supporting the use of decorin to control the progression of glomerulosclerosis in kidney diseases *(113)*. Finally, ex vivo transfer of the decorin gene has been achieved by injecting decorin-transfected rat MCs into the renal artery of Sprague-Dawley rats *(114)*. The glomeruli of the injected kidney showed high levels of decorin expression, significantly decreasing TGF-β_1 expression and attenuating fibronectin and collagen IV in the rat model of antithymocyte serum glomerulonephritis *(114)*.

THERAPY WITH SOLUBLE TGF-β TYPE-II RECEPTOR

Using soluble TGF-β receptors is another effective way to block the TGF-β system. These receptors bind to extracellular TGF-β but do not transduce a signal. Investigators have used soluble forms of each of the three TGF-β receptors, but most have used the soluble TGF-β type-II receptor (TβRII). This choice probably relates to the fact that the type II receptor is the primary ligand-binding receptor and that it initiates the first step in TGF-β signaling. Soluble type-II receptor is commercially available from R&D Systems (Minneapolis, Minnesota) or can be mass produced by recombinant techniques *(115)*. It can then be administered exogenously to cultured cells in vitro or systemically/locally in vivo *(116–118)*. Gene delivery is another feasible way of achieving therapeutic levels of soluble TβRII systemically. An adenoviral vector that encoded the extracellular domain of TβRII was injected into the muscle of a rodent, resulting in detectable blood levels of the receptor protein, and this prevented TGF-β-mediated gliosis of the retina *(119)*, corneal opacification from ECM accumulation *(120)*, and liver fibrosis caused by dimethylnitrosamine *(121)*. Similarly, transduction with a recombinant retrovirus encoding soluble TβRII dramatically reduced the tumorigenicity of EL4, a mouse thymoma cell line that secretes a large amount of TGF-β *(122)*. Related to gene delivery, transgenic expression of a soluble TβRII:F_c chimera *(123)* or even a dominant-negative TβRII *(124–126)* can also abrogate the effects of TGF-β.

THERAPY WITH SOLUBLE TGF-β TYPE-III RECEPTOR

In addition to TβRII, the type-III receptor (also called betaglycan) binds to the TGF-β ligand. Betaglycan presents TGF-β directly to the type-II receptor, facilitating TGF-β signaling *(127)*. It has been shown that the effects of TGF-β are strongly inhibited by a recombinant, soluble type-III receptor that binds TGF-β but is unable to shepherd the ligand to the type-II receptor *(128–130)*. Without resorting to the competitive binding strategy of soluble receptors, one novel way to inhibit TGF-β signaling involves the glycosaminoglycan (GAG) modifications of betaglycan. When rat betaglycan is artificially expressed in the LLC-PK_1 cell (porcine proximal tubule epithelial cell that does not normally express β-glycan), high-molecular-weight GAG chains are added to betaglycan that physically prevent TGF-β type-II–type-I receptor interactions, through a mechanism not involving ligand sequestration or increased production of soluble betaglycan *(131)*. Mutations to remove the GAG attachment sites restored the type-II–type-I receptor association in co-immunoprecipitation assays, proving that the GAG was responsible for the inhibitory behavior of betaglycan on TGF-β signaling *(131)*.

EFFECT OF SOLUBLE TGF-β TYPE I RECEPTOR

Finally, the soluble form of TGF-β type-I receptor (TβRI) has rarely been used. This may relate to the fact that TβRI does not bind directly to the TGF-β ligand but rather to the type-II receptor after it has bound TGF-β. Therefore, a soluble type-I receptor probably cannot bind and sequester TGF-β. As a matter of fact, soluble TβRI seems to potentiate the effect of TGF-β, measured by the TGF-β-inducible luciferase reporter assay, 3TP-Lux *(132)*. The mechanism of action is unknown, but soluble TβRI may act like a chaperone that stabilizes the ligand-bound type-II receptor, facilitating the recruitment of membrane-anchored TβRI and the formation of a heteromeric signaling complex *(132)*. Not surprisingly then, when soluble TβRI was added to the mink lung epithelial cell (Mv1Lu), it mimicked TGF-β-induced transcriptional and growth responses, even in the absence of TGF-β1 *(133)*. Although the soluble TGF-β receptors have been used to treat many different diseases in a wide variety of disciplines, none of them have yet been tried in diabetes or specifically in diabetic nephropathy.

THERAPEUTIC APPLICATIONS OF ACTIVIN-LIKE KINASE 5 INHIBITION

Perhaps a better way to target the TGF-β type-I receptor is to block its signaling activity. Recently, a chemical compound was discovered that inhibits the serine/threonine kinase activity of the type-I receptor (TβRI is also called activin-like kinase [ALK]5). This ALK5 inhibitor, dubbed SB-431,542, was originally identified from a panel of candidate imidazole inhibitors against p38 MAP kinase, but it has negligible activity as a p38 inhibitor *(134,135)*. More importantly, in cell culture applications, SB-431,542 was able to prevent the phosphorylation of Smad3 by the type-I receptor, at an IC_{50} of 94 n*M* *(136)*. Furthermore, SB-431,542 blocked the TGF-β_1-induced mRNA expression of both fibronectin and α1(I) collagen *(136)*, suggesting that this inhibitor of TGF-β signaling can attenuate the accumulation of ECM in DN.

A related ALK5 inhibitor, SB-525,334, has a longer half-life than SB-431,542, is more potent (IC_{50} = 58.5 n*M* vs 94 n*M*), and can be used in vivo *(137)*. In the rat model of puromycin aminonucleoside (PAN) renal injury, a form of nephritis-induced renal fibrosis, orally administered doses of SB-525,334 for 11 d significantly reduced the renal mRNA expression of plasminogen activator inhibitor-1, a protein that would be strongly induced by TGF-β *(138)*. The compound also produced dose-dependent decreases in renal procollagen α1(I) and procollagen α1(III) mRNA, which reached statistical significance at the 10-mg/kg/d dose when compared with the PAN controls. Furthermore, PAN-induced proteinuria was significantly inhibited at the 10-mg/kg/d dose level. These results provide further evidence for the involvement of TGF-β_1 in the profibrotic changes that occur in the PAN model and demonstrate the ability of a small-molecule inhibitor of ALK5 to block several of the markers that are predictive of fibrosis and renal injury *(138)*. Whether ALK5 inhibition will be therapeutic for DN remains to be tested.

ANTI-TGF-β ANTIBODY AS AN EFFECTIVE THERAPEUTIC AGENT

One final way to target extracellular TGF-β and interfere with the binding to its receptors is to use a panselective, neutralizing anti-TGF-β antibody. Studies employing a neutralizing anti-TGF-β antibody have provided convincing evidence that the pro-sclerotic and hypertrophic effects of high-ambient glucose on cultured renal cells are largely mediated by autocrine production and activation of TGF-β. In particular, such studies have involved glomerular MCs *(14,23)*, glomerular epithelial cells *(139)*, proximal tubular cells *(15,140,141)*, and renal cortical fibroblasts *(25)*. Neutralizing anti-TGF-β antibodies also reverse the downregulation of collagenase activity in rat MCs grown in high glucose *(142)*.

In experimental diabetic kidney disease, the central importance of TGF-β has also been demonstrated with a neutralizing anti-TGF-β antibody. Short-term treatment of the STZ diabetic mouse with the anti-TGF-β antibody prevented glomerular hypertrophy, reduced the increment in kidney weight by 50%, and significantly attenuated the increase in TGF-β_1, α1(IV) collagen, and fibronectin mRNAs without affecting glycemic control *(6)*. The results of this study suggested a cause-and-effect relationship between the renal TGF-β system and the development of early structural changes in DN.

To expand on these findings, we conducted a similar study on the db/db mouse to examine whether long-term anti-TGF-β antibody treatment would ameliorate the late structural changes and functional consequences of DN *(8)*. We found that systemic anti-TGF-β therapy for 8 wk prevented the mesangial matrix expansion of diabetic glomerulosclerosis and, most important, preserved the creatinine clearance, showing for the first time that neutralization of TGF-β activity could prevent the progression of renal failure in diabetes. However, the anti-TGF-β antibody did not reduce albuminuria, which itself may promote the progression of renal insufficiency *(143)*. The paradox of preserved renal function in the face of persistent albuminuria may perhaps be explained by postulating that the deleterious downstream effects of proteinuria in promoting tubulointerstitial injury are themselves mediated by the TGF-β system *(144)*.

Having established that anti-TGF-β antibody prevents DN, the current challenge lies in adapting the antibody treatment for human use. Certainly, the usual tests should be performed to establish the route of delivery, measure the pharmacokinetics, determine the efficacy, and watch for side effects, but one of the bigger hurdles will be to develop a human or humanized form of the anti-TGF-β antibody. The monoclonal anti-TGF-β antibody (Genentech, S. San Francisco, CA) that we used in our studies is a mouse antibody *(26,145)*, and its use in humans might trigger the development of antimouse antibodies that will greatly shorten the half-life and therefore the usefulness of any nonhuman anti-TGF-β antibody.

TARGETING THE POSTRECEPTOR SIGNALING CASCADES

Because the TGF-β type-II receptor acts as a primary ligand-binding receptor and the TGF-β type-I receptor acts as a signaling receptor that uses its kinase activity to propagate a signal, intracellular proteins that interact with the type-I receptor are likely to play important roles in TGF-β signaling.

Serine–Threonine Kinase Receptor-Associated Protein

An example of such a protein that interacts with TGF-β type-I receptor was confirmed by a yeast two-hybrid system, found to contain a novel WD domain, and has been designated as STRAP (serine–threonine kinase receptor-associated protein) *(146)*. Overexpression of STRAP inhibited TGF-β-mediated transcriptional activation. It also showed synergistic inhibition of TGF-β signaling with Smad7 (an inhibitory Smad detailed next) *(146,147)*. STRAP recruits Smad7 to the activated type-I receptor and forms a complex, stabilizing the association between Smad7 and the activated receptor and assisting Smad7 in preventing Smad2 and Smad3 access to the receptor. STRAP interacts with Smad2 and Smad3 but does not cooperate functionally with these Smads to transactivate TGF-β-dependent transcription. Thus, STRAP may potentially be a molecular means to inhibit TGF-β. This has not been tried in DN.

Smad7

Smad7 is an inhibitory Smad (I-Smad) that may have some utility in blocking the TGF-β signal and hence extracellular matrix buildup. This discussion will focus mostly on Smad7, because another I-Smad, termed Smad6, inhibits TGF-β signaling less effectively and may be involved in functions independent of TGF-β/Smad signaling *(148,149)*.

It was first reported in 1997 that Smad7 interacts stably with the activated TGF-β type-I receptor and thus blocks the phosphorylation of the receptor-regulated Smads (R-Smads) that are downstream of the TGF-β pathway *(150)*. In the absence of TGF-β, Smad7 is predominantly localized in the nucleus, but on TGF-β receptor activation, Smad7 is mobilized into the cytoplasm in which it can associate with the type-I receptor *(151)*. In addition, Smad7 can export out of the nucleus with an E3 ubiquitin-ligase, either Smurf1 or Smurf2, that causes degradation of the activated TGF-β type-I receptor via proteasomal and lysosomal pathways *(152–154)*. One final mechanism of action of the I-Smads (especially Smad6) may take place in the nucleus rather than the cytoplasm and involve the direct repression of gene transcription by Smad6 via the recruitment of histone deacetylases, which can negatively regulate transcription *(155,156)*.

Interestingly, Smad7 expression is induced by TGF-β itself, perhaps at the transcriptional level by AP-1, Smad2–Smad4, and Smad3–Smad4 *(157–163)*, in what appears to be a negative feedback loop to control TGF-β responses *(164,165)*. The ability of Smad7 to extinguish the TGF-β signal has made it an attractive target for antifibrotic therapies. Stable or transient transfection or recombinant viral vector techniques to achieve Smad7 overexpression have been used to limit fibrosis in various models of kidney disease, but the experience with Smad7 in diabetic nephropathy is limited. From our work, murine mesangial cells in culture were transiently transfected with a fibronectin promoter–luciferase construct, pGL2F1900, which contains the –1908-bp flanking region upstream of the rat fibronectin gene *(166,167)*. Exposure of these transfected cells to either high glucose or exogenous TGF-β_1 increased fibronectin promoter activity, but the combination of high glucose and TGF-β_1 resulted in an even greater increase than either stimulus alone, demonstrating that high glucose can act synergistically with TGF-β1 and that TGF-β stimulates fibronectin gene transcription. When the mesangial cells were concurrently transfected with a Smad7 expression vector, pFlag-Smad7 *(164)*, the increase in fibronectin–luciferase activity owing to TGF-β_1 treatment was totally prevented *(168)*. Smad7 has potential efficacy in attenuating the extracellular matrix production by the mesangium in DN.

However, it must be remembered that the inhibitory Smads are not specific for the TGF-β pathway. They block the activation of other R-Smads that are regulated by other members of the TGF-β superfamily such as the bone morphogenetic proteins and the activins *(169–171)*. As a result of this somewhat indiscriminate inhibition of pathways, the use of Smad7 as a therapy may have unintended consequences. Furthermore, Smad7 does not appear to have an effect on TGF-β-induced growth inhibition *(172)*, meaning that overexpression of Smad7 may not prevent the renal hypertrophy characteristic of DN. Finally, there is some evidence that Smad7 may mediate the apoptotic effects of TGF-β; so purposeful expression of Smad7 may exacerbate the tendency toward cellular apoptosis *(173–175)*. This last point, however, is controversial as some studies have found that Smad7 inhibits TGF-β-mediated apoptosis *(176,177)*. Perhaps the potential dangers of Smad7 overexpression are best illustrated by the Smad7 transgenic mouse. The K5.Smad7 mice exhibited pathological changes in multiple epithelial tissues (open eyelids, corneal defects, aberrant hair follicle morphogenesis, epidermal hyperproliferation, and thymic atrophy) and died within 10 d after birth *(178)*.

Yes-Associated Protein 65

A recently discovered protein that interacts with Smad7 was found by a yeast two-hybrid screen and has been named Yes-Associated Protein (YAP) 65 *(179)*. This Smad7 partner, YAP65, appears to augment the inhibitory activity of Smad7 against the TGF-β-induced, Smad3/Smad4-dependent gene activation by strengthening the association of Smad7 with the activated TGF-β type-I receptor. Thus, YAP65 may one day be another treatment to block the deleterious effects of TGF-β in DN.

SMADS 2 AND 3

Besides the inhibitory Smads, the receptor-regulated Smads (R-Smads) that can transduce a TGF-β signal are Smad2 and Smad3. In particular, Smad3 may be involved in the stimulatory effect of high glucose on ECM expression. In mouse MCs, high glucose stimulates the transcription of fibronectin and potentiates the transcriptional activation of fibronectin by TGF-β_1 *(168)*. This effect of TGF-β_1 appears to be mediated by Smad3, because overexpression of Smad3 was able to induce fibronectin promoter activity by itself. Smad3 overexpression also increased fibronectin synergistically in conjunction with exogenous TGF-β_1, as if the extra Smad3 had increased the efficiency of TGF-β signaling. More importantly, transfection of a Smad3-dominant-negative construct was able to inhibit TGF-β_1 from stimulating the promoter activity of fibronectin *(168)*. However, part of the TGF-β_1-induced fibronectin expression may also be mediated in parallel by the p38 mitogen-activated protein kinase (MAPK) pathway *(136)*. Finally, there is evidence to suggest that Smad3 predominantly mediates the effect of TGF-β_1 to increase the mRNA expression of α1(I) collagen *(136)*.

Little information is available, however, regarding Smad2 as a therapeutic target in DN. However, Smad2 has been shown to be increased in protein expression and to be activated in the kidney of the Otsuka Long-Evans Tokushima Fatty rat, a model of spontaneous type-2 diabetes *(180)*. In the model of type 1 diabetes induced by STZ, Smad2 signaling was also activated in the glomerular cells, evidenced by immunostaining for phosphorylated Smad2 *(181)*.

In contrast, blockade of Smad3 as a therapeutic tool in diabetic kidney disease is becoming feasible in vivo. In one study, Smad3-null mice, created on a CL57/Bl6J strain background, were made diabetic by STZ *(182)*. After 4 wk of diabetes, glomerular expression of TGF-β_1, as assessed by RTPCR, was not enhanced in Smad3-null mice vs wild-type, indicating that the absence of Smad3 did not result in a compensatory increase of the TGF-β message. Matrix expression was inhibited, however, in the kidneys of the Smad3-null mice; mRNA levels of fibronectin and the α3 chain of type IV collagen were increased in the diabetic wild-type mice (compared with the nondiabetic controls), but not in the diabetic Smad3-null mice *(182)*. Along with the increase in α3(IV) collagen in diabetes, glomerular basement membrane thickening had occurred in the wild-type mice but was significantly prevented in the diabetic Smad3-null mice. Thus, Smad3 seems to function in the diabetes-induced upregulation of fibronectin and α3(IV) collagen, and thereby may play a critical role in the early phase of diabetic glomerulopathy *(182)*.

CONCLUSIONS

TGF-β clearly plays an important role in the pathogenesis of DN, and investigative research has come a long way in elucidating the inner workings and key players of the TGF-β signaling system. By stepping through the TGF-β pathway from the gene expression to protein processing to receptor binding to the effectors of signaling, one can envision ample opportunities to design a rational and novel intervention to treat DN.

REFERENCES

1. Ziyadeh FN. Evidence for the involvement of transforming growth factor-b in the pathogenesis of diabetic kidney disease: are Koch's postulates fulfilled? Curr Pract Med 1998;1:87–89.
2. Iwano M, Kubo A, Nishino T, et al. Quantification of glomerular TGF-β1 mRNA in patients with diabetes mellitus. Kidney Int 1996;49:1120–1126.
3. Yamamoto T, Nakamura T, Noble N, Ruoslahti E, Border W. Expression of transforming growth factor beta is elevated in human and experimental diabetic nephropathy. Proc Natl Acad Sci USA 1993;90:1814–1818.

4. Yamamoto T, Noble NA, Cohen AH, et al. Expression of transforming growth factor-β isoforms in human glomerular diseases. Kidney Int 1996;49:461–469.
5. Yoshioka K, Takemura T, Murakami K, et al. Transforming growth factor-β protein and mRNA in glomeruli in normal and diseased human kidneys. Lab Invest 1993;68:154–163.
6. Sharma K, Jin Y, Guo J, Ziyadeh FN. Neutralization of TGF-β by anti-TGF-β antibody attenuates kidney hypertrophy and the enhanced extracellular matrix gene expression in STZ-induced diabetic mice. Diabetes 1996;45:522–530.
7. Sharma K, Ziyadeh FN. Renal hypertrophy is associated with upregulation of TGF-β1 gene expression in diabetic BB rat and NOD mouse. Am J Physiol 1994;267:F1094–F1101.
8. Ziyadeh FN, Hoffman BB, Han DC, et al. Long-term prevention of renal insufficiency, excess matrix gene expression, and glomerular mesangial matrix expansion by treatment with monoclonal anti-transforming growth factor-beta antibody in db/db diabetic mice. Proc Natl Acad Sci USA 2000;97:8015–8020.
9. Hong SW, Isono M, Chen S, et al. Increased glomerular and tubular expression of transforming growth factor-beta1, its type II receptor, and activation of the Smad signaling pathway in the db/db mouse. Am J Pathol 2001;158:1653–1663.
10. Houlihan CA, Akdeniz A, Tsalamandris C, Cooper ME, Jerums G, Gilbert RE. Urinary transforming growth factor-beta excretion in patients with hypertension, type 2 diabetes, and elevated albumin excretion rate: effects of angiotensin receptor blockade and sodium restriction. Diabetes Care 2002;25:1072–1077.
11. Agarwal R, Siva S, Dunn SR, Sharma K. Add-on angiotensin II receptor blockade lowers urinary transforming growth factor-beta levels. Am J Kidney Dis 2002;39:486–492.
12. Mogyorosi A, Kapoor A, Isono M, Kapoor S, Sharma K, Ziyadeh FN. Utility of serum and urinary transforming growth factor-beta levels as markers of diabetic nephropathy. Nephron 2000;86: 234–235.
13. Sharma K, Ziyadeh FN, Alzahabi B, et al. Increased renal production of transforming growth factor-β1 in patients with type II diabetes. Diabetes 1997;46:854–859.
14. Ziyadeh FN, Sharma K, Ericksen M, Wolf G. Stimulation of collagen gene expression and protein synthesis in murine mesangial cells by high glucose is mediated by autocrine activation of transforming growth factor-β. J Clin Invest 1994;93:536–542.
15. Ziyadeh FN, Snipes ER, Watanabe M, Alvarez RJ, Goldfarb S, Haverty TP. High glucose induces cell hypertrophy and stimulates collagen gene transcription in proximal tubule. Am J Physiol 1990;259:F704–F714.
16. Wolf G, Haberstroh U, Neilson EG. Angiotensin II stimulates the proliferation and biosynthesis of type I collagen in cultured murine mesangial cells. Am J Pathol 1992;140:95–107.
17. Chen S, Cohen MP, Lautenslager GT, Shearman CW, Ziyadeh FN. Glycated albumin stimulates TGF-beta 1 production and protein kinase C activity in glomerular endothelial cells. Kidney Int 2001;59:673–681.
18. Han DC, Isono M, Chen S, et al. Leptin stimulates type I collagen production in db/db mesangial cells: glucose uptake and TGF-beta type II receptor expression. Kidney Int 2001;59:1315–1323.
19. Wolf G, Hamann A, Han DC, et al. Leptin stimulates proliferation and TGF-b expression in renal glomerular endothelial cells: Potential role in glomerulosclerosis. Kidney Int 1999;56:860–872.
20. Hoffman BB, Ziyadeh FN. The role of growth factors in the development of diabetic nephropathy. Curr Opin Endocrinol Diabetes 1996;3:322–329.
21. Abboud HE. Growth factors and diabetic nephrology: an overview. Kidney Int Suppl 1997;60: S3–S6.
22. Chen S, Iglesias-de la Cruz MC, Isono M, Ziyadeh FN. Transforming growth factor-beta and other cytokines in experimental and human nephropathy. The Kidney and Hypertension in Diabetes Mellitus, 5th ed. Mogensen CE, 2000;313–338.
23. Wolf G, Sharma K, Chen Y, Ericksen M, Ziyadeh FN. High glucose-induced proliferation in mesangial cells is reversed by autocrine TGF-beta. Kidney Int 1992;42:647–656.
24. Wolf G, Schroeder R, Ziyadeh FN, Thaiss F, Zahner G, Stahl RA. High glucose stimulates expression of p27Kip1 in cultured mouse mesangial cells: relationship to hypertrophy. Am J Physiol 1997;273:F348–F356.
25. Han DC, Isono M, Hoffman BB, Ziyadeh FN. High glucose stimulates proliferation and collagen type I synthesis in renal cortical fibroblasts: mediation by autocrine activation of TGF-b. J Am Soc Nephrol 1999;10:1891–1899.
26. Lucas C, Bald L, Fendly BM, et al. The autocrine production of transforming growth factor-b during lymphocyte activation. A study with a monoclonal antibody-based ELISA. J Immunol 1990;145: 1415–1422.

27. Wolf G, Mueller E, Stahl RAK, Ziyadeh FN. Angiotensin II-induced hypertrophy of cultured murine proximal tubular cells is mediated by endogenous transforming growth factor-b. J Clin Invest 1993;92:1366–1372.
28. Ziyadeh FN, Han DC, Cohen JA, Guo J, Cohen MP. Glycated albumin stimulates fibronectin gene expression in glomerular mesangial cells: involvement of the transforming growth factor-beta system. Kidney Int 1998;53:631–638.
29. MacKay K, Kondaiah P, Danielpour D, Austin HA, Brown PD. Expression of transforming growth factor-β1 and β2 in rat glomeruli. Kidney Int 1990;38:1095–1100.
30. Roberts AB, Kim S-J, Noma T, et al. Multiple forms of TGF-β: distinct promoters and differential expression. In: Sporn MB, Roberts AB, eds. Clinical Applications of TGF-β. Ciba Foundation Symposium, Chichester, UK, 1991, pp. 7–28.
31. Sharma K, Ziyadeh FN. Biochemical events and cytokine interactions linking glucose metabolism to the development of diabetic nephropathy. Semin Nephrol 1997;17:80–92.
32. Thompson NL, Flanders KC, Smith JM, Ellingsworth LR, Roberts AB, Sporn MB. Expression of transforming growth factor-βl in specific cells and tissues of adult and neonatal mice. J Cell Biol 1989;108:661–669.
33. Hoffman M. Researchers get a first look at the versatile TGF-β family. Science 1992;257:332.
34. Miyazono K, Heldin CH: Latent forms of TGF-β: Molecular structure and mechanisms of activation. In: Bock GR, Marsh J, eds. Clinical Applications of TGF-β. Wiley, Chichester, UK, 1991, pp. 81–92.
35. Paralkar VM, Vukicevic S, Reddi AH. Transforming growth factor β type 1 binds to collagen IV of basement membrane matrix: implications for development. Dev Biol 1991;143:303–308.
36. Wakefield LM, Winokur TS, Hollands RS, Christopherson K, Levinson AD, Sporn MB. Recombinant latent transforming growth factor β1 has a longer plasma half-life in rats than active transforming growth factor β1, and a different tissue distribution. J Clin Invest 1990;86:1976–1984.
37. Ando T, Okuda S, Tamaki K, Yoshitomi K, Fujishima M. Localization of transforming growth factor-β and latent transforming growth factor-β binding protein in rat kidney. Kidney Int 1995;47:733–739.
38. Flaumenhaft R, Abe M, Mignatti P, Rifkin DB. Basic fibroblast growth factor-induced activation of latent transforming growth factor beta in endothelial cells: regulation of plasminogen activator activity. J Cell Biol 1992;118:901–909.
39. ten Dijke P, Miyazono K, Heldin CH. Signaling via hetero-oligomeric complexes of type I and type II serine/threonine kinase receptors. Curr Opin Cell Biol 1996;8:139–145.
40. Derynck R, Feng XH. TGF-beta receptor signaling. Biochim Biophys Acta 1997;1333:F105–F150.
41. Massague J. Receptors for the TGF-β family. Cell 1992;69:1067–1070.
42. Huse M, Chen YG, Massague J, Kuriyan J. Crystal structure of the cytoplasmic domain of the type I TGF beta receptor in complex with FKBP12. Cell 1999;96:425–436.
43. Wrana JL, Attisano L, Wieser R, Ventura F, Massague J. Mechanism of activation of the TGF-beta receptor. Nature 1994;370:341–347.
44. Massague J, Wotton D. Transcriptional control by the TGF-beta/Smad signaling system. EMBO J 2000;19:1745–1754.
45. Shi Y, Wang YF, Jayaraman L, Yang H, Massague J, Pavletich NP. Crystal structure of a Smad MH1 domain bound to DNA: insights on DNA binding in TGF-beta signaling. Cell 1998,94.585–594.
46. Kim J, Johnson K, Chen HJ, Carroll S, Laughon A. Drosophila Mad binds to DNA and directly mediates activation of vestigial by Decapentaplegic. Nature 1997;388:304–308.
47. Attisano L, Wrana JL. Smads as transcriptional co-modulators. Curr Opin Cell Biol 2000;12: 235–243.
48. Laiho M, Saksela O, Andreasen PA, Keski-Oja J. Enhanced production and extracellular deposition of the endothelial-type plasminogen activator inhibitor in cultured human lung fibroblasts by transforming growth factor-beta. J Cell Biol 1986;103:2403–2410.
49. Kim SJ, Jeang KT, Glick AB, Sporn MB, Roberts AB. Promoter sequences of the human transforming growth factor-beta 1 gene responsive to transforming growth factor-beta 1 autoinduction. J Biol Chem 1989;264:7041–7045.
50. Kim S-J, Denhez F, Kim K-Y, Holt JT, Sporn MB, Roberts AB. Activation of the second promoter of the transforming growth factor-β1 gene by transforming growth factor-β1 and phorbol ester occurs through the same target sequences. J Biol Chem 1989;264:19,373–19,378.
51. Han DC, Hoffman BB, Hong SW, Guo J, Ziyadeh FN. Therapy with antisense TGF-beta1 oligodeoxynucleotides reduces kidney weight and matrix mRNAs in diabetic mice. Am J Physiol Renal Physiol 2000;278:F628–F634.
52. Ihn H, Yamane K, Kubo M, Tamaki K. Blockade of endogenous transforming growth factor beta signaling prevents up-regulated collagen synthesis in scleroderma fibroblasts: association with

increased expression of transforming growth factor beta receptors. Arthritis Rheum 2001;44: 474–480.
53. Arias M, Lahme B, Van De Leur E, Gressner AM, Weiskirchen R. Adenoviral Delivery of an Antisense RNA Complementary to the 3′ Coding Sequence of Transforming Growth Factor-beta1 Inhibits Fibrogenic Activities of Hepatic Stellate Cells. Cell Growth Differ 2002;13:265–273.
54. Fernandez T, Amoroso S, Sharpe S, et al. Disruption of transforming growth factor beta signaling by a novel ligand-dependent mechanism. J Exp Med 2002;195:1247–1255.
55. Gambaro G, Weigert C, Ceol M, Schleicher ED. Inhibition of transforming growth factor-beta 1 gene overexpression as a strategy to prevent fibrosis. Contrib Nephrol 2001;107–113.
56. Weiss RH, Randour CJ. Attenuation of matrix protein secretion by antisense oligodeoxynucleotides to the cyclin kinase inhibitor p21(Waf1/Cip1). Atherosclerosis 2002;161:105–112.
57. Derynck R, Jarrett JA, Chen EY, et al. Human transforming growth factor-beta complementary DNA sequence and expression in normal and transformed cells. Nature 1985;316:701–705.
58. Dubois CM, Blanchette F, Laprise MH, Leduc R, Grondin F, Seidah NG. Evidence that furin is an authentic transforming growth factor-beta1-converting enzyme. Am J Pathol 2001;158:305–316.
59. Gentry LE, Lioubin MN, Purchio AF, Marquardt H. Molecular events in the processing of recombinant type 1 pre-pro-transforming growth factor beta to the mature polypeptide. Mol Cell Biol 1988;8:4162–4168.
60. Seidah NG, Chretien M. Eukaryotic protein processing: endoproteolysis of precursor proteins. Curr Opin Biotechnol 1997;8:602–607.
61. Steiner DF. The proprotein convertases. Curr Opin Chem Biol 1999;2:31–39.
62. Dubois CM, Laprise MH, Blanchette F, Gentry LE, Leduc R. Processing of transforming growth factor beta 1 precursor by human furin convertase. J Biol Chem 1995;270:10,618–10,624.
63. Jean F, Stella K, Thomas L, et al. Alpha1-antitrypsin Portland, a bioengineered serpin highly selective for furin: application as an antipathogenic agent. Proc Natl Acad Sci USA 1998;95:7293–7298.
64. Benjannet S, Savaria D, Laslop A, et al. Alpha1-antitrypsin Portland inhibits processing of precursors mediated by proprotein convertases primarily within the constitutive secretory pathway. J Biol Chem 1997;272:26,210–26,218.
65. Anderson ED, Thomas L, Hayflick JS, Thomas G. Inhibition of HIV-1 gp160-dependent membrane fusion by a furin-directed alpha 1-antitrypsin variant. J Biol Chem 1993;268:24,887–24,891.
66. Benjannet S, Rondeau N, Paquet L, et al. Comparative biosynthesis, covalent post-translational modifications and efficiency of prosegment cleavage of the prohormone convertases PC1 and PC2: glycosylation, sulphation and identification of the intracellular site of prosegment cleavage of PC1 and PC2. Biochem J 1993;294(Pt 3):735–743.
67. Blanchette F, Day R, Dong W, Laprise MH, Dubois CM. TGFbeta1 regulates gene expression of its own converting enzyme furin. J Clin Invest 1997;99:1974–1983.
68. Blanchette F, Rivard N, Rudd P, Grondin F, Attisano L, Dubois CM. Cross-talk between the p42/p44 MAP kinase and Smad pathways in transforming growth factor beta 1-induced furin gene transactivation. J Biol Chem 2001;276:33,986–33,994.
69. Blanchette F, Rudd P, Grondin F, Attisano L, Dubois CM. Involvement of Smads in TGF-beta1-induced furin (fur) transcription. J Cell Physiol 2001;188:264–273.
70. Nakayama K. Furin: a mammalian subtilisin/Kex2p-like endoprotease involved in processing of a wide variety of precursor proteins. Biochem J 1997;327(Pt 3):625–635.
71. Constam DB, Robertson EJ. Regulation of bone morphogenetic protein activity by pro domains and proprotein convertases. J Cell Biol 1999;144:139–149.
72. Constam DB, Robertson EJ. Tissue-specific requirements for the proprotein convertase furin/SPC1 during embryonic turning and heart looping. Development 2000;127:245–254.
73. Roebroek AJ, Umans L, Pauli IG, et al. Failure of ventral closure and axial rotation in embryos lacking the proprotein convertase Furin. Development 1998;125:4863–4876.
74. van de Ven WJ, Voorberg J, Fontijn R, et al. Furin is a subtilisin-like proprotein processing enzyme in higher eukaryotes. Mol Biol Rep 1990;14:265–275.
75. Bresnahan PA, Leduc R, Thomas L, et al. Human fur gene encodes a yeast KEX2-like endoprotease that cleaves pro-beta-NGF in vivo. J Cell Biol 1990;111:2851–2859.
76. Robertson BJ, Moehring JM, Moehring TJ. Defective processing of the insulin receptor in an endoprotease-deficient Chinese hamster cell strain is corrected by expression of mouse furin. J Biol Chem 1993;268:24,274–24,277.
77. Komada M, Hatsuzawa K, Shibamoto S, Ito F, Nakayama K, Kitamura N. Proteolytic processing of the hepatocyte growth factor/scatter factor receptor by furin. FEBS Lett 1993;328:25–29.

78. Crawford SE, Stellmach V, Murphy-Ullrich JE, et al. Thrombospondin-1 is a major activator of TGF-beta1 in vivo. Cell 1998;93:1159–1170.
79. Bornstein P. Thrombospondins as matricellular modulators of cell function. J Clin Invest 2001;107:929–934.
80. Murphy-Ullrich JE, Schultz-Cherry S, Hook M. Transforming growth factor-beta complexes with thrombospondin. Mol Biol Cell 1992;3:181–188.
81. Schultz-Cherry S, Murphy-Ullrich JE. Thrombospondin causes activation of latent transforming growth factor-beta secreted by endothelial cells by a novel mechanism. J Cell Biol 1993;122: 923–932.
82. Schultz-Cherry S, Ribeiro S, Gentry L, Murphy-Ullrich JE. Thrombospondin binds and activates the small and large forms of latent transforming growth factor-beta in a chemically defined system. J Biol Chem 1994;269:26,775–26,782.
83. Schultz-Cherry S, Lawler J, Murphy-Ullrich JE. The type 1 repeats of thrombospondin 1 activate latent transforming growth factor-beta. J Biol Chem 1994;269:26,783–26,788.
84. Schultz-Cherry S, Chen H, Mosher DF, et al. Regulation of transforming growth factor-beta activation by discrete sequences of thrombospondin 1. J Biol Chem 1995;270:7304–7310.
85. Ribeiro SM, Poczatek M, Schultz-Cherry S, Villain M, Murphy-Ullrich JE. The activation sequence of thrombospondin-1 interacts with the latency-associated peptide to regulate activation of latent transforming growth factor-beta. J Biol Chem 1999;274:13,586–13,593.
86. Murphy-Ullrich JE, Poczatek M. Activation of latent TGF-beta by thrombospondin-1: mechanisms and physiology. Cytokine Growth Factor Rev 2000;11:59–69.
87. Yevdokimova N, Wahab NA, Mason RM. Thrombospondin-1 is the key activator of TGF-beta1 in human mesangial cells exposed to high glucose. J Am Soc Nephrol 2001;12:703–712.
88. Guo NH, Krutzsch HC, Inman JK, Shannon CS, Roberts DD. Antiproliferative and antitumor activities of D-reverse peptides derived from the second type-1 repeat of thrombospondin-1. J Pept Res 1997;50:210–221.
89. Miao WM, Seng WL, Duquette M, Lawler P, Laus C, Lawler J. Thrombospondin-1 type 1 repeat recombinant proteins inhibit tumor growth through transforming growth factor-beta-dependent and -independent mechanisms. Cancer Res 2001;61:7830–7839.
90. Poczatek MH, Hugo C, Darley-Usmar V, Murphy-Ullrich JE. Glucose stimulation of transforming growth factor-beta bioactivity in mesangial cells is mediated by thrombospondin-1. Am J Pathol 2000;157:1353–1363.
91. Bailly S, Brand C, Chambaz EM, Feige JJ. Analysis of small latent transforming growth factor-beta complex formation and dissociation by surface plasmon resonance. Absence of direct interaction with thrombospondins. J Biol Chem 1997;272:16,329–16,334.
92. Grainger DJ, Frow EK. Thrombospondin 1 does not activate transforming growth factor beta1 in a chemically defined system or in smooth-muscle-cell cultures. Biochem J 2000;350(Pt 1):291–298.
93. Abdelouahed M, Ludlow A, Brunner G, Lawler J. Activation of platelet-transforming growth factor beta-1 in the absence of thrombospondin-1. J Biol Chem 2000;275:17,933–17,936.
94. Bayraktar M, Dundar S, Kirazli S, Teletar F. Platelet factor 4, beta-thromboglobulin and thrombospondin levels in type I diabetes mellitus patients. J Int Med Res 1994,22.90–94.
95. Tschoepe D, Driesch E, Schwippert B, Lampeter EF. Activated platelets in subjects at increased risk of IDDM. DENIS Study Group. Deutsche Nikotinamid Interventionsstudie. Diabetologia 1997;40: 573–577.
96. Murphy M, Godson C, Cannon S, et al. Suppression subtractive hybridization identifies high glucose levels as a stimulus for expression of connective tissue growth factor and other genes in human mesangial cells. J Biol Chem 1999;274:5830–5834.
97. Tada H, Isogai S. The fibronectin production is increased by thrombospondin via activation of TGF-b in cultured human mesangial cells. Nephron 1998;79:38–43.
98. Tada H, Kuboki K, Nomura K, Inokuchi T. High glucose levels enhance TGF-beta1-thrombospondin-1 pathway in cultured human mesangial cells via mechanisms dependent on glucose-induced PKC activation. J Diabetes Complications 2001;15:193–197.
99. Hugo C, Shankland SJ, Pichler RH, Couser WG, Johnson RJ. Thrombospondin 1 precedes and predicts the development of tubulointerstitial fibrosis in glomerular disease in the rat. Kidney Int 1998;53: 302–311.
100. Hugo C, Kang DH, Johnson RJ. Sustained expression of thrombospondin-1 is associated with the development of glomerular and tubulointerstitial fibrosis in the remnant kidney model. Nephron 2002;90: 460–470.

101. Border WA, Noble NA, Yamamoto T, et al. Natural inhibitor of transforming growth factor-beta protects against scarring in experimental kidney disease. Nature 1992;360:361–364.
102. Isaka Y, Brees DK, Ikegaya K, et al. Gene therapy by skeletal muscle expression of decorin prevents fibrotic disease in rat kidney. Nat Med 1996;2:418–423.
103. Vleming LJ, Baelde JJ, Westendorp RG, Daha MR, van Es LA, Bruijn JA. Progression of chronic renal disease in humans is associated with the deposition of basement membrane components and decorin in the interstitial extracellular matrix. Clin Nephrol 1995;44:211–219.
104. Diamond JR, Levinson M, Kreisberg R, Ricardo SD. Increased expression of decorin in experimental hydronephrosis. Kidney Int 1997;51:1133–1139.
105. Wahab NA, Harper K, Mason RM. Expression of extracellular matrix molecules in human mesangial cells in response to prolonged hyperglycaemia. Biochem J 1996;316(Pt 3):985–992.
106. Mogyorosi A, Ziyadeh FN. Increased decorin mRNA in diabetic mouse kidney and in mesangial and tubular cells cultured in high glucose. Am J Physiol 1998;275:F827–F832.
107. Demoor-Fossard M, Galera P, Santra M, Iozzo RV, Pujol JP, Redini F. A composite element binding the vitamin D receptor and the retinoic X receptor alpha mediates the transforming growth factor-beta inhibition of decorin gene expression in articular chondrocytes. J Biol Chem 2001;276:36,983–36,992.
108. Mogyorosi A, Ziyadeh FN. What is the role of decorin in diabetic kidney disease? Nephrol Dial Transplant 1999;14:1078–1081.
109. Fukui N, Fukuda A, Kojima K, Nakajima K, Oda H, Nakamura K. Suppression of fibrous adhesion by proteoglycan decorin. J Orthop Res 2001;19:456–462.
110. Fukushima K, Badlani N, Usas A, Riano F, Fu F, Huard J. The use of an antifibrosis agent to improve muscle recovery after laceration. Am J Sports Med 2001;29:394–402.
111. Fischer JW, Kinsella MG, Levkau B, Clowes AW, Wight TN. Retroviral overexpression of decorin differentially affects the response of arterial smooth muscle cells to growth factors. Arterioscler Thromb Vasc Biol 2001;21:777–784.
112. Kolb M, Margetts PJ, Galt T, et al. Transient transgene expression of decorin in the lung reduces the fibrotic response to bleomycin. Am J Respir Crit Care Med 2001;163:770–777.
113. Costacurta A, Priante G, D'Angelo A, Chieco-Bianchi L, Cantaro S. Decorin transfection in human mesangial cells downregulates genes playing a role in the progression of fibrosis. J Clin Lab Anal 2002;16:178–186.
114. Huijun W, Long C, Zhigang Z, Feng J, Muyi G. Ex vivo transfer of the decorin gene into rat glomerulus via a mesangial cell vector suppressed extracellular matrix accumulation in experimental glomerulonephritis. Exp Mol Pathol 2005;78:17–24.
115. Glansbeek HL, van Beuningen HM, Vitters EL, van der Kraan PM, van den Berg WB. Expression of recombinant human soluble type II transforming growth factor-beta receptor in Pichia pastoris and Escherichia coli: two powerful systems to express a potent inhibitor of transforming growth factor-beta. Protein Expr Purif 1998;12:201–207.
116. George J, Roulot D, Koteliansky VE, Bissell DM. In vivo inhibition of rat stellate cell activation by soluble transforming growth factor beta type II receptor: a potential new therapy for hepatic fibrosis. Proc Natl Acad Sci USA 1999;96:12,719–12,724.
117. Muraoka RS, Dumont N, Ritter CA, et al. Blockade of TGF-beta inhibits mammary tumor cell viability, migration, and metastases. J Clin Invest 2002;109:1551–1559.
118. Scharstuhl A, Glansbeek HL, van Beuningen HM, Vitters EL, van der Kraan PM, van den Berg WB. Inhibition of endogenous TGF-beta during experimental osteoarthritis prevents osteophyte formation and impairs cartilage repair. J Immunol 2002;169:507–514.
119. Hisatomi T, Sakamoto T, Yamanaka I, et al. Photocoagulation-induced retinal gliosis is inhibited by systemically expressed soluble TGF-beta receptor type II via adenovirus mediated gene transfer. Lab Invest 2002;82:863–870.
120. Sakamoto T, Ueno H, Sonoda K, et al. Blockade of TGF-beta by in vivo gene transfer of a soluble TGF-beta type II receptor in the muscle inhibits corneal opacification, edema and angiogenesis. Gene Ther 2000;7:1915–1924.
121. Ueno H, Sakamoto T, Nakamura T, et al. A soluble transforming growth factor beta receptor expressed in muscle prevents liver fibrogenesis and dysfunction in rats. Hum Gene Ther 2000; 11:33–42.
122. Won J, Kim H, Park EJ, Hong Y, Kim SJ, Yun Y. Tumorigenicity of mouse thymoma is suppressed by soluble type II transforming growth factor beta receptor therapy. Cancer Res 1999;59: 1273–1277.
123. Yang YA, Dukhanina O, Tang B, et al. Lifetime exposure to a soluble TGF-beta antagonist protects mice against metastasis without adverse side effects. J Clin Invest 2002;109:1607–1615.

124. Piccirillo CA, Letterio JJ, Thornton AM, et al. CD4(+)CD25(+) regulatory T cells can mediate suppressor function in the absence of transforming growth factor beta1 production and responsiveness. J Exp Med 2002;196:237–246.
125. Bouche M, Canipari R, Melchionna R, Willems D, Senni MI, Molinaro M. TGF-beta autocrine loop regulates cell growth and myogenic differentiation in human rhabdomyosarcoma cells. FASEB J 2000;14:1147–1158.
126. Oft M, Heider KH, Beug H. TGFbeta signaling is necessary for carcinoma cell invasiveness and metastasis. Curr Biol 1998;8:1243–1252.
127. Lopez-Casillas F, Wrana JL, Massague J. Betaglycan presents ligand to the TGFβ signaling receptor. Cell 1993;73:1435–1444.
128. Lopez-Casillas F, Payne HM, Andres JL, Massague J. Betaglycan can act as a dual modulator of TGF-beta access to signaling receptors: mapping of ligand binding and GAG attachment sites. J Cell Biol 1994;124:557–568.
129. Liu M, Suga M, Maclean AA, St George JA, Souza DW, Keshavjee S. Soluble transforming growth factor-beta type III receptor gene transfection inhibits fibrous airway obliteration in a rat model of Bronchiolitis obliterans. Am J Respir Crit Care Med 2002;165:419–423.
130. Bandyopadhyay A, Zhu Y, Malik SN, et al. Extracellular domain of TGFbeta type III receptor inhibits angiogenesis and tumor growth in human cancer cells. Oncogene 2002;21:3541–3551.
131. Eickelberg O, Centrella M, Reiss M, Kashgarian M, Wells RG. Betaglycan inhibits TGF-beta signaling by preventing type I-type II receptor complex formation. Glycosaminoglycan modifications alter betaglycan function. J Biol Chem 2002;277:823–829.
132. Choi ME. Cloning and characterization of a naturally occurring soluble form of TGF-beta type I receptor. Am J Physiol 1999;276:F88–F95.
133. Docagne F, Colloc'h N, Bougueret V, et al. A soluble transforming growth factor-beta (TGF-beta) type I receptor mimics TGF-beta responses. J Biol Chem 2001;276:46,243–46,250.
134. Callahan JF, Burgess JL, Fornwald JA, et al. Identification of novel inhibitors of the transforming growth factor beta1 (TGF-beta1) type 1 receptor (ALK5). J Med Chem 2002;45:999–1001.
135. Inman GJ, Nicolas FJ, Callahan JF, et al. SB-431542 is a potent and specific inhibitor of transforming growth factor-beta superfamily type I activin receptor-like kinase (ALK) receptors ALK4, ALK5, and ALK7. Mol Pharmacol 2002;62:65–74.
136. Laping NJ, Grygielko E, Mathur A, et al. Inhibition of transforming growth factor (TGF)-beta1-induced extracellular matrix with a novel inhibitor of the TGF-beta type I receptor kinase activity: SB-431542. Mol Pharmacol 2002;62:58–64.
137. Laping NJ. ALK5 inhibition in renal disease. Curr Opin Pharmacol 2003;3:204–208.
138. Grygielko ET, Martin WM, Tweed C, et al. Inhibition of gene markers of fibrosis with a novel inhibitor of transforming growth factor-beta type I receptor kinase in puromycin-induced nephritis. J Pharmacol Exp Ther 2005;313:943–951.
139. van Det NF, Verhagen NA, Tamsma JT, et al. Regulation of glomerular epithelial cell production of fibronectin and transforming growth factor-β by high glucose, not by angiotensin II. Diabetes 1997;46:834–840.
140. Ziyadeh FN, Simmons DA, Snipes ER, Goldfarb S. Effect of myo-inositol on cell proliferation and collagen transcription and secretion in proximal tubule cells cultured in elevated glucose. J Am Soc Nephrol 1991;1:1220–1229.
141. Rocco MV, Chen Y, Goldfarb S, Ziyadeh FN. Elevated glucose stimulates TGF-β gene expression and bioactivity in proximal tubule. Kidney Int 1992;41:107–114.
142. Song RH, Singh AK, Alavi N, Leehey DJ. Decreased collagenase activity of mesangial cells incubated in high glucose media is reversed by neutralizing antibody to transforming growth factor-beta. J Am Soc Nephrol 1994;5:972 (abstract).
143. Remuzzi G, Bertani T. Pathophysiology of progressive nephropathies. N Engl J Med 1998;339:1448–1456.
144. Reeves WB, Andreoli TE. Transforming growth factor beta contributes to progressive diabetic nephropathy. Proc Natl Acad Sci USA 2000;97:7667–7669.
145. Lucas C, Fendly BM, Mukku VR, Wong WL, Palladino MA. Generation of antibodies and assays for transforming growth factor beta. Methods Enzymol 1991;198:303–316.
146. Datta PK, Chytil A, Gorska AE, Moses HL. Identification of STRAP, a novel WD domain protein in transforming growth factor-beta signaling. J Biol Chem 1998;273:34,671–34,674.
147. Datta PK, Moses HL. STRAP and Smad7 synergize in the inhibition of transforming growth factor beta signaling. Mol Cell Biol 2000;20:3157–3167.

148. Hanyu A, Ishidou Y, Ebisawa T, Shimanuki T, Imamura T, Miyazono K. The N domain of Smad7 is essential for specific inhibition of transforming growth factor-beta signaling. J Cell Biol 2001;155: 1017–1027.
149. Schiffer M, Schiffer LE, Gupta A, et al. Inhibitory smads and tgf-Beta signaling in glomerular cells. J Am Soc Nephrol 2002;13:2657–2666.
150. Hayashi H, Abdollah S, Qiu Y, et al. The MAD-related protein Smad7 associates with the TGFbeta receptor and functions as an antagonist of TGFbeta signaling. Cell 1997;89:1165–1173.
151. Itoh S, Landstrom M, Hermansson A, et al. Transforming growth factor beta1 induces nuclear export of inhibitory Smad7. J Biol Chem 1998;273:29,195–29,201.
152. Ebisawa T, Fukuchi M, Murakami G, et al. Smurf1 interacts with transforming growth factor-beta type I receptor through Smad7 and induces receptor degradation. J Biol Chem 2001;276:12,477–12,480.
153. Kavsak P, Rasmussen RK, Causing CG, et al. Smad7 binds to Smurf2 to form an E3 ubiquitin ligase that targets the TGF beta receptor for degradation. Mol Cell 2000;6:1365–1375.
154. Suzuki C, Murakami G, Fukuchi M, et al. Smurf1 regulates the inhibitory activity of Smad7 by targeting Smad7 to the plasma membrane. J Biol Chem 2002;277:39,919–39,925.
155. Bai S, Cao X. A nuclear antagonistic mechanism of inhibitory Smads in transforming growth factor-beta signaling. J Biol Chem 2002;277:4176–4182.
156. Bai S, Shi X, Yang X, Cao X. Smad6 as a transcriptional corepressor. J Biol Chem 2000;275: 8267–8270.
157. Nagarajan RP, Zhang J, Li W, Chen Y. Regulation of Smad7 promoter by direct association with Smad3 and Smad4. J Biol Chem 1999;274:33,412–33,418.
158. Denissova NG, Pouponnot C, Long J, He D, Liu F. Transforming growth factor beta inducible independent binding of SMAD to the Smad7 promoter. Proc Natl Acad Sci USA 2000;97:6397–6402.
159. Brodin G, Ahgren A, ten Dijke P, Heldin CH, Heuchel R. Efficient TGF-beta induction of the Smad7 gene requires cooperation between AP-1, Sp1, and Smad proteins on the mouse Smad7 promoter. J Biol Chem 2000;275:29,023–29,030.
160. Stopa M, Anhuf D, Terstegen L, Gatsios P, Gressner AM, Dooley S. Participation of Smad2, Smad3, and Smad4 in transforming growth factor beta (TGF-beta)-induced activation of Smad7. THE TGF-beta response element of the promoter requires functional Smad binding element and E-box sequences for transcriptional regulation. J Biol Chem 2000;275:29,308–29,317.
161. Hua X, Miller ZA, Benchabane H, Wrana JL, Lodish HF. Synergism between transcription factors TFE3 and Smad3 in transforming growth factor-beta-induced transcription of the Smad7 gene. J Biol Chem 2000;275:33,205–33,208.
162. von Gersdorff G, Susztak K, Rezvani F, Bitzer M, Liang D, Bottinger EP. Smad3 and Smad4 mediate transcriptional activation of the human Smad7 promoter by transforming growth factor beta. J Biol Chem 2000;275:11,320–11,326.
163. Uchida K, Suzuki H, Ohashi T, Nitta K, Yumura W, Nihei H. Involvement of MAP kinase cascades in Smad7 transcriptional regulation. Biochem Biophys Res Commun 2001;289:376–381.
164. Nakao A, Afrakhte M, Moren A, et al. Identification of Smad7, a TGFbeta-inducible antagonist of TGF-beta signalling. Nature 1997;389:631–635.
165. Afrakhte M, Moren A, Jossan S, et al. Induction of inhibitory Smad6 and Smad7 mRNA by TGF-beta family members. Biochem Biophys Res Commun 1998;249:505–511.
166. Lee BH, Kim MS, Rhew JH, Park RW, de Crombrugghe B, Kim IS. Transcriptional regulation of fibronectin gene by phorbol myristate acetate in hepatoma cells: a negative role for NF-kappaB. J Cell Biochem 2000;76:437–451.
167. Nakajima T, Nakamura T, Tsunoda S, Nakada S, Oda K. E1A-responsive elements for repression of rat fibronectin gene transcription. Mol Cell Biol 1992;12:2837–2846.
168. Isono M, Chen S, Hong SW, Iglesias-de la Cruz MC, Ziyadeh FN. Smad pathway is activated in the diabetic mouse kidney and Smad3 mediates TGF-beta-induced fibronectin in mesangial cells. Biochem Biophys Res Commun 2002;296:1356–1365.
169. Souchelnytskyi S, Nakayama T, Nakao A, et al. Physical and functional interaction of murine and *Xenopus* Smad7 with bone morphogenetic protein receptors and transforming growth factor-beta receptors. J Biol Chem 1998;273:25,364–25,370.
170. Bilezikjian LM, Corrigan AZ, Blount AL, Chen Y, Vale WW. Regulation and actions of Smad7 in the modulation of activin, inhibin, and transforming growth factor-beta signaling in anterior pituitary cells. Endocrinology 2001;142:1065–1072.
171. Itoh F, Asao H, Sugamura K, Heldin CH, ten Dijke P, Itoh S. Promoting bone morphogenetic protein signaling through negative regulation of inhibitory Smads. EMBO J 2001;20:4132–4142.

172. Zhu HJ, Iaria J, Sizeland AM. Smad7 differentially regulates transforming growth factor beta-mediated signaling pathways. J Biol Chem 1999;274:32,258–32,264.
173. Landstrom M, Heldin NE, Bu S, et al. Smad7 mediates apoptosis induced by transforming growth factor beta in prostatic carcinoma cells. Curr Biol 2000;10:535–538.
174. Schiffer M, Bitzer M, Roberts IS, et al. Apoptosis in podocytes induced by TGF-beta and Smad7. J Clin Invest 2001;108:807–816.
175. Mazars A, Lallemand F, Prunier C, et al. Evidence for a role of the JNK cascade in Smad7-mediated apoptosis. J Biol Chem 2001;276:36,797–36,803.
176. Patil S, Wildey GM, Brown TL, Choy L, Derynck R, Howe PH. Smad7 is induced by CD40 and protects WEHI 231 B-lymphocytes from transforming growth factor-beta -induced growth inhibition and apoptosis. J Biol Chem 2000;275:38,363–38,370.
177. Yamamura Y, Hua X, Bergelson S, Lodish HF. Critical role of Smads and AP-1 complex in transforming growth factor-beta-dependent apoptosis. J Biol Chem 2000;275:36,295–36,302.
178. He W, Li AG, Wang D, et al. Overexpression of Smad7 results in severe pathological alterations in multiple epithelial tissues. Embo J 2002;21:2580–2590.
179. Ferrigno O, Lallemand F, Verrecchia F, et al. Yes-associated protein (YAP65) interacts with Smad7 and potentiates its inhibitory activity against TGF-beta/Smad signaling. Oncogene 2002;21: 4879–4884.
180. Furuse Y, Hashimoto N, Maekawa M, et al. Activation of the Smad pathway in glomeruli from a spontaneously diabetic rat model, OLETF rats. Nephron Exp Nephrol 2004;98:e100–e108.
181. Kim HW, Kim BC, Song CY, Kim JH, Hong HK, Lee HS. Heterozygous mice for TGF-betaIIR gene are resistant to the progression of streptozotocin-induced diabetic nephropathy. Kidney Int 2004;66:1859–1865.
182. Fujimoto M, Maezawa Y, Yokote K, et al. Mice lacking Smad3 are protected against streptozotocin-induced diabetic glomerulopathy. Biochem Biophys Res Commun 2003;305:1002–1007.

I

Basic Pathophysiology and Biochemistry of Diabetic Nephropathy

H. New Approaches to the Study of Diabetic Nephropathy

13 Hepatocyte Growth Factor

Physiological and Therapeutic Ligand to Attenuate Diabetic Nephropathy

Shinya Mizuno, PhD
and Toshikazu Nakamura, PhD

CONTENTS

INTRODUCTION

Chronic renal disease (CRD) has been considered to be irreversible *(1)*. Renal fibrosis, a histological diagnosis of end-stage CRD, is characterized by a loss of renal parenchymal cells that are replaced by extracellular matrix (ECM) proteins, a common final pathway leading to renal dysfunction *(1,2)*. The number of patients affected with CRD is on the increase, and dialysis market estimates indicate that more than 1 million patients worldwide have undergone maintenance dialysis. Thus, many nations are burdened with social and financial problems associated with funding health services for the dialysis of CRD patients *(3)*. Diabetes is now the leading cause of end-stage renal disease (ESRD) in many developed countries, and diabetic nephropathy (DN) has emerged as a silent epidemic worldwide *(2,3)*. This is certainly the case in Japan, in which diabetic kidney disease accounted for 35% of all new patients undergoing dialysis in 2003. To maintain replacement therapy, it now costs nearly \$10 million per year in Japan for public financial support. Likewise, in the United States, DN accounted for 35% of all new cases of ESRD in 1997. The physical and monetary costs of diabetic kidney disease to both the patient and society are now enormous.

Histopathologically, DN is characterized by glomerular hypertrophy, followed by sclerotic lesions, in which ECM protein is overaccumulated in the mesangial interstitium *(3)*.

From: *Contemporary Diabetes: The Diabetic Kidney*
Edited by: P. Cortes and C. E. Mogensen © Humana Press Inc., Totowa, NJ

This sclerogenic event is associated with glomerular hyperfiltration and hypertension, and such a local hemodynamic change is followed by the onset of glomerular injury and albuminuria *(1–3)*. Induction of tubular inflammation by albuminuria accelerates progression of renal fibrosis and dysfunction under diabetic conditions. Especially in the progressive stage of DN, "resolution" of glomerular and peritubular fibrosis may be a promising target for reducing the renal disease. Of importance, these pathological changes are the final pathway not only in DN but also in other CRD, regardless of the initial cause *(1,3)*. Thus, many investigators have studied the common mechanisms whereby DN occurs, focusing on fibrogenic events in the different nephron components. Nevertheless, to this date, it is still difficult to arrest the onset and progression of diabetic kidney diseases.

Hepatocyte growth factor (HGF) was discovered and molecularly cloned as a long-thought hepatotropic factor *(4,5)*. In contrast to its name, HGF is now known to be a multifunctional cytokine with mitogenic, motogenic, and morphogenic activities in almost all organs and tissues. Regarding the kidney, HGF acts as a renotrophic, renoprotective, and angiogenic factor during embryonic and disease processes. Thus, HGF-mediated biological effects results in morphological as well as functional renal repair in the presence of acute injury *(6–8)*. We have accumulated evidence indicating that suppression of HGF production allows the rapid progression of renal fibrosis and dysfunction in CRD, whereas supplementing HGF reverses the progression of renal fibrosis, especially via regenerating tubular components *(9–11)*. Recently, we found that HGF targets glomerular cells and reduces mesangial fibrosis, a final common pathway of chronic glomerular injury. More recently, using a mouse model of diabetes we have obtained evidence that both glomerular and tubulo-interstitial fibrogenic events are attenuated by HGF and associated with improvements in albuminuria and renal dysfunction *(12)*.

In this chapter, we summarize recent outcomes, focusing on therapeutic mechanisms of HGF in DN as well as other CRD, with emphasis on the role of HGF for interrupting the common pathway leading to renal fibrosis. Based on recent results, we wish to postulate that DN progresses in part via impairment of endogenous HGF production, whereas supplementing HGF (or its gene) seems to be a new therapeutic strategy to improve hyperglycemia-induced renal disease, even in advanced stages of CRD.

HGF AND ITS UNIQUE BIOACTIVITY

Physiologically, HGF has an organotrophic role in the regeneration and protection of various organs, including the liver, lung, stomach, pancreas, heart, neurons, and kidney *(13–16)*. HGF levels increase in tissues and blood in response to various parenchymal injuries and diseases *(10,17)*, whereas inhibition of HGF activity by anti-HGF immunoglobulin (Ig)G or its receptor deletion leads to impaired tissue repair *(18–21)*. For a better understanding of the intrinsic repair system, we will describe the role of HGF and its receptor, c-Met, as well as the c-Met intracellular signaling events.

HGF and Its Receptor, c-Met

HGF was partially isolated in 1984 as a mitogen for fully differentiated hepatocytes, on the basis of DNA synthesis in a primary culture system *(4)*. Thereafter, HGF was completely purified from rat platelets and its biological properties were well characterized *(22)*. Based on purified HGF protein, cDNA encoding human HGF was successfully cloned in 1989 *(5)*. As a result, its molecular structure was demonstrated to be unique

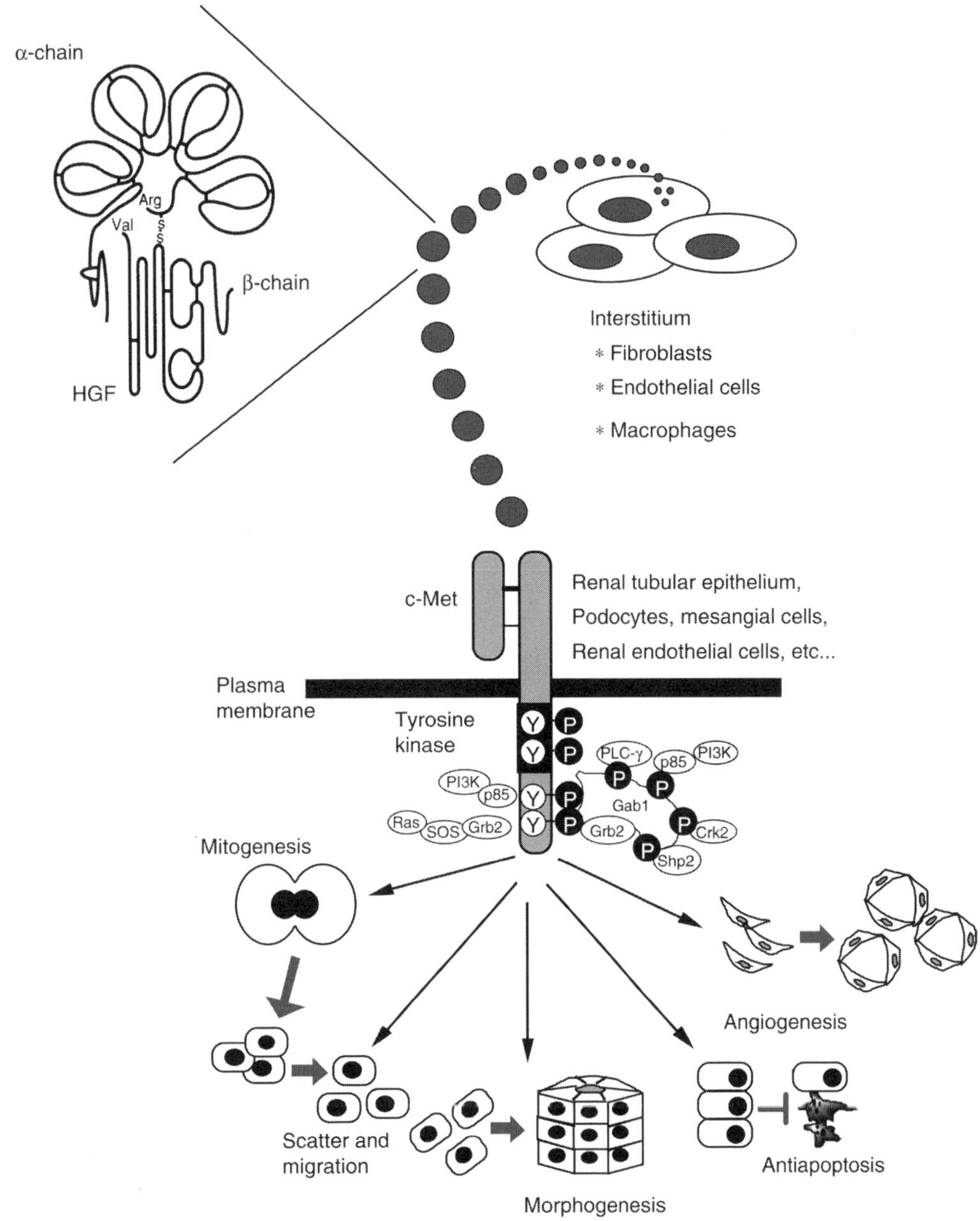

Fig. 1. Interstitium to ephithelium hemostatic and regenerative system through a HGF/Met signaling. HGF is produced by interstitial cells, such as fibroblasts, endothelial cells, and possibly infiltrated macrophages. Met/HGF receptor is expressed in kidney mainly on renal tubular epithelial cells, glomerular podocytes, mesangial cells, and endothelial cells. Binding of HGF to Met leads to phosphorylation of tyrosine kinase in intracellular domains of Met, followed by onset of multiple bioactivities, such as mitogenesis, migration, morphogenesis, and angiogenesis. HGF has anti-apoptotic and hyperfunctional activities (such as enhancing tubular Na^+-K^+-ATPase). Each activity is produced via combinations of intracellular signaling molecules, recruited by phosphorylated tyrosine kinase.

as a heterodimer composed of a 69 kDa α-chain and a 34 kDa β-chain *(5,23)*. The α-chain contains the N-terminal hairpin domain and the subsequent four kringle domains, and the β-chain contains a serine protease-like domain (Fig. 1, top). The kringle domain was initially found in serine proteases involved in blood coagulation or thrombolysis, and HGF has a 38% amino acid sequence homology to plasminogen.

On the other hand, c-Met, a protooncogene product, was identified as a receptor specific for HGF *(24)*. The c-Met/HGF-receptor is composed of a 50 kDa α-chain and a 145 kDa β-chain *(24)*. The α-chain is exposed extracellularly, whereas the β-chain is a transmembrane subunit containing an intracellular tyrosine kinase domain. Binding of HGF to c-Met induces activation of tyrosine kinase, which results in biological actions in a wide variety of cells, including mitogenic, motogenic, morphogenic, and anti-apoptotic activities, via subsequent phosphorylation of C-terminally clustered tyrosine residues *(25–27)* (Fig. 1). Phosphorylation of these tyrosine residues recruits intracellular signaling molecules containing the src homology domain, including Gab-1, phospholipase C-γ, Ras-GTPase-activating protein, phosphatidylinositol 4,5-bisphosphate 3-kinase, c-Src, Shp-2, Crk-2, and Grb-2. Although the intracellular signaling pathways driven by HGF that lead to the specific or preferential activation of biological responses (i.e., mitogenic, motogenic, morphogenic, or anti-apoptotic) have yet to be fully defined, the unique activation of signaling molecules responsible for specific cellular responses is evident. For example, phosphotyrosine-dependent recruitment of the Grb-2/SOS complex activates Ras and phosphorylation events, including extracellular signal-regulated kinase (ERK). Activation of the Ras-ERK pathway is required for cell proliferation *(27)*. On the other hand, the association and tyrosine phosphorylation of Gab-1, a docking protein that couples c-Met with multiple signaling proteins such as PI-3 kinase, PLC, Shp-2, and Crk-2, plays a definite role in HGF-induced morphogenesis and cellular motion *(26,27)*. These specific actions on the activity of diverse intracellular pathways explain the multi-functional effects of HGF.

Role of HGF During Organ Repair and Development

HGF is produced and secreted from nonparenchymal cells (such as resident fibroblasts, infiltrated macrophages as well as endothelial cells), whereas c-Met is mainly expressed on the side of parenchymal areas *(9,10,17)* (Fig. 1). The c-Met level is upregulated in response to injurious stresses and activated specifically in diseased tissues *(10,28)*. This mesenchyme-to-parenchyme humoral signal(s) is essential for organ tissue repair, development as well as organ protection.

Tissue Repair

In injured sites of parenchymal organs, HGF elicits mitogenic and motogenic activities in order to restore the integrity of the parenchymal components *(9,10,17)* (Fig. 1, bottom). HGF has a morphogenic function toward replicated cells to create tubular duct formation via controlling cell arrangement and polarity *(9,10,27)*. Furthermore, HGF controls metabolic events in parenchymal epithelial cells, for example HGF stimulates production and secretion of albumin in hepatocytes *(29)* and of insulin in pancreatic β-cells *(30)*, hence there is a role of HGF for inducing and sustaining homeostasis within physiological limits. In repair processes, vascular endothelial cell proliferation is a prerequisite for delivery of oxygen and nutrition to injured sites. Because HGF is a potent mitogen for vascular endothelium *(31,32)*, its activity contributes to maintain aerobic conditions in injured sites.

Organ Development

The multiple functions mediated by HGF/c-Met coupling are critical also for organogenesis in an embryonic stage. We prepared c-Met-deficient zenopus embryo, using a c-Met dominant negative mutant, and showed that HGF signal is required for development of the kidney, liver, and intestines *(33)*. During lung development, branching tubulogenesis becomes evident in parenchymal areas at E13.5 d of the mouse embryo, and is associated with increased HGF expression in meschenchymal areas *(34)*. When this HGF activity is neutralized by an antibody specific to HGF, branching tubulogenesis is diminished, hence HGF plays a key role for lung development *(34)*. Furthermore, studies with the c-Met-deficient mouse strain delineated an essential role of HGF/c-Met signaling in placental, hepatic, and muscular development *(35–37)*. Given that meschenchymal stromal cells (such as fibroblasts) are a major source of HGF, HGF/c-Met axis confers a mesenchyme-to-parenchyme system for organ development.

Organ Protection

In addition to such morphogenic bioactivities, HGF has a protective function in a variety of organs *(10,17,38)*. In fact, HGF is anti-apoptotic and completely blocks the onset of fulminant hepatitis *(39)*, myocardial infarction *(40)*, and ischemic neuron cell death in rodents *(41)*. Inducing anti-apoptotic signals (such as Bcl-xL/Bcl-2 and Bag-1) *(39–43)* as well as sequestration of Fas by activated c-Met *(44)* is involved in this anti-apoptotic process. Such protective effects are now widely demonstrated in numerous organs during parenchymal injury *(45–47)*. Overall, HGF is identified as a key ligand not only to induce regenerative responses but also to reduce parenchymal damage.

RENOTROPHIC ROLE OF HGF

HGF plays multiple roles in various organs *(10,17)*, as determined in the following studies. Initially, we found in 1991 that HGF is a potent mitogen for renal tubular epithelial cells, using a primary culture system *(48)* (Fig. 2A-I). In the same year, Montesano's and our group identified a soluble factor capable of inducing renal tubulogenesis in fibroblast-conditioned medium as HGF *(49)* (Fig. 2A-II). Furthermore, HGF targets renal tubular cells and upregulates expression of Na^+-K^+ATPase *(50)*, a key enzyme for regulating a balance of plasma and urinary Na^+/K^+ levels. Thus, HGF is important for maturation of renal tubules. In addition to the tubular epithelium, HGF may be also critically involved in repair and protection of glomerular cells, based on the following:

1. HGF is an anti-apoptotic factor toward mesangial cells (MCs) and podocytes *(51,52)*.
2. HGF is a mitogen for glomerular endothelial cells in vivo *(53)*, and
3. HGF is a negative regulator of glomerular hyperfiltration *(54)*, a pathogenic event accelerating glomerular injury.

These potential renotrophic effects of HGF on the diverse renal cellular components are summarized in Table 1.

Physiological Effects of HGF in Renal Growth and Repair

In the adult kidney, the number of nephrons remains constant and demonstrate little proliferative activity under physiological conditions. However, the kidney shows great potential for regeneration in order to restore normal size or function once renal mass, morphology, or function are impaired *(55)*. For example, renal regeneration is induced by nephrectomy or cell death caused by toxins. A humoral factor(s) is involved in renal enlargement after unilateral nephrectomy *(55)*, named "renotropine." Although the existence of such renotrophic factor(s) seems well documented, their identity and initial

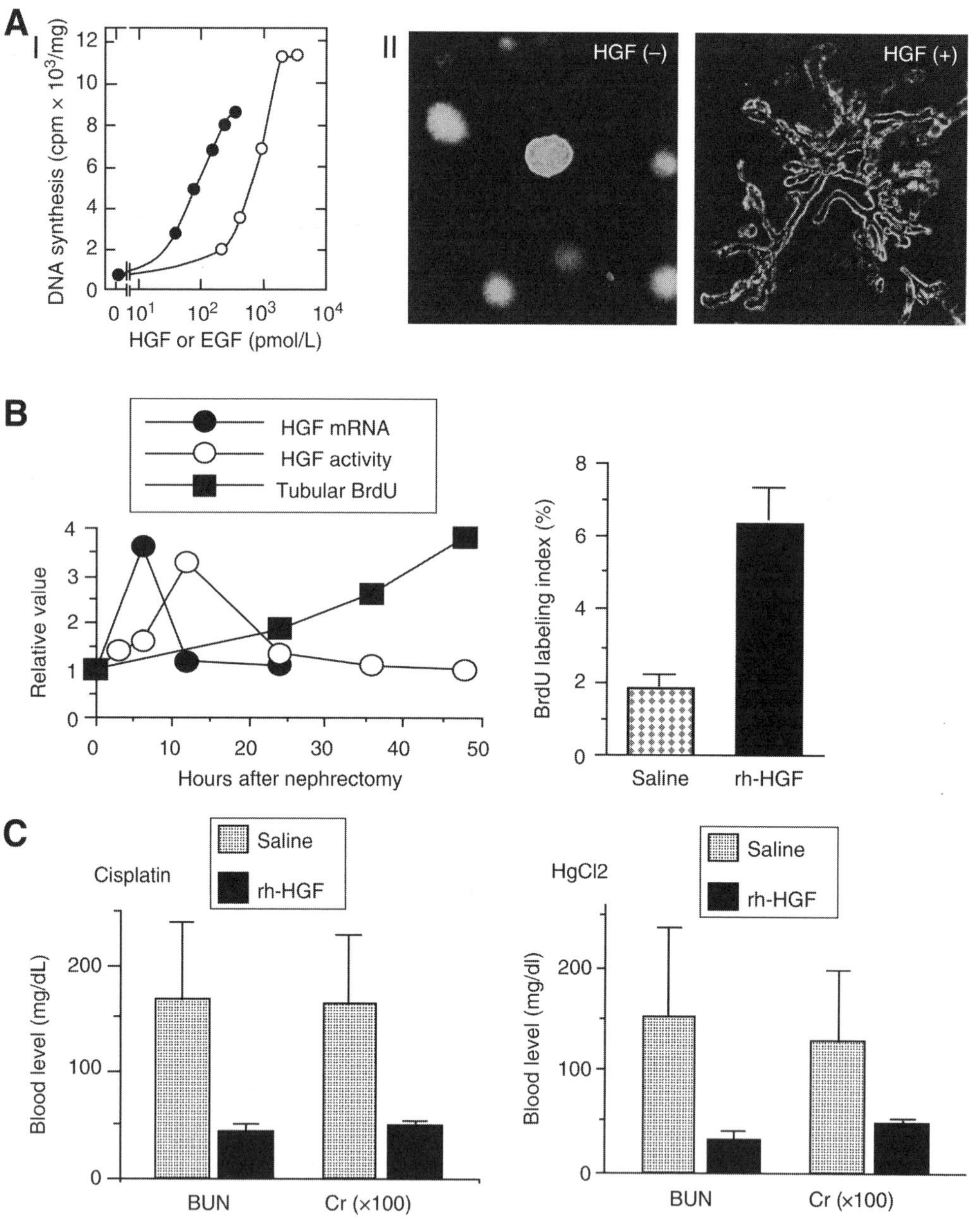

Fig. 2. Renotrophic roles of HGF in vitro and in vivo. **(A)** In vitro activity of HGF toward renal tubular epithelium. (I) Mitogenic action of HGF (closed circle) and of epidermal growth factor (open circle) on cultured rabbit renal epithelial cells. DNA synthesis of renal tubular cells cultured with or without HGF or epidermal growth factor was measured. (II) Induction of branching tubulogenesis by HGF in Mardin-Darby Canine Kidney renal tubular cells grown in a collagen gel. **(B)** Renotrophic roles of HGF in compensatory renal growth in rodents undergone unilateral nephrectomy (left). Changes of HGF mRNA, HGF protein activity, and tubular proliferation, as evidenced by BrdU intake (right). Tubular proliferation, as evaluated by BrdU intake, at 48 h after the left nephrectomy is markedly increased in mice by rh-HGF administration. **(C)** Preventive effect of rh-HGF on onsets of acute renal failure in mice, caused by a single injection of renal toxins such as cisplatin and $HgCl_2$.

Table 1
Renotropic Roles of HGF in Nephron Component Cells

Targets	*Bioactivity*	*Respected outcomes*	*References*
1. Glomeruli			
Mesangial cells	Anti-prolifcration, suppressed ECM deposition	Inhibition of glomerulonephritis	*51, 86*
		inhibition of truft sclerosis	*10, 12, 101*
Podocytes	Anti-apoptosis, enhanced outgrowth	Protection of proteinuria inhibition of tuft sclerosis	*11, 12, 52*
Endothelium	Proliferation	Inhibition of tuft sclerosis	*53*
2. Tubules			
	Proliferation,	Tubular repair	*6–8, 11*
	anti-apoptosis,		*61, 78*
	migration and	Tubular repair	*10*
	scattering, morphoenesis,	tubular repair and development	*49, 71*
	induction of Na+-K+ ATP-ase	functional improvement	*50*
	supressed transdifferentiation	anti-fibrosis	*72, 73*
3. Interstitium			
Endothelium	Anti-inflammation	Inhibition of leucocyte attack	*61, 93*
		induction of immune tolerance	*78*
(Myo) fibroblasts	ECM degradation, myofibroblast death	Resolution of fibrosis	*103, 115, 118*

HGF, hepatocyte growth factor; ECM, extracellular matrix.

origins have remained unclear. In rats with unilateral nephrectomy, HGF mRNA and protein levels rapidly increases in the remaining kidney as well as in distant organs. In the kidney, this change is followed by compensatory growth of tubular cells *(56)* (Fig. 2B, left). When recombinant human HGF (rh-HGF) is administrated into mice immediately after unilateral nephrectomy or $HgCl_2$ exposure, tubular epithelial proliferation, evidenced by the uptake of bromodeoxyuridine (BrdU), is significantly enhanced *(6,7)* (Fig. 2B, right), hence demonstrating HGF to be a renotrophic factor. Furthermore, HGF is required for renal development at the embryogenic stage when tubules develop from the metanephron via branching tubulogenesis with mesenchyme-to-epithelial differentiation. Treatment with anti-HGF IgG blocks tubular formation and epithelization in an embryonic renal organ culture *(57)*, indicating an essential role of HGF for renal tubular development. Together with the in vitro findings that HGF is a mitogenic and morphogenic factor *(6,11,48,49)*, the rapid production of HGF after renal damage indicates the presence of an intrinsic renotrophic switch that drives nephron repair.

Therapeutic Effects of HGF in Acute Renal Failure

Based on the renotrophic actions of HGF, the potential application of HGF for the treatment of renal diseases has been tested in various experimental models. In a clinical setting, acute renal failure is often caused by nephrotoxic drug administration (e.g., cisplatin, cyclosporine A, tacrolimus, and antibiotics) and renal ischemia. Administration of cisplatin caused acute renal failure in mice, whereas HGF administration prevented histological damage of renal tubules and suppressed renal dysfunction *(6)* (Fig. 2C). Similarly, HGF prevented the renal histological damage and acute renal dysfunction caused by $HgCl_2$ administration, while enhancing regeneration of tubular epithelial cells *(7)*. The protective effects of HGF in acute tubular injury and renalfailure were also seen in cases of immunosuppressant toxicity *(58,59)* and in the crush syndrome *(60)*. Likewise, as compared with controls, rodents administered HGF postischemia had better renal function, reduced mortality, and a lesser degree of histological damage after renal ischemia was induced by renal artery occlusion *(8,61)*. All of these results suggest that HGF is promising as a drug for a cure-oriented therapy in acute renal injury *(62)*.

Anti-Fibrotic Function of HGF in Chronic Renal Diseases

Tubular and tubulo-interstitial damage is the key determinant for outcome of renal dysfunction in CRD *(63)*. It is now widely accepted that HGF is a potent regenerative and renoprotective factor, especially toward renal tubular cells *(10,64,65)*. HGF is antifibrotic in liver and lung *(66,67)*, and the molecular pathogenesis of these conditions is similar to that of renal fibrosis *(68)*. This led us to determine if the renotrophic action of HGF could improve the loss of renal function in CRD through the regeneration of tubular epithelial cells.

Nephrotic Syndrome

The fact that HGF is anti-fibrotic in CRD is first demonstrated in a murine model of nephrotic syndrome *(11,18)*. The ICGN mouse is a unique model of progressive albuminuria, owing to congenital alteration of the glomerular barrier *(69)*. In this model, tubulo-interstitial fibrosis, rather than glomerular injury, is the cause of a renal dysfunction that is characteristically associated with decreased renal HGF content *(18)*. We hypothesized that renal function could be preserved if tubular growth (compensatory renal growth) is elicited, using a renotrophic factor, HGF. To test this hypothesis, we administered rh-HGF to 14-wk-old ICGN mice, in which renal function was impaired with loss of tubular regeneration *(69)*. As a result, rh-HGF increased BrdU-positive tubular cells and this was associated with recovery from renal dysfunction, as evaluated by blood urea nitrogen (BUN) and creatinine (Cr) levels *(11)* (Fig. 3A). In addition, fibrotic events, such as myofibroblast hyperplasia and ECM overaccumulation, were strongly inhibited in the ICGN mice by rh-HGF administration. Furthermore, this was associated with a significant decrease in the renal content of transforming growth factor (TGF)-β_1 *(11)*, a key fibrogenic cytokine. Conversely, administration of anti-HGF IgG accelerated renal dysfunction and fibrosis, and this was associated with increased renal TGF-β_1 *(18)*. These findings indicate that deficient HGF production favors renal fibrosis and dysfunction, whereas replacement of endogenous HGF by rh-HGF administration prevents TGF-β_1-driven fibrogenic events in CRD.

Obstructive Nephropathy

Obstructive nephropathy occurs as a result of urinary retention, caused by obstructive causes (such as congenital hypoplasia, and urinary calculi) *(70)*. Ureteral obstruction and tubulo-interstitial fibrosis is one of the most frequent causes of end-stage CRD in children *(70)*. Unilateral ureter-ligation obstruction (UUO) in rodents mimics human obstructive nephropathy. Using this UUO model, we found that HGF supplementation suppressed renal TGF-β_1 expression, associated with repressed infiltration of macrophages, a source of TGF-β_1 *(71)*. This was followed by inhibition of interstitial fibrosis (i.e., myofibroblast hyperplasia and ECM overdeposition). In this process, HGF

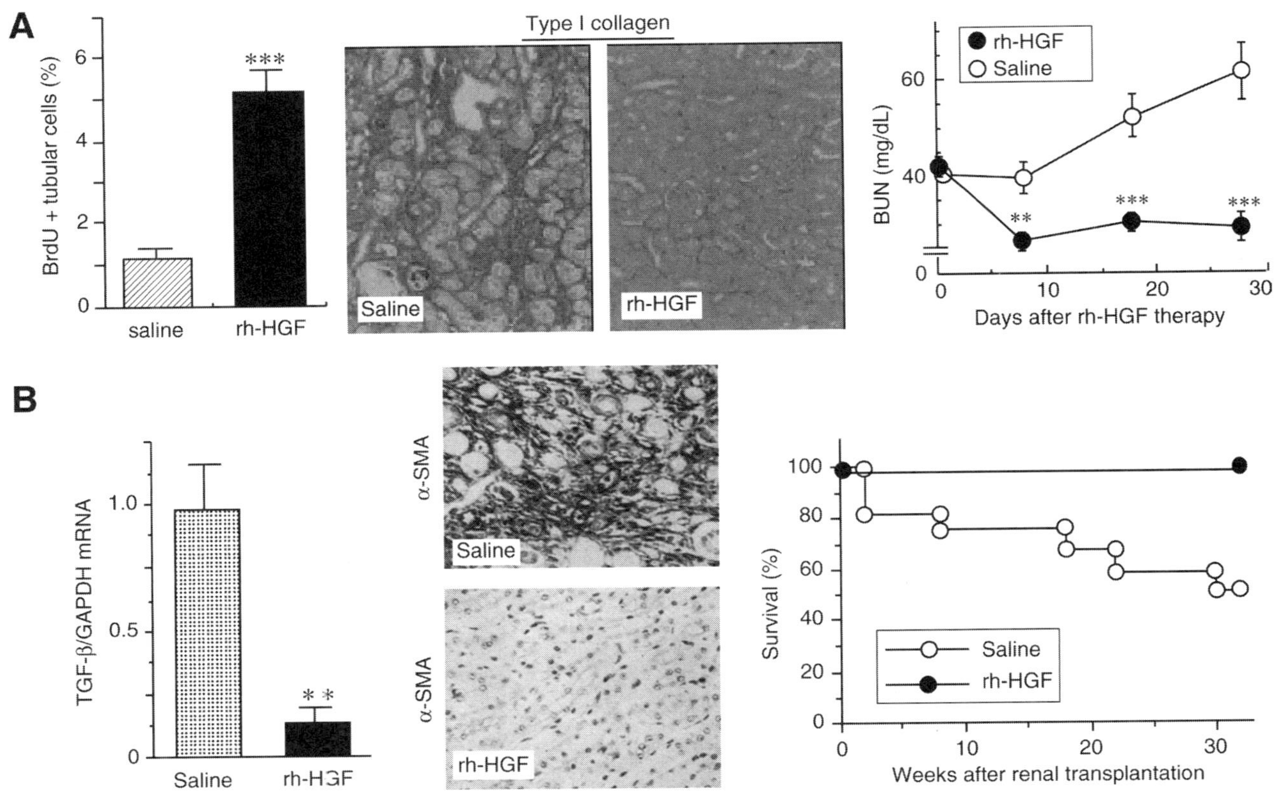

Fig. 3. Anti-fibrotic effect of HGF in chronic renal diseases. **(A)** Anti-fibrotic and therapeutic effects of HGF on nephrotic syndrome. Administration of rh-HGF into nephrotic ICGN mice enhanced tubular regeneration (as evidenced by BrdU intake) (left), whereas interstitial fibrosis was markedly suppressed in the mice undergoing rh-HGF supplement therapy (middle: collagen I staining). As a result, renal dysfunction (evaluated by the increase in BUN levels) was significantly attenuated by rh-HGF (right). **(B)** Suppression of renal fibrogenesis and individual death by HGF after renal allograft between F344 and Lewis rats. Serial injections of rh-HGF into recipient rats for 4 wk strongly suppressed renal TGF-β_1 production levels, followed by reduced myofibroblast accumulation at 32 wk after allograft transplantation. Consistently with histological results, HGF rescued the recipient rats from death, caused by the graft rejection. **, $P < 0.01$; ***, $P < 0.001$ vs same time-point of the saline control.

maintained tubular morphology and function via inducing tubular cell proliferation and inhibiting apoptotic cell death *(71)*. Using the same model, Liu et al. *(72,73)* also demonstrated that HGF suppresses TGF-β-mediated differentiation of tubular cells to myofibroblasts and identified this growth factor as an important anti-fibrosis mechanism in the kidney.

Other CRD

Such a reciprocal balance between HGF and TGF-β_1 is noted in various CRDs, independently of the primary underlying disorder *(18,71,74)*. In 5/6-nephrectomized rodents, evident renal fibrosis is associated with increased renal TGF-β_1 levels, whereas endogenous and exogenous HGF sustained nephronal integrity and inhibited interstitial fibrogenesis *(75,76)*. Likewise, renal *HGF* cDNA transfection led to prevention of chronic allograft nephropathy, associated with reduced TGF-β_1 levels and diminished renal fibrosis *(77)*. It is noteworthy that in a rat model of chronic allograft nephropathy administration of rh-HGF for the first 4 wk inhibited immunological damage, renal dysfunction, and proteinuria *(78)* (Fig. 3B). In this process, renal TGF-β_1 levels in the recipient rats were strongly suppressed by HGF, resulting in long-term maintenance of allograft function *(78)*.

HGF AS A PHYSIOLOGICAL LIGAND IN DIABETIC NEPHROPATHY

There is now ample evidence that TGF-β plays a fibrotic role during a progression of CRD, including diabetic nephropathy *(68,79,80)*. Overexpression of TGF-β induces fibrogenic lesions in normal kidneys *(81)*, whereas inhibiting TGF-β production or its function by anti-TGF-β IgG suppresses fibrosis in renal tissues under diabetic conditions *(68,79)*. However, the role of HGF in diabetic disease has remained undefined. Morishita et al. *(82)* described that elevated levels of glucose induce reduction of the renal production of HGF by increasing TGF-β_1. Liu et al. *(83)* showed in vitro and in vivo that hyperglycemia alters the renal expression of HGF and c-Met, suggesting that HGF could play a protective role. In clinical reports, variable levels of endogenous HGF have been reported in patients with diabetes *(84,85)*. These different findings may be a reflection of a changing HGF expression, perhaps owing to the stage of the disease. In fact, in murine models of other forms of CRD we reported that renal HGF levels increase at an early stage, decreasing below basal levels at late periods, in inverse correlation with both TGF-β_1 and ECM expression *(18,71)*. To demonstrate the role of HGF in diabetic nephropathy, we studied a mouse model of diabetes to examine whether HGF is involved in the protection of high glucose-induced renal injury.

Streptozotocin (STZ) is toxic specifically to pancreatic β-cells and causes insulin-dependent diabetes in mice. In mice given STZ injections, blood glucose levels increased within 7 d, to a threefold level over the control, associated with polyuria and glycosuria (not shown). Renal morphometry demonstrated that glomerular hypertrophy and sclerosis, as evidenced by increases in tuft size and collagen deposition, became evident between 6 and 10 wk after STZ administration. In addition, this was associated with increased renal TGF-β content *(12)* (Fig. 4A-I and III). In this process, renal HGF levels transiently increased at 2 wk, followed by a significant decrease at 10 wk after induction of the disease (Fig. 4A-II). The degree of glomerular HGF expression negatively correlated with the glomerular collagen IV score or with glomerular tuft size during progression of DN *(12)*. To elucidate the significance of glomerular HGF we injected during 2 wk anti-rodent HGF IgG in 4-wk diabetic mice. As compared with a control group, HGF-neutralized mice demonstrated evident glomerular sclerosis (i.e., type IV collagen

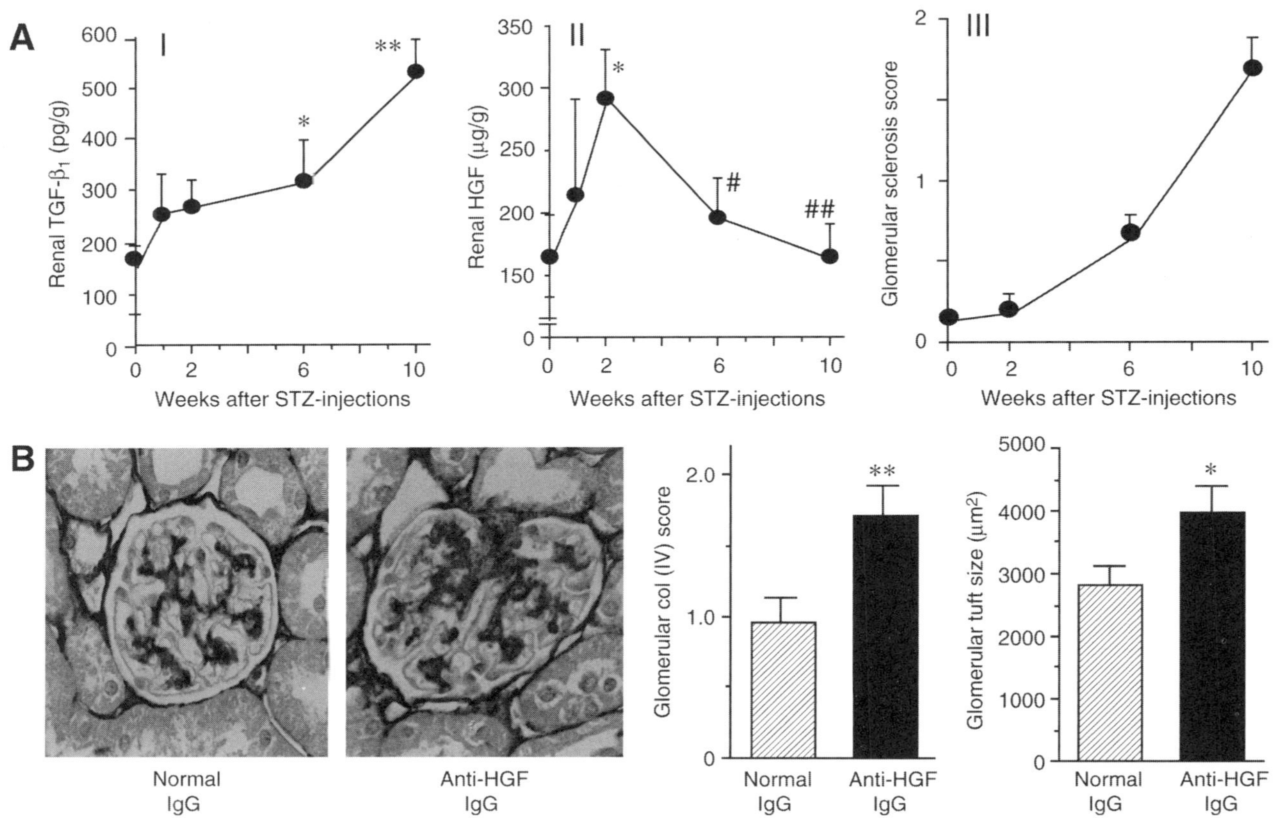

Fig. 4. A loss in endogenous HGF is pathogenic for manifestation of diabetic glomerulopathy in STZ-treated mice. **(A)** Time-course changes in renal TGF-β_1 (I), and HGF levels (II) as well as glomerular sclerosis score (III), during the natural course of diabetic nephropathy. *, $P < 0.05$; **, $P < 0.01$ vs pretreatment 0W. #, $P < 0.05$; ##, $P < 0.01$ vs 2W **(B)** Acceleration of diabetic glomerulopathy in the mice after anti-HGF IgG injections. The anti-HGF IgG was injected from 4 wk after STZ injections for 14 d. As a result, glomerular sclerosis and hypertrophy were both accelerated by the HGF-neutralizing treatment.

deposition and tuft size expansion) (Fig. 4B). The glomerular type IV collagen score was 1.8-fold higher in HGF-neutralized mice than in control mice *(12)*. Likewise, glomerular fibronectin and type I collagen deposition in diabetic mice was enhanced by anti-HGF IgG, as compared with treatment with irrelevant IgG (not shown). Furthermore, the size of the glomerular area was significantly increased after anti-HGF IgG treatment. These findings suggest the following:

1. Glomerular HGF is anti-fibrotic as well as antihypertrophic.
2. Failure to sustain endogenous HGF levels seems responsible for the development of diabetic glomerulophaty *(10,12,18)*.

Because we have demonstrated that HGF is a critical determinant of DN, it is important to discuss how HGF expression levels are controlled under diabetic conditions. At the initial stages of diabetes, plasma and renal HGF increase, especially at 2 wk after STZ injection *(12)*. In the early stages of diabetes, renal HGF is mainly localized in intra-glomerular cells and in only partially in peri-tubular interstitial cells. With regard to this, glomerular hyperfiltration and hypertension may elicit HGF production in mesangial and endothelial cells, as we have previously reported *(86,87)*. We will next discuss the mechanisms by which glomerular HGF declines in association with progressive glomerular hypertrophy and sclerosis. It is well documented that HGF and TGF-β_1 inhibit the synthesis of each other *(10,12,18,88)*. Mesangial (and in part endothelial) cells are the source of glomerular HGF formation *(10,86)*. In cultured MCs it has been shown that angiotensin-II (Ang-II) inhibits HGF production via induction of TGF-β_1 *(89)*. Furthermore, high glucose downregulates HGF expression in the vascular endothelium also via increasing TGF-β_1 levels *(82)*. Taken together, inhibition of HGF production by upregulated Ang-II and/or TGF-β_1 may be a fundamental mechanism whereby DN occurs and progresses in hyperglycemic conditions.

THERAPEUTIC POTENTIAL OF HGF IN DIABETIC NEPHROPATHY

Given that a loss in endogenous HGF production by hyperglycemia may be causative for the histological and clinical manifestations of diabetic renal disease, administration of exogenous HGF (or its gene) would inhibit or reverse the progression of diabetic renal injury. Using a model of DN, we obtained evidence that HGF may be a therapeutic factor for inhibiting TGF-β upregulation and renal fibrosis. We will discuss herein the relationship among molecular, histological, and clinical changes to understand the therapeutic effect of HGF in DN.

Glomerular Injury

Glomerular alterations, characterized by tuft hypertrophy and sclerosis, are the initial events in the diabetic kidney constituting the diabetic glomerulopathy *(3)*. As mentioned earlier, STZ-treated mice show glomerular lesions (i.e., expansion of glomerular tuft and overdeposition of ECM), which are similar to events in human diabetic glomeruropathy. Using this experimental model, we first focused on the effect of rh-HGF treatment during the progression of glomerulopathy. In the STZ-injected mice, glomerular hypertrophy became evident between 6 and 10 wk after the induction of diabetes. Of note, administration of rh-HGF (800 μg/kg/d, sc) significantly ameliorated the expansion of the tuft area that was evident in saline-injected diabetic controls *(12)* (Fig. 5A). TGF-β_1 is a key factor in the pathogenesis of DN. Ziyadeh et al. *(79)* reported

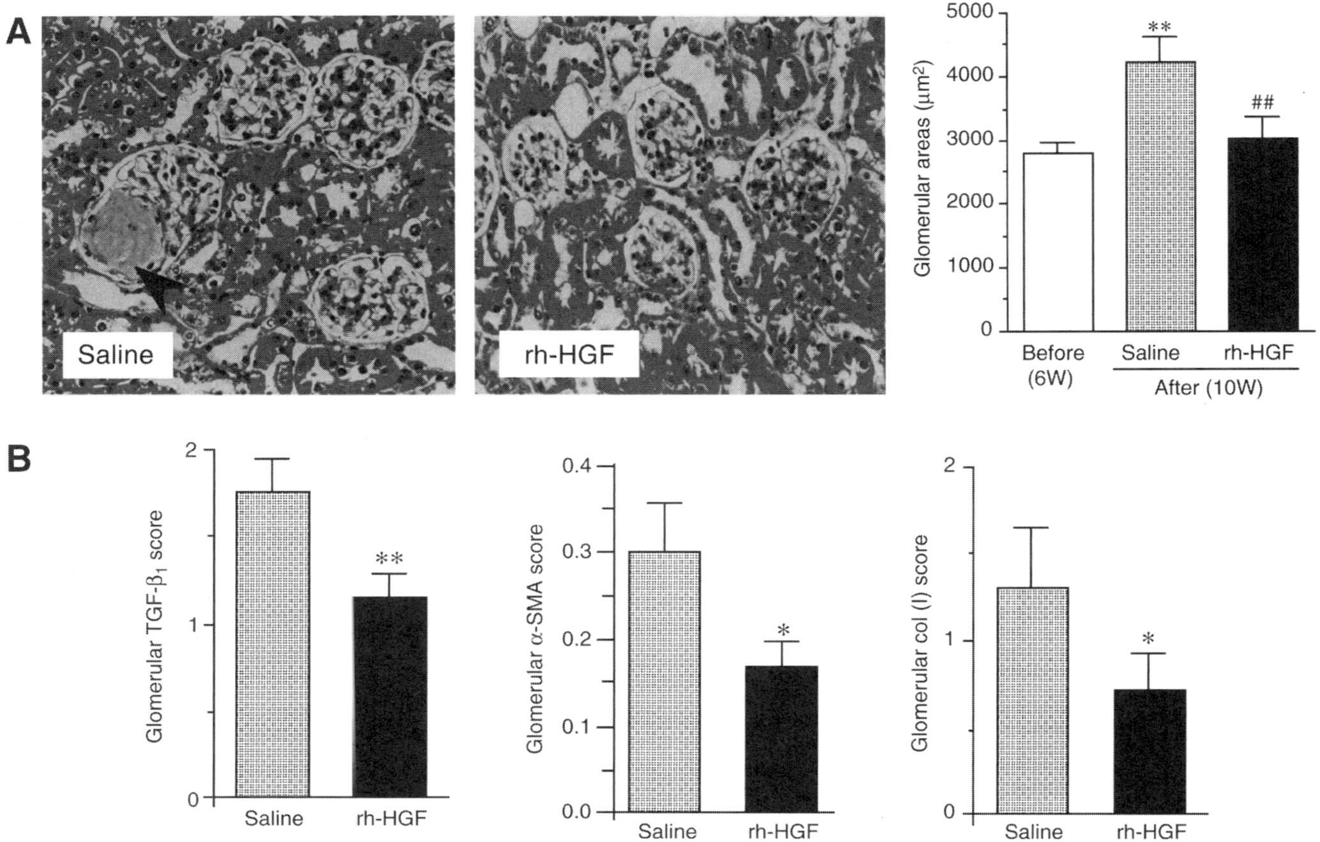

Fig. 5. Inhibitory effects of rh-HGF therapy on progression of diabetic glomerulopathy in mice. The mice were treated with rh-HGF between 6 and 10 wk after STZ injections. **(A)** HGF mediated prevention of glomerular hypertrophy, as determined by size of tuft areas. **(B)** Suppression of glomerular fibrotic events in mice by rh-HGF treatment. During progression of glomerular injuries, glomerular TGF-β_1 expression levels increased, followed by myofibroblast accumulation and sclerosis, as evaluated by increased α-SMA and collagen staining, respectively. By contrast, HGF suppressed the glomerular fibrogenic events. *, $p < 0.05$; **, $p < 0.01$ vs 6W (in A) or saline control (in B). ##, $p < 0.01$ vs saline (10W).

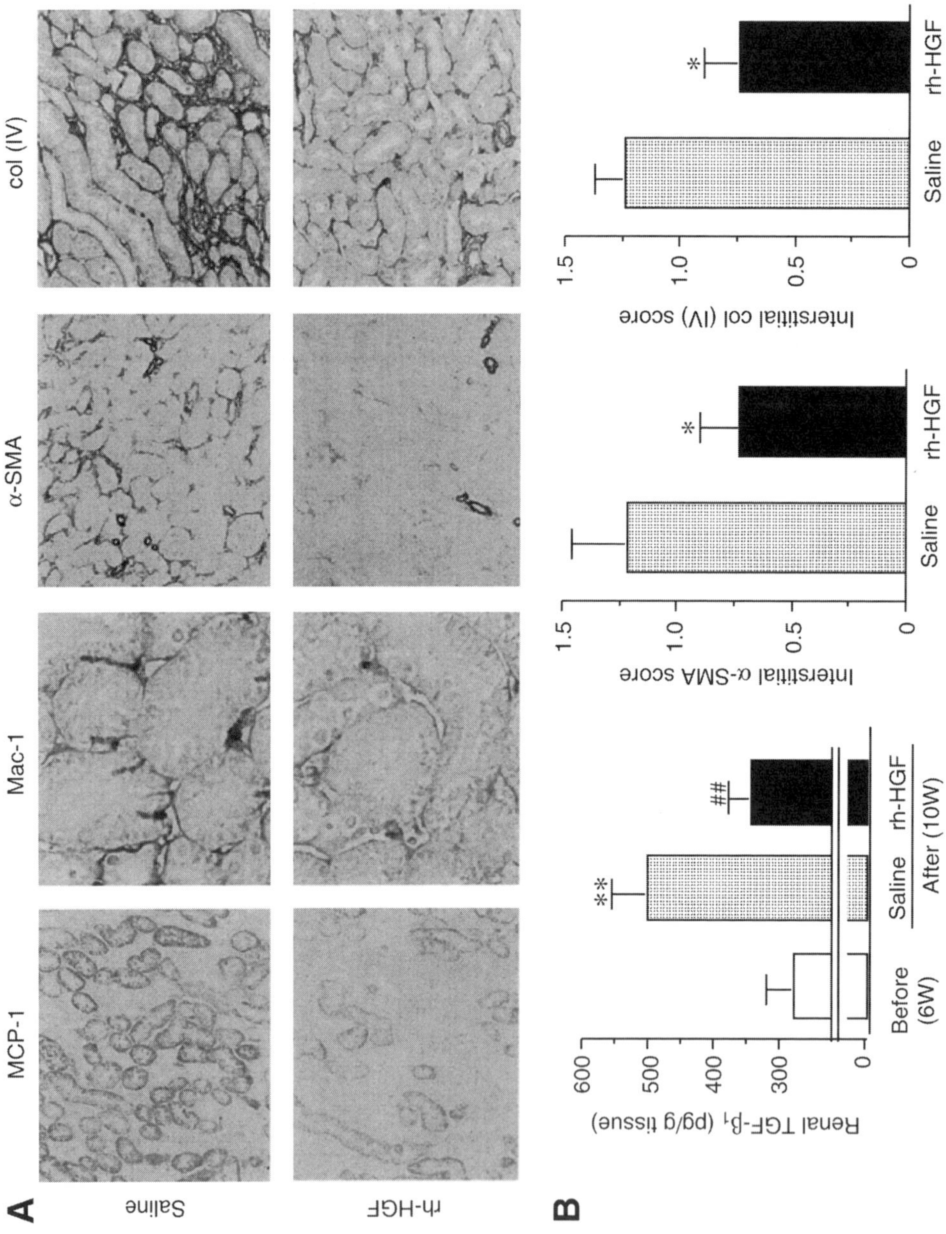
A
MCP-1
Mac-1
α-SMA
col (IV)
Saline
rh-HGF
B
Renal TGF-β1 (pg/g tissue)
600
500
400
300
0
**
##
Before (6W)
Saline
rh-HGF
After (10W)
Interstitial α-SMA score
1.5
1.0
0.5
0
*
Saline
rh-HGF
Interstitial col (IV) score
1.5
1.0
0.5
0
*
Saline
rh-HGF

that TGF-β_1 expression becomes evident in diabetic glomeruli, whereas anti-TGF-β_1 IgG administration inhibits these pathological events. Of importance, administration of rh-HGF to diabetic mice diminished TGF-β_1 production in MCs and partially in peri-tubular cells *(12)* (Fig. 5B). This seemed to be a direct effect, because in cultured MCs rh-HGF dose-dependently suppressed the induction of TGF-β_1 by high glucose *(12)*. Concomitantly with the decrease in mesangial TGF-β_1 expression in vivo, glomerular sclerotic events, such as myofibroblast formation and ECM accumulation, were repressed by HGF supplementation therapy (Fig. 5B). These findings indicate that the inhibitory effects of HGF on hyperglycemia-mediated TGF-β_1 overexpression may be the major mechanism whereby HGF therapy effectively inhibits diabetic glomerulopathy.

Tubular and Interstitial Injury

Tubulo-interstitial fibrosis is the most important predictor of renal insufficiency in CRD of diverse etiology *(63)*. In DN, the degree of tubular and tubulo-interstitial change (rather than glomerulopathy) accurately reflect the progression of renal dysfunction *(90)*. Thus, our attention was directed to effects of rh-HGF treatment on tubular and interstitial lesions. Monocyte chemoattractant factor (MCP)-1 is a key cytokine needed for recruiting inflammatory cells such as macrophages, which are a major source of TGF-β_1 and linked to subsequent fibrogenesis *(91,92)*. Shimizu et al. *(92)* reported that inhibition of the *MCP-1* gene repressed renal inflammation and fibrosis in a rat model of CRD. However, whether MCP-1 expression is modulated by HGF under diabetic conditions was unclear. In our diabetic mice, MCP-1 was mainly detected on proximal tubular cells, followed by interstitial macrophage infiltration. The administration of HGF suppressed the interstitial macrophage infiltration in association with a significant decrease of renal MCP-1 levels (Fig. 6). In contrast to treated animals, control diabetic mice demonstrated significant macrophage infiltration, accumulation of myofibroblasts (identified as the α-SMA marker) that was followed by interstitial fibrosis. Treatment with rh-HGF decreased the number of TGF-β-positive macrophages, lowered renal TGF-β_1 levels, and attenuated fibrogenesis. Given that HGF is directly capable of suppressing tubular inflammation in vivo *(61,93)*, these anti-inflammatory effects (i.e., inhibition of chemokine expression and macrophage influx) of HGF will contribute to the reduction in TGF-β_1 levels and TGF-β-mediated fibrogenesis.

Clinical Outcomes

We have shown that glomerular injury and interstitial fibrosis are preventable by exogenous HGF. The former lesion is linked to proteinuria and the later to renal dysfunction *(1,90)*. Here, we discuss the relationship between histological and clinical changes, focusing on the cytokine network(s) and its/their modulation by HGF.

Fig. 6. (*See opposite page*) Suppression of tubular and peri-tubular fibrotic lesions by HGF in diabetic mice. **(A)** Immunohistochemical evidence that HGF reduces tubular MCP-1 expression level, leading to suppressions of macrophage infiltration (i.e., Mac-1 staining), myofibroblast accumulation (i.e., α-SMA staining), and fibrosis (i.e., collagen staining). **(B)** Quantification of fibrogenic events in diabetic nephropathy and its modification by rh-HGF. Renal TGF-β_1 levels increased by diabetes, whereas rh-HGF suppressed such TGF-β_1 upregulation (left). As a result, α-SMA and type IV collagen scores were significantly lower in the HGF treated mice than in saline-treated mice (middle and right). Statistical analysis is same as in Fig. 5.

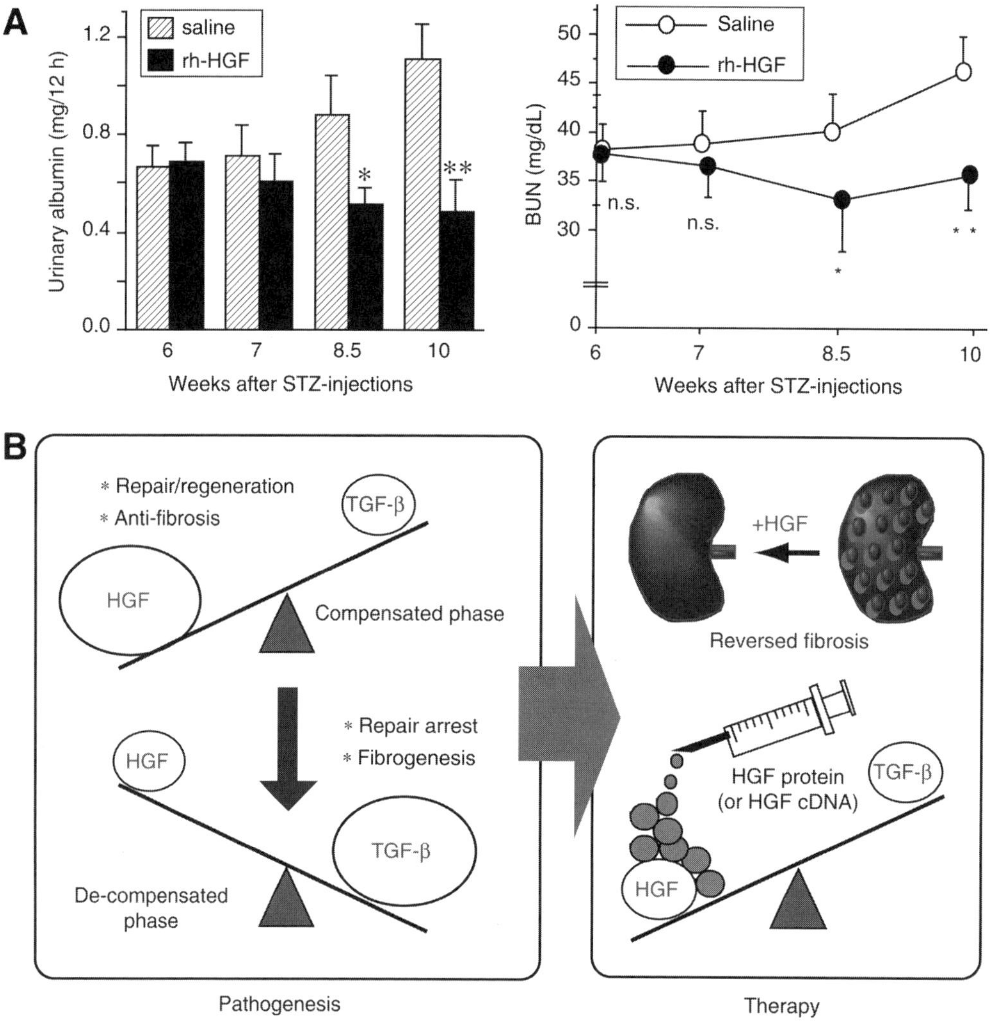

Fig. 7. Improvement of clinical findings by rh-HGF in diabetic mice and its therapeutic principal. **(A)** Amelioration of albuminuria and renal dysfunction by HGF in STZ-induced diabetic mice. The albumin and BUN and levels were determined in saline-injected mice and rh-HGF-treated mice (mean ± S.D., $n = 6$). Statistical analysis: n.s.; not significant, *; $p < 0.05$ and **; $p < 0.01$ vs same time-point of the saline group. **(B)** A hypothetical model for pathogenesis and therapy of diabetic nephropathy by HGF. A reciprocal balance between HGF and TGF-β_1 is involved in determining the fates of diabetic nephropathy. To reverse the fibrosis-progressed balance, supplement with HGF (or its gene) could be considered to attenuate fibrosis, a common pathway leading to end-stage CRD.

Albuminuria

Proteinuria is widely recognized as a risk factor for renal fibrosis and dysfunction in various CRDs, including DN *(1,3)*. In DN, albuminuria is a sensitive marker to predict prognosis *(1–3)*. Regarding this, it is noteworthy that albuminuria upregulates chemokines such MCP-1 with the onset and progression of tubular inflammation and fibrosis *(91–93)*. HGF treatment reduces urinary albumin levels in diabetic mice throughout the entire period of its administration (Fig. 7A, left), without changing blood glucose levels *(12)*. Therefore, this effect may explain the reduction of renal MCP-1 levels in HGF-treated mice.

Proteinuria occurs in part owing to persistent glomerular hyperfiltration and hypertension, caused by hyperglycemia *(1)*. Regarding this, HGF reduces systemic blood pressure, whereas attenuation of hypertension restores the HGF production *(94,95)*. Furthermore, HGF attenuates glomerular hyperfiltration *(11,54)*. An additional mechanism explaining the beneficial action of HGF is its effects on podocytes. Podocyte injury occurs in DN being manifested as albuminuria *(96)*. In our animal study *(12)*, podocyte injury, which was progressive up to 10 wk after induction of diabetes, was suppressed with rh-HGF therapy (unpublished data). In fact, HGF protects podocytes from apoptosis in vitro *(52)*. HGF is capable of promoting foot process extension (i.e., outgrowth) in podocytes in tissue culture (Dr. N. Kobayashi, personal communication). Together, antihypertension, podocyte protection, and possibly process outgrowth may be mechanisms responsible for the reduction in albuminuria in diabetic mice during rh-HGF therapy.

Renal Dysfunction

As described earlier, tubulo-interstitial fibrosis is the most reliable finding to predict renal dysfunction in diabetes *(63,90)*. Consistent with the histological findings that HGF prevents tissue fibrosis, renal function was improved by rh-HGF treatment (Fig. 7A, right). These findings indicate that tubular protection is a "practical" target of HGF to minimize the clinical manifestations of diabetic nephropathy, although prevention of glomerular damage (including albuminuria) by HGF may also contribute as an upstream mechanism.

Another possible mechanism is a direct effect of HGF on the tubular epithelium, as reported for other CRDs *(11,18,72,75)*. rh-HGF administration enhances tubular epithelial cell regeneration in STZ-injected diabetic mice *(12)*. It is known that tubular Na^+-K^+-ATPase activity is critical to maintain normal renal function by regulating glomerular filtration rate. Tubular Na^+-K^+-ATPase expression is increased in diabetes *(97)*, probably as a compensatory response to maintain Na^+/K^+ balance. HGF is a positive regulator for Na^+-K^+-ATPase expression *(50)* and more importantly, HGF therapy promotes the expression of tubular Na^+-K^+-ATPase in our STZ model (unpublished data). Thus, we predict that enhancement of Na^+-K^+-ATPase by HGF may lead to improved renal function in DN.

Molecular Basis

There are sequential pathological steps during the establishment of DN *(1,3)*. In these, multifunctional activities driven via HGF/c-Met coupling are needed to induce protective, regenerative and antifibrotic functions. A possible main sequence of events is as follows:

1. HGF initially targets glomerular cells and reduces hyperfiltration;
2. albuminuria is then attenuated, possibly associated with podocyte protection;
3. suppression of albuminuria leads to inhibiting MCP-1 expression and reduction in the number of macrophages (a major source of TGF-β_1); and
4. as a result, renal TGF-β levels decline then interstitial myofibroblastosis and fibrosis are inhibited.

TGF-β and HGF are counteracting in many multipotent biological actions. TGF-β induces growth arrest and/or apoptosis in epithelial and endothelial cells, and HGF exhibits mitogenic and anti-apoptotic activities in these same cell types *(98–100)*. HGF-induced regenerative responses are inhibited by TGF-β, and vice versa in cases of TGF-β-mediated fibrogenic events *(72,98–101)*. HGF stimulates or induces proteases involved in the breakdown of ECMs in several types of cells, including MT1-matrix metalloproteases (MMPs), uPA, and MMPs *(75,102–104)*. In contrast, TGF-β stimulates the synthesis of ECM and the production of inhibitors of proteases involved in ECM breakdown *(68)*. Consistently, HGF increases the expression of MMP-9, whereas HGF decreases the expression of tissue inhibitors of matrix metalloproteinase (TIMP)-1 and TIMP-2 in proximal tubular cells *(75,104)*. Together, we predict that such a balance between HGF vs TGF-β regulates a threshold to inhibit or foster renal tissue fibrosis (Fig. 7B). Thus, administration of HGF is a pathogenesis-based therapy for DN and other CRDs.

It is noteworthy that administration of exogenous HGF leads to restoration of endogenous HGF production *(18,71)*, associated with suppressed TGF-β_1 levels. In fact, exogenous HGF is capable of enhancing HGF production in an auto-inductive manner *(82,89,105)*. Considering that endogenous HGF is essential to minimize renal fibrogenesis in CRDs *(18,71,75)*, restoration of HGF production by exogenous HGF also participates in the attenuation of renal fibrosis. For example, blockade of Ang-II action with an Ang-II receptor antagonist delays progression of renal fibrosis, and this is associated with the increase in HGF production *(106)*. More importantly, HGF and Ang-II receptor antagonist synergistically improved renal fibrosis in a model of UUO *(107)*. These findings mean that restoration of the pathologically suppressed HGF production or its exogenous administration can be a sound strategy for treating CRDs.

ANTI-FIBROTIC MECHANISMS COMMON TO PARENCHYMAL ORGANS

Thus far, we have discussed how HGF prevents or improves renal fibrosis in DN and other CRDs. We have also accumulated evidence that HGF is anti-fibrotic in other chronic nonrenal diseases, such as liver cirrhosis *(66,105)*, pulmonary fibrosis *(67,103)*, cardiomyopathy *(108)*, and scleroderma *(109)*, thus suggesting common mechanisms of fibrosis and its counteraction. Hyperplasia of interstitial myofibroblasts is the common denominator in multiple tissues, and the degree of myofibroblast hyperplasia reflects the severity and course of fibrosis in diseases including the kidney *(110)*, liver *(111)*, and lung *(112)*. To understand the extensive actions of HGF, we will further discuss the role of HGF in myofibroblastosis, the common pathology in multiple disease states.

Induction of Myofibroblast Cell Death by HGF

Overdeposition of ECM by myofibroblasts is a compensatory response following the loss of parenchymal cells *(110–112)*. This extensive ECM deposition limits epithelial cell regeneration, resulting in progressive tissue damage. Under chronic conditions, progression of fibrosis is regulated via a balance between myofibroblast survival vs apoptosis *(111,112)*. Myofibroblast apoptosis is evident during matrix removal (i.e., "resolution" of fibrosis) in renal and hepatic fibrosis *(113,114)*, suggesting a key role for myofibroblast reduction to reverse the fibrotic process. Thus, how myofibroblast death occurs will be addressed below.

Recently, we demonstrated that myofibroblasts acquire the c-Met/HGF receptor during the HGF-induced apoptosis. This is associated with resolution of disease in animal models of liver and pulmonary fibrosis *(103,115)*. Contrary to its actions in a variety of cells *(18,39–41,61)*, HGF induces apoptosis in lung and liver myofibroblasts in vitro and in vivo. This effect is contingent on the HGF activation of MMPs. We have shown that MMP-9 induced in myofibroblasts by HGF leads to degradation of RGD-containing fibronectin and dephosphorylation of focal adhesion kinase *(103)*. Because fibronectin and focal adhesion kinase activation are essential for fibroblast survival *(116)*, HGF may induce anoikis-like cell death following the loss of ECM-cell attachment. Therefore, HGF is critical for reducing interstitial fibrosis by its concomitant action on myofibroblast cell death and ECM degradation during regression of tissue fibrosis, as noted elsewhere *(113,114)*.

Inhibition of Myofibroblast Differentiation and Hyperplasia by HGF

Another important role of HGF toward myofibroblasts is inhibition of the cellular proliferation and differentiation that is induced by fibrogenic cytokines *(11,72,86,115)*. Platelet-derived growth factor (PDGF) is a major mitogen for myofibroblasts. Overexpression of PDGF in the normal kidney leads to lesions mimicking mesangial proliferative glomerulonephritis (MPGN) *(81)*, whereas anti-PDGF antibody treatment suppresses myofibroblast overgrowth in an experimental model of MPGN *(117)*. Of interest, PDGF-mediated proliferation of MCs in culture is inhibited by HGF via inactivation of ERK-42/44 *(86)*. Similarly, HGF inhibited the PDGF-mediated proliferation of mesangium-derived myofibroblasts in association with early de-phosphorylation of ERK in a rat model of Thy-1 nephritis (i.e., MPGN). As a result, glomerular fibrosis was attenuated in HGF-treated rats *(86)*. This effect was also reproduced in the case of experimental hepatic cirrhosis *(115)* and in the atherosclerosis of pulmonary hypertension *(118)* in which myofibroblast hyperplasia is prominent.

Liu et al. *(119)* reported that the transdifferentiation of resident fibroblasts to myofibroblasts induced via TGF-β signaling was suppressed by HGF through inhibition of smad-2/3 nuclear translocation. HGF also inhibits the production of connective tissue growth factor (CTGF), another key ligand for fibrosis *(68)*, contributing to the prevention of CRDs, including DN *(76,120)*. The synthesis of decorin, a proteoglycan that suppresses TGF-β activity and fibrosis *(68)*, has been shown to be upregulated by HGF in myofibroblasts *(121)*. Overall, TGF-β, PDGF, and CTGF are all critical for tissue fibrosis and scar formation, whereas HGF has counteractive effects against the production and/or function of these fibrogenic ligands. Such inhibitory effects of HGF may be an event common to multiple disease conditions (Fig. 8).

Deletion of myofibroblasts and matix breakdown via HGF/c-Met activation would provide a mechanism to restore tissue integrity, even when parenchymal areas had been replaced by myofibroblasts. This is supported by the observation that parenchymal cell proliferation is enhanced by HGF in animal models of CRDs *(11,71)*, liver cirrhosis *(66)*, and lung fibrosis *(103)* in association with resolution of fibrosis. Together, our studies provide a molecular basis explaining how regression vs progression of tissue fibrosis is regulated and how it may be reversed in chronic conditions.

Specificity of HGF's Effects to Diseased Tissues

As mentioned earlier, HGF has a broad potential to produce regenerative and antifibrogenic outcomes in chronically diseased tissues. The systemic or local therapeutic administration of HGF will depend more on the degree and anatomical location of the

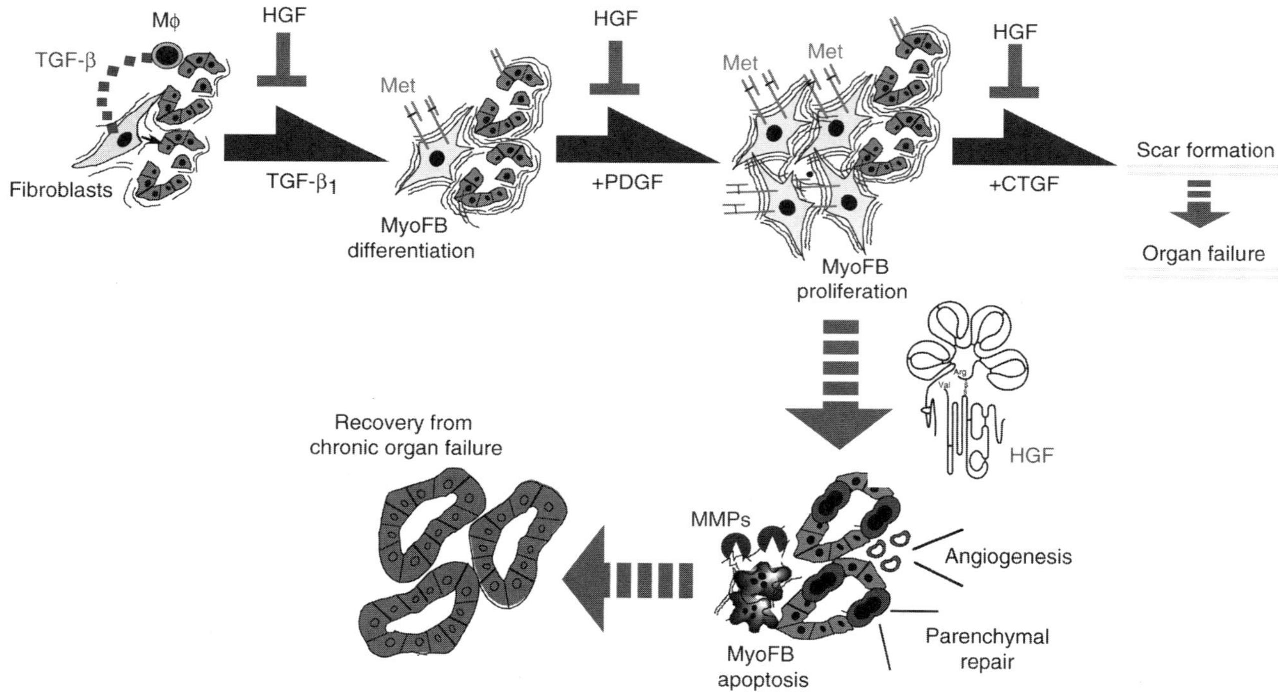

Fig. 8. Putative mechanisms for therapeutic effects of HGF against tissue fibrosis. There are sequential steps for pathogenesis of tissue fibrosis: (1) under chronic injuries, interstitial macrophages (Mϕ) are activated and overproduce TGF-β, then peri-tubular fibroblasts converts to ECM-producing myofibroblasts (MyoFB); (2) the myofibroblasts show overgrowth in response to PDGF, followed by hyperplasia of myofibroblasts (so called, myofibroblastosis); and (3) under such fibrotic conditions, CTGF and TGF-β further accelerate interstitial ECM accumulation, whereas epithelial cells undergo cell death. In this pathological process, (1) HGF inhibits TGF-β-mediated differentiation to myofibroblasts; (2) PDGF-mediated overgrowth is inhibited by HGF; (3) HGF suppresses production of fibrogenic cytokines (such as CTGF and TGF-β); and of note (4) HGF targets myofibroblasts and induces MMP-dependent anoikis-like cell death in myofibroblasts along with ECM degradation, followed by subsequent parenchymal repair and angiogenesis. Overall, HGF-mediated fibrotic resolution and parenchymal reconstruction lead to recovery from chronic organ dysfunction, noted in renal sclerosis, liver cirrhosis, pulmonary fibrosis and so on.

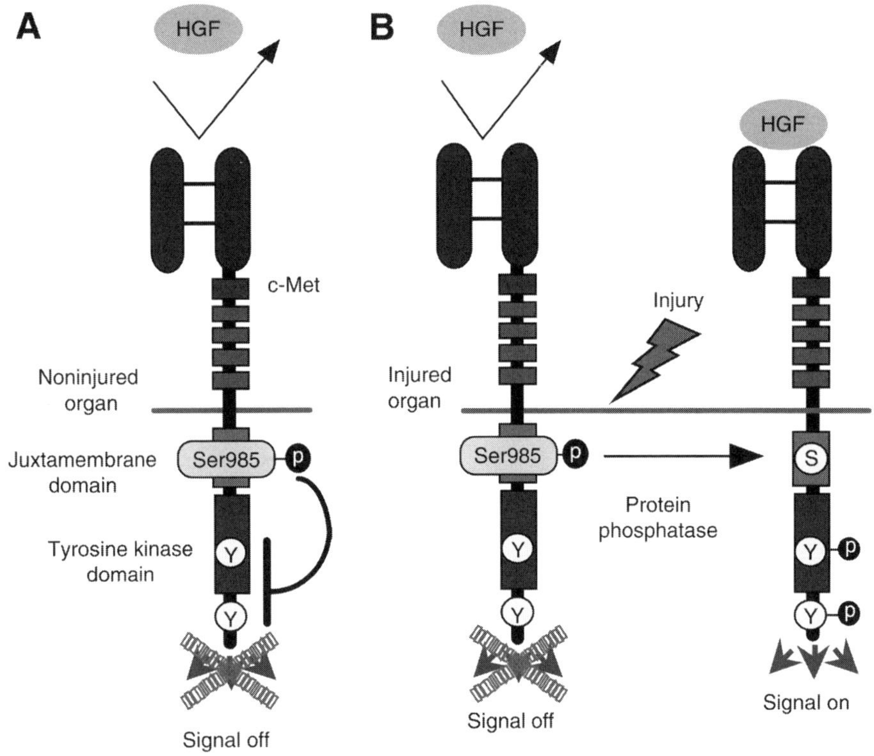

Fig. 9. A hypothetical model for injury-specific HGF/c-Met intracellular signaling. **(A)** In noninjurious (i.e., normal) organ tissues, a serine residue site at position 985 (Ser-985) in the juxtamembrane of c-Met/HGF receptor is constitutively phosphorylated and functions as a negative regulator to inhibit HGF/Met signaling (i.e., switch OFF). **(B)** Once organ tissues undergo injuries, Ser-985 site is "de"phosphorylated, probably via recruitment of intracellular protein phosphatases. As a result, c-Met tyrosine sites are phosphorylated, then pleiotropic activities are delivered (i.e., switch ON).

disease process rather than on the potential limitation from side effects *(10,17)*. The systemic administration of HGF in dosages resulting in physiological plasma levels (3–5 ng/ml) is not associated with significant side effects in any animal model or in humans *(61,122)*. This lack of side effects may be explained by the specific and limited HGF activation of c-Met to diseased tissues *(123)*. In this context, we have recently obtained evidence that a serine residue at position 985 (Ser-985) in the juxtamembrane of c-Met acts as a "negative regulator" to limit HGF/c-Met signaling *(124)*. Ser-985-phosphorylation prevents the HGF-induced mitogenesis and migration of lung carcinoma cells, whereas Ser-985 de-phosphorylation by protein phosphatases restores HGF activity. These findings were confirmed in a mouse model of acute hepatic injury (our unpublished data). Together, we predict that the reciprocal balance between Ser-985 and tyrosine phosphorylation may be a key event to regulate HGF/Met signaling. In healthy tissues, Ser-985 is always phosphorylated for preventing c-Met tyrosine phosphorylation even in the presence of ligand HGF. However, during tissue damage Ser-985 is de-phosphorylated owing to increased phosphatase activity. Concomitant with this change, c-Met tyrosine is phosphorylated in the presence of HGF to trigger biological activity, including mitogenesis, migration and antifibrosis effects (Fig. 9). This regulatory system explains the lack of untoward effects of HGF after its systemic or local administration *(12,77,120,125)*.

Table 2
Potential Uses of HGF (or Its Gene) in Chronic Renal Diseases and Respected Outcomes

Target disease	*Outcomes*	*Model*	*References*	*Respected approach*
Diabetic nephropathy	Reduced glomerulopathy, ECM degration, increased Na^+K^+ATPase, reduced albuminuria, reduced podocyte injury, restration of dysfunction	STZ	*12,120,125*	rh-HGF: im, sc, iv, DDS (with ACE inhibition) *HGF* cDNA: iv, im, local
Nephrotic syndrome	Tubular repair and protection, resolution of fibrosis, myofibroblasts deletion, restration of dysfunction, prevention of albuminuria	Spontaneous (ICGN mice)	*11,18*	rh-HGF: im, sc, local DDS *HGF* cDNA: im, local
Obstructive nephropathy	Tubular repair and protection, inhibited transdifferentiation of tubular cells, resolution of fibrosis	Surgical ligation (UUO)	*71,72*	rh-HGF: im, sc rh-HGF: im, sc, iv, DDS
Renal hypertension	Compensatory growth, tubular proliferation, reduced ECM deposit, restration of dysfunction	5/6-nephrectomy	*75,76,93*	*HGF* cDNA: local, rh-HGF: im, sc, iv, DDS
Mesangial proliferative glomerulonephritis (MPGN)	Inhibition of mesangial over-growth, suppressed tuft scar, endothelial repair	Anti-Thy-1 antibody	*86* *53*	rh-HGF: im, sc, local DDS
Chronic allograft nephropathy (CAN)	Induction of immunne tolerance, prevention of ischemia	Renal allograft (rats, pig)	*77,78*	rh-HGF: im, sc *HGF* cDNA: local
Cycrosporine nephropathy	Tubular protection, anti-apoptosis, tubular repair, anti-fibrosis, reduced ECM deposit	Repeated expose to cyclosporine	*69,78*	*HGF* cDNA: local, im rh-HGF: im, sc, DDS
Herb tea nephropathy	Tubular protection, tubular repair, anti-fibrosis	Aristolochic acid	*128*	rh-HGF: sc, im *HGF* cDNA: local

DDS, drug delivery system; ACE, angiorension-converting enzyme; iv, intravenous injection; im, intramuscular injection; sc, subcutaneous injection, for all other abbreviations, *see* text.

PERSPECTIVE

The pathology of DN involves a complex interplay between glomerular hemodynamics, albuminuria, tubular inflammatory, and fibrogenic processes. Using such a complex renal disease as model, we demonstrated that HGF mediates epithelial–stromal and endothelial–mesangial interactions for the recovery and maintenance of renal function even under consistent diabetic conditions, strengthening the renotrophic roles of HGF. The dominant expression of TGF-β over HGF is associated with progression of diabetic nephropathy, whereas HGF replacement by exogenous administration has preventive and therapeutic effects by enhancing the reorganization of renal tissue following regression of fibrosis. More importantly, fibroblasts are a major source of HGF, whereas myofibroblasts (i.e., smooth muscle cell-like fibroblasts) lose the ability to produce HGF *(88,103)*. Thus, chronic organ failure may be defined as a HGF-deficient disease, wherein the parenchymal area is replaced with numerous myofibroblasts.

To overcome the loss or insufficient levels of endogenous HGF, recombinant HGF protein as well as *HGF* gene delivery are now available, and the therapeutic modality to be used may depend on the clinical situation. For example, ischemia reperfusion injury occurs within a few hours and thus intravenous injection of rh-HGF seems suitable according to the acuity of the condition *(40,61)*. However, *HGF* gene delivery may be useful to sustain effective HGF levels for a long-term, without repeated injections. In particular, a single intra-renal injection of a naked HGF cDNA-containing plasmid may be a promising method to inhibit renal fibrogenesis in specific circumstances, i.e., after renal transplantation *(77)*. Furthermore, restoration of endogenous HGF with an anti-TGF-β antibody or after Ang-II blockade would be synergistic with the HGF supplementation therapy. Potential uses of HGF in CRDs are summarized in Table 2 that includes anticipated outcomes.

In addition to DN, HGF has potential to improve the primary cause of diabetes (i.e., pancreatic β-cell protection and repair) *(46,126)* and prevent diabetic complications *(16,122,127)*. Thus, clinical trials of rh-HGF or *HGF* gene therapy for treating patients with diabetes can be designed if a careful evaluation of side effects is established. The first clinical trials of *HGF* gene therapy for patients with arteriosclerosis obliterans is now ongoing in Japan *(122)*, and data on safety and effectiveness of HGF in humans are now accumulating. Based on the clinical and experimental data *(77,78,122)*, a study to suppress tissue fibrosis by HGF administration in renal allografts is now in the planning stage. Future basic and clinical studies will provide a better understanding of the renal effects of HGF and provide a paradigm concerning tissue regeneration in biological defense systems.

CONCLUSIONS

Diabetes is now the leading cause of ESRD in many developed countries, and DN has emerged as a silent epidemic worldwide. The pathology of DN involves a complex interplay between glomerular hemodynamics, albuminuria, tubular inflammatory, and fibrogenic processes. Using such a multipathological renal disease in mice, we demonstrated that HGF mediates epithelial–stromal and endothelial–mesangial interactions for recovery and maintenance of renal function under consistent diabetic injuries. In the diabetic mice, endogenous HGF had an essential role in minimizing clinical and histological manifestations of DN, whereas loss in HGF production results in rapid progression of renal fibrosis and renal dysfunction, associated with the increased levels of TGF-β.

More importantly, supplement therapy with HGF led to the decrease in renal TGF-β levels, followed by the arrest of glomerular and peritubular fibrotic lesions during diabetes. Overall, HGF supplement therapy inhibited the onset of renal dysfunction in the diabetic mice. The reciprocal balance between TGF-β and HGF levels is noted not only in DN but also in other chronic renal diseases. Taken together, restoration of endogenous HGF production levels as well as the supplementation of exogenous HGF could be a common target to arrest or reverse renal fibrosis and dysfunction, caused by chronic renal disease.

ACKNOWLEDGMENTS

The work in the authors' laboratory was supported by research grants from the Ministry of Education, Science, Sports, and Culture of Japan, the Ministry of Health and Welfare of Japan, and by a research grant from the Osaka Kidney Foundation. We are also grateful to M. Ohara (Fukuoka) for helpful comments.

REFERENCES

1. Ong A, Fine LG. Loss of glomerular function and tubulointerstitial fibrosis: cause or effect? Kidney Int 1994;45:345–351.
2. Akmal M. Hemodialysis in diabetic patients. Am J Kidney Dis 2001;38:S195–S199.
3. Parving HH. Initiation and progression of diabetic nephropathy. N Engl J Med 1996;335:1682–1683.
4. Nakamura T, Nawa K, Ichihara A. Partial purification and characterization of hepatocyte growth factor from serum of hepatectomized rats. Biochem Biophys Res Commun 1984;122:1450–1459.
5. Nakamura T, Nishizawa T, Hagiya M, et al. Molecular cloning and expression of human hepatocyte growth factor. Nature 1989;342:440–443.
6. Kawaida K, Matsumoto K, Shimazu H, Nakamura T. Hepatocyte growth factor prevents acute renal failure and accelerates renal regeneration in mice. Proc Natl Acad Sci 1994;91:4357–4361.
7. Igawa T, Matsumoto K, Kanda S, Saito Y, Nakamura T. Hepatocyte growth factor may function as a renotropic factor for regeneration in rats with acute renal injury. Am J Physiol 1993;265:F61–F69.
8. Miller SB, Martin DR, Kissane J, Hammerman MR. Hepatocyte growth factor accelerates recovery from acute ischemic renal injury in rats. Am J Physiol 1994;266:F129–F134.
9. Matsumoto K, Mizuno S, Nakamura T. Hepatocyte growth factor in renal regeneration, renal disease, and potential therapeutics. Curr Opin Nephrol Hypertens 2000;9:395–402.
10. Matsumoto K, Nakamura T. Hepatocyte growth factor: renotropic role and potential therapeutics for renal diseases. Kidney Int 2001;59:2023–2038.
11. Mizuno S, Kurosawa T, Matumoto K, Mizuno-Horikawa Y, Okamoto M, Nakamura T. Hepatocyte growth factor prevents renal fibrosis and dysfunction in a mouse model of chronic renal disease. J Clin Invest 1998;101:1827–1834.
12. Mizuno S, Nakamura T. Suppressions of chronic glomerular injuries and TGF-β_1 production by HGF in attenuation of murine diabetic nephropathy. Am J Physiol 2004;286:F134–F143.
13. Ishiki Y, Ohnishi H, Muto Y, Matsumoto K, Nakamura T. Direct evidence that hepatocyte growth factor is a hepatotrophic factor for liver regeneration and has a potent antihepatitis effect in vivo. Hepatology 1992;16:1227–1235.
14. Ohmichi H, Matsumoto K, Nakamura T. In vivo mitogenic action of HGF on lung epithelial cells: pulmotrophic role in lung regeneration. Am J Physiol 1996;270:L1031–L1039.
15. Takahashi M, Ota S, Terano A, et al. Hepatocyte growth factor is the most potent endogenous stimulant of rabbit gastric epithelial cell proliferation and migration in primary culture. J Clin Invest 1995;95:1994–2003.
16. Yoshida S, Matsumoto K, Tomioka D, et al. Recombinant hepatocyte growth factor accelerates cutaneous wound healing in diabetic mouse model. Growth Factors 2004;22:111–119.
17. Funakoshi H, Nakamura T. Hepatocyte growth factor: from diagnosis to clinical applications. Clin Chim Acta 2003;327:1–23.
18. Mizuno S, Matsumoto K, Kurosawa T, Mizuno-Horikawa Y, Nakamura T. Reciprocal balance of hepatocyte growth factor and transforming growth factor-β_1 in renal fibrosis in mice. Kidney Int 2001;57:937–948.

19. Sakamaki Y, Matsumoto K, Mizuno S, Miyoshi S, Matsuda H, Nakamura T. Hepatocyte growth factor stimulates proliferation of respiratory epithelial cells during postpneumonectomy compenbatory lung growth in mice. Am J Respir Cell Mol Biol 2002;26:525–533.
20. Yoshida S, Yamaguchi Y, Itami S, et al. Neutralization of hepatocyte growth factor leads to retarded cutaneous wound healing associated with decreased neovascularization and granulation tissue formation. J Invest Dermatol 2003;120:335–343.
21. Huh CG, Factor VM, Sanchez A, Uchida K, Conner EA, Thorgeisson SS. Hepatocyte growth factor/c-Met signaling pathway is required for efficient liver regeneration and repair. Proc Natl Acad Sci 2004;101:4477–4482.
22. Nakamura T, Nawa K, Ichihara A, Kaise N, Nishino T. Purification and subunit structure of hepatocyte growth factor from rat platelets. FEBS Lett 1987;224:311–316.
23. Miyazawa K, Tsubouchi H, Naka D, et al. Molecular cloning and sequence analysis of cDNA for human hepatocyte growth factor. Biochem Biophys Res Commun 1989;163:967–973.
24. Bottaro DP, Rubin JS, Faletto DL, et al. Identification of hepatocyte growth factor receptor as the c-met proto-oncogene product. Science 1991;251:802–804.
25. Ponzetto C, Bardelli A, Zhen Z, et al. A multifunctional docking site mediates signaling and transformation by the hepatocyte growth factor/scatter factor receptor family. Cell 1994;77:261–271.
26. Schaeper U, Gehring NH, Fuchs KP, et al. Coupling of gab1 to c-met, grb2, and shp2 mediates biological responses. J Cell Biol 2000;149:1419–1432.
27. Birchmeier C, Birchmeier W, Gherardi E, Vande-Woude GF. Met, metastasis, motility, and more. Nature Rev Mol Cell Biol 2003;4:915–925.
28. Liu Y, Tolbert EM, Lin L, et al. Up-regulation of hepatocyte growth factor receptor: an amplification and targeting mechanism for hepatocyte growth factor action in acute renal failure. Kidney Int 1999;55:442–453.
29. Takehara T, Matsumoto K, Nakamura T. Cell density-dependent regulation of albumin synthesis and DNA synthesis in rat hepatocytes by hepatocyte growth factor. J Biochem 1992;112:330–334.
30. Otonkoski T, Beattie GM, Rubin JS, Lopez AD, Baird A, Hayek A. Hepatocyte growth factor/scatter factor has insulinotropic activity in human fetal pancreatic cells. Diabetes 1994;43:947–953.
31. Bussolino F, Direnzo MF, Ziche M, et al. Hepatocyte growth factor is a potent angiogenic factor which stimulates endothelial cell motility and growth. J Cell Biol 1992;119:629–641.
32. Nakamura Y, Morishita R, Higaki J, et al. Expression of local hepatocyte growth factor system in vascular tissue. Biochem Biophys Res Commun 1995;215:483–488.
33. Aoki S, Takahashi K, Matsumoto K, Nakamura T. Activation of Met tyrosine kinase by hepatocyte growth factor is essential for internal organogenesis in Xenopus embryo. Biochem Biophys Res Commun 1997;234:8–14.
34. Ohmichi H, Koshimizu U, Matsumoto K, Nakamura T. Hepatocyte growth factor (HGF) acts as a mesenchyme-derived morphogenic factor during fetal lung development. Development 1998;125: 1315–1324.
35. Schmidt C, Bladt F, Goedecke S, et al. Scatter factor/hepatocyte growth factor is essential for liver development. Nature 1995;373:699–702.
36. Uehara Y, Minowa O, Mori C, et al. Placental defect and embryonic lethality in mice lacking hepatocyte growth factor/scatter factor. Nature 1995;373:702–705.
37. Bladt F, Riethmacher D, Isenmann S, Aguzzi A, Birchmeier C. Essential role for the c-met receptor in the migration of myogenic precurcor cells into the limb bud. Nature 1995;376:768–771.
38. Takehara T, Nakamura T. Protective effect of hepatocyte growth factor on in vitro hepatitis in primary cultured hepatocytes. Biomed Res 1991;12:335–338.
39. Kosai K, Matsumoto K, Nagata S, Tsujimoto Y, Nakamura T. Abrogation of Fas-induced fulminant hepatic failure in mice by hepatocyte growth factor. Biochem Biophys Res Commun 1998;244:683–690.
40. Nakamura T, Mizuno S, Matsumoto K, Sawa Y, Matsuda H, Nakamura T. Myocardial protection from infarction by endogenous and exogenous hepatocyte growth factor. J Clin Invest 2000;106:1511–1519.
41. Miyazawa T, Matsumoto K, Ohmichi H, Yamashima T, Chigasaki H, Nakamura T. Protection of hippocampal neurons from ischemia-induced delayed neuronal death by hepatocyte growth factor: a novel neurotrophic factor. J Celebral Blood Flow Metabolism 1998;18:345–348.
42. Yamamoto K, Morishita R, Hayashi S, et al. Contribution of Bcl-2, but not Bcl-xL and Bax, to antiapoptotic actions of hepatocyte growth factor in hypoxia-conditioned human endothelial cells. Hypertension 2001;37:1341–1348.
43. Bardelli A, Longati P, Comoglio PM, et al. HGF receptor associates with the anti-apoptotic protein BAG-1 and prevents cell death. EMBO J. 1996;22:6205–6212.

44. Wang X, DeFrances MC, Dai Y, et al. A mechanism of cell survival: sequestration of Fas by the HGF receptor Met. Mol Cell 2002;9:411–421.
45. Oshima K, Shimamura M, Mizuno S, et al. HGF gene transfer in cerebrospinal fluid can prevent hearing impairment in rats. FASEB J 2004;18:212–214.
46. Nakano M, Yasunami Y, Maki T, et al. Hepatocyte growth factor is essential for amelioration of hyperglycemia in streptozotocin-induced diabetic mice receiving a marginal mass of intrahepatic islet grafts. Transplantation 2000;69:214–222.
47. Warzecha Z, Dembinski A, Ceranowicz P, et al. Inhibition of cyclooxygenase-2 reduces the protective effect of hepatocyte growth factor in experimenal pancreatitis. Eur J Pharmacol 2004;486:107–119.
48. Igawa T, Kanda S, Kanetake H, et al. Hepatocyte growth factor is a potent mitogen for cultured rabbit renal tubular epithelial cells. Biochem Biophys Res Commun 1991;174:831–838.
49. Montesano R, Matsumoto K, Nakamura T, Orci L. Identification of a fibroblast-derived epithelial morphogen as hepatocyte growth factor. Cell 1991;67:901–908.
50. Ishibashi K, Sasaki S, Sakamoto H, et al. Hepatocyte growth factor is a paracrine factor for renal epithelial cells: Stimulation of DNA synthesis and Na,K-ATPase activity. Biochem Biophys Res Commun 1992;182:960–965.
51. Yo Y, Morishita R, Nakamura S, et al. Potential role of hepatocyte growth factor in the maintenance of renal structure: anti-apototic action of HGF on epithelial cells. Kidney Int 1998;54:1128–1138.
52. Fornoni A, Li H, Foschi A, Striker GE, Striker LJ. Hepatocyte growth factor, but not insulin-like growth factor I, protects podocytes against cyclosporin A-induced apoptosis. Am J Pathol 2001;158:275–280.
53. Mori T, Shimizu A, Masuda Y, Fukuda Y, Yamanaka N. Hepatocyte growth factor-stimulating endothelial cell growth and accelerating glomerular capillary repair in experimental progressive glomerulonephritis. Nephron Exp Nephrol 2003;94:44–54.
54. Biswas P, Roy A, Gong R, et al. Hepatocyte growth factor induces an endothelin-mediated decline in glomerular filtration rate. Am J Physiol 2005;288:F8–F15.
55. Lowenstein LM, Stern A. Serum factor in renal compensatory hyperplasia. Science 1963;142:1479.
56. Nagaike M, Hirao S, Tajima H, et al. Renotropic functions of hepatocyte growth factor in renal regeneration after unilateral nephrectomy. J Biol Chem 1991;266:22,781–22,784.
57. Barros EJG, Santos OFP, Matsumoto K, Nakamura T, Nigam SK. Differential tubulogenic and branching morphogenetic activities of growth factors: Implications for epithelial tissue development. Proc Natl Acad Sci 1995;92:4412–4416.
58. Amaike H, Matsumoto K, Oka T, Nakamura T. Human recombinant HGF prevents lethal side effects of cyclosporin A in mice. Cytokine 1996;8:387–394.
59. Takada S, Takahara S, Nishimura K, et al. Effect of hepatocyte growth factor on tacrolimus-induced nephrotoxicity in spontaneously hypertensive rats. Transpl Int 1999;12:27–32.
60. Nagano T, Mori-Kudo I, Kawamura T, Taiji M, Noguchi H. Pre- or post-treatment with hepatocyte growth factor prevents glycerol-induced acute renal failure. Renal Fail 2004;26:5–11.
61. Mizuno S, Nakamura T. Prevention of neutrophil extravasation by HGF leads to attenuations of tubular apoptosis and renal dysfunction in mouse ischemic kidneys. Am J Pathol 2005;166:1895–1905.
62. Matsumoto K, Nakamura T. Hepatocyte growth factor as a renotropic factor and therapeutic potential for acute renal failure. In: M. S. Goligorosky, ed. Acute Renal Failure: Emerging New Concepts and Therapeutic Strategies. Churchill Livingstone, 1995, pp. 450–474.
63. Risdon RA, Sloper JC, Wardener WH. Relationship between renal function and histological changes found in renal-biopsy specimens from patients with persistent glomerular nephritis. Lancet 1968;2:363–366.
64. Kopp JB. Hepatocyte growth factor: Mesenchymal signal for epithelial homeostasis. Kidney Int 1998;54:1392–1393.
65. Balkovetz DF, Lipschutz JH. Hepatocyte growth factor and the kidney: it is not just for the liver. Int Rev Cytol 1999;186:225–260.
66. Matsuda Y, Matsumoto K, Tsuchida T, Nakamura T. Hepatocyte growth factor prevents liver cirrhosis caused by dimethylnitrosamine in rats. J Biochem 1995;118:643–649.
67. Yaekashiwa M, Nakamura S, Ohnuma K, et al. Simultaneous or delayed administration of hepatocyte growth factor equally represses the fibrotic changes in murine lung injury induced by bleomycin: a morphologic study. Am J Respir Crit Care Med 1997;156:1937–1944.
68. Border WA, Noble NA. Transforming growth factor-β in tissue fibrosis. N Engl J Med 1994;331:1286–1292.

69. Mizuno S, Yue BF, Okamoto M, Horikawa Y, Kurosawa T. Diffuse glomerulosclerosis without tubular injury does not manifest renal dysfunction in nephrotic mice (ICGN strain). Exp Nephrol 1997;5:498–507.
70. Klahr S. Obstructive nephropathy. Kidney Int 1998;54:286–300.
71. Mizuno S, Matsumoto K, Nakamura T. Hepatocyte growth factor suppresses interstitial fibrosis in a mouse model of obstructive nephropathy. Kidney Intl 2001;59:1304–1314.
72. Yang J, Liu Y. Blockage of tubular epithelial to myofibroblast transition by hepatocyte growth factor prevents renal interstitial fibrosis. J Am Soc Nephrol 2002;13:96–107.
73. Liu Y. Hepatocyte growth factor in kidney fibrosis: therapeutic potential and mechanisms of action. Am J Physiol 2004;287:F7–F16.
74. Florquin S, Rouschop KM. Reciprocal functions of hepatocyte growth factor and transforming growth factor-β_1 in the progression of renal diseases: a role for CD44? Kidney Int 2003;86:S15–S20.
75. Liu Y, Raju K, Tolbert E, Dworkin LD. Endogenous hepatocyte growth factor ameliorates chronic renal injury by activating matrix degradation pathways. Kidney Int 2000;58:2028–2043.
76. Inoue T, Okada H, Kobayashi T, et al. Hepatocyte growth factor counteracts transforming growth factor-β_1, through attenuation of connective tissue growth factor induction, and prevents renal fibrogenesis in 5/6 nephrectomized mice. FASEB J 2003;17:268–270.
77. Isaka Y, Yamada K, Takabatake Y, et al. Electroparation-mediated HGF gene transfection protected the kidney against graft injury. Gene Ther 2005;12:815–820.
78. Azuma H, Takahara S, Matsumoto K, et al. Hepatocyte growth factor prevents the development of chronic allograft nephropathy in rats. J Am Soc Nephrol 2001;12:1280–1292.
79. Ziyadeh FN, Hoffman BB, Han CC, et al. Long-term prevention of renal insufficiency, excess matrix gene expression, and glomerular mesangial matrix expansion by treatment with monoclonal anti-transforming growth factor-β antibody in db/db diabetic mice. Proc Natl Acad Sci 2000;97: 8015–8020.
80. Goldfar S, Ziyadeh FN. TGF-β: a crucial component of the pathogenesis of diabetic nephropathy. Trans Am Clin Climatol Assoc 2001;112:27–32.
81. Isaka Y, Fujiwara Y, Ueda N, Kaneda Y, Kamada T, Imai E. Glomerulosclerosis induced by in vivo transfection of transforming growth factor-β or platelet-derived growth factor gene into the rat kidney. J Clin Invest 1993;92:2597–2601.
82. Morishita R, Nakamura S, Nakamura Y, et al. Potential role of an endothelium specific growth factor, hepatocyte growth factor, on endothelial damage in diabetes. Diabetes 1997;46:138–142.
83. Liu Y, Tolbert EM, Sun AM, Dworkin LD. In vivo and in vitro evidence for increased expression of HGF receptor in kidney of diabetic rats. Am J Physiol 1996;271:F1202–F1210.
84. Nakamura S, Morishita R, Moriguchi A, et al. Hepatocyte growth factor as a potential index of complication in diabetes mellitus. J Hypertensions 1998;16:2019–2026.
85. Kulseng B, Borset M, Espevik T, Sundan A. Elevated hepatocyte growth factor in sera from patients with insulin-dependent diabetes mellitus. Acta Diabetol 1998;35:77–80.
86. Bessho K, Mizuno S, Matsumoto K, Nakamura T. Counteractive effects of HGF on PDGF-induced mesangial cell proliferation in a rat model of glomerulonephritis. Am J Physiol 2003,284.F1171–F1180.
87. Nakamura Y, Morishita R, Higaki J, et al. A vascular modulator, hepatocyte growth factor (HGF), is associated with systolic blood pressure. Hypertension 1996;28:409–413.
88. Matsumoto K, Tajima H, Okazaki H, Nakamura T. Negative regulation of hepatocyte growth factor gene expression in human lung fibroblasts and leukemic cells by transforming growth factor-β_1 and glucocorticoids. J Biol Chem 1992;267:24,917–24,920.
89. Yo Y, Morishita R, Yamamoto K, et al. Actions of hepatocyte growth factor as a local modulator in the kidney: potential role in pathogenesis of renal disease. Kidney Int 1998;53:50–58.
90. Gilbert RE, Cooper ME. The tubulointerstitium in progressive diabetic kidney disease: More than an aftermath of glomerular injury? Kidney Int 1999;56:1627–1637.
91. Eddy AA. Molecular insights into renal interstitial fibrosis. J Am Soc Nephrol 1996;7:2495–2508.
92. Shimizu H, Maruyama S, Yuzawa Y, et al. Anti-monocyte chemoattractant protein-1 gene therapy attenuates renal injuries induced by protein-overload proteinuria. J Am Soc Nephrol 2003;14: 1496–1505.
93. Gong R, Rifai A, Tolbert EM, Biswas P, Centracchio JN, Dworkin LD. Hepatocyte growth factor ameliorates renal interstitial inflammation in rat remnant kidney by modulating tubular expression of macrophage chemoattractant protein-1 and RANTES. J Am Soc Nephrol 2004;15:2868–2881.
94. Matsumoto K, Morishita R, Tomita N, et al. Improvement of endothelial dysfunction by angiotensin II blockade accompanied by induction of vascular hepatocyte growth factor system in diabetic spontaneously hypertensive rats. Heart Vessels 2003;18:18–25.

95. Yang R, Bunting S, Ko A, Schwall R, Jin H. Hemodynamic effects of scatter factor in conscious rats. J Cardiovasc Pharm 1997;30:294–301.
96. Kriz W, Lemley KV. The role of the podocyte in glomerulosclerosis. Curr Opin Nephrol Hypertens 1999;8:489–497.
97. Wald H, Scherzer P, Rasch R, Popovtzer MM. Renal tubular Na^+-K^+-ATPase in diabetes mellitus: relationship to metabolic abnormality. Am J Physiol 1993;265:E96–E101.
98. Nakamura T, Tomita Y, Hirai R, Yamaoka K, Kaji K, Ichihara A. Inhibitory effect of transforming growth factor-β on DNA synthesis of adult rat hepatocytes in primary culture. Biochem Biophys Res Commun 1985;133:1042–1050.
99. Taipale J, Keski OJ. Hepatocyte growth factor releases epithelial andendothelial cells from growth arrest induced by transforming growth factor-β_1. J Biol Chem 1996;271:4342–4348.
100. Santos OFP, Nigam SK. HGF-induced tubulogenesis and branching of epithelial cells is modulated by extracellular matrix and TGF-β. Dev Biol 1993;160:293–302.
101. Dai C, Liu Y. Hepatocyte growth factor antagonizes the profibrotic action of TGF-β_1 in mesangial cells by stabilizing Smad transcriptional corepressor TGIF. J Am Soc Nephrol 2004;15:1402–1412.
102. Pepper MS, Matsumoto K, Nakamura T, Orci L, Montesano R. Hepatocyte growth factor induces urokinase-type plasminogen activator and plasminogen activator inhibitor-1 in MDCK epithelial cells. J Biol Chem 1992;267:20,493–20,496.
103. Mizuno S, Matsumoto K, Li MY, Nakamura T. HGF reduces advancing lung fibrosis in mice: a potential role for MMP-dependent myofibroblast apoptosis. FASEB J 2005;19:580–582.
104. Dworkin LD, Gong R, Tolbert E, et al. Hepatocyte growth factor ameliorates progression of interstitial fibrosis in rats with established renal injury. Kidney Int 2004;65:409–419.
105. Ueki T, Kaneda Y, Tsutsui H, et al. Hepatocyte growth factor gene therapy of liver cirrhosis in rats. Nat Med 1999;5:226–230.
106. Matsumoto K, Morishita R, Moriguchi A, et al. Prevention of renal damage by Angiotensin II blockade, accompanied by increased renal hepatocyte growth factor in experimental hypertensive rats. Hypertension. 1999;34,279–34,284.
107. Yang J, Dai C, Liu Y. Hepatocyte growth factor gene therapy and angiotensin-II blockade synergiastically attenuate renal interstitial fibrosis in mice. J Am Soc Nephrol 2002;13:2464–2477.
108. Nakamura T, Matsumoto K, Mizuno S, Sawa Y, Matsuda H, Nakamura T. Hepatocyte growth factor prevents tissue fibrosis, remodeling and dysfunction in cardiomyopathic hamster hearts. Am J Physiol 2005;288:H2131–H2139.
109. Wu MH, Yokozeki H, Takagawa S, et al. Hepatocyte growth factor both prevents and ameliorates the symptoms of dermal sclerosis in a mouse model of scleroderma. Gene Ther 2004;11:170–180.
110. Nahas AMEL, Muchaneta-Kubara H, Essawy M, Soylemezoglu O. Renal fibrosis: Insights into pathogenesis and treatment. Int J Biochem Cell Biol 1997;29:55–56.
111. Gressner AM. Cytokines and cellular crosstalk involved in the activation of fat-storing cells. J Hepatol 1995;22:28–36.
112. Phan SH. The myofibroblast in pulmonary fibrosis. Chest 2002;122(6):286S–289S.
113. Baker AJ, Mooney A, Hughes J, Lombardi D, Johnson RJ, Savill J. Mesangial cell apoptosis: the major mechanism for resolution of glomerular cellularity in experimental mesangial proliferative nephritis. J Clin Invest 1994;94:2105–2116.
114. Iredale JP, Benyon RC, Pickering J, et al. Mechanisms of spontaneous resolution of rat liver fibrosis: Hepatic stellate cell apoptosis and reduced hepatic expression of metalloproteinase inhibitors. J Clin Invest 1998;102:538–549.
115. Kim HW, Matsumoto K, Bessho K, Nakamura T. Growth inhibition and apoptosis in liver myofibroblasts promoted by hepatocyte growth factor leads to resolution from liver cirrhosis. Am J Pathol 2005;166:1017–1028.
116. Almeida EA, Ilic D, Han Q, et al. Matrix survival signaling: from fibronectin via focal adhesion kinase to c-Jun NH(2)-terminal kinase. J Cell Biol 2000;149:741–754.
117. Johnson RJ, Raines EW, Floege J, et al. Inhibition of mesangial cell proliferation and matrix expansion in glomerulo- nephritis in the rat by antibody to platelet-derived growth factor. J Exp Med 1992;175:1413–1416.
118. Ono M, Sawa Y, Mizuno S, et al. Hepatocyte growth factor suppresses vascular medial hyperplasia and matrix accumulation in advanced pulmonary hypertension of rats. Circulation 2004;110:2896–2902.
119. Yang J, Dai C, Liu Y. Hepatocyte growth factor suppresses renal interstitial myofibroblast activation and intercepts smad signal transduction. Am J Pathol 2003;163:621–632.

120. Cruzado JM, Lloberas N, Torras J, et al. Regression of advanced diabetic nephropathy by hepatocyte growth factor gene therapy in rats. Diabetes 2004;53:1119–1127.
121. Kobayashi E, Sasamura H, Mifune M, et al. Hepatocyte growth factor regulates proteoglycan synthesis in interstitial fibroblasts. Kidney Int 2003;64:1179–1188.
122. Morishita R, Aoki M, Hashiya N, et al. Safety evaluation of clinical gene therapy using hepatocyte growth factor to treat peripheral arterial disease. Hypertension 2004;44:203–209.
123. Tajima H, Higuchi O, Mizuno K, Nakamura T. Tissue distribution of hepatocyte growth factor receptor and its exclusive down-regulation in a regenerating organ after injury. J Biochem 1992;111: 401–406.
124. Hashigasako A, Machide M, Nakamura T, Matsumoto K, Nakamura T. Bi-directional regulation of c-Met Ser 985 phosphorylation via PKC and protein phosphatase 2A involves c-Met activation and cellular responsiveness to HGF. J Biol Chem 2004;279:26,445–26,452.
125. Dai C, Yang J, Bastacky S, Xia J, Li Y, Liu Y. Intravenous administration of hepatocyte growth factor gene ameliorates diabetic nephropathy in mice. J Am Soc Nephrol 2004;15:2637–2647.
126. Dai C, Li Y, Yang J, Liu Y. Hepatocyte growth factor preserves beta cell mass and mitigates hyperglycemia in streptozotocin-induced diabetic mice. J Biol Chem 2003;278:27,080–27,087.
127. Kato N, Nemoto K, Nakanishi K, et al. Nonviral gene transfer of human hepatocyte growth factor improves streptozotocin-induced diabetic neuropathy in rats. Diabetes 2005;54:846–854.
128. Okada H, Watanabe Y, Inoue T, et al. Transgene-derived hepatocyte growth factor attenuates reactive renal fibrosis in aristolochic acid nephrotoxicity. Nephrol Dial Transplant 2003;18:2515–2523.

14 Proteomics in the Investigation of Diabetic Nephropathy

Visith Thongboonkerd, MD *(Hon),* FRCPT

Contents

INTRODUCTION

Diabetic nephropathy (DN) remains the major complication of diabetes and the leading cause of end-stage renal disease (ESRD) despite adequate treatment with current available drugs. Better understanding of its pathogenesis and pathophysiology as well as earlier diagnosis is crucial to achieve better therapeutic outcome and to prevent this diabetic complication. Microalbuminuria is the best available noninvasive predictor for the risk of DN *(1)*. However, some patients with microalbuminuria have advanced renal histopathological changes *(2–4)*. Additionally, the conventional assay to detect microalbuminuria measures only immunoreactive form of albumin, whereas the immuno-unreactive albumin is not detectable *(5)*. Therefore, the more sensitive biomarker(s) and/or other laboratory test(s) that can detect all of the albumin isoforms are crucially required.

The pathogenic mechanisms of diabetic renal injury are most likely the effects of multiple pathways. Metabolic mechanisms interplay with hemodynamic processes via common intermediate pathways. The final results are glomerular injury, tubulo-interstitial damage, proteinuria, and ultimately renal failure. Molecular genetics and genomics have been applied in an attempt to identify genes that may involve in the development

From: *Contemporary Diabetes: The Diabetic Kidney*
Edited by: P. Cortes and C. E. Mogensen © Humana Press Inc., Totowa, NJ

of DN. There are several evidences that support the hypothesis of genetic susceptibility in both type 1 *(6,7)* and type 2 DN *(8–11)*. However, the information obtained from genetic or genomic study provides rather the static information than the dynamic image of the disease pathophysiology. Indeed, proteins, not genes, directly govern cellular function. One gene can be modified to be several different translation products (proteins) by the process called posttranslational modifications (PTMs), which are very important to determine differential functions of proteins derived from the same gene *(12)*. The correlation of altered expression of genes and transcripts and change in protein expression levels has been evaluated, but the results remain inconclusive. Some studies have shown that mRNA levels correlated well with the protein levels *(13,14)*, whereas the others have demonstrated a poor correlation or even the opposite direction of changes *(15,16)*. Therefore, the data obtained from protein analysis are complementary to those obtained from analyses of genes and transcripts, and a combination of different analytical approaches (i.e., genomics, transcriptomics, proteomics, and others) is likely to fulfill the dynamic image of the pathogenesis and pathophysiology of diabetic renal complication. This chapter focuses on proteomics in the investigation of DN and provides some perspectives of integrating all of the "omics" sciences to complete such investigation.

PROTEOMICS: AN EMERGING DISCIPLINE IN THE POSTGENOMIC BIOMEDICAL RESEARCH

Conventional analysis of proteins in biological samples has been conducted mainly with immunological methods (i.e., Western blotting, ELISA, and radioimmunoassay). These methods, however, have some limitations. For example, a relatively small number of proteins can be examined in a single experiment. It may take several months to years to study a large number of proteins using these methods. Additionally, specific antibodies for the proteins to be examined must be existing and available. Moreover, the proteins of interest are based on *a priori* assumption. To better understand the pathogenesis and pathophysiology of medical diseases, an effective method for global analysis of proteins is required. This ideal technique should have the capability of simultaneous exploring both known (previously determined) and unknown (previously undetermined) components of the "protein universe" in the cell, tissue, organ, or biofluid *(17)*. There had been no satisfactory tool available for simultaneous analysis of multiple proteins until 1975, when O'Farrell *(18)* and Klose *(19)* first introduced two-dimensional polyacrylamide gel electrophoresis (2D PAGE) to separate a large complement of proteins. This technique permits separation of proteins in a complex mixture into hundreds to thousands of components (or spots) in a single 2D gel. Even with the success in protein separation science, the global analysis of proteins during the late 1970s through the 1980s was handicapped because of limitations in the high-throughput protein identification and quantitative analysis of separated proteins at that time.

In the postgenomic era, especially when the Human Genome Project is complete and genome projects for other species are on-going, there is a flood of genomic information leading to the development of several biotechnologies, which utilize the invaluable genome data to explain the complexity of biology, physiology, and pathophysiology. Mass spectrometry (MS) has become an important tool to identify proteins on the genomic scale *(20)*. This technological development makes the high-throughput, global analysis of proteins more feasible. Because of the usefulness and success of MS in biomedical research, John B. Fenn, who developed electrospray ionization (ESI) and Koichi Tanaka,

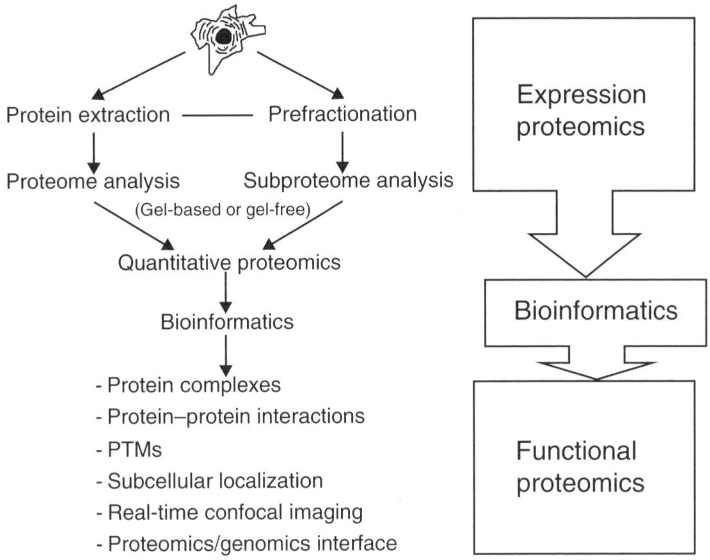

Fig. 1. Expression and functional proteomics. Proteins are extracted from cell, tissue, organ, or biofluid and subjected to either gel-based or gel-free proteomic analysis. Quantitative analysis is then performed to define differential protein expression between samples. Bioinformatics is utilized to obtain additional protein information for further functional study.

who developed matrix-assisted laser desorption/ionization (MALDI) shared the 2002 Nobel Prize in Chemistry for their great contributions in the development of MS *(21)*.

With the strengths of protein separation science and mass spectrometric protein identification, Marc Wilkins first coined the term "proteome" (set of proteins encoded by the genome) during the Siena electrophoresis conference in 1994 *(22)*. The field of science to study the proteome is called "proteomics," which has been defined as "the systematic analysis of proteins for their identity, quantity, and function" *(23)*. Protein identification in proteomics is based primarily on mass analysis of proteolytic peptide fragments and does not rely on *a priori* assumption and the availability of the specific antibody. Both expected (previously determined) and unexpected (previously undetermined) proteins can be examined simultaneously. Therefore, proteomic analysis is a suitable tool for the high-throughput, large-scale, postgenomic study of proteins.

Proteomics should be distinguished from protein chemistry, which is another field of protein science. Protein chemistry is to examine protein structure and physical and chemical properties of each protein in details, whereas proteomics is to examine the overall expression profile of proteins (or the entire proteome), protein–protein interactions, their complexes, and PTMs in a complex mixture of biological samples *(24)*. Both of them are aimed to better understand the cellular biology and physiology, and to determine functional significance of proteins in normal and disease states. Therefore, these two fields are different but complementary. Proteomics can be divided into two broad categories: expression and functional proteomics. Expression proteomics is directed to define normal proteome profile and differential protein expression among different sets of biological samples, and to determine alterations in protein expression caused by experimental interventions, physiological stimuli, or pathogenic conditions. Functional proteomics is aimed to define functional significance of the protein of interest; for example, its complexes, protein–protein interactions, and PTMs *(25)*. Figure 1

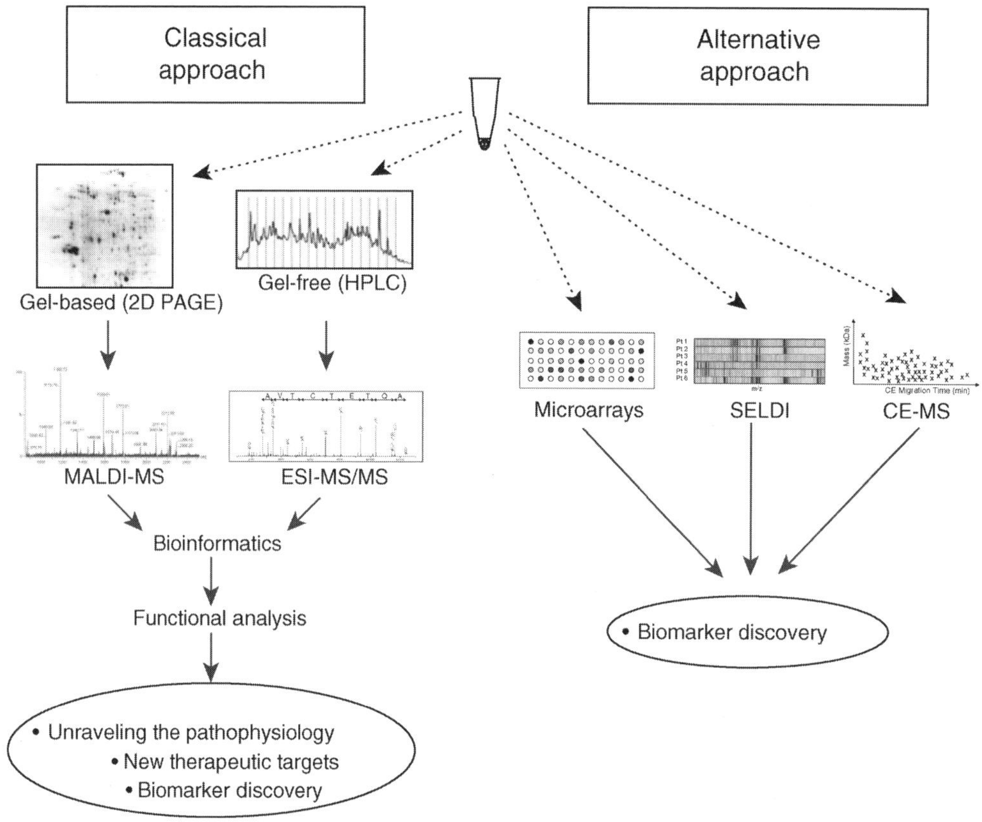

Fig. 2. Classical vs alternative proteomics approach. The classical approach is to extensively and systematically examine protein expression and function to better understand the pathophysiology of medical diseases. Although biomarker discovery can be attained via this approach, most clinical proteomics studies aiming to diagnostics employ the alternative one, which bypasses complicated analytical procedures in the classical proteomics. The alternative approach is to examine "profiles" or "patterns" of protein expression in various samples to differentiate types or groups of different samples (i.e., normal vs diseases) without any detailed characterization of proteins (identity, PTMs, interactions, etc.). The latter is suitable for multifactorial diseases for which multiple proteins may serve as the biomarkers and examining them all together may offer more precise information than looking only for a single marker. (Copyright © 2005 Future Drugs Ltd., London, UK; modified with permission from ref. *26*.)

demonstrates the relationship between expression and functional proteomics. Commonly, expression proteomics is applied at the initial step to identify the set of candidate proteins for further functional study. Bioinformatics serves as a link between expression and functional proteomics.

ANALYTICAL APPROACHES FOR PROTEOMIC ANALYSIS

Classical vs Alternative Approach

Based on the study purposes, analytical approaches for proteomic analysis can be classified into two main types (Fig. 2). The "classical approach" extensively and systematically examines protein expression and function to better understand the pathophysiology of medical diseases *(26)*. The analytical procedures in this approach involve expression proteomics, bioinformatics, quantitative analysis, and functional proteomics as described in details in Fig. 1. The "alternative approach" examines the proteome profiles or patterns of protein expression in biological samples to differentiate types or groups of samples (i.e., normal vs diseases; a specific disease vs others), rather than focusing on a specific protein *(26)*. Common analytical methods used in the latter approach are microarrays *(27)*, surface-enhanced laser desorption/ionization *(28)*, and capillary electrophoresis (CE) coupled to MS *(29)*. The advantage of this approach is that detailed characterizations (identity, PTMs, interactions, etc.) of a specific protein are unnecessary. This approach is, therefore, suitable for clinical diagnostics and biomarker discovery, especially in cases of multifactorial diseases for which one marker may not be sufficient for effective detection or diagnosis. In addition, information about dynamic changes of the proteome profile during or after treatment may be useful to predict therapeutic outcome and/or prognosis of the disease. The alternative approach also offers an opportunity of its use as a complementary diagnostic tool for some medical diseases in which clinical diagnosis relies only on invasive procedures that may be limited in some occasions. For example, renal biopsy, which remains the gold standard for the diagnosis of glomerular diseases, may not be possible in patients whose indications for this invasive procedure are not fulfilled and those with bleeding tendency or flank skin infection, thereby delayed diagnosis. In these cases, urinary and serum/plasma proteomics via the alternative approach may potentially be useful in the clinical diagnostics.

Global Analysis vs Highly Focused Study

Analysis of the entire proteome of any cell, tissue, organ, or biofluid can be done at either macro (global analysis) or micro (highly focused study) level (Fig. 3). Proteomic analysis of the kidney is a model used herein for the discussion. Analysis of the entire renal proteome is suitable for screening for "global changes" of renal proteins affected by an experimental condition or disease state. The global analysis, however, does not provide precise information of each identified protein, especially its locale(s), although bioinformatics can be applied to predict the localization. Additionally, low abundant proteins may be obscured by major abundant components making the analysis more difficult. In these cases, the highly focused study is required. "Subproteome analysis" is a concept of examining the selected compartment of cell or organ, based on microstructures (plasma membranes, cytosol, or individual intrarenal microstructures such as glomeruli, mesangial cells, podocytes, afferent/efferent arterioles, tubules, etc.) *(30,31)*. Another type of the highly focused proteomic analysis is "targeted proteomics" study. This type of the highly focused proteomic analysis refers to "the highly focused study, targeting on an interesting set of proteins" *(26)*. In some instances, this term may be confused with the subproteome analysis and used interchangeably. Although the strategy of subproteome analysis is to selectively examine a particular microstructure of cell or organ *(30,31)*, selection strategy of targeted proteomics has a wider spectrum: for example, selection of protein abundance (i.e., removal of albumin and other high-abundant plasma proteins prior to proteomic analysis) *(32)*; hydropathicity (hydrophilic vs hydrophobic proteins) *(33–35)*; peptides with specific amino acid (Cys, His, Met, etc.) *(36–38)*; N- or C-terminal peptides *(39,40)*; posttranslationally modified proteins (glycosylation, phosphorylation, oxidation, nitration, etc.) *(12)*; and affinity-purified proteins (lectin affinity, coimmunoprecipitation, tandem affinity purification, etc.) *(41)*. In addition to these selection strategies, targeted proteomics study in the nephrology field can be referred to as the study of a particular set of renal salt and water transport proteins using immunoblotting *(42–45)*.

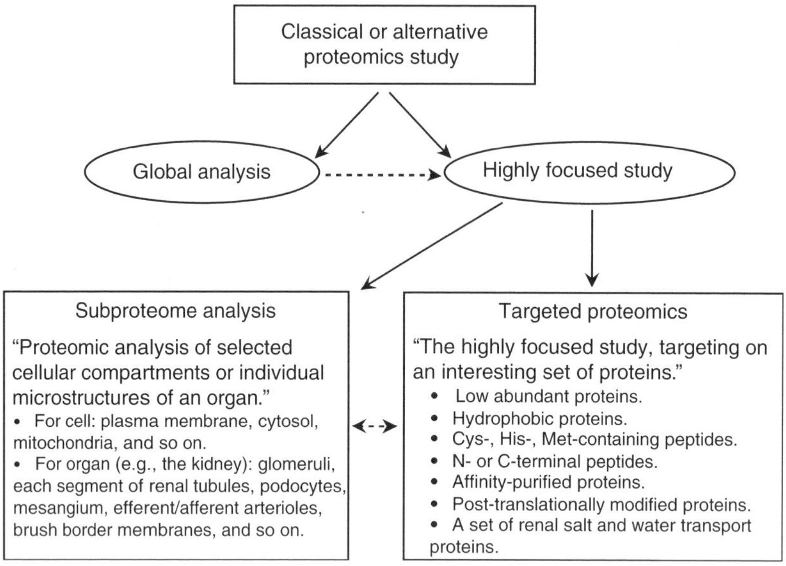

Fig. 3. Global analysis vs highly focused study. Both classical and alternative proteomics studies can be conducted at two different levels. The global analysis is to screen for overall changes of the entire proteome, whereas the highly focused study is to examine a particular set of proteins using the concepts of "subproteome analysis" and "targeted proteomics." (Copyright © 2005 Future Drugs Ltd., London, UK; modified with permission from ref. *26*.)

Gel-Based vs Gel-Free Proteomic Analysis

Gel-Based Proteomic Analysis

Gel-based analysis is the most commonly used method in current proteomic studies. Proteins are first extracted from cell, tissue, organ, or biofluid and then separated by 2D PAGE. The first dimensional separation resolves proteins on the basis of differential pH or charges, using immobilized pH-gradient strips or mobiline ampholytes tube gels *(46)*. During the electrophoresis, acidic proteins (anions) migrate toward the anode, whereas basic proteins (cations) migrate toward the cathode. At a point where the dynamic net charge is zero, a protein will stop migration. This point of pH value is called "isoelectric point" and this process is called "isoelectric focusing" *(47)*. After completion of the isoelectric focusing, proteins are subjected to further separation in the vertical axis (2D) by sodium dodecyl sulfate-PAGE that resolves proteins on the basis of differential molecular sizes (M_r). Separated proteins in the 2D gel can be visualized by various types of staining (Coomassie blue, silver, fluorescence, etc.). The visualized spots are then excised, in-gel digested with proteolytic enzymes (trypsin, chymotrypsin, Arg-C, Asp-N, Lys-C, PepsinA, V8-E, V8-DE, etc.), and identified by MALDI-MS followed by peptide mass fingerprinting (Fig. 4).

MALDI-MS provides a high-throughput manner of protein identification; hundreds of proteins can be identified within a day *(48)*. In MALDI analysis, proteins, or tryptic peptide fragments are mixed with chemical matrix, which has the property of facilitating ion activation by laser beam. The most commonly used matrix in MALDI is α-cyano-4-hydroxycinnamic acid for peptide analysis and *trans*-3,5-dimethoxy-4-hydroxycinnamic acid (sinapinic acid) for protein analysis *(49)*. The mixture of analytes

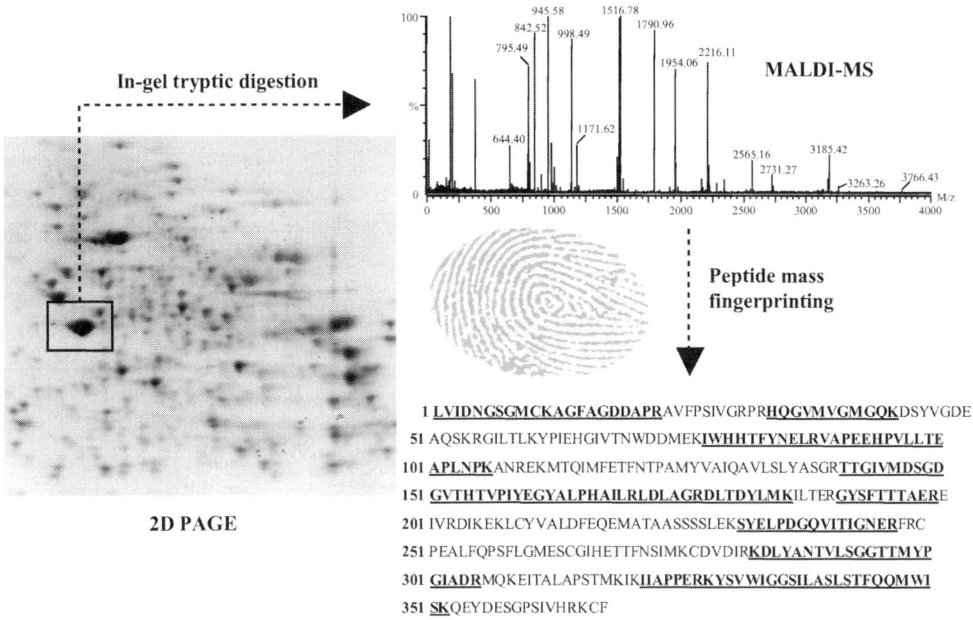

Fig. 4. Gel-based proteomic analysis: the most commonly used method in proteomic studies. Proteins derived from cell, tissue, organ, or biofluid are resolved by 2D PAGE, which separates proteins on the basis of differential isoelectric point (*x*-axis) and M_r (*y*-axis). Separated protein spots are visualized by various types of staining. After spot matching and quantitative intensity analysis, the interesting spots are excised, in-gel digested with proteolytic enzymes (mostly trypsin), and then identified by MALDI-MS followed by peptide mass fingerprinting.

and matrix is spotted onto the target plate and allowed to air-dry. Thereafter, crystals of matrix are formed together with the analytes. The target plate is then placed into the MS instrumentation, which is equipped with a laser-beam generator. After laser firing, the matrix adsorbs the energy from laser and then undergoes rapid solid-to-gas phase transition or the exciting state. The analytes embedded in the matrix crystals are then ionized by the excited matrix with a poorly understood process. Most of ions formed in the activated analytes are single-charged ions *(50)*. These ions are then ejected from the target plate to the mass analyzer. The most common type of mass analyzer employed in MALDI analysis is time-of-flight (TOF). With a fixed distance of ion passage, the time to the target of the activated ions is different because of variations in mass per charge (*m/z*) values of the ionized peptides. Various peptide fragments can then be distinguished and identified by peptide mass fingerprinting, based on differential *m/z* values *(51)* (Fig. 4).

Gel-Free Proteomic Analysis

The major limitation in gel-based proteomic analysis is the difficulty in identifying low abundant, transmembrane, and highly hydrophobic proteins. Reverse-phase high-performance liquid chromatography coupled to ESI-tandem MS (ESI-MS/MS) has gained a wide acceptance for gel-free proteomic analysis and become a method of choice for analysis of membrane and low-abundant proteins *(52–54)*. ESI is the process of ionization from electrospray source, whereas tandem MS refers to the strategy of multistep mass analyses. The analyte solution is pumped through the high-voltage capillary and electrostatic force of this high-voltage field exceeds surface tension of the solution, leading to the spray of highly charged droplets from the capillary tip. Desolvation process of these droplets can be accomplished by either passing through a heated capillary or passing across a stream of heated gas. The peptide ions then enter into the mass analyzer. There are several types of mass analyzers (e.g., quadrupole, ion trap, and TOF) that can be used in tandem MS in various combinations *(55)*. Although these combinations operate differently, all of them have similar strategy to analyze peptide masses in the tandem manner (multisteps of mass analysis) to produce more accurate data than the analysis with only a single path of mass analyzer. Recent advance in gel-free proteomic analysis is an approach namely multidimensional protein identification technology or "shotgun proteomics" *(56)*. Multidimensional protein identification technology takes advantage of the high resolution capacity of protein separation using 2D liquid chromatography (which resolves proteins on the basis of electrostatic charge and hydrophobicity) and the powerful peptide characterization of tandem MS to analyze proteins in a complex mixture *(57)*. It provides higher sensitivity and shorter analytical time when compared with gel-based proteomic analysis, but requires a more complicated instrumentation. Other types of gel-free proteomic technologies include microarrays *(27)*, surface-enhanced laser desorption/ionization *(28)*, and CE-MS *(29)* that are commonly used in the alternative proteomics approach.

DIABETES RESEARCH IN THE ERA OF PROTEOMICS

During the past few years, proteomics has been extensively applied to diabetes research. The main objectives of proteomic applications to diabetes are not only to better understand the pathophysiology of this metabolic disease and its complications, but also to define novel biomarkers and new therapeutic targets. Recent proteomic studies applied to diabetes research are summarized in Table 1.

Construction of 2D reference maps and proteome databases of pancreas *(58,59)* and mitochondria *(60–64)* will be useful for future diabetes research. Because proteins have already been identified in these maps, MS analysis may not be further required in the next study that examines the same organ/organelle using the exactly same protocols of sample preparation and separation. There are several additional 2D reference maps and proteome databases for other specific organs and organelles that have not been included in Table 1 but may potentially be useful in diabetes research and can be found at the WORLD-2D PAGE (http://www.expasy.org/ch2d/2d-index.html). Differential proteomics has been applied to diabetes research to determine differentially expressed proteins in different sets of biological samples and to define alterations in protein expression or proteome profiles during experimental intervention and disease state. Among these applications, differential proteomic analysis of pancreatic islets and β-cells has been mostly applied *(65–71)*. These studies have investigated the altered protein expression of differentiating β-cells, islets exposed to cytokine (IL-1β) and drug (rosiglitazone), dietary-manipulated islets, and transplanted islets. Finally, examination of PTMs related to diabetes provides significant functional information of the identified proteins although only few PTMs, to date, have been explored in the proteomic investigation of diabetes. With the strength of proteomic technologies and the availability of genomic information, proteomics will be more widely applied in diabetes research in the coming years and will lead to lots more information to unravel the pathophysiology of diabetes and its complications.

Table 1
Summary of Recent Proteomic Studies in the Investigation of Diabetes

Type of study	*Reference(s)*
Two-dimensional reference maps and proteome databases	
Human pancreas	*58*
Mouse pancreatic islets, adipose tissue, liver, and muscle	*59*
Human, rat, and mouse mitochondria	*60–62*
Metabolic network in human mitochondria	*63,64*
Differential proteomics	
Pancreatic islets and β-cells	*65–71*
Heart	*72*
Kidney	*73–77*
Liver	*78–80*
Muscle	*79*
Adipose tissue	*79*
Red blood cell membranes	*81*
Serum	*82,83*
Urine	*84,85*
Vitreous fluid	*86*
Proteomic analysis of posttranslational modifications	
Glycation	*87–91*
Oxidation	*92*
Nitration	*93*
Phosphorylation	*94*

PROTEOMICS IN THE INVESTIGATION OF DIABETIC NEPHROPATHY

Even with the extensive applications of proteomics to diabetes research during the past few years, proteomics in the investigation of DN is in its infancy phase and the number of such studies is relatively small. These studies can be summarized as follows.

Classical Proteomics Approach to Define Alterations in Renal Protein Expression in Diabetic Nephropathy Using Animal Models of Type 1 and Type 2 Diabetes

The author and colleagues *(73–75,95)* have performed the classical, gel-based proteomic analysis (using 2D PAGE, SYPRO Ruby staining, quantitative intensity analysis, and MALDI–TOF MS) of DN in the OVE26 transgenic mouse model for type 1 diabetes *(96–98)* and the *db/db* mouse model for type 2 diabetes *(99)*. Differential proteomics has been performed using these two mouse models compared with their respective background strains. A total of 41 (30 identified and 11 unidentified) and 39 (20 identified and 19 unidentified) proteins are differentially expressed proteins observed in diabetic kidneys of type 1 and 2, respectively *(73,74,95)*. The altered proteins include proteases, protease inhibitors, apoptosis-associated proteins, regulators for oxidative tolerance, Ca^{2+}-binding proteins, transport regulators, cell-signaling proteins, and smooth muscle contractile elements. Some of the altered proteins have been previously shown to be regulated during diabetes; whereas roles for the other altered proteins have not previously been established, suggesting that they may be involved in the novel mechanisms of DN. These data may provide a new roadmap for diabetes research.

Among the altered proteins that have been identified, changes in the renal elastin–elastase pathway *(73,95)* and increased calbindin-D28k expression *(75)* are consistent among the two types of diabetes. In the renal elastin–elastase system, expression of elastase inhibitor is increased, whereas elastase expression is decreased (Fig. 5A). These coordinated changes suggest the hypothesis that elastin, a protein degraded by elastase, should be accumulated in the diabetic kidney. The hypothesis has been addressed by an immunohistochemical study of elastin on mouse kidney sections and human renal biopsy specimens. The elastin expression is markedly increased in renal tubular epithelial cells (early stage) and in the interstitium (advanced stage) of diabetic kidneys (Fig. 5B). Elastin is an extracellular matrix (ECM) protein, which plays an important role in maintaining vascular elasticity and glomerular integrity. The increase in elastin expression, however, is localized in renal tubular epithelial cells, not the vessels nor the glomeruli. This change occurs in parallel with an increase of vimentin, a marker of cells derived from mesenchymal tissues *(100)*. These data are consistent with those reported in a previous study *(101)*, indicating that renal tubular epithelial cells can produce ECM proteins and directly intervene in the fibrotic process via a mechanism namely "epithelial–mesenchymal transdifferentiation." Additionally, expression of a myofibroblast protein (fibroblast tropomyosin) and proteins associated with proliferation, modulation and differentiation of myofibroblasts, and fibrogenesis (calmodulin and cellular retinol-binding protein) *(102,103)* are also upregulated in diabetic kidneys. Taken together, these data suggest that elastin may play an important role in tubular disorders and interstitial fibrosis of DN.

The other consistent finding in the kidney of both types of diabetes is the increase in renal Calbindin-D28k expression (Fig. 6A) *(75)*. Calbindin-D28k is generally known as a vitamin-D-dependent Ca^{2+}-binding protein that plays an important role in renal tubular Ca^{2+} reabsorption *(104)*. In the normal kidney, calbindin-D28k distributes along distal convoluted tubules (DCT), connecting tubules and collecting ducts (CD) *(105,106)*, and colocalizes with epithelial Ca^{2+} channel, plasma membrane Ca^{2+}-ATPase, and Na^+/Ca^{2+} exchanger along $1,25(OH)_2D_3$-responsive nephron segments *(107)*. These proteins regulate tubular Ca^{2+} reabsorption via an active transcellular Ca^{2+} transport process in the distal nephron *(108)*. The results from a previous study *(109)* indicate that renal calbindin-D28k expression is probably the best marker for the $1,25(OH)_2D_3$ activity. Renal calbindin-D28k appears to enhance tubular Ca^{2+} reabsorption, and reduction of renal calbindin-D28k is associated with hypercalciuria *(110–114)*. Findings from a recent in vivo study using a gene-knockout model confirm the critical role of calbindin-D28k in maintaining renal Ca^{2+} homeostasis *(115)*.

Hypercalciuria is commonly associated with diabetes *(116–121)*. However, there are a limited number of studies to address the pathophysiology of the altered Ca^{2+} homeostasis during diabetes *(119–122)*. The results from these studies clearly indicate that diabetic animals have hypercalciuria, decreased circulating $1,25(OH)_2D_3$, and reduced bone mass. Although hypercalciuria occurs, plasma levels of ionized and total Ca^{2+} can be maintained at the normal levels in several study models *(119,121,122)*. These data implicate that a compensatory mechanism for diabetes-induced renal Ca^{2+} loss exists. The increased calbindin-D28k expression is prominent at DCT and CD of the OVE26 diabetic mice (Fig. 6B) *(75)*. Both DCT and CD are the $1,25(OH)_2D_3$-responsive nephron segments. Considered together, these data

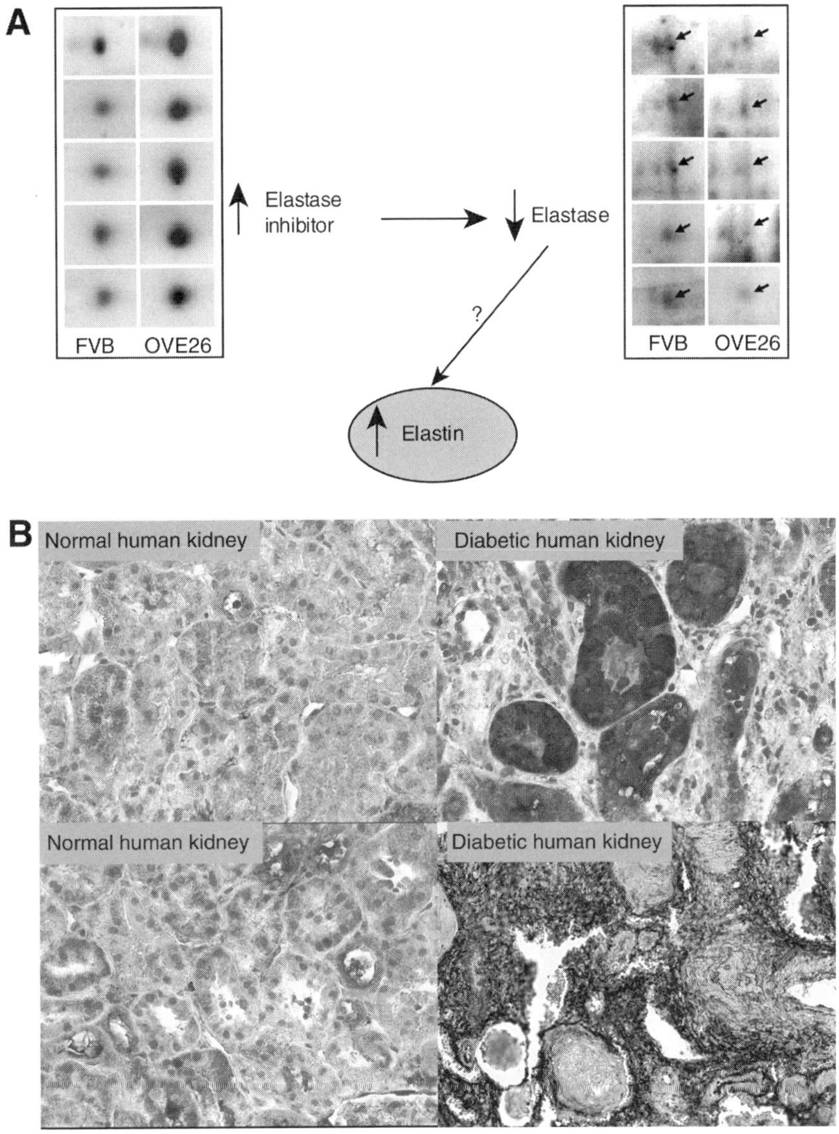

Fig. 5. Alterations in the renal elastin–elastase system in diabetic nephropathy identified by proteomic analysis. **(A)** Classical proteomics approach (using 2D PAGE, SYPRO Ruby staining, quantitative intensity analysis, and MALDI–TOF MS) has been applied to screen for average changes of proteins in diabetic mouse kidney. Among several altered proteins, elastase inhibitor is upregulated, whereas elastase is downregulated in diabetic kidney. These coordinated changes have led to the hypothesis that elastin, a protein degraded by elastase, should be accumulated in diabetic kidney. The hypothesis has been addressed by immunohistochemical study on human renal biopsies. **(B)** Elastin is markedly increased in renal tubular epithelial cells (early stage; right upper panel) and the interstitium (late stage; right lower panel) of diabetic kidney. These findings have led to the new hypothesis that elastin may play role in a process namely "tubular epithelial–mesenchymal transdifferentiation" in the fibrogenesis pathway of diabetic nephropathy. Magnification power in **(B)** is ×100 for the right lower panel and ×400 for the others. (Modified from ref. *73* with permission.)

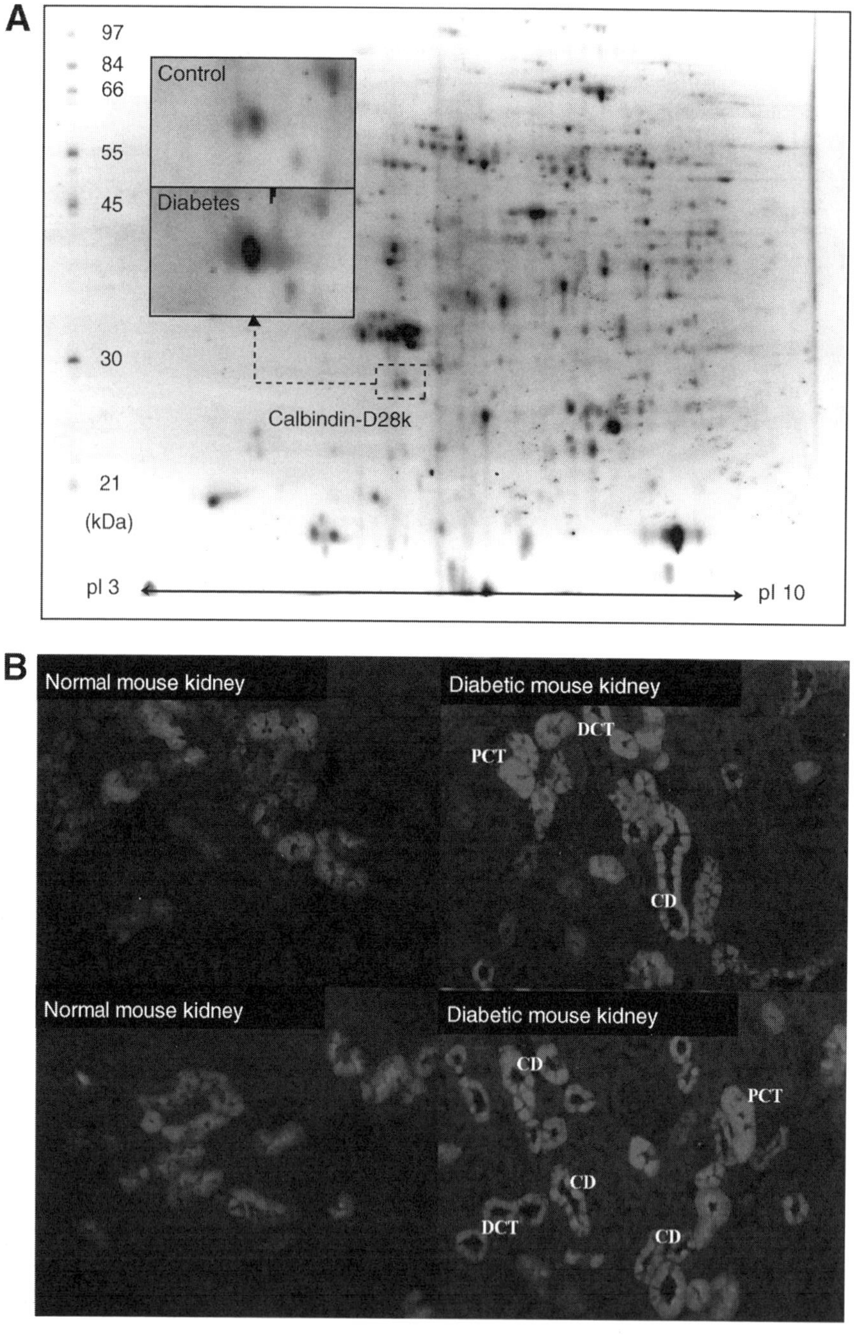

Fig. 6. Proteomic identification and immunolocalization of increased calbindin-D28k in diabetic kidney. **(A)** Classical proteomics approach (using 2D PAGE, SYPRO Ruby staining, quantitative intensity analysis, and MALDI–TOF MS) has been applied to screen for average changes of proteins in diabetic mouse kidney. Among several altered proteins, renal calbindin-D28k expression is markedly increased in animal models of type 1 and 2 diabetes. **(B)** Immunohistochemistry has confirmed the proteomic data and demonstrated the increase of renal calbindin-D28k at DCT, CD, and proximal convoluted tubules . Magnification power in **(B)** is ×200. (Modified from ref. *75* with permission.)

suggest the hypothesis that the increase in renal calbindin-D28k in diabetic kidney may be one of the compensatory mechanisms responsive to diabetes-induced abnormal Ca^{2+} homeostasis *(116–121)*.

Interestingly, the increase in renal calbindin-D28k expression in diabetic kidney appears not only in the distal nephron, in which calbindin-D28k facilitates active Ca^{2+} reabsorption, but also in proximal convoluted tubules, in which a role for calbindin-D28k is not clear (Fig. 6B) *(75)*. There is an evidence demonstrating that transfection of calbindin-D28k gene into murine proximal tubular epithelial cells provides protective effects against chemical hypoxic injury *(123)*. Several other lines of inquiry indicate that calbindin-D28k has a cytoprotective role in preventing various cell types from cellular degeneration and apoptosis via a Ca^{2+}-buffer mechanism *(124–127)*. Therefore, it is speculated that calbindin-D28k may have another potential role in preventing apoptotic tubular cell death induced by diabetes.

Alternative Proteomics Approach to Define Alterations in Urinary Proteome Profile in Patients With Diabetic Nephropathy

In addition to the classical proteomics approach described above, the alternative proteomics approach has also been applied to DN using CE-TOF MS to differentiate urinary proteome profile of patients with type 2 diabetes from that of the healthy controls *(84)*. The urinary polypeptide pattern of patients with diabetes significantly differs from the normal. Moreover, there is a specific polypeptide pattern of "diabetic renal damage" in patients with high-grade albuminuria (urine albumin >100 mg/L). The urinary polypeptide profiles in diabetic patients can be classified into four types. Type A pattern is typically found in the diabetic state and the occurrence in healthy subjects is low. Type B pattern represents polypeptide profile observed mainly in healthy subjects and the frequency in patients with diabetes is low. Types C and D are the typical patterns of markers for diabetic renal damage of which the frequency in diabetes is increased and decreased, respectively *(84)*. These data underscore the usefulness of the alternative proteomics approach in clinical diagnostics and biomarker discovery.

Targeted Proteomics Approach to Define Alterations in Renal Salt and Water Transport Proteins in Diabetic Nephropathy

Only few studies have applied targeted proteomics using immunoblotting to define alterations in renal salt and water transport proteins during diabetes. The evaluation of type 1 diabetes has been performed in streptozotocin (STZ)-induced diabetic rats *(77)*. STZ administration results in increased expression of type 3 Na^+/H^+ exchanger, thiazide-sensitive Na^+-Cl^- cotransporter, epithelial Na^+ channel subunits α, β, and γ, aquaporin (AQP)-2, and AQP-3 *(77)*. For the evaluation of type 2 diabetes, lean and obese Zucker rats have been employed *(76)*. Obese rats are significantly heavier and have larger kidneys with increased plasma creatinine, abnormal high glucose levels, and elevated blood pressure. Furthermore, they have a marked decrease in abundance of several renal transport proteins; i.e., Na^+-P^- cotransporter-2, type-3 Na^+/H^+ exchanger, bumetanide-sensitive Na^+-K^+-$2Cl^-$ contransporter, AQP2, AQP3, AQP4, and apical urea transporter *(76)*. These findings may reflect the pathophysiology of renal salt and water retention and hypertension associated with DN.

PROTEIN BIOINFORMATICS IN THE INVESTIGATION OF DIABETIC NEPHROPATHY

Bioinformatics can be applied to obtain additional protein information including:

1. protein identities using MS or MS/MS data;
2. protein characterization and structure prediction;
3. homology and sequence alignment;
4. motifs and domains;
5. protein interactions and networks;
6. potential PTMs;
7. predicted transmembrane regions;
8. subcellular localization; and
9. miscellaneous *(51)*.

There are numerous on-line analytical tools that are freely accessible in the websites for bioinformatic analysis (http://www.expasy.org/tools/). The data obtained from bioinformatic analysis are very helpful to predict the correlation between "protein expression" and "protein function" and make functional studies more focused.

An obvious example of the usefulness of bioinformatics in the investigation of DN has been demonstrated in a recent proteomic study, which has identified an unnamed protein product (gi|12841975; BAB25424) as a highly regulated protein in the kidney of the OVE26 diabetic mice *(51,73,74)*. The MS-based protein identification frequently provides the identities that are designated as "unknown protein," "unnamed protein," "putative protein," "hypothetical protein," "unnamed gene product," and so on. All of these terms refer to the proteins that have been submitted to the database without detailed characterizations or those, whose sequences have been predicted from DNA sequences but their other information is limited or unknown. When this occurs, the investigators frequently ignore the proteins and the data may be of limited usefulness.

Bioinformatic analysis is of substantial assistance in characterizing hypothetical proteins identified by mass spectrometric analysis. It can "unmask" those unknown proteins, which may turn out to be common or well-known proteins. Using data mining, the unnamed protein (gi|12841975; BAB25424) that is upregulated in diabetic mouse kidney has been finally unmasked *(51)*. The data indicate that this unknown protein is, indeed, phosphatidylethanolamine-binding protein. Additionally, motif scanning shows that this unknown protein contains several kinase motifs, especially protein kinase C that plays an important role in the pathogenesis of diabetic nephropathy. Therefore, this protein phosphatidylethanolamine-binding protein should have a potential functional role in protein kinase C-dependent pathogenic mechanisms of diabetic nephropathy.

The same group of the investigators, who have applied the classical proteomics approach to DN *(51,73–75,95)*, have also performed bioinformatic analysis of the altered proteins identified from the OVE26 diabetic mice, integrating with literature search to make a correlation between the altered proteins and the pathogenesis and pathophysiology of DN. A model of renal protein trafficking that occurs in DN has been proposed (Fig. 7). The pathogenic mechanisms that are involved in this model are apoptosis, vasculopathy, glomerulopathy, and fibrogenesis. However, it should be noted that this model represents only the phenomena occur in an animal model of type 1 diabetes and has not yet been examined in humans. Moreover, the data do not cover all of the known proteins that have previously been shown to be regulated during diabetes.

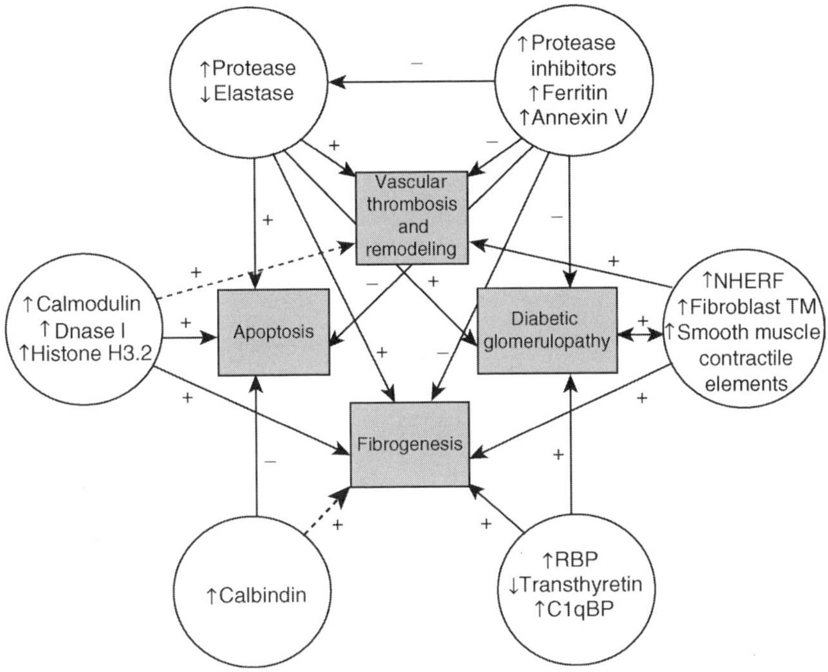

Fig. 7. The model of renal protein trafficking in type 1 diabetic nephropathy. This model has been created by extensive bioinformatic analysis and literature search of the data obtained from a proteomic analysis of the kidney in the OVE26 model of type 1 diabetes *(73)*. All of the altered proteins that have been identified in this model play important roles in apoptosis, vasculopathy, glomerulopathy, and fibrogenesis. Abbreviations used: +, activation or stimulation; –, inhibition; TM, tropomyosin; RBP, retinol-binding protein; C1qBP, Complement 1q-binding protein. (Modified from ref. *131* with permission.)

This model will be more valuable when a systematic functional study is designed to address all of these multiplexed mechanisms globally, not just a particular pathway.

CONCLUSIONS

Proteomic analysis has become an important tool for the investigation of DN. With more extensive applications in the coming years, proteomics will add up lots more information and knowledge to better understand the pathogenesis and pathophysiology of diabetic renal complication. In addition, proteomics will make also biomarker discovery and identification of novel therapeutic targets for DN more feasible. The ultimate goal of improved therapeutic outcome and successful prevention of the disease can then be achieved.

CURRENT PERSPECTIVES AND FUTURE DIRECTIONS

Diabetes Research: From Individual Omics to Integrative Omics and Systems Biology

The suffix—omics—has been used frequently for the nomenclature of several fields in biomedical research (i.e., genomics, transcriptomics, proteomics, lipomics, metabolomics, interactomics, and several others). Current diabetes research applies each of these omics sciences, separately, for individual study project. It is unlikely that the complexity of diabetes will be completely understood by a single omics study. Integrating all of these omics fields is required in future diabetes research. With the strength of bioinformatics, each omics field is complementary to the others and serves as an individual piece of the jigsaw to fulfill the dynamic image of the pathogenesis and pathophysiology of diabetes and its complications. Recently, the concept of "systems biology" has been emerging for the global evaluation of biological systems and has included integrative omics as one of analytical procedures *(128,129)*. Systems biology has been defined by Weston and Hood *(130)* as "the analysis of the relationships among the elements in a system in response to genetic or environmental perturbations, with the goal of understanding the system or the emergent properties of the system." A system may be a few protein molecules carrying out a particular task such as galactose metabolism (termed a biomodule), a complex set of proteins and other molecules working together as a molecular machine such as the ribosome, a network of proteins operating together to carry out an important cellular function such as giving the cell shape (protein network), or a cell or group of cells carrying out particular phenotypic functions. Thus, a biological system may encompass molecules, cells, organs, individuals, or even ecosystems *(130)*.

The major keys that make systems biology being the ideal approach for future biomedical research are as follow:

1. The successfulness of the genome projects and the availability of databases.
2. The emergence of cross-disciplinary biology that allows biologists, chemists, physiologists, computer scientists, engineers, mathematicians, statisticians, physicians, and health care professionals to work closely together.
3. The availability of bioinformatics that serves as a link for a cross-talk among different fields.
4. Advances in the high-throughput platforms of biotechnologies that permit simultaneous study of a large complement of genes, transcripts, proteins, lipids, or other elements.

Systems biology is therefore the ideal approach for future diabetes research and should result in the following:

1. Better understanding of the pathogenesis and pathophysiology of diabetes and its complications.
2. Identification of new therapeutic targets.
3. Discovery of novel drugs and biomarkers.
4. Better therapeutic outcomes.
5. Prevention of the disease and its complications.

REFERENCES

1. Caramori ML, Fioretto P, Mauer M. The need for early predictors of diabetic nephropathy risk: is albumin excretion rate sufficient? Diabetes 2000;49:1399–1408.
2. Chavers BM, Bilous RW, Ellis EN, Steffes MW, Mauer SM. Glomerular lesions and urinary albumin excretion in type I diabetes without overt proteinuria. N Engl J Med 1989;320:966–970.
3. Fioretto P, Steffes MW, Mauer M. Glomerular structure in nonproteinuric IDDM patients with various levels of albuminuria. Diabetes 1994;43:1358–1364.
4. Bangstad HJ, Osterby R, Dahl-Jorgensen K, et al. Early glomerulopathy is present in young, type 1 (insulin-dependent) diabetic patients with microalbuminuria. Diabetologia 1993;36:523–529.
5. Comper WD, Osicka TM, Jerums G. High prevalence of immuno-unreactive intact albumin in urine of diabetic patients. Am J Kidney Dis 2003;41:336–342.

6. Seaquist ER, Goetz FC, Rich S, Barbosa J. Familial clustering of diabetic kidney disease. Evidence for genetic susceptibility to diabetic nephropathy. N Engl J Med 1989;320:1161–1165.
7. Borch-Johnsen K, Norgaard K, Hommel E, et al. Is diabetic nephropathy an inherited complication? Kidney Int 1992;41:719–722.
8. Pettitt DJ, Saad MF, Bennett PH, Nelson RG, Knowler WC. Familial predisposition to renal disease in two generations of Pima Indians with type 2 (non-insulin-dependent) diabetes mellitus. Diabetologia 1990;33:438–443.
9. Faronato PP, Maioli M, Tonolo G, et al. Clustering of albumin excretion rate abnormalities in Caucasian patients with NIDDM. The Italian NIDDM Nephropathy Study Group. Diabetologia 1997;40:816–823.
10. Vijay V, Snehalatha C, Shina K, Lalitha S, Ramachandran A. Familial aggregation of diabetic kidney disease in type 2 diabetes in south India. Diabetes Res Clin Pract 1999;43:167–171.
11. Canani LH, Gerchman F, Gross JL. Familial clustering of diabetic nephropathy in Brazilian type 2 diabetic patients. Diabetes 1999;48:909–913.
12. Mann M, Jensen ON. Proteomic analysis of post-translational modifications. Nat Biotechnol 2003;21:255–261.
13. Tooyama I, Sato H, Yasuhara O, et al. Correlation of the expression level of C1q mRNA and the number of C1q- positive plaques in the Alzheimer Disease temporal cortex. analysis of C1q mRNA and its protein using adjacent or nearby sections. Dement Geriatr Cogn Disord 2001;12:237–242.
14. Tong X, Kawabata H, Koeffler HP. Iron deficiency can upregulate expression of transferrin receptor at both the mRNA and protein level. Br J Haematol 2002;116:458–464.
15. Gygi SP, Rochon Y, Franza BR, Aebersold R. Correlation between protein and mRNA abundance in yeast. Mol Cell Biol 1999;19:1720–1730.
16. Ji P, Xuan JW, Onita T, et al. Correlation study showing no concordance between EPAS-1/HIF-2alpha mRNA and protein expression in transitional cellcancer of the bladder. Urology 2003;61:851–857.
17. Aebersold R. Constellations in a cellular universe. Nature 2003;422:115, 116.
18. O'Farrell PH. High resolution two-dimensional electrophoresis of proteins. J Biol Chem 1975;250:4007–4021.
19. Klose J. Protein mapping by combined isoelectric focusing and electrophoresis of mouse tissues. A novel approach to testing for induced point mutations in mammals. Humangenetik 1975;26:231–243.
20. Aebersold R, Mann M. Mass spectrometry-based proteomics. Nature 2003;422:198–207.
21. Cho A, Normile D. Nobel Prize in Chemistry. Mastering macromolecules. Science 2002;298: 527–528.
22. Wasinger VC, Cordwell SJ, Cerpa-Poljak A, et al. Progress with gene-product mapping of the Mollicutes: Mycoplasma genitalium. Electrophoresis 1995;16:1090–1094.
23. Peng J, Gygi SP. Proteomics: the move to mixtures. J Mass Spectrom 2001;36:1083–1091.
24. Patterson SD. Proteomics: the industrialization of protein chemistry. Curr Opin Biotechnol 2000;11:413–418.
25. Yanagida M. Functional proteomics; current achievements. J Chromatogr B Analyt Technol Biomed Life Sci 2002;771:89–106.
26. Thongboonkerd V. Proteomic analysis of renal diseases: Unraveling the pathophysiology and biomarker discovery. Expert Rev Proteomics 2005;2:349–366.
27. Templin MF, Stoll D, Schwenk JM, Potz O, Kramer S, Joos TO. Protein microarrays: promising tools for proteomic research. Proteomics 2003;3:2155–2166.
28. Fung E, Diamond D, Simonsesn AH, Weinberger SR. The use of SELDI Protein Chip array technology in renal disease research. Methods Mol Med 2003;86:295–312.
29. Weissinger EM, Wittke S, Kaiser T, et al. Proteomic patterns established with capillary electrophoresis and mass spectrometry for diagnostic purposes. Kidney Int 2004;65:2426–2434.
30. Nouwens AS, Cordwell SJ, Larsen MR, et al. Complementing genomics with proteomics: the membrane subproteome of Pseudomonas aeruginosa PAO1. Electrophoresis 2000;21:3797–3809.
31. Neverova I, Van Eyk JE. Application of reversed phase high performance liquid chromatography for subproteomic analysis of cardiac muscle. Proteomics 2002;2:22–31.
32. Govorukhina NI, Keizer-Gunnink A, van der Zee AG, de Jong S, de Bruijn HW, Bischoff R. Sample preparation of human serum for the analysis of tumor markers. Comparison of different approaches for albumin and gamma-globulin depletion. J Chromatogr A 2003;1009:171–178.
33. Rabilloud T. Solubilization of proteins in 2-D electrophoresis. An outline. Methods Mol Biol 1999;112:9–19.
34. Santoni V, Rabilloud T, Doumas P, et al. Towards the recovery of hydrophobic proteins on two-dimensional electrophoresis gels. Electrophoresis 1999;20:705–711.

35. Seigneurin-Berny D, Rolland N, Garin J, Joyard J. Technical Advance: Differential extraction of hydrophobic proteins from chloroplast envelope membranes: a subcellular-specific proteomic approach to identify rare intrinsic membrane proteins. Plant J 1999;19:217–228.
36. Gevaert K, Ghesquiere B, Staes A, et al. Reversible labeling of cysteine-containing peptides allows their specific chromatographic isolation for non-gel proteome studies. Proteomics 2004;4:897–908.
37. Ren D, Penner NA, Slentz BE, Mirzaei H, Regnier F. Evaluating immobilized metal affinity chromatography for the selection of histidine-containing peptides in comparative proteomics. J Proteome Res 2003;2:321–329.
38. Gevaert K, Van Damme J, Goethals M, et al. Chromatographic isolation of methionine-containing peptides for gel-free proteome analysis: identification of more than 800 Escherichia coli proteins. Mol Cell Proteomics 2002;1:896–903.
39. Gevaert K, Goethals M, Martens L, et al. Exploring proteomes and analyzing protein processing by mass spectrometric identification of sorted N-terminal peptides. Nat Biotechnol 2003;21: 566–569.
40. Kumazaki T, Terasawa K, Ishii S. Affinity chromatography on immobilized anhydrotrypsin: general utility for selective isolation of C-terminal peptides from protease digests of proteins. J Biochem (Tokyo) 1987;102:1539–1546.
41. Mirzaei H, Regnier F. Structure specific chromatographic selection in targeted proteomics. J Chromatogr B Analyt Technol Biomed Life Sci 2005;817:23–34.
42. Knepper MA, Masilamani S. Targeted proteomics in the kidney using ensembles of antibodies. Acta Physiol Scand 2001;173:11–21.
43. Knepper MA. Proteomics and the kidney. J Am Soc Nephrol 2002;13:1398–1408.
44. Ecelbarger CA. Targeted proteomics using immunoblotting technique for studying dysregulation of ion transporters in renal disorders. Expert Rev Proteomics 2004;1:219–227.
45. Ecelbarger CA. Proteomics and sodium transport. In: Thongboonkerd V, Klein JB, eds. Proteomics in Nephrology. Basel: Karger, 2004:124–141.
46. Klein E, Klein JB, Thongboonkerd V. Two-dimensional gel electrophoresis: A fundamental tool for expression proteomics studies. In: Thongboonkerd V, Klein JB, eds. Proteomics in Nephrology. Basel: Karger, 2004:25–39.
47. Righetti PG, Bossi A. Isoelectric focusing in immobilized pH gradients: an update. J Chromatogr B Biomed Sci Appl 1997;699:77–89.
48. Henzel WJ, Watanabe C, Stults JT. Protein identification: the origins of peptide mass fingerprinting. J Am Soc Mass Spectrom 2003;14:931–942.
49. Pierce WM, Cai J. Applications of mass spectrometry in proteomics. In: Thongboonkerd V, Klein JB, eds. Proteomics in Nephrology. Basel: Karger, 2004:40–58.
50. Karas M, Gluckmann M, Schafer J. Ionization in matrix-assisted laser desorption/ionization: singly charged molecular ions are the lucky survivors. J Mass Spectrom 2000;35:1–12.
51. Thongboonkerd V, Klein JB. In: Practical bioinformatics for proteomics. Thongboonkerd V, Klein JB, eds. Proteomics in Nephrology. Basel: Karger, 2004:79–92.
52. McCormack AL, Schieltz DM, Goode B, et al. Direct analysis and identification of proteins in mixtures by LC/MS/MS and database searching at the low-femtomole level. Anal Chem 1997;69:767–776.
53. Wu CC, MacCoss MJ, Howell KE, Yates JR, III. A method for the comprehensive proteomic analysis of membrane proteins. Nat Biotechnol 2003;21:532–538.
54. Gygi SP, Rist B, Griffin TJ, Eng J, Aebersold R. Proteome analysis of low-abundance proteins using multidimensional chromatography and isotope-coded affinity tags. J Proteome Res 2002;1: 47–54.
55. Griffiths WJ, Jonsson AP, Liu S, Rai DK, Wang Y. Electrospray and tandem mass spectrometry in biochemistry. Biochem J 2001;355:545–561.
56. Link AJ, Eng J, Schieltz DM, et al. Direct analysis of protein complexes using mass spectrometry. Nat Biotechnol 1999;17:676–682.
57. Liu H, Lin D, Yates JR, III. Multidimensional separations for protein/peptide analysis in the post-genomic era. Biotechniques 2002;32:898, 900, 902.
58. Hu L, Evers S, Lu ZH, Shen Y, Chen J. Two-dimensional protein database of human pancreas. Electrophoresis 2004;25:512–518.
59. Sanchez JC, Chiappe D, Converset V, et al. The mouse SWISS-2D PAGE database: a tool for proteomics study of diabetes and obesity. Proteomics 2001;1:136–163.
60. Taylor SW, Fahy E, Zhang B, et al. Characterization of the human heart mitochondrial proteome. Nat Biotechnol 2003;21:281–286.

61. Lopez MF, Kristal BS, Chernokalskaya E, et al. High-throughput profiling of the mitochondrial proteome using affinity fractionation and automation. Electrophoresis 2000;21:3427–3440.
62. Mootha VK, Bunkenborg J, Olsen JV, et al. Integrated analysis of protein composition, tissue diversity, and gene regulation in mouse mitochondria. Cell 2003;115:629–640.
63. Vo TD, Greenberg HJ, Palsson BO. Reconstruction and functional characterization of the human mitochondrial metabolic network based on proteomic and biochemical data. J Biol Chem 2004;279:39,532–39,540.
64. Thiele I, Price ND, Vo TD, Palsson BO. Candidate metabolic network states in human mitochondria: Impact of diabetes, ischemia, and diet. J Biol Chem 2005;280:11,683–11,695.
65. Andersen HU, Fey SJ, Larsen PM, et al. Interleukin-1beta induced changes in the protein expression of rat islets: a computerized database. Electrophoresis 1997;18:2091–2103.
66. Larsen PM, Fey SJ, Larsen MR, et al. Proteome analysis of interleukin-1beta-induced changes in protein expression in rat islets of Langerhans. Diabetes 2001;50:1056–1063.
67. Sparre T, Bjerre CU, Mose LP, et al. IL-1beta induced protein changes in diabetes prone BB rat islets of Langerhans identified by proteome analysis. Diabetologia 2002;45:1550–1561.
68. Nielsen K, Sparre T, Larsen MR, et al. Protein expression changes in a cell system of beta-cell maturation reflect an acquired sensitivity to IL-1beta. Diabetologia 2004;47:62–74.
69. Sparre T, Reusens B, Cherif H, et al. Intrauterine programming of fetal islet gene expression in rats—effects of maternal protein restriction during gestation revealed by proteome analysis. Diabetologia 2003;46:1497–1511.
70. Christensen UB, Larsen PM, Fey SJ, et al. Islet protein expression changes during diabetes development in islet syngrafts in BB-DP rats and during rejection of BB-DP islet allografts. Autoimmunity 2000;32:1–15.
71. Sanchez JC, Converset V, Nolan A, et al. Effect of rosiglitazone on the differential expression of diabetes- associated proteins in pancreatic islets of C57Bl/6 lep/lep mice. Mol Cell Proteomics 2002;1:509–516.
72. Shen X, Zheng S, Thongboonkerd V, et al. Cardiac mitochondrial damage and biogenesis in a chronic model of type 1 diabetes. Am J Physiol Endocrinol Metab 2004;287:E896–E905.
73. Thongboonkerd V, Barati MT, McLeish KR, et al. Alterations in the renal elastin-elastase system in type 1 diabetic nephropathy identified by proteomic analysis. J Am Soc Nephrol 2004;15:650–662.
74. Thongboonkerd V, Barati MT, McLeish KR, Pierce WM, Epstein PN, Klein JB. Proteomics and diabetic nephropathy. In: Proteomics in Nephrology. Thongboonkerd V, Klein JB, eds. Basel: Karger, 2004:142–154.
75. Thongboonkerd V, Zheng S, McLeish KR, Epstein PN, Klein JB. Proteomic identification and immunolocalization of increased renal calbindin-D28k expression in OVE26 diabetic mice. Rev Diab Stud 2005;2:17–24.
76. Bickel CA, Knepper MA, Verbalis JG, Ecelbarger CA. Dysregulation of renal salt and water transport proteins in diabetic Zucker rats. Kidney Int 2002;61:2099–2110.
77. Song J, Knepper MA, Verbalis JG, Ecelbarger CA. Increased renal ENaC subunit and sodium transporter abundances in streptozotocin-induced type 1 diabetes. Am J Physiol Renal Physiol 2003;285: F1125–F1137.
78. Edvardsson U, Alexandersson M, Brockenhuus vL, et al. A proteome analysis of livers from obese (ob/ob) mice treated with the peroxisome proliferator WY14,643. Electrophoresis 1999;20: 935–942.
79. Sanchez JC, Converset V, Nolan A, et al. Effect of rosiglitazone on the differential expression of obesity and insulin resistance associated proteins in lep/lep mice. Proteomics 2003;3:1500–1520.
80. Edvardsson U, Brockenhuus vL, Panfilov O, Nystrom AC, Nilsson F, Dahllof B. Hepatic protein expression of lean mice and obese diabetic mice treated with peroxisome proliferator-activated receptor activators. Proteomics 2003;3:468–478.
81. Jiang M, Jia L, Jiang W, et al. Protein disregulation in red blood cell membranes of type 2 diabetic patients. Biochem Biophys Res Commun 2003;309:196–200.
82. Tsuneki H, Ishizuka M, Terasawa M, Wu JB, Sasaoka T, Kimura I. Effect of green tea on blood glucose levels and serum proteomic patterns in diabetic (db/db) mice and on glucose metabolism in healthy humans. BMC Pharmacol 2004;4:18.
83. Zhang R, Barker L, Pinchev D, et al. Mining biomarkers in human sera using proteomic tools. Proteomics 2004;4:244–256.
84. Mischak H, Kaiser T, Walden M, et al. Proteomic analysis for the assessment of diabetic renal damage in humans. Clin Sci (Lond) 2004;107:485–495.

85. Thongboonkerd V, Klein JB, Jevans AW, McLeish KR. Urinary proteomics and biomarker discovery for glomerular diseases. In: Thongboonkerd V, Klein JB, eds. Proteomics in Nephrology. Basel: Karger, 2004:292–307.
86. Yamane K, Minamoto A, Yamashita H, et al. Proteome analysis of human vitreous proteins. Mol Cell Proteomics 2003;2:1177–1187.
87. Brock JW, Hinton DJ, Cotham WE, et al. Proteomic analysis of the site specificity of glycation and carboxymethylation of ribonuclease. J Proteome Res 2003;2:506–513.
88. Lapolla A, Gerhardinger C, Baldo L, et al. A study on in vitro glycation processes by matrix-assisted laser desorption ionization mass spectrometry. Biochim Biophys Acta 1993;1225:33–38.
89. Lapolla A, Fedele D, Aronica R, et al. A highly specific method for the characterization of glycation and glycol-oxidation products of globins. Rapid Commun Mass Spectrom 1997;11:613–617.
90. Lapolla A, Fedele D, Aronica R, et al. Evaluation of IgG glycation levels by matrix-assisted laser desorption/ionization mass spectrometry. Rapid Commun Mass Spectrom 1997;11:1342–1346.
91. Lapolla A, Fedele D, Plebani M, et al. Evaluation of glycated globins by matrix-assisted laser desorption/ionization mass spectrometry. Clin Chem 1999;45:288–290.
92. Oh-Ishi M, Ueno T, Maeda T. Proteomic method detects oxidatively induced protein carbonyls in muscles of a diabetes model Otsuka Long-evans Tokushima Fatty (OLETF) rat. Free Radic Biol Med 2003;34:11–22.
93. Turko IV, Li L, Aulak KS, Stuehr DJ, Chang JY, Murad F. Protein tyrosine nitration in the mitochondria from diabetic mouse heart. Implications to dysfunctional mitochondria in diabetes. J Biol Chem 2003;278:33,972–33,977.
94. Hojlund K, Wrzesinski K, Larsen PM, et al. Proteome analysis reveals phosphorylation of ATP synthase beta -subunit in human skeletal muscle and proteins with potential roles in type 2 diabetes. J Biol Chem 2003;278:10,436–10,442.
95. Thongboonkerd V, Barati MT, McLeish KR, et al. Altered elastase inhibitor and elastin expression in type 2 diabetic kidneys defined by proteomic analysis. J Am Soc Nephrol 2003;14(Suppl):600A.
96. Carlson EC, Audette JL, Klevay LM, Nguyen H, Epstein PN. Ultrastructural and functional analyses of nephropathy in calmodulin- induced diabetic transgenic mice. Anat Rec 1997;247:9–19.
97. Epstein PN, Overbeek PA, Means AR. Calmodulin-induced early-onset diabetes in transgenic mice. Cell 1989;58:1067–1073.
98. Zheng S, Noonan WT, Metreveli NS, et al. Development of Late-Stage Diabetic Nephropathy in OVE26 Diabetic Mice. Diabetes 2004;53:3248–3257.
99. Sharma K, McCue P, Dunn SR. Diabetic kidney disease in the db/db mouse. Am J Physiol Renal Physiol 2003;284:F1138–F1144.
100. Geisler N, Plessmann U, Weber K. Amino acid sequence characterization of mammalian vimentin, the mesenchymal intermediate filament protein. FEBS Lett 1983;163:22–24.
101. Rastaldi MP, Ferrario F, Giardino L, et al. Epithelial–mesenchymal transition of tubular epithelial cells in human renal biopsies. Kidney Int 2002;62:137–146.
102. Dalley A, Smith JM, Reilly JT, Neil SM. Investigation of calmodulin and basic fibroblast growth factor (bFGF) in idiopathic myelofibrosis: evidence for a role of extracellular calmodulin in fibroblast proliferation. Br J Haematol 1996;93:856–862.
103. Uchio K, Tuchweber B, Manabe N, Gabbiani G, Rosenbaum J, Desmouliere A. Cellular retinol-binding protein-1 expression and modulation during in vivo and in vitro myofibroblastic differentiation of rat hepatic stellate cells and portal fibroblasts. Lab Invest 2002;82:619–628.
104. Sooy K, Kohut J, Christakos S. The role of calbindin and 1,25dihydroxyvitamin D3 in the kidney. Curr Opin Nephrol Hypertens 2000;9:341–347.
105. Borke JL, Caride A, Verma AK, Penniston JT, Kumar R. Plasma membrane calcium pump and 28-kDa calcium binding protein in cells of rat kidney distal tubules. Am J Physiol 1989;257:F842–F849.
106. Biner HL, Arpin-Bott MP, Loffing J, et al. Human cortical distal nephron: distribution of electrolyte and water transport pathways. J Am Soc Nephrol 2002;13:836–847.
107. Hoenderop JG, Hartog A, Stuiver M, Doucet A, Willems PH, Bindels RJ. Localization of the epithelial Ca(2+) channel in rabbit kidney and intestine. J Am Soc Nephrol 2000;11:1171–1178.
108. Hoenderop JG, Nilius B, Bindels RJ. Molecular mechanism of active Ca^{2+} reabsorption in the distal nephron. Annu Rev Physiol 2002;64:529–549.
109. Christakos S, Gabrielides C, Rhoten WB. Vitamin D-dependent calcium binding proteins: chemistry, distribution, functional considerations, and molecular biology. Endocr Rev 1989;10:3–26.
110. Koster HP, Hartog A, van Os CH, Bindels RJ. Calbindin-D28K facilitates cytosolic calcium diffusion without interfering with calcium signaling. Cell Calcium 1995;18:187–196.

111. Yang CW, Kim J, Kim YH, et al. Inhibition of calbindin D28K expression by cyclosporin A in rat kidney: the possible pathogenesis of cyclosporin A-induced hypercalciuria. J Am Soc Nephrol 1998;9:1416–1426.
112. Grenet O, Bobadilla M, Chibout SD, Steiner S. Evidence for the impairment of the vitamin D activation pathway by cyclosporine A. Biochem Pharmacol 2000;59:267–272.
113. Grenet O, Varela MC, Staedtler F, Steiner S. The cyclosporine A-induced decrease in rat renal calbindin-D28kDa protein as a consequence of a decrease in its mRNA. Biochem Pharmacol 1998;55:1131–1133.
114. Aicher L, Meier G, Norcross AJ, et al. Decrease in kidney calbindin-D 28kDa as a possible mechanism mediating cyclosporine A- and FK-506-induced calciuria and tubular mineralization. Biochem Pharmacol 1997;53:723–731.
115. Zheng W, Xie Y, Li G, Kong J, Feng JQ, Li YC. Critical role of calbindin-D28k in calcium homeostasis revealed by mice lacking both vitamin D receptor and calbindin-D28k. J Biol Chem 2004;279: 52,406–52,413.
116. Chau DL, Edelman SV, Chandran M. Osteoporosis and diabetes. Curr Diab Rep 2003;3:37–42.
117. Selby PL. Osteopenia and diabetes. Diabet Med 1988;5:423–428.
118. Malone JI, Lowitt S, Duncan JA, Shah SC, Vargas A, Root AW. Hypercalciuria, hyperphosphaturia, and growth retardation in children with diabetes mellitus. Pediatrics 1986;78:298–304.
119. Verhaeghe J, Van Herck E, Visser WJ, et al. Bone and mineral metabolism in BB rats with long-term diabetes. Decreased bone turnover and osteoporosis. Diabetes 1990;39:477–482.
120. Stone LA, Weaver VM, Bruns ME, Christakos S, Welsh J. Vitamin D receptors and compensatory tissue growth in spontaneously diabetic BB rats. Ann Nutr Metab 1991;35:196–202.
121. Ward DT, Yau SK, Mee AP, et al. Functional, molecular, and biochemical characterization of streptozotocin-induced diabetes. J Am Soc Nephrol 2001;12:779–790.
122. Anwana AB, Garland HO. Renal calcium and magnesium handling in experimental diabetes mellitus in the rat. Acta Endocrinol (Copenh) 1990;122:479–486.
123. Wu MJ, Lai LW, Lien YH. Cytoprotective effects of calbindin-D(28k) against antimycin-A induced hypoxic injury in proximal tubular cells. Life Sci 2002;71:559–569.
124. Rabinovitch A, Suarez-Pinzon WL, Sooy K, Strynadka K, Christakos S. Expression of calbindin-D(28k) in a pancreatic islet beta-cell line protects against cytokine-induced apoptosis and necrosis. Endocrinology 2001;142:3649–3655.
125. Christakos S, Barletta F, Huening M, et al. Vitamin D target proteins: function and regulation. J Cell Biochem 2003;88:238–244.
126. Chard PS, Bleakman D, Christakos S, Fullmer CS, Miller RJ. Calcium buffering properties of calbindin D28k and parvalbumin in rat sensory neurones. J Physiol 1993;472:341–357.
127. Guo Q, Sopher BL, Furukawa K, et al. Alzheimer's presenilin mutation sensitizes neural cells to apoptosis induced by trophic factor withdrawal and amyloid beta-peptide: involvement of calcium and oxyradicals. J Neurosci 1997;17:4212–4222.
128. Morel NM, Holland JM, van der GJ, et al. Primer on medical genomics. Part XIV: Introduction to systems biology—a new approach to understanding disease and treatment. Mayo Clin Proc 2004;79:651–658.
129. Ge H, Walhout AJ, Vidal M. Integrating 'omic' information: a bridge between genomics and systems biology. Trends Genet 2003;19:551–560.
130. Weston AD, Hood L. Systems biology, proteomics, and the future of health care: toward predictive, preventative, and personalized medicine. J Proteome Res 2004;3:179–196.
131. Thongboonkerd V, Klein E, Klein JB. Renal and urinary proteomics. In: Handbook of Proteomics Methods. Conn PM, ed. Humana Press Inc., Totowa, New Jersey: 2003:375–395.

15 Gene Expression Profiling in the Investigation of Diabetic Nephropathy

Katalin Susztak, PhD, MD, *Erwin Bottinger,* MD, *and Kumar Sharma,* MD

CONTENTS

INTRODUCTION

Diabetic nephropathy (DN) develops in about one-third of patients with diabetes, with genetic and environmental factors both contributing to the development of the disease. Clinical studies have established that hypertension, poor glycemic and lipid control, and smoking *(1)* increase the risk of the development of the disease. It is clear however, that environmental factors alone are not sufficient for the development of this complication *(2)*. In contrast, the prevalence of diabetic retinopathy continues to rise with the duration of diabetes in most populations. Family studies among type 1 diabetics have shown that if one sibling develops nephropathy, the other sibling has a fourfold increased risk of developing it *(3)*. These observations have clearly established the importance of genetic risk factors in the development of DN. It is likely that the genetic response to hyperglycemia varies among individuals and patients who develop a pattern of excessive regulation of nephropathy-related genes will be the ones at greatest risk of developing DN.

Current clinical practice lacks powerful diagnostic and predictive molecular approaches for accurate assessment of the risk for DN in individuals diagnosed with diabetes. Because both environmental and genetic factors play an important role in the disease, nonbiased approaches such as gene expression profiling may be particularly

From: *Contemporary Diabetes: The Diabetic Kidney*
Edited by: P. Cortes and C. E. Mogensen © Humana Press Inc., Totowa, NJ

useful to develop a gene expression profile of nephropathy-related genes and to identify new markers for progressive DN.

Apart from accurate diagnostic assessments, there is a paucity of directed therapies to arrest DN. The available therapies are able to slow the rate of progression, but do not arrest or reverse the disease. For example, the Diabetes Control and Complications trial and the UK Prospective Diabetes study showed the importance of strict glucose and blood pressure control in delaying diabetic complications *(2,4)*. Recently completed large studies showed that inhibition of the renin–angiotensin system by either angiotensin-converting enzyme inhibitors or angiotensin receptor blockers slows the progression of DN *(5)*. With gene expression profiling, novel and specific molecular drug targets may be developed with the potential to arrest the progression of DN altogether.

FUNCTIONAL GENOMICS

Functional genomics is the study of gene function through parallel expression measurements of a genome. The most common tools used to carry out these measurements include DNA microarrays, consisting of either oligonucleotide microarrays or serial analysis of gene expression (SAGE). Microarrays are artificially constructed grids of DNA, such that each element of the grid probes for a specific RNA sequence (i.e., each holds a DNA sequence that is a reverse complement to the target RNA sequence). The basic concept behind all microarrays is the precise positioning of DNA fragments (probes) at high density on a solid support so that they can act as molecular detectors. In practice, microarrays vary according to the solid support used (such as glass or filters), the surface modifications with various substrates, the type of DNA fragments on the array (such as cDNA, oligonucleotides, or genomic fragments), whether the gene fragments are presynthesized and deposited or synthesized *in situ*, and the machinery used to place the fragments on the array (such as ink-jet printing, spotting, mask, or micromirror-based *in situ* synthesis). Currently, combinations of these variables are used to generate three main types of microarray: filter arrays, spotted glass slide arrays, and *in situ*-synthesized oligonucleotide arrays. Both filter and spotted arrays are produced readily in academic facilities; they can also be purchased from commercial vendors. By contrast, arrays of oligonucleotides that are synthesized *in situ*, such as the Affymetrix GeneChip, require complex equipment and are only produced in commercial settings.

In gene expression microarrays, either synthetic oligonucleotides or cDNA fragments are used as probes. For most researchers, the ideal microarray for expression profiling would be a complex array of sequence-validated probes, in which each sequence is unique, shows minimal cross-hybridization to related sequences, and provides, collectively, a comprehensive representation of the expressed fraction of the genome including splice variants. In a similar way, a nonredundant set of fragments that provide a comprehensive representation of a genome would be ideal for carrying out comparative genomic hybridization. The sources of probe fragments used for arrays have been bacterial cDNA and bacterial artificial chromosome (BAC) clone sets, along with sets of long oligonucleotides. Considerable progress has been made in the past few years in improving the complexity and reliability of the cDNA and BAC clone sets. Frequently, these libraries contain a certain amount of redundancy, misannotation, and contamination. The production of complex, spotted oligonucleotide microarrays has become progressively more accessible as the cost of oligonucleotide synthesis has fallen and the yield of full-length long oligonucleotides or "longmers" has improved. Because oligonucleotide sets, unlike cDNA sets, are not limited by the availability of physical clones, in principle, sets could be generated in-house from sequence information. But the design of oligonucleotides is a complicated procedure and in practice, most investigators use commercially available oligonucleotide sets that encompass large numbers of genes ascertained from the latest draft of the relevant genomic sequence. The situation regarding purchase of arrays has changed markedly in the past few years as the price of commercial arrays has tumbled. Affymetrix GeneChip arrays have increased in complexity and in the number of species represented, and the unit cost per probe has decreased several-fold; thus, GeneChip arrays are now within the reach of academic users. Affymetrix has also introduced new arrays for single-nucleotide polymorphism analysis.

Although there are many protocols and types of systems available, the basic technique involves extraction of RNA from biological samples in either normal or interventional states. The RNA (or in some protocols isolated messenger RNA) is then copied, while incorporating either fluorescent nucleotides or a tag that is later stained with fluorescence. The labeled RNA is then hybridized to a microarray for a period of time, after which the excess is washed off and the microarray is scanned under laser light. With oligonucleotide microarrays, for which all probes have been designed to be theoretically similar regarding hybridization temperature and binding affinity, each microarray measures a single sample and provides an absolute measurement level for each RNA molecule. However, this absolute measurement may not correlate exactly with concentration in terms of micrograms per unit volume. With cDNA microarrays, for which each probe has its own hybridization characteristic, each microarray measures two samples, and provides a relative measurement level for each RNA molecule. Regardless of the technique, the end result is 4000–50,000 measurements of gene expression per biological sample.

Similar to microarrays, SAGE is a high-throughput expression profiling technique well suited to gene discovery. It provides a quantifiable inventory of all transcripts in a cell or tissue at one point in time, requiring no *a priori* assumptions about gene expression.

As the cost of microarrays continues to drop, it is clear that microarrays are becoming more integral to the drug discovery process. In addition to the obvious use of functional genomics in basic research and target discovery, there are many other specific uses in this domain. These include biomarker determination, to find genes that correlate with and presage disease progression, but are easier to measure and follow in clinical trials; pharmacology, to determine differences in gene expression in tissues exposed to various doses of compounds; toxicogenomics, to find gene expression patterns in a model tissue or organism exposed to a compound and their use as early predictors of adverse events in humans; prognostic tests, to find a set of genes that accurately distinguishes one disease from another; and disease subclass determination, to find multiple subcategories of a disease process within a single clinical diagnosis.

Methodological Issues in Gene Profiling With Kidney Tissue

To date, the feasibility of finding diagnostic and outcome predictor "biomarker genes" of human diseases based on gene expression profiling have been demonstrated for various malignancies, including acute leukemia *(6)*, breast cancer *(6)*, and lung cancer *(7)*. In comparison with studies on tumor material, the application of microarray studies to human DN poses different challenges *(8)*. Highly sensitive and reproducible methods are needed to assess gene expression profiles in limited amount of available tissue.

The standard normal vs diseased tissue type of comparison, which is currently the basic design principle of profiling studies, carries the limitation that gene expression profile in "normal" tissue is still not well characterized. Garonne et al. *(9)* performed pioneering work on gene expression analysis along the human nephron. The transcriptome of isolated glomeruli and seven different nephron segments via microdissection from fresh tissue specimens was characterized using the SAGE method. More than 400,000 mRNA SAGE tags were sequenced, making it possible to detect transcripts present at 18 copies per cell with a 95% confidence level. Expression of genes responsible for ion transport and permeability was evidenced, as were transcripts for 119 solute carriers, 84 channels, 43 ion-transport ATPases, and 12 claudins. Searching for differences between the transcriptomes, 998 transcripts were found to greatly vary in abundance from one nephron segment to another. Clustering analysis of these transcripts demonstrated different extents of similarity between the nephron portions. Approximately 75% of the differentially distributed transcripts corresponded to cDNAs of known or unknown function that are accurately mapped in the human genome. This systematic large-scale analysis of individual structures of a complex human tissue reveals sets of genes underlying the function of well-defined nephron portions. It also provides quantitative expression data for a variety of genes mutated in hereditary diseases and helps in sorting candidate genes for renal diseases that affect specific portions of the human nephron. However, gene expression in normal tissue is likely to be dependent on several factors, including the patient's sex, age, and genetic background. Therefore, larger studies will be necessary to describe gene expression profiles in the range of "normal/healthy" gene expression levels.

Hsiao et al. created a compendium of gene expression in normal human tissues, including the kidney, suitable as a reference for defining basic organ systems biology *(10)*. Using oligonucleotide microarrays, they analyzed 59 samples representing 19 distinct tissue types. Their compendium reveals similarities and differences among organs and tissues and also provides a publicly available resource (Human Gene Expression Index, the HuGE Index, http://www.hugeindex.org). A recent study by Higgins et al. *(11)* characterized gene expression in discrete human nephron compartments. Using a custom cDNA microarray, cluster of genes expressed in glomerulus, tubules, medulla, papilla, and pelvis were tabulated. The identification of the specific gene expression profiles in each compartment will be invaluable for future comparisons and for identifying novel functional roles of each compartment in physiology and pathophysiology.

A major limitation for studies of human diabetic renal disease at a molecular level is that current clinical practice usually does not require tissue analysis to establish the diagnosis of DN. In cases in which kidney biopsy material is available, interpretation may be confounded by tissue heterogeneity. The proportion of glomeruli and different tubular segments present in the biopsy material can vary significantly; therefore different cell types can be present in different proportion among different samples. Pioneering studies by Kretzler et al. *(8)* have established that manual microdissection of fresh renal biopsy cores is an effective approach that allows efficient separation of glomeruli and tubuli in experienced hands. Laser capture microdissection (LCM) technology *(12,13)* is a powerful alternative to manual microdissection. LCM allows accurate identification and procurement of glomerular or tubular cells from tissue samples under direct microscopic visualization. Archived samples can also be analyzed with LCM, however, a major drawback of this technique is the low amount and often inadequate quality of mRNA that is extracted from fixed or frozen tissue. Thus, adequate quality control for

RNA integrity is paramount for each sample obtained by LCM. Because renal biopsies represent a minute fraction of the diseased organ, considerable sample bias is also inevitable. A representative number of glomeruli are required to obtain adequate profiles. Detailed histopathological examination of the biopsy material, including light and electron microscopic analysis, can help to overcome these difficulties.

Technical challenges pose significant additional problems. A major issue is the stability of the mRNA. Several promising technical innovations have been developed to overcome this problem. A new class of RNAse inhibitors provided in commercial reagents (i.e., RNALater from Ambion™) allows good preservation of RNA. New column-based RNA extraction methods provide high-quality RNA quickly with minimal loss during extraction. RNA quantification and quality measurements are critical steps for gene expression studies. A new technology (Lab-on-Chip) *(14)*, which is based on capillary gel electrophoresis, has revolutionized this field and as little as picogram quantities of RNA can now be accurately analyzed.

Another major limitation for DNA array-based technologies was that earlier assays required a large amount (20–100 μg) of high-quality total RNA as a starting material. Recently, new technologies with improved RNA amplification and labeling have become available *(15,16)*. A major concern is the linearity of the amplification across different mRNA species. With highly effective amplification, even small differences in amplification efficiencies can result in significantly distorted representation of individual transcripts. It is now generally recommended that microarray analysis also employ a "universal standard" that is the same among the different array studies. This allows for a more reliable comparison of data and decreases technical variations from experiment to experiment.

Microarrays deliver massive amounts of data on 10s of 1000s of genes. The result is an immense quantity of biological information that needs to be analyzed, presented, and archived in a meaningful way. Therefore, functional genomic studies should be combined with advanced computational and biostatistical approaches. The gene expression data have to be analyzed in conjunction with patient and sample variables. Additionally, potential gene candidates must be assessed for relevance to disease using parallel technologies, methods at the RNA and protein level, and more importantly in functional studies. Many such programs now exist for meaningful analysis of microarray data, and the comparison of these are beyond the scope of the current manuscript. Genespring™, GeneTraffic, and BioConductor are some of the most frequently used ones. Standard approaches include cluster analysis, hierarchical clustering, *K* nearest neighborhood analysis, and predictive modeling.

A key issue is the adequate prospective design of a microarray-based study. Adequate samples should be analyzed initially based on the likely number of genes that will be deregulated and the range of expression. Subsequent to the discovery mode, and after data analysis, predictive gene expression profiles should be evaluated in a separate cohort of samples. However, most of the published studies using microarray-based expression analysis have included only a limited numbers of replicates. In fact, many studies conduct the experiment only once. Considering the potential sources of assay variation, the need for sufficiently replicated studies is underscored.

On statistically identifying a list of relevant genes, a validation step is necessary. Typically, real-time polymerase chain reaction analysis is performed on the genes of interest in the same pool of RNA that was subjected to microarray analysis. After validation, it is optimal to then use statistical modeling to use the key classifier genes to predict disease phenotype in a separate cohort of samples. Various approaches can be employed to fulfill these pathways.

GENE EXPRESSION PROFILING IN HUMAN DIABETIC NEPHROPATHY

Bruijn and colleagues *(17)* were able to overcome some of the limitations and had published gene expression analysis of kidneys from healthy patients and those with DN. They determined gene expression levels in two morphologically normal kidneys and in two kidneys from patients with DN. Glomerular RNA was hybridized in duplicate on Human Genome U95Av2 Arrays (Affymetrix, Santa Clara, CA). They found that 96 genes were upregulated in diabetic glomeruli, whereas 519 genes were downregulated. The list of overexpressed genes in DN included aquaporin 1, calpain 3, hyaluronoglucosidase, and platelet/endothelial cell adhesion molecule. The list of downregulated genes included bone morphogenetic protein 2, vascular endothelial growth factor, fibroblast growth factor 1, insulin-like growth factor binding protein 2, and nephrin. A decrease in vascular endothelial growth factor and nephrin was validated at the protein level and also at the RNA level in renal biopsy specimens from five additional patients with diabetes. One of the limitations of their study was that it was performed in kidneys from a total of four patients, therefore analysis of gene expression heterogeneity in "healthy" and "diseased" tissue was not possible. In addition, because the study was performed on cadaveric kidneys it raised concern whether it added unnecessary bias to the results.

FUNCTIONAL GENOMIC STUDIES OF KIDNEYS IN EXISTING RODENT MODELS OF DIABETES

Because of the difficulties that researchers encountered with gene expression studies on human diabetic kidney biopsy materials, a number of investigators have performed gene expression studies in animal models of DN. One of the earliest studies was from Wada et al. *(18)*. This group analyzed gene expression in the kidneys of streptozotocin (STZ)-induced diabetic mice using high-density DNA filter arrays. They had four experimental groups: controls (CD-1 mice), unilaterally nephrectomized mice, STZ-induced diabetic (STZ) mice, and STZ mice with unilateral renal ablation. Pathological changes were examined at 24 wk after the induction of diabetes. The gene expression profile was compared between the control and STZ-treated mice by a cDNA arrays. The uninephrectomized mouse kidney showed prominent glomerular hypertrophy with minimal mesangial matrix accumulation. Both the STZ-treated and the uninephrectomized STZ-treated mice had significant glomerular hypertrophy and glomerulosclerosis, and the lesions were not enhanced by renal ablation. The comparison between control and STZ mice identified 16 clones with increased in expression with the induction of diabetes and 65 clones that decreased in diabetic kidneys were identified. The 37 known genes were related to glucose and lipid metabolism, ion transport, transcription factors, signaling molecules, and extracellular matrix (ECM)-related molecules. The genes known to be involved in cell differentiation and organogenesis in various tissues (i.e., Unc-18 homolog, POU domain transcription factor 2, lunatic fringe gene homolog, fibrous sheath component 1, Sox-17, fibulin 2, and MRJ) were found to be differentially expressed in the early phase of diabetic kidneys.

Simonson et al. *(19)* published gene expression profiling of whole kidneys of newly diabetic and long-standing diabetic db/db mice on BKLS background. They had found significant mesangial expansion in this model by 16 wk of age. By using Affymetrix expression arrays they had found 639 RNA transcripts differentially regulated in control vs 16-wk-old diabetic animals. Interestingly, diabetic kidneys specifically expressed several genes normally found in adipocytes, including adipocyte differentiation-regulated protein (ADRP; or adipophilin in humans). ADRP mRNA was specifically upregulated 5.4-fold in 16-wk db/db kidneys. This finding was confirmed at the protein level by Western blotting, and immunohistochemistry localized ADRP diffusely to tubular epithelium throughout the cortex. ADRP is a perilipin family protein that forms lipid storage vesicles and controls triglyceride utilization; they showed that accumulation of lipid storage droplets correlated with the magnitude and localization of ADRP in db/db kidneys. Other genes involved in lipid transport, oxidation, and storage were differentially regulated in db/db kidneys, and peroxisome proliferator-activated receptor (PPAR)α has been shown to regulate their expression in adipocytes. PPARα mRNA was elevated in db/db diabetic kidneys, and PPARα protein was upregulated in glomeruli, cortical tubules, and renal arterial vessels of db/db mice.

Wilson et al. *(20)* performed gene expression profiling of cDNA arrays (containing 5760 clones) in the kidneys of three groups of non-obese diabetic (NOD) mice: nondiabetic, new-onset, and long-term diabetic. A total of 27 genes had lower expression and 1 gene (Gpx3) had higher expression in the new-onset diabetic mice compared with nondiabetic control NOD mice ($p < 0.001$). Similarly, 19 of the above 27 genes and 7 additional genes had higher expression and the Gpx3 gene had lower expression in long-term diabetic mice compared with controls ($p < 0.001$). Interestingly, only three genes were different between new-onset and long-term diabetic mice ($p < 0.0004$). These genes are from diverse functional groups, including oxidative phosphorylation, free radical neutralization, channels, pumps, lipid processing, transcription, and translation machinery, protein trafficking, constitutive protein processing, and immune function. The majority of these genes fall into four signaling pathways: insulin, transforming growth factor-β, tumor necrosis factor-α, and peroxisome proliferator-activated receptor. The most significant expression change was found for the stearoyl-coenzyme A desaturase 1 gene ($p < 10^{-7}$). The lower expression levels of the stearoyl-coenzyme A desaturase 1 gene in both diabetic groups compared with controls were further confirmed by Northern blot analysis and immunohistochemistry.

An interesting study by Feng et al. *(21)* aimed to combine gene expression profiling and quantitative trait loci (QTL) analysis to identify susceptibility genes for DN. They used the Affymetrix GeneChip® Expression Analysis system to survey the gene expression profile of diabetic KK/Ta mouse kidneys. Profiling was performed in kidneys from three KK/Ta and two BALB/c mice at 20 wk of age. The gene expression profile was compared between KK/Ta and BALB/c mice using GeneChip expression analysis software. Out of 12,490 probe pairs present on GeneChip, 98 known genes and 31 expressed sequence tags (ESTs) were found to be differentially expressed between KK/Ta and BALB/c kidneys. Twenty-one known genes and 7 ESTs that increased in expression and 77 known genes and 24 ESTs that decreased in KK/Ta kidneys were identified. The differentially expressed genes are related to renal function, ECM expansion and degradation, signal transduction, transcription regulation, ion transport, glucose and lipid metabolism, and protein synthesis and degradation. In the vicinity of UA-1 (QTL for the development of albuminuria in KK/Ta mice), candidate genes that showed differential expression were identified, including the *Sdc4* gene for syndecan-4, *Ahcy* gene for *S*-adenosylhomocysteine hydrolase, *Sstr4* gene for somatostatin receptor 4, and *MafB* gene for Kreisler leucine zipper protein.

One of the major limitations of these studies was that a single animal model was compared with control nondiabetic mice and in some studies small number of microarrays was used. As there are multiple phenotypic differences that can be observed in the various diabetic animal models (i.e., presence or absence of obesity, presence or absence of STZ, high or low insulin levels, presence or absence of albuminuria, mesangial expansion, and so on), it is difficult to select gene sets from microarray datasets that are associated with a single phenotypic outcome (i.e., albuminuria or development of diabetic glomerulosclerosis). In addition, most investigators use inbred mice to avoid genetic and phenotypic heterogeneity, which allows the investigator to use fewer numbers of chips, but the lack of the spectrum of the disease makes it difficult to associate single phenotypic outcome with gene expression profile changes.

Gene Expression Profiling in Diabetic Nephropathy With Structure–Function Correlation

To screen for genes that show correlation with different phenotypic outcome in diabetic mouse models, we used a cross-sectional design and performed microarray analysis on 24-wk-old STZ-treated C57B6J and 129svJ mice and db/db mice with established renal pathology *(22)*. In parallel with functional genomics characterization, each individual mouse underwent a detailed renal phenotype analysis. Mice treated with low-dose STZ (50 mg/kg ipx5 doses) developed diabetes and moderately severe albuminuria (twice the control). In mice with C57B6/J background, the mesangial changes were mild or absent. Mice with 129SvJ genetic background, developed significant glomerular changes. However, these were not significantly different from the age-matched controls. The db/db mice are insulin resistant and developed type 2 diabetes at 8 wk of age. Albuminuria was detected as early as 3–4 wk after the development of hyperglycemia. The glomerular histology was characterized by severe diffuse mesangial expansion, as previously reported *(23,24)*.

This experimental design allowed for grouping of animals based on the phenotypic outcome rather than on their underlying genotype. To identify genes with correlation to certain phenotypes, statistical analysis of microarray data was performed *(25)*. We used supervised data-mining algorithms to find genes with high discriminative value for a certain phenotypic outcome (hyperglycemia and mesangial pathology). This method is based on the *K* nearest-neighborhood algorithm. The nearest-neighborhood supervised method first constructs hypothetical gene expression profile that best fit the desired pattern (e.g., a gene with high expression in hyperglycemic animals and low expression in animals with normal glucose values, or vice versa). The technique then identifies individual genes that are most similar to the hypothetical gene expression profile. Other supervised methods are based on support vector machines and artificial neuronal networks *(6,26–28)*. Unsupervised methods can also be used to answer different questions. The main advantage of these methods is that they could uncover new unexpected subclasses within the same diseased group. However, in general they are less intuitive. From these methods, we used hierarchical clustering in the initial phase of the analysis. It sorted all genes (or samples), such that similar genes appear near each other. The number and size of expression patterns within a data set can be estimated quickly, although the division of the tree into actual clusters is often performed visually.

Functional genomic analysis on different diabetic mouse models provided a global view into the pathomechanisms of DN. We identified hydroxysteroid dehydrogenase-3β isotype 4, and osteopontin as lead classifier genes in relation to the mesangial matrix expansion phenotype. We used the expression levels of these genes in the kidney to classify a separate group of animals for the absence or presence of diabetic glomerulopathy with a high degree of precision. Immunohistochemical analysis of murine and human diabetic kidney samples showed that both markers were expressed in podocytes in the glomeruli and followed regulation similar to that observed in the microarray. A similar type of analysis led to the identification of CD36 as a lead classifier in relation to hyperglycemia and albuminuria. CD36 was recently found to be increased in proximal tubular cells in human DN and mediate tubular cell apoptosis advanced glycosylation endproducts and free fatty acids *(29)*. Thus, the application of phenotype-based statistical modeling approaches with microarray may lead to the identification of new markers for the development of diabetic kidney disease.

CONCLUSIONS

Functional genomic approaches combined with advanced phenotypic characterization and computational algorithms are new powerful methods. Application of these methods for DN shows great promise but also poses challenges for investigators. Microarrays make it possible to investigate differential gene expression in normal vs diseased tissue, in treated vs nontreated tissue, and in different stages during the natural course of a disease, all on a genomic scale. Gene expression profiles may help to unlock the molecular basis of phenotype, response to treatment, and heterogeneity of disease. They may also help to define patterns of expression that will aid in diagnosis as well as define susceptibility loci that may lead to the identification of individuals at risk. Finally, as specific genes are identified and their functional roles in the development and course of disease are characterized, new targets for therapy should emerge. The overall goal is to obtain complementary information that allows a stringent prediction concerning the diagnosis, prognosis and differential therapy of DN.

REFERENCES

1. Parving HH. Diabetic nephropathy: prevention and treatment. Kidney Int 2001;60:2041–2055.
2. Group TDCaCDR. Effect of intensive therapy on the development and progression of diabetic nephropathy in the Diabetes Control and Complications Trial. Kidney Int 1995;47:1703–1720.
3. Seaquist ER, Goetz FC, Rich S, Barbosa J. Familial clustering of diabetic kidney disease. Evidence for genetic susceptibility to diabetic nephropathy. N Eng J Med 1989;320:1161–1165.
4. Group UPDS. Tight blood pressure control and risk of macrovascular and microvascular complications in type 2 diabetes. BMJ 1998;317:703–713.
5. Lewis E, Hunsicker L, Bain R, Rohde R. The effect of angiotensin-converting-enzyme inhibition on diabetic nephropathy. N Eng J Med 1993;329:1456–1462.
6. Golub T, Slonim D, Tamayo P, et al. Molecular classification of cancer: class discovery and class prediction by gene expression. Science 1999;286:531–537.
7. van de Vijver M, He Y, van't Veer L, et al. A gene-expression signature as a predictor of survival in breast cancer. N Eng J Med 2002;13:1961–1972.
8. Kretzler M, Cohen C, Doran P, et al. Repuncturing the renal biopsy: strategies for molecular diagnosis in nephrology. J Am Soc Nephrol 2002;13:1961–1972.
9. Chabardes-Garrone D, Mejean A, Aude J, et al. A panoramic view of gene expression in the human kidney. Proc Natl Acad Sci USA 2003;100:13,710–13,715.
10. Hsiao L, Dangond F, Yoshida T, et al. A compendium of gene expression in normal human tissues. Physiol Genomics. 2001;7:97–104.
11. Higgins J, Wang L, Kambham N, et al. Gene expression in the normal adult human kidney assessed by complementary DNA microarray. Mol Biol Cell 2004;15:649–656.

12. Bonner R, Emmert-Buck M, Cole K, et al. Laser capture microdissection: molecular analysis of tissue. Science 1997;278:1481–1483.
13. Aaltonen P, Luimula P, Astrom E, et al. Changes in the expression of nephrin gene and protein in experimental diabetic nephropathy. Lab Invest 2001;81:1185–1190.
14. Gottwald E, Muller O, Polten A. Semiquantitative reverse transcription-polymerase chain reaction with the Agilent 2100 bioanalyzer. Electrophoresis 2001;22:4016–4022.
15. Xiang C, Kozhich O, Chen M, et al. Amine-modified random primers to label probes for DNA microarrays. Nat Biotechnol 2002;20:738–742.
16. Iscove N, Barbara M, Gu M, Gibson M, Modi C, Winegarden N. Representation is faithfully preserved in global cDNA amplified exponentially from sub-picogram quantities of mRNA. Nat Biotechnol 2002;20:940–943.
17. Baelde H, Eikmans M, Doran P, Lappin D, de Heer E, Brujin J. Gene expression profiling in glomeruli from human kidneys with diabetic nephropathy. Am J Kidney Disease 2004;43:636–650.
18. Wada J, Zhang H, Tsuchiyama Y, et al. Gene expression profile in streptozotocin-induced diabetic mice kidneys undergoing glomerulosclerosis. Kidney Int 2001;59:1363–1373.
19. Mishra R, Emancipator S, Miller C, Kern T, Simonson M. Adipose differentiation-related protein and regulators of lipid homeostasis identified by gene expression profiling in the murine db/db diabetic kidney. Am J Physiol Renal Physiol 2004;286:F913–F921.
20. Wilson K, Eckenrode S, Li Q, et al. Microarray analysis of gene expression in the kidneys of new- and post-onset diabetic NOD mice. Diabetes 2003;52:2151–2159.
21. Fan Q, Shike T, Shigihara T, et al. Gene expression profile in diabetic KK/Ta mice. Kidney Int 2003;64:1978–1985.
22. Susztak K, Bottinger E, Novetsky A, et al. Molecular profiling of diabetic mouse kidney reveals novel genes linked to glomerular disease. Diabetes 2004;53:784–794.
23. Sharma K, McCue P, Dunn SR. Diabetic kidney disease in the db/db mouse. Am J Physiol Renal Physiol 2003;284:F1138–F1144.
24. Ziyadeh F, Hoffman B, Han D, et al. Long-term prevention of renal insufficiency, excess matrix gene expression, and glomerular mesangial matrix expansion by treatment with monoclonal anti-transforming growth factor-beta antibody in db/db diabetic mice. Proc Natl Acad Sci USA 2000;97:8015–8020.
25. Tusher V, Tibshirani R, Chu G. Significance analysis of microarrays applied to the ionizing radiation response. Proc Natl Acad Sci USA 2001;98:5116–5121.
26. Khan J, Wei J, Ringner M, et al. Classification and diagnostic prediction of cancers using gene expression profiling and artificial neural networks. Nat Med 2001;7:673–679.
27. Butte A. The use and analysis of microarray data. Nat Rev Drug Discov 2002;1:951–960.
28. Yang Y, Speed T. Design issues for cDNA microarray experiments. Nat Rev Genet 2002;3: 579–588.
29. Susztak K, Ciccone E, McCue P, Sharma K, Bottinger E. Multiple metabolic hits converge on CD36 as novel mediator of tubular epithelial apoptosis in diabetic nephropathy. PLoS Med 2005;2:e45.

SUGGESTED READINGS

1. Parving HH: Diabetic nephropathy: prevention and treatment. Kidney Int 2001;60:2041–2055.
2. Effect of intensive therapy on the development and progression of diabetic nephropathy in the Diabetes Control and Complications Trial. The Diabetes Control and Complications (DCCT) Research Group. Kidney Int 1995;47:1703–1720.
3. Seaquist ER, Goetz FC, Rich S, Barbosa J. Familial clustering of diabetic kidney disease. Evidence for genetic susceptibility to diabetic nephropathy. N Engl J Med 1989;320:1161–1165.
4. Tight blood pressure control and risk of macrovascular and microvascular complications in type 2 diabetes. UKPDS 38. UK Prospective Diabetes Study Group. BMJ 1998;317:703–713.
5. Brenner BM, Cooper ME, de Zeeuw D, et al. Effects of losartan on renal and cardiovascular outcomes in patients with type 2 diabetes and nephropathy. N Engl J Med 2001;345:861–869.
6. Lewis EJ, Hunsicker LG, Bain RP, Rohde RD. The effect of angiotensin-converting-enzyme inhibition on diabetic nephropathy. The Collaborative Study Group. N Engl J Med 1993;329: 1456–1462.
7. Golub TR, Slonim DK, Tamayo P, et al. Molecular classification of cancer: class discovery and class prediction by gene expression monitoring. Science 1999;286:531–537.

8. Perou CM, Sorlie T, Eisen MB, et al. Molecular portraits of human breast tumours. Nature 2000;406:747–752.
9. van de Vijver MJ, He YD, van't Veer LJ, et al. A gene-expression signature as a predictor of survival in breast cancer. N Engl J Med 2002;347:1999–2009.
10. Kretzler M, Cohen CD, Doran P, et al. Repuncturing the renal biopsy: strategies for molecular diagnosis in nephrology. J Am Soc Nephrol 2002;13:1961–1972.
11. Chabardes-Garonne D, Mejean A, Aude JC, et al. A panoramic view of gene expression in the human kidney. Proc Natl Acad Sci USA 2003;100:13,710–13,715.
12. Serra A, Romero R, Bayes B, Lopez D, Bonet J. Is there a need for changes in renal biopsy criteria in proteinuria in type 2 diabetes? Diabetes Res Clin Pract 2002;58:149.
13. Bonner RF, Emmert-Buck M, Cole K, et al. Laser capture microdissection: molecular analysis of tissue. Science 1997;278:1481–1483.
14. Aaltonen P, Luimula P, Astrom E, et al. Changes in the expression of nephrin gene and protein in experimental diabetic nephropathy. Lab Invest 2001;81:1185–1190.
15. Gottwald E, Muller O, Polten A. Semiquantitative reverse transcription-polymerase chain reaction with the Agilent 2100 Bioanalyzer. Electrophoresis 2001;22:4016–4022.
16. Xiang CC, Kozhich OA, Chen M, et al. Amine-modified random primers to label probes for DNA microarrays. Nat Biotechnol 2002;20:738–742.
17. Iscove NN, Barbara M, Gu M, Gibson M, Modi C, Winegarden N. Representation is faithfully preserved in global cDNA amplified exponentially from sub-picogram quantities of mRNA. Nat Biotechnol 2002;20:940–943.
18. Baelde HJ, Eikmans M, Doran PP, Lappin DW, de Heer E, Bruijn JA. Gene expression profiling in glomeruli from human kidneys with diabetic nephropathy. Am J Kidney Dis 2004;43:636–650.
19. Mauer SM, Steffes MW, Ellis EN, Sutherland DE, Brown DM, Goetz FC. Structural-functional relationships in diabetic nephropathy. J Clin Invest 1984;74:1143–1155.
20. Velasquez MT, Kimmel PL, Michaelis OE. Animal models of spontaneous diabetic kidney disease. FASEB J 1990;4:2850–2859.
21. Sharma K, Jin Y, Guo J, Ziyadeh FN: Neutralization of TGF-beta by anti-TGF-beta antibody attenuates kidney hypertrophy and the enhanced extracellular matrix gene expression in STZ-induced diabetic mice. Diabetes 1996;45:522–530.
22. Hall-Craggs M, Brenner DE, Vigorito RD, Sutherland JC: Acute renal failure and renal tubular squamous metaplasia following treatment with streptozotocin. Hum Pathol 1982;13:597–601.
23. Sharma K, Ziyadeh FN. Renal hypertrophy is associated with upregulation of TGF-beta 1 gene expression in diabetic BB rat and NOD mouse. Am J Physiol 1994;267:F1094–F1101.
24. Haseyama T, Fujita T, Hirasawa F, et al. Complications of IgA nephropathy in a non-insulin-dependent diabetes model, the Akita mouse. Tohoku J Exp Med 2002;198:233–244.
25. Doolittle, DP. Mouse Locus Catalog. http//www.informatics.jax.orgJune. 1998. ref type: generic
26. Wehner H. Sequence of changes in KK mouse nephropathy. Adv Exp Med Biol 1988;246:147–156.
27. Yamamoto Y, Kato I, Doi T, et al. Development and prevention of advanced diabetic nephropathy in RAGE- overexpressing mice. J Clin Invest 2001;108:261–268.
28. Pugliese G, Pricci F, Iacobini C, et al. Accelerated diabetic glomerulopathy in galectin-3/AGE receptor 3 knockout mice. FASEB J 2001;15:2471–2479.
29. Sun L, Halaihel N, Zhang W, Rogers T, Levi M. Role of sterol regulatory element-binding protein 1 in regulation of renal lipid metabolism and glomerulosclerosis in diabetes mellitus. J Biol Chem 2002;277:18,919–18,927.
30. Wada J, Zhang H, Tsuchiyama Y, et al. Gene expression profile in streptozotocin-induced diabetic mice kidneys undergoing glomerulosclerosis. Kidney Int 2001;59:1363–1373.
31. Mishra R, Emancipator SN, Miller C, Kern T, Simonson MS. Adipose differentiation-related protein and regulators of lipid homeostasis identified by gene expression profiling in the murine db/db diabetic kidney. Am J Physiol Renal Physiol 2004;286:F913–F921.
32. Wilson KH, Eckenrode SE, Li QZ, et al. Microarray analysis of gene expression in the kidneys of new- and post-onset diabetic NOD mice. Diabetes 2003;52:2151–2159.
33. Susztak K, Bottinger E, Novetsky A, et al. Molecular profiling of diabetic mouse kidney reveals novel genes linked to glomerular disease. Diabetes 2004;53:784–794.
34. Ziyadeh FN, Hoffman BB, Han DC, et al. Long-term prevention of renal insufficiency, excess matrix gene expression, and glomerular mesangial matrix expansion by treatment with monoclonal anti-transforming growth factor-beta antibody in db/db diabetic mice. Proc Natl Acad Sci USA 2000;97:8015–8020.

35. Tusher VG, Tibshirani R, Chu G. Significance analysis of microarrays applied to the ionizing radiation response. Proc Natl Acad Sci USA 2001;98:5116–5121.
36. Khan J, Wei JS, Ringner M, et al. Classification and diagnostic prediction of cancers using gene expression profiling and artificial neural networks. Nat Med 2001;7:673–679.
37. Butte A. The use and analysis of microarray data. Nat Rev Drug Discov 2002;1:951–960.
38. Yang YH, Speed T. Design issues for cDNA microarray experiments. Nat Rev Genet 2002;3:579–588.

16 PPAR-γ Ligands and Diabetic Nephropathy

Keiji Isshiki, MD, PhD, *Daisuke Koya,* MD, PhD, *and Masakazu Haneda,* MD, PhD

Contents

INTRODUCTION

Peroxisome proliferator-activated receptors (PPARs), originally cloned in an attempt to identify the molecular mediators of peroxisome proliferation in the liver of rodents, are ligand-activated transcription factors belonging to the nuclear hormone receptor superfamily *(1,2)*. To date, three isoforms (PPAR-α, -β/δ, and -γ) have been cloned and characterized by their unique expression patterns, different ligand-binding specificity, and distinct metabolic functions *(3)*. On ligand binding, PPARs form heterodimers with retinoid X receptor (RXR) proteins and bind to PPAR response elements within the promoter regions of target genes. A variety of natural and synthetic ligands for PPARs have been identified. As natural ligands for PPAR-α, some polyunsaturated fatty acids (FAs), oxidized phospholipids, and lipoprotein can activate PPAR-α *(4)*. 15-Deoxy-δ-12, 14-prostaglandin J_2 (15dPGJ_2) derived from prostaglandin D_2 can activate PPAR-γ as a natural ligand *(5)*. Among synthetic ligands, the hypolipidemic fibrate drugs such as fenofibrate and gemfibrozil bind to PPAR-α *(6,7)*. Thiazolidinediones (TZDs) such as troglitazone, pioglitazone, and rosiglitazone, are well-known synthetic ligands for PPAR-γ *(8)*. PPARs have been reported to regulate diverse cell functions, including FA metabolism, adipocyte differentiation, inflammation, atherosclerosis, and cell cycle *(9–12)*. PPAR-α has an important role in lipid metabolism, especially in the liver *(7)*. It is suggested that PPAR-β/δ carries out the effects in cell survival and carcinogenesis in the colon *(13)*. PPAR-γ plays a pivotal role in adipogenesis and its activation by TZDs improves insulin sensitivity through adipocyte differentiation *(14)*. TZDs have been

From: *Contemporary Diabetes: The Diabetic Kidney*
Edited by: P. Cortes and C. E. Mogensen © Humana Press Inc., Totowa, NJ

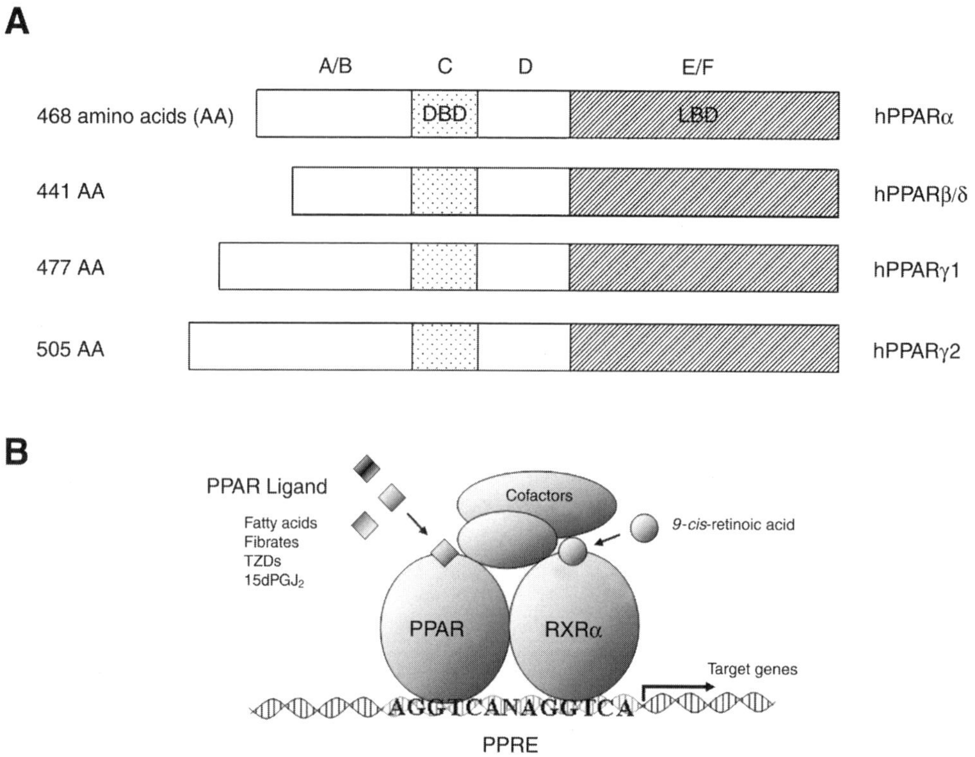

Fig. 1. Structure and action of PPARs. **(A)** Domain structure of human PPARs. **(B)** Molecular mechanism of PPAR activation. After ligand binding, PPARs undergo conformational changes with association of RXR and cofactors.

widely used as oral antidiabetic agents for treatment of type 2 diabetes *(14,15)*. Therefore, many basic investigators and clinical researches are engaged in clarifying the role of PPARs the physiology and pathophysiology of multiple diseases such as diabetes, obesity, hypertension, atherosclerosis, and cancer.

In this chapter, evidence regarding the role of PPARs and their ligands, especially PPAR-γ ligands and diabetic nephropathy, will be briefly reviewed.

STRUCTURE OF PPARs

Since the first identification of PPAR from mouse cDNA library in 1990 *(2)*, three isoforms of PPAR have been cloned: PPAR-α, -β/δ, and -γ (Fig. 1) *(3)*. Although there are no splicing variants of PPAR-α and PPAR-β/δ mRNA, PPAR-γ mRNA has three splicing forms derived from a single gene in human *(16)*. As result of the translation of each of three PPAR-γ mRNA, two PPAR-γ protein isoforms exist; PPAR-γ1 and -γ2 *(17)*. PPAR-γ1 and PPAR-γ3 mRNA give rise to the same protein, PPAR-γ1. PPAR-γ2 protein is bigger than PPAR-γ1 with 30 additional amino acids in N-terminal. Because of different promoters, each PPAR-γ isoform has a different expression pattern *(18)*.

All three isoforms of PPARs possess four domain structures similar to other nuclear hormone receptors *(1,19)*; the NH_2-terminal ligand-independent transactivation domain (activation function-1) which regulates PPAR activity *(20,21)* (A/B domain), the DNA-binding domain, which consists of 70 amino acids (two zinc fingers) (DNA-binding domain, C domain), the docking domain for cofactors (D domain), and the COOH-terminal region, which contains the ligand-binding domain (LBD) and activation function-2 domain (E/F domain). DNA-binding domain and LBD will share about 70% homology among three PPAR isoforms.

LIGANDS FOR PPARs

PPARs are ligand-activated transcriptional factors similar to other members of the nuclear hormone receptor superfamily. The modulation of the target gene transcription depends on the binding of ligands to the receptor. PPARs form heterodimers with the 9-*cis* retinoic acid receptor, RXR-α. Activation of heterodimers, PPAR: RXR-α by PPAR ligands and/or RXR ligands triggers the conformational change of these receptors, resulting in binding of the heterodimers to PPAR response elements with the sequence AGGTCANAGGTCA in the promoter region of the target genes and modulate gene transcription (Fig. 1).

Ligands have been identified for each PPAR isoform in both functional (cell-based transactivation efficiency) and in vitro interaction assay *(11,22)*. The different amino acid sequences in LBD of each PPAR isoform provide the molecular basis for ligand specificity. Each PPAR can accommodate several structurally diverse compounds as ligands because PPARs have the large ligand-binding pocket *(23)*. Many compounds including the natural or synthetic agents are identified as ligands for each PPAR. PPAR-α binds unsaturated FAs with the highest affinity of the three isoforms *(24–27)*; saturated FAs have lower affinity for PPAR-α. Among natural ligands for PPAR-γ, several unsaturated FAs including oleate, linoleate, eicosapentaenoic and arachidonic acids, and $15dPGJ_2$, can bind PPAR-γ *(11,24,28,29)*. TZD compounds such as troglitazone (the first agent of this class on the market, withdrawn because of liver toxicity), ciglitazone, pioglitazone, and rosiglitazone act as synthetic PPAR-γ ligands (Fig. 2) and promote adipocyte differentiation through of PPAR-γ activation *(22,30–34)*. Interestingly, TZD compounds were developed without knowing that they were ligands for PPAR-γ. TZDs are specific PPAR-γ ligands with high-affinity KD in the 100 nmol/l range *(8,22,35)*. FAs also act as PPAR-α ligands or -β/δ ligands with low-affinity KD in the micromolar range *(35,36)*. Rosiglitazone has greater selectivity for PPAR-γ than those of troglitazone in several cell types *(37)*. The effects of each TZD on diverse cell functions depend on its binding selectivity for PPAR-γ. However, the relationship between the level of PPAR-γ activity and insulin-sensitizing properties is complex and not completely clarified. TZDs super physiologically activate PPAR-γ and reduce insulin resistance and hyperglycemia in type 2 diabetes, and cause weight gain through the promotion of adipocyte differentiation. Unexpectedly, a moderate reduction of PPAR-γ activity, obtained in heterozygous PPAR-γ-deficient mice, or a Pro12Ala polymorphism in human PPAR-γ prevent insulin resistance and the obesity induced by a high-fat diet *(38–40)*. Moderate reduction of PPAR-γ with PPAR-γ antagonist or RXR antagonist ameliorates specific abnormalities such as obesity and insulin resistance that are related to type 2 diabetes *(41)*. Paradoxically, inducing a severe reduction of PPAR-γ in the heterozygous PPAR-γ-deficient mouse by treatment with PPAR-γ antagonists results in depletion of white adipose tissue and the re-emergence of insulin resistance *(41)* Appropriate functional antagonism of PPAR-γ may be a logical approach to protect against obesity and related diseases such as type 2 diabetes. Recently, telmisartan, one of angiotensin II type-1 receptor blockers (ARB), was demonstrated to bind to PPAR-γ and reduce the level of blood glucose *(42,43)*.

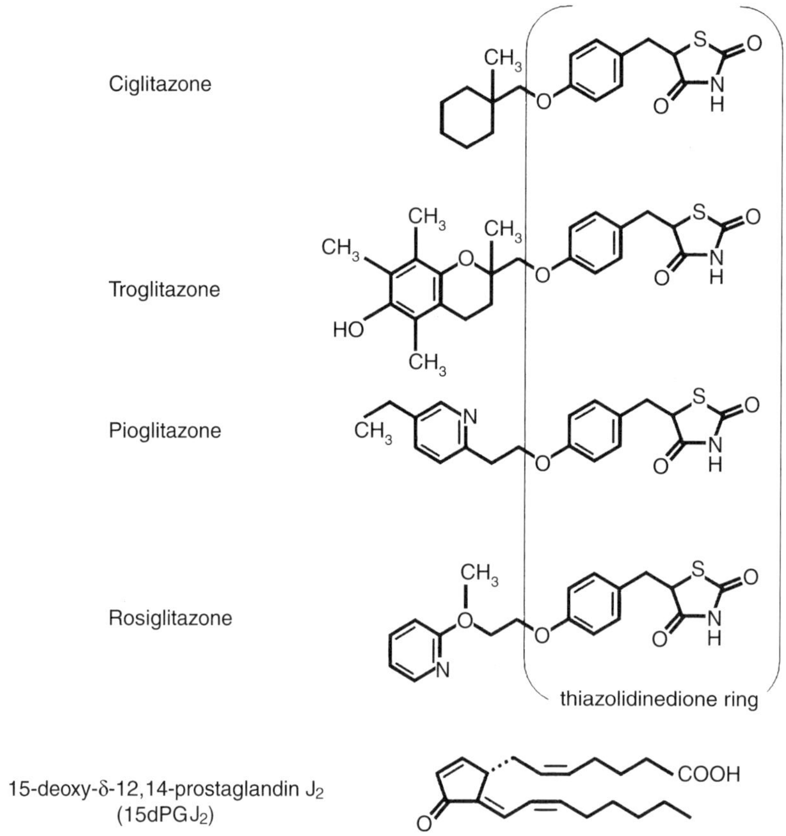

Fig. 2. Synthetic and natural PPAR-γ ligands. Synthetic ligands; thiazolidinedione compounds. Pioglitazone and rosiglitazone have been used as oral antidiabetic agents in clinical practice. Natural ligands; $15dPGJ_2$.

DISTRIBUTION OF PPARs IN THE KIDNEY

Expression of the three PPAR isoforms has been examined in many species, including Xenopus, rat, mouse, rabbit, and human. PPAR-α is mainly expressed in tissues exhibiting high catabolic rates of FAs such as adipose tissue, liver, heart, and skeletal muscle *(44,45)* PPAR-β/δ is ubiquitously expressed isoform. PPAR-γ is highly expressed in white and brown adipose tissues that store large amounts of FAs as well as in other tissues such as heart, liver, immune cells (monocytes and macrophages), placenta, and colon at low levels *(46–48)*.

In kidney, all three PPAR isoforms are expressed *(44,47–50)*. Renal expression of PPAR-γ mRNA has been reported in medullary collecting ducts and pelvic urothelium *(51)*. In isolated glomeruli and cultured mesangial cells (MCs), mRNA expression of PPAR-γ was also identified *(52,53)*. Especially, the protein expression of PPAR-α and -γ1 (not γ2) was demonstrated in the kidney by immunoblot analysis using specific anti-PPARs antibodies. Using immunohistochemical analysis, PPAR-α and -γ1 proteins were shown to be expressed in the nuclei of mesangial and epithelial cells in glomeruli, proximal and distal tubules, the loop of Henle, medullary collecting ducts and in the intima/media of renal vessels *(54)*. In contrast to PPAR-α, PPAR-γ is highly expressed in the distal nephron, predominantly collecting ducts. These findings suggest that the PPAR-γ isoform may contribute to water and sodium retention *(55,56)*.

INVOLVEMENT OF PPAR-γ IN DIABETIC NEPHROPATHY

The TZD class of PPAR-γ ligands, including troglitazone, pioglitazone, and rosiglitazone have been extensively used as antidiabetic agents in clinical practice for type 2 diabetes. Accumulating evidence has also suggested a therapeutic benefit of PPAR-γ ligands in diabetic nephropathy (DN). However, the molecular mechanisms by which PPAR-γ ligands may ameliorate the abnormalities of DN appear to be multiple and complex.

The Effect of PPAR-γ Ligands on the Enhancement of Insulin-Sensitizing Action

Via Improving Hyperglycemia

The Diabetes Control and Complications Trial and the United Kingdom Prospective Diabetes Study reported that the strict maintenance of euglycemia by intensive insulin treatment can delay the onset and slow the progression of DN in patients with type 1 and type 2 diabetes mellitus *(57,58)*. These studies suggested that the adverse effects of hyperglycemia are the main cause for the development of long-term complications in diabetes such as kidney disease.

TZDs as PPAR-γ ligands are a new class of oral antidiabetic agents that are used widely and improve insulin resistance, hyperinsulinemia, and hyperglycemia in patients with type 2 diabetes *(59–62)*. Because amelioration of hyperglycemia can prevent the development and progression of DN, TZDs could be renoprotective in patients with type 2 diabetes and in the corresponding animal models of the disease by their insulin sensitizing ability *(63)*. In *fa/fa* rats, one of type 2 diabetic models, treatment with TZDs reduced albuminuria, improved glomerular hyperfiltration, and inhibited the histological alterations of nephropathy such as mesangial expansion and glomerulosclerosis *(56,64,65)*. In MCs cultured in high-glucose conditions, troglitazone and $15dPGJ_2$ suppress the expression of α-smooth muscle actin, i.e., preventing the de-differentiation of MCs from a quiescent phenotype to a proliferative myofibroblast-like phenotype *(52)*. Furthermore, TZDs inhibited proliferation of MCs in a dose-dependent manner *(52)*. Taken together, these observations indicate that PPAR-γ activators significantly lower blood glucose concentration and protect the kidney against hyperglycemic damage in type 2 diabetic patients and animal models.

Via Lowering Blood Pressure With or Without Improvement of Insulin Resistance

Blood pressure control is important in the treatment of chronic kidney diseases including DN *(66)*. Hypertension is commonly linked to obesity and insulin resistance *(67)*. This syndrome, in which insulin resistance, hypertension, obesity, dyslipidemia, and microalbuminuria are associated has been termed "the metabolic syndrome" *(68,69)*. TZDs have the ability to lower blood pressure as well as to enhance of insulin sensitivity both in type 2 diabetic patients and animal models *(70–74)*. Therefore, TZDs could also be effective agents in the treatment of the metabolic syndrome *(75)*. It has been suggested that the antihypertensive effect of TZDs is a result of improved insulin resistance because insulin sensitivity has been found to be related to blood pressure levels both in diabetic animals and humans *(56,71–74)*. On the other hand, PPAR-γ ligands may also have direct effects on vascular function because PPAR-γ is expressed in endothelial cells and vascular smooth muscle cells (VSMCs) *(76–78)*. Indeed, pioglitazone lowers blood pressure in 5/6 nephrectomized hypertensive rats, without an associated change in insulin resistance *(79,80)* The antihypertensive effects of TZDs could involve release of vasodilators such as nitric oxide and prostaglandins *(81)*, decrease in FAs levels, and alterations in vasoactive peptides synthesis such as endothelin-1 *(82)*. Recently PPAR-γ was shown to downregulate the expression of angiotensin II type-1 receptor and decrease VSMC tone, thereby reducing vascular contractility *(83)*.

In contrast, it has been suggested that PPAR-γ could contribute to water and sodium retention as this isoform is predominantly expressed in collecting ducts *(48)*. In clinical practice, caution must be paid when TZD agents are prescribed in patients with edema or congestive heart failure. Although the precise mechanisms still remain unclear, PPAR-γ expression participates in blood pressure regulation via multiple mechanisms.

Effects of PPAR-γ Ligands Independent of Changes in Blood Glucose Levels

TZD treatment could ameliorate renal abnormalities in streptozotocin (STZ)-induced diabetic rats, a type 1 model of diabetes, without changing blood glucose levels *(84,85)*. This finding suggests that the beneficial effects of PPAR-γ ligands in preventing diabetes-induced renal dysfunction are independent of their insulin-sensitizing properties. Multiple biochemical mechanisms have been proposed to explain the adverse effects of hyperglycemia including activation of the diacylglycerol (DAG)–protein kinase C (PKC) pathway *(86,87)*, enhancement of the polyol pathway related with myoinositol depletion *(88)*, alteration of redox state *(89)*, overproduction of advanced glycation endproducts *(90)*, increased oxidative stress *(91)*, and augmented growth factor and cytokine production *(92)*. The effect of PPAR-γ ligands on individual biochemical alteration induced by hyperglycemia will be discussed later.

Via Amelioration of the Activation of DAG Kinase–DAG–PKC Pathway

DAG–PKC–extracellular signal-regulated kinase (ERK) pathway is enhanced in MCs cultured with high glucose conditions and in glomeruli isolated from STZ-induced diabetic rats *(93–96)*. D-α-Tocopherol (vitamin E), a well-known antioxidant agent, has been reported to reverse diabetic-induced renal dysfunction by modulating the activity of PKC signal transduction pathway and preventing the increased glomerular filtration and albumin excretion associated with diabetes *(93)*. This effect was also thought to be owing to its antioxidant action in addition to the modulation of DAG kinase (DGK) activity *(93,97)*.

Because troglitazone has the α-tocopherol moiety, the chromane ring, in its structure, the effects of troglitazone and α-tocopherol have been compared in STZ-induced diabetic rats. Troglitazone also ameliorated the increase in glomerular filtration rate, urinary albumin excretion, and mRNA expression of extracellular matrix proteins (fibronectin and type IV collagen) and transforming growth factor (TGF)-β associated with diabetes without changing the blood glucose levels (Fig. 3A) *(85)*. These findings demonstrate for the first time that PPAR-γ ligands can protect glomerular function independently of their insulin-sensitizing action. In MCs cultured in high-glucose conditions and in isolated glomeruli from diabetic rats, it was also confirmed that the mechanism of TZDs action is via activation of DGK, that metabolizes DAG to phosphatidic acid

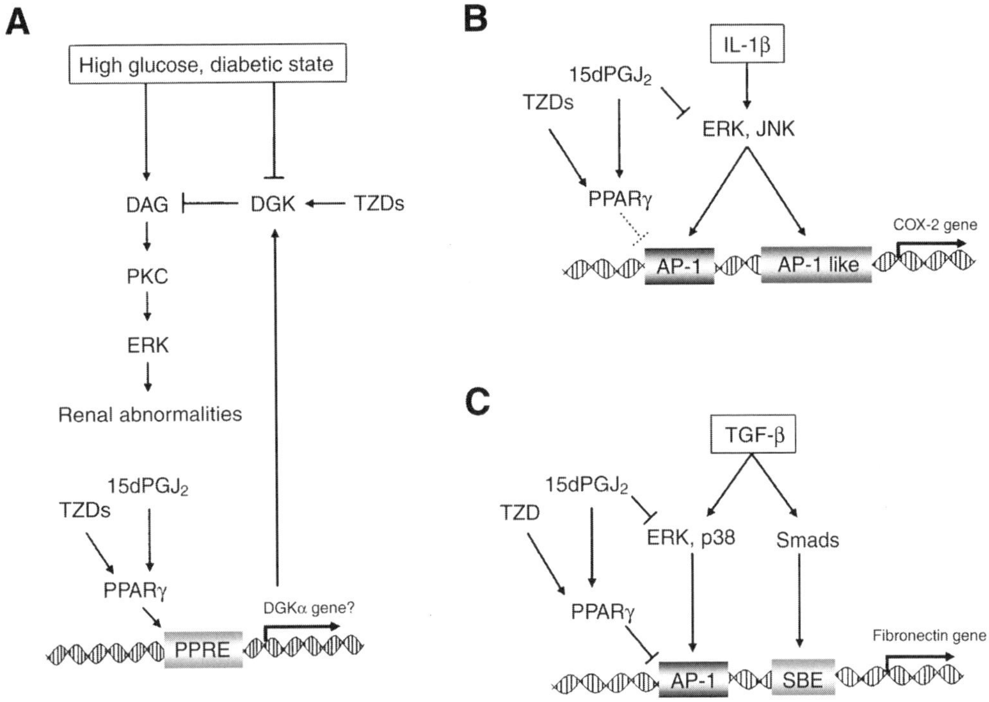

Fig. 3. Effects of PPAR-γ ligands. **(A)** under conditions of high-glucose concentration and diabetes *(85)*, **(B)** on IL-1β stimulation *(125)* and **(C)** on TGF-β stimulation *(139)*.

and therefore prevents the accumulation of DAG and the subsequent activation of the PKC–ERK pathway. Furthermore, another TZD, pioglitazone, which does not have the α-tocopherol moiety, also could prevent the enhancement of DAG–PKC–ERK pathway in MCs exposed to high glucose (Fig. 3A) *(85)*. Recently, TZDs and $15dPGJ_2$ have been reported to be able to increase the protein expression of DGK-α and prevent DAG–PKC pathway activation in endothelial cells (Fig. 3A) *(98)*.

Via Attenuating Oxidative Stress

Increase in oxidative stress is observed in renal glomeruli and a variety of the vascular and nonvascular tissues exposed to hyperglycemia *(99–101)*. Emerging evidence suggests that oxidative stress may contribute to the development of diabetic complications, possibly through activating DAG–PKC pathways. As stated before, D-α-tocopherol can inhibit the diabetes-induced activation of DAG–PKC pathway in addition of its antioxidant properties *(102)*. Troglitazone, which has D-α-tocopherol moiety, has potent antioxidant effects in suppression of phosphoenolpyruvate gene expression in vitro and in scavenging reactive oxygen species in vivo *(103)*. It also normalizes the decrease of plasma lipid hydroperoxide concentration and increase of superoxide dismutase activity in Otsuka Long-Evans Tokushima Fatty rats, a type 2 diabetes animal model, and improves decreased skin blood flow in STZ-induced diabetic rats *(81,104,105)*. Pioglitazone also can reduce renal oxidative stress in alloxan-induced diabetic rabbits although this compound does not share the D-α-tocopherol moiety *(106,107)*. In addition, pioglitazone reduces renal oxidative stress such as renal lipid peroxides, urinary isoprostane excretion, and expression of p47*phox* and gp91*phox* in high-fat diet-induced obesity rats *(108)*.

Via Suppressing Inflammation

Hyperglycemia and the diabetic state induce the production of cytokines *(92)* and the glomerular and interstitial infiltration with macrophages *(109,110)*. It is, therefore, relevant that both PPAR-γ and -α have potent anti-inflammatory effects in macrophages *(111,112)*.

IL-1β is one of proinflammatory cytokines produced in response to diverse extracellular stimuli *(113)*. IL-1β, formed by both infiltrating macrophages and activated MCs, is able to stimulate the production of prostaglandins and nitric oxide in MCs *(114,115)*. In addition, cyclooxygenase-2 (COX-2), a key enzyme in the synthesis of prostaglandins, is induced in MCs in response to IL-1β *(116,117)*. A potent endogenous PPAR-γ ligand, $15dPGJ_2$, is a natural metabolite derived from prostaglandin D2, which is the most abundant prostaglandin in normal tissues, and has the highest binding affinity to PPAR-γ in the J-series prostaglandins *(118)*. Several studies have shown that the anti-inflammatory effect of $15dPGJ_2$ or TZDs appears to be regulated through transcriptional inhibition by not only a PPAR-γ-dependent *(111,112,119)* but also via PPAR-γ-independent mechanisms *(120–122)*. Nuclear factor-κB, a well-known inflammatory transcription factor, is repressed by $15dPGJ_2$ in a PPAR-γ-independent manner *(123,124)*. It has been previously reported that $15dPGJ_2$ inhibits IL-1β-induced COX-2 expression and PGE_2 production, independent of PPAR-γ activation, by suppression of ERK and c-Jun NH_2-terminal kinase pathways and activator protein (AP)-1 activation in MCs (Fig. 3B) *(125)*. Ciglitazone, an additional TZD compound, prevents platelet-derived growth factor-induced MC proliferation, without altering ERK activation, by directly inhibiting the activation of serum response element *(126)*. In the renal ischemia and reperfusion model, PPAR-γ expression increases in MCs and endothelial cells *(127)* and PPAR-γ agonists ameliorate renal dysfunction *(128)* and neutrophil accumulation *(129)*.

Via Modifying Atherosclerotic Change

Atherosclerotic changes such as renovascular stenosis and atheroembolism are common in elderly diabetic patients and contribute to acceleration of renal insufficiency *(130,131)*. PPAR-γ activation also may modify the progression of atherosclerosis through multiple mechanisms including those related to foam cell differentiation, inflammatory reaction, and cell proliferation *(132)*. The infiltrating monocytes take up oxidized low-density lipoprotein (OxLDL) via scavenger receptors, resulting in accumulation of intracellular lipids and generation of foam cells *(132)*. OxLDL scavenger receptor, CD36, is under direct control of PPAR-γ *(28,29)*. OxLDL contains natural PPAR-γ agonists, such as 9-hydroxyoctadecadienoic acids and 13-hydroxyoctadecadienoic. Furthermore, OxLDL induces the expression of PPAR-γ *(112)*, which demonstrates anti-inflammatory properties by reducing the monocyte production of cytokines *(111)*. The decrease in cytokine production is mediated by inhibition of the activity of proinflammatory transcription factors such as nuclear factor-κB, AP-1, and signal transducer and activator of transcription (STAT) *(112)*. Furthermore, PPAR-γ has additional effects in atherosclerosis including induction of monocyte apoptosis *(133)*, inhibition of VSMCs proliferation *(77,134)*, and suppression of matrix metalloproteinase-9 expression *(135)*.

The Effect of PPAR-γ Ligands in Tubular Tissue

Nephrotic syndrome is a common occurrence in patients with DN. In nephrotic syndrome, large quantities of albumin enter the tubule carrying a heavy load of FAs.

Albumin-bound FAs can activate PPAR-γ and induce apoptosis in proximal tubular cells. Activation of PPAR-γ by specific agonists is associated with inhibition of tubular cell proliferation, whereas activation by albumin-bound FAs is accompanied by increased proliferation *(136)*. However, the net result of these opposing effects is the decrease in the number of cells. Interestingly, whereas pioglitazone increases the tubular cell albumin uptake it reverses the expression of inflammatory and profibrotic markers, monocyte chemoattractant protein-1 and TGF-β *(137)*.

The Effect of PPAR-γ Ligands in Nondiabetic Renal Disease

In nondiabetic models of glomerulosclerosis, PPAR-γ ligands are also effective in preventing renal dysfunction. In the 5/6 nephrectomized rat, treatment with troglitazone significantly reduced proteinuria, serum creatinine level, and glomerulosclerosis through the inhibition of glomerular cell proliferation and reduction of glomerular and tubular TGF-β expression *(138)*. In cultured mouse MCs, pioglitazone inhibits TGF-β-induced fibronectin expression by inhibiting the PPAR-γ dependent activation of AP-1, whereas $15dPGJ_2$ also inhibits TGF-β-induced fibronectin expression through a dual mechanism that is both dependent on and independent of PPAR-γ activation (Fig. 3C) *(139)*.

INVOLVEMENT OF PPAR-α AND -β/δ IN DIABETIC NEPHROPATHY

PPAR-α is highly expressed in renal proximal tubules in which it influences metabolic activity *(140)*. PPAR-α plays a role in lipid metabolism in renal cortex because its activation by clofibrates induces expression of β-oxidation enzymes *(141)*. Clinical evidence also suggests a beneficial effect of PPAR-α ligands on DN *(142,143)*. In type 2 diabetic patients, treatment of dyslipidemia with gemfibrozil, one of antidyslipidemic agents and PPAR-α activators, stabilizes the increase in urinary albumin excretion *(143)*. In *db/db* type 2 diabetic mice, treatment with fenofibrate, another of PPAR-α activator, improves urinary albumin excretion rate and glomerular mesangial expansion *(144)*. One possible mechanism of PPAR-α action on the mesangial matrix production may be related to TGF-β signaling *(145)*. Clofibrate directly inhibits oxidant stress-induced TGF-β expression in MCs *(145)*. In addition, fenofibrate also downregulates TGF-β and TGF-β receptor type-2 expression decreasing type-IV collagen accumulation in diabetic glomeruli *(144)*.

PPAR-β/δ is equally expressed in renal cortex and medulla as well as other tissues *(48)*. However, the role of PPAR-β/δ in the kidney remains poorly understood. Overexpression of this isoform protects cultured medullary interstitial cells from hypertonicity-induced cell death, suggesting that PPAR-β/δ is an important survival factor for these cells exposed to the hypertonic environment of the renal medulla *(146)*. Further studies are necessary to clarify the effect of PPAR-β/δ in kidney.

CONCLUSIONS

PPARs are ligand-activated transcription factors belonging to the nuclear hormone receptor superfamily. Three PPAR isoforms (α, β/δ, and γ) identified and detected in several tissues and cells including kidney have a pivotal role in the glucose and lipid metabolism, cell differentiation, inflammation, and cell cycle control. PPAR-γ is a key player in adipogenesis and insulin sensitivity mainly and its specific synthetic ligands, TZDs are used as oral antidiabetic agents in clinical practice all over the world. In addition to its insulin-sensitizing action, TZD compounds are protective against diabetic nephropathy through multiple pathways such as antihypertensive agents, PKC inhibitors via DGK activation, antioxidant and anti-inflammatory agents, and antiatherosclerogenic compounds without altering blood glucose levels. A natural PPAR-γ ligand, $15dPGJ_2$ also play a beneficial role in diabetic nephropathy dependently or independently of PPAR-γ. Accumulating evidence regarding the role of PPAR-γ in DN indicates the therapeutic potential of PPAR-γ ligands and the possibilities of developing newer agents for treatment of DN.

REFERENCES

1. Corton JC, Anderson SP, Stauber A. Central role of peroxisome proliferator-activated receptors in the actions of peroxisome proliferators. Annu Rev Pharmacol Toxicol 2000;40:491–518.
2. Issemann I, Green S. Activation of a member of the steroid hormone receptor superfamily by peroxisome proliferators. Nature 1990;347:645–650.
3. Dreyer C, Krey G, Keller H, Givel F, Helftenbein G, Wahli W. Control of the peroxisomal beta-oxidation pathway by a novel family of nuclear hormone receptors. Cell 1992;68:879–887.
4. Ziouzenkova O, Perrey S, Asatryan L, et al. Lipolysis of triglyceride-rich lipoproteins generates PPAR ligands: evidence for an antiinflammatory role for lipoprotein lipase. Proc Natl Acad Sci USA 2003;100:2730–2735.
5. Kliewer SA, Lenhard JM, Willson TM, Patel I, Morris DC, Lehmann JM. A prostaglandin J2 metabolite binds peroxisome proliferator-activated receptor gamma and promotes adipocyte differentiation. Cell 1995;83:813–819.
6. Forman BM, Chen J, Evans RM. Hypolipidemic drugs, polyunsaturated fatty acids, and eicosanoids are ligands for peroxisome proliferator-activated receptors alpha and delta. Proc Natl Acad Sci USA 1997;94:4312–4317.
7. Staels B, Dallongeville J, Auwerx J, Schoonjans K, Leitersdorf E, Fruchart JC. Mechanism of action of fibrates on lipid and lipoprotein metabolism. Circulation 1998;98:2088–2093.
8. Lehmann JM, Moore LB, Smith-Oliver TA, Wilkison WO, Willson TM, Kliewer SA. An antidiabetic thiazolidinedione is a high affinity ligand for peroxisome proliferator-activated receptor gamma (PPAR gamma). J Biol Chem 1995;270:12,953–12,956.
9. Guan Y, Breyer MD. Peroxisome proliferator-activated receptors (PPARs): novel therapeutic targets in renal disease. Kidney Int 2001;60:14–30.
10. Willson TM, Lambert MH, Kliewer SA. Peroxisome proliferator-activated receptor gamma and metabolic disease. Annu Rev Biochem 2001;70:341–367.
11. Desvergne B, Wahli W. Peroxisome proliferator-activated receptors: nuclear control of metabolism. Endocr Rev 1999;20:649–688.
12. Fajas L, Debril MB, Auwerx J. Peroxisome proliferator-activated receptor-gamma: from adipogenesis to carcinogenesis. J Mol Endocrinol 2001;27:1–9.
13. Wu GD. A nuclear receptor to prevent colon cancer. N Engl J Med 2000;342:651–653.
14. Auwerx J. PPARgamma, the ultimate thrifty gene. Diabetologia 1999;42:1033–1049.
15. Jones AB. Peroxisome proliferator-activated receptor (PPAR) modulators: diabetes and beyond. Med Res Rev 2001;21:540–552.
16. Fajas L, Fruchart JC, Auwerx J. PPARgamma3 mRNA: a distinct PPARgamma mRNA subtype transcribed from an independent promoter. FEBS Lett 1998;438:55–60.
17. Rosen ED, Spiegelman BM. PPARgamma: a nuclear regulator of metabolism, differentiation, and cell growth. J Biol Chem 2001;276:37,731–37,734. Epub 2001 Jul 17.
18. Fajas L, Auboeuf D, Raspe E, et al. The organization, promoter analysis, and expression of the human PPARgamma gene. J Biol Chem 1997;272:18,779–18,789.
19. Escher P, Wahli W. Peroxisome proliferator-activated receptors: insight into multiple cellular functions. Mutat Res 2000;448:121–138.
20. Juge-Aubry CE, Hammar E, Siegrist-Kaiser C, et al. Regulation of the transcriptional activity of the peroxisome proliferator-activated receptor alpha by phosphorylation of a ligand-independent trans-activating domain. J Biol Chem 1999;274:10,505–10,510.
21. Shao D, Rangwala SM, Bailey ST, Krakow SL, Reginato MJ, Lazar MA. Interdomain communication regulating ligand binding by PPAR-gamma. Nature 1998;396:377–380.

22. Kliewer SA, Xu HE, Lambert MH, Willson TM. Peroxisome proliferator-activated receptors: from genes to physiology. Recent Prog Horm Res 2001;56:239–263.
23. Moras D, Gronemeyer H. The nuclear receptor ligand-binding domain: structure and function. Curr Opin Cell Biol 1998;10:384–391.
24. Kliewer SA, Sundseth SS, Jones SA, et al. Fatty acids and eicosanoids regulate gene expression through direct interactions with peroxisome proliferator-activated receptors alpha and gamma. Proc Natl Acad Sci USA 1997;94:4318–4323.
25. Ellinghaus P, Wolfrum C, Assmann G, Spener F, Seedorf U. Phytanic acid activates the peroxisome proliferator-activated receptor alpha (PPARalpha) in sterol carrier protein 2-/ sterol carrier protein x-deficient mice. J Biol Chem 1999;274:2766–2772.
26. Moya-Camarena SY, Vanden Heuvel JP, Blanchard SG, Leesnitzer LA, Belury MA. Conjugated linoleic acid is a potent naturally occurring ligand and activator of PPARalpha. J Lipid Res 1999; 40:1426–1433.
27. Lin Q, Ruuska SE, Shaw NS, Dong D, Noy N. Ligand selectivity of the peroxisome proliferator-activated receptor alpha. Biochemistry 1999;38:185–190.
28. Tontonoz P, Nagy L, Alvarez JG, Thomazy VA, Evans RM. PPARgamma promotes monocyte/ macrophage differentiation and uptake of oxidized LDL. Cell 1998;93:241–252.
29. Nagy L, Tontonoz P, Alvarez JG, Chen H, Evans RM. Oxidized LDL regulates macrophage gene expression through ligand activation of PPARgamma. Cell 1998;93:229–240.
30. Lambe KG, Tugwood JD. A human peroxisome-proliferator-activated receptor-gamma is activated by inducers of adipogenesis, including thiazolidinedione drugs. Eur J Biochem 1996;239:1–7.
31. Lowell BB. PPARgamma: an essential regulator of adipogenesis and modulator of fat cell function. Cell 1999;99:239–242.
32. Rosen ED, Sarraf P, Troy AE, et al. PPAR gamma is required for the differentiation of adipose tissue in vivo and in vitro. Mol Cell 1999;4:611–617.
33. Wu Z, Rosen ED, Brun R, et al. Cross-regulation of C/EBP alpha and PPAR gamma controls the transcriptional pathway of adipogenesis and insulin sensitivity. Mol Cell 1999;3:151–158.
34. Spiegelman BM, Hu E, Kim JB, Brun R. PPAR gamma and the control of adipogenesis. Biochimie 1997;79:111,112.
35. Forman BM, Tontonoz P, Chen J, Brun RP, Spiegelman BM, Evans RM. 15-Deoxy-delta 12,14-prostaglandin J2 is a ligand for the adipocyte determination factor PPAR gamma. Cell 1995;83:803–812.
36. Xu HE, Lambert MH, Montana VG, et al. Molecular recognition of fatty acids by peroxisome proliferator-activated receptors. Mol Cell 1999;3:397–403.
37. Camp HS, Li O, Wise SC, et al. Differential activation of peroxisome proliferator-activated receptor-gamma by troglitazone and rosiglitazone. Diabetes 2000;49:539–547.
38. Kubota N, Terauchi Y, Miki H, et al. PPAR gamma mediates high-fat diet-induced adipocyte hypertrophy and insulin resistance. Mol Cell 1999;4:597–609.
39. Hara K, Okada T, Tobe K, et al. The Pro12Ala polymorphism in PPAR gamma2 may confer resistance to type 2 diabetes. Biochem Biophys Res Commun 2000;271:212–216.
40. Kadowaki T. Insights into insulin resistance and type 2 diabetes from knockout mouse models. J Clin Invest 2000;106:459–465.
41. Yamauchi T, Waki H, Kamon J, et al. Inhibition of RXR and PPARgamma ameliorates diet-induced obesity and type 2 diabetes. J Clin Invest 2001;108:1001–1013.
42. Benson SC, Pershadsingh HA, Ho CI, et al. Identification of telmisartan as a unique angiotensin II receptor antagonist with selective PPARgamma-modulating activity. Hypertension 2004;43:993–1002.
43. Schupp M, Janke J, Clasen R, Unger T, Kintscher U. Angiotensin type 1 receptor blockers induce peroxisome proliferator-activated receptor-gamma activity. Circulation 2004;109:2054–2057.
44. Braissant O, Foufelle F, Scotto C, Dauca M, Wahli W. Differential expression of peroxisome proliferator-activated receptors (PPARs): tissue distribution of PPAR-alpha, -beta, and -gamma in the adult rat. Endocrinology 1996;137:354–366.
45. Su JL, Simmons CJ, Wisely B, Ellis B, Winegar DA. Monitoring of PPAR alpha protein expression in human tissue by the use of PPAR alpha-specific MAbs. Hybridoma 1998;17:47–53.
46. Auboeuf D, Rieusset J, Fajas L, et al. Tissue distribution and quantification of the expression of mRNAs of peroxisome proliferator-activated receptors and liver X receptor-alpha in humans: no alteration in adipose tissue of obese and NIDDM patients. Diabetes 1997;46:1319–1327.
47. Mukherjee R, Jow L, Croston GE, Paterniti JR, Jr. Identification, characterization, and tissue distribution of human peroxisome proliferator-activated receptor (PPAR) isoforms PPARgamma2 versus

PPARgamma1 and activation with retinoid X receptor agonists and antagonists. J Biol Chem 1997;272:8071–8076.
48. Guan Y, Zhang Y, Davis L, Breyer MD. Expression of peroxisome proliferator-activated receptors in urinary tract of rabbits and humans. Am J Physiol 1997;273:F1013–F1022.
49. Kliewer SA, Forman BM, Blumberg B, et al. Differential expression and activation of a family of murine peroxisome proliferator-activated receptors. Proc Natl Acad Sci USA 1994;91:7355–7359.
50. Jain S, Pulikuri S, Zhu Y, et al. Differential expression of the peroxisome proliferator-activated receptor gamma (PPARgamma) and its coactivators steroid receptor coactivator-1 and PPAR-binding protein PBP in the brown fat, urinary bladder, colon, and breast of the mouse. Am J Pathol 1998;153:349–354.
51. Yang T, Michele DE, Park J, et al. Expression of peroxisomal proliferator-activated receptors and retinoid X receptors in the kidney. Am J Physiol 1999;277:F966–F973.
52. Asano T, Wakisaka M, Yoshinari M, et al. Peroxisome proliferator-activated receptor gamma1 (PPARgamma1) expresses in rat mesangial cells and PPARgamma agonists modulate its differentiation. Biochim Biophys Acta 2000;1497:148–154.
53. Iwashima Y, Eto M, Horiuchi S, Sano H. Advanced glycation end product-induced peroxisome proliferator-activated receptor gamma gene expression in the cultured mesangial cells. Biochem Biophys Res Commun 1999;264:441–448.
54. Sato K, Sugawara A, Kudo M, Uruno A, Ito S, Takeuchi K. Expression of peroxisome proliferator-activated receptor isoform proteins in the rat kidney. Hypertens Res 2004;27:417–425.
55. Gorson DM. Significant weight gain with rezulin therapy. Arch Intern Med 1999;159:99.
56. Yoshimoto T, Naruse M, Nishikawa M, et al. Antihypertensive and vasculo- and renoprotective effects of pioglitazone in genetically obese diabetic rats. Am J Physiol 1997;272:E989–E996.
57. The diabetes control and complications trial research group. The effect of intensive treatment of diabetes on the development and progression of long-term complications in insulin-dependent diabetes mellitus. N Engl J Med 1993;329:977–986.
58. UK prospective diabetes study group. Intensive blood–glucose control with sulphonylureas or insulin compared with conventional treatment and risk of complications in patients with type 2 diabetes (UKPDS 33). Lancet 1998;352:837–853.
59. Kumar S, Boulton AJ, Beck-Nielsen H, et al. Troglitazone, an insulin action enhancer, improves metabolic control in NIDDM patients. Troglitazone Study Group. Diabetologia 1996;39:701–709.
60. Prigeon RL, Kahn SE, Porte D, Jr. Effect of troglitazone on B cell function, insulin sensitivity, and glycemic control in subjects with type 2 diabetes mellitus. J Clin Endocrinol Metab 1998;83:819–823.
61. Fonseca VA, Valiquett TR, Huang SM, Ghazzi MN, Whitcomb RW. Troglitazone monotherapy improves glycemic control in patients with type 2 diabetes mellitus: a randomized, controlled study. The Troglitazone Study Group. J Clin Endocrinol Metab 1998;83:3169–3176.
62. Spencer CM, Goa KL, Gillis JC. Tacrolimus. An update of its pharmacology and clinical efficacy in the management of organ transplantation. Drugs 1997;54:925–975.
63. Imano E, Kanda T, Nakatani Y, et al. Effect of troglitazone on microalbuminuria in patients with incipient diabetic nephropathy. Diabetes Care 1998;21:2135–2139.
64. McCarthy KJ, Routh RE, Shaw W, Walsh K, Welbourne TC, Johnson JH. Troglitazone halts diabetic glomerulosclerosis by blockade of mesangial expansion. Kidney Int 2000;58:2341–2350.
65. Buckingham RE, Al-Barazanji KA, Toseland CD, et al. Peroxisome proliferator-activated receptor-gamma agonist, rosiglitazone, protects against nephropathy and pancreatic islet abnormalities in Zucker fatty rats. Diabetes 1998;47:1326–1334.
66. Bakris GL. Protecting renal function in the hypertensive patient: Clinical guidelines. Am J Hypertens 2005;18:112–119.
67. Ferrari P, Weidmann P. Insulin, insulin sensitivity and hypertension. J Hypertens 1990;8:491–500.
68. Reaven GM. Banting lecture 1988. Role of insulin resistance in human disease. Diabetes 1988;37:1595–1607.
69. Kereiakes DJ, Willerson JT. Metabolic syndrome epidemic. Circulation 2003;108:1552,1553.
70. Inzucchi SE, Maggs DG, Spollett GR, et al. Efficacy and metabolic effects of metformin and troglitazone in type II diabetes mellitus. N Engl J Med 1998;338:867–872.
71. Uchida A, Nakata T, Hatta T, et al. Reduction of insulin resistance attenuates the development of hypertension in sucrose-fed SHR. Life Sci 1997;61:455–464.
72. Grinsell JW, Lardinois CK, Swislocki A, et al. Pioglitazone attenuates basal and postprandial insulin concentrations and blood pressure in the spontaneously hypertensive rat. Am J Hypertens 2000;13:370–375.

73. Walker AB, Chattington PD, Buckingham RE, Williams G. The thiazolidinedione rosiglitazone (BRL-49653) lowers blood pressure and protects against impairment of endothelial function in Zucker fatty rats. Diabetes 1999;48:1448–1453.
74. Sung BH, Izzo JL, Jr, Dandona P, Wilson MF. Vasodilatory effects of troglitazone improve blood pressure at rest and during mental stress in type 2 diabetes mellitus. Hypertension 1999;34:83–88.
75. Guan Y. Peroxisome proliferator-activated receptor family and its relationship to renal complications of the metabolic syndrome. J Am Soc Nephrol 2004;15:2801–2815.
76. Iijima K, Yoshizumi M, Ako J, et al. Expression of peroxisome proliferator-activated receptor gamma (PPARgamma) in rat aortic smooth muscle cells. Biochem Biophys Res Commun 1998;247: 353–356.
77. Law RE, Goetze S, Xi XP, et al. Expression and function of PPARgamma in rat and human vascular smooth muscle cells. Circulation 2000;101:1311–1318.
78. Marx N, Schonbeck U, Lazar MA, Libby P, Plutzky J. Peroxisome proliferator-activated receptor gamma activators inhibit gene expression and migration in human vascular smooth muscle cells. Circ Res 1998;83:1097–1103.
79. Zhang HY, Reddy SR, Kotchen TA. Antihypertensive effect of pioglitazone is not invariably associated with increased insulin sensitivity. Hypertension 1994;24:106–110.
80. Zhang F, Sowers JR, Ram JL, Standley PR, Peuler JD. Effects of pioglitazone on calcium channels in vascular smooth muscle. Hypertension 1994;24:170–175.
81. Fujiwara T, Ohsawa T, Takahashi S, et al. Troglitazone, a new antidiabetic agent possessing radical scavenging ability, improved decreased skin blood flow in diabetic rats. Life Sci 1998;63: 2039–2047.
82. Satoh H, Tsukamoto K, Hashimoto Y, et al. Thiazolidinediones suppress endothelin-1 secretion from bovine vascular endothelial cells: a new possible role of PPARgamma on vascular endothelial function. Biochem Biophys Res Commun 1999;254:757–763.
83. Sugawara A, Takeuchi K, Uruno A, et al. Transcriptional suppression of type 1 angiotensin II receptor gene expression by peroxisome proliferator-activated receptor-gamma in vascular smooth muscle cells. Endocrinology 2001;142:3125–3134.
84. Fujii M, Takemura R, Yamaguchi M, et al. Troglitazone (CS-045) ameliorates albuminuria in streptozotocin-induced diabetic rats. Metabolism 1997;46:981–983.
85. Isshiki K, Haneda M, Koya D, Maeda S, Sugimoto T, Kikkawa R. Thiazolidinedione compounds ameliorate glomerular dysfunction independent of their insulin-sensitizing action in diabetic rats. Diabetes 2000;49:1022–1032.
86. King GL, Ishii H, Koya D. Diabetic vascular dysfunctions: a model of excessive activation of protein kinase C. Kidney Int Suppl 1997;60:S77–S85.
87. Derubertis FR, Craven PA. Activation of protein kinase C in glomerular cells in diabetes. Mechanisms and potential links to the pathogenesis of diabetic glomerulopathy. Diabetes 1994;43:1–8.
88. Greene DA, Lattimer SA, Sima AA. Sorbitol, phosphoinositides, and sodium-potassium-ATPase in the pathogenesis of diabetic complications. N Engl J Med 1987;316:599–606.
89. Williamson JR, Chang K, Frangos M, et al. Hyperglycemic pseudohypoxia and diabetic complications. Diabetes 1993;42:801–813.
90. Brownlee M, Cerami A, Vlassara H. Advanced glycosylation end products in tissue and the biochemical basis of diabetic complications. N Engl J Med 1988;318:1315–1321.
91. Nishikawa T, Edelstein D, Du XL, et al. Normalizing mitochondrial superoxide production blocks three pathways of hyperglycaemic damage. Nature 2000;404:787–790.
92. Sharma K, Ziyadeh FN. Hyperglycemia and diabetic kidney disease. The case for transforming growth factor-beta as a key mediator. Diabetes 1995;44:1139–1346.
93. Koya D, Lee IK, Ishii H, Kanoh H, King GL. Prevention of glomerular dysfunction in diabetic rats by treatment with d-alpha-tocopherol. J Am Soc Nephrol 1997;8:426–435.
94. Koya D, Jirousek MR, Lin YW, Ishii H, Kuboki K, King GL. Characterization of protein kinase C beta isoform activation on the gene expression of transforming growth factor-beta, extracellular matrix components, and prostanoids in the glomeruli of diabetic rats. J Clin Invest 1997;100:115–126.
95. Kikkawa R, Haneda M, Uzu T, Koya D, Sugimoto T, Shigeta Y. Translocation of protein kinase C alpha and zeta in rat glomerular mesangial cells cultured under high glucose conditions. Diabetologia 1994;37:838–841.
96. Haneda M, Araki S, Togawa M, Sugimoto T, Isono M, Kikkawa R. Mitogen-activated protein kinase cascade is activated in glomeruli of diabetic rats and glomerular mesangial cells cultured under high glucose conditions. Diabetes 1997;46:847–853.

97. Lee IK, Koya D, Ishi H, Kanoh H, King GL. d-Alpha-tocopherol prevents the hyperglycemia induced activation of diacylglycerol (DAG)-protein kinase C (PKC) pathway in vascular smooth muscle cell by an increase of DAG kinase activity. Diabetes Res Clin Pract 1999;45:183–190.
98. Verrier E, Wang L, Wadham C, et al. PPARgamma agonists ameliorate endothelial cell activation via inhibition of diacylglycerol-protein kinase C signaling pathway: role of diacylglycerol kinase. Circ Res 2004;94:1515–1522.
99. Dandona P, Thusu K, Cook S, et al. Oxidative damage to DNA in diabetes mellitus. Lancet 1996;347:444,445.
100. Leinonen J, Lehtimaki T, Toyokuni S, et al. New biomarker evidence of oxidative DNA damage in patients with non-insulin-dependent diabetes mellitus. FEBS Lett 1997;417:150–152.
101. Baynes JW, Thorpe SR. Role of oxidative stress in diabetic complications: a new perspective on an old paradigm. Diabetes 1999;48:1–9.
102. Bursell SE, Clermont AC, Aiello LP, et al. High-dose vitamin E supplementation normalizes retinal blood flow and creatinine clearance in patients with type 1 diabetes. Diabetes Care 1999;22: 1245–1251.
103. Davies GF, Khandelwal RL, Wu L, Juurlink BH, Roesler WJ. Inhibition of phosphoenolpyruvate carboxykinase (PEPCK) gene expression by troglitazone: a peroxisome proliferator-activated receptor-gamma (PPARgamma)-independent, antioxidant-related mechanism. Biochem Pharmacol 2001;62: 1071–1079.
104. Inoue I, Katayama S, Takahashi K, et al. Troglitazone has a scavenging effect on reactive oxygen species. Biochem Biophys Res Commun 1997;235:113–116.
105. Fukui T, Noma T, Mizushige K, Aki Y, Kimura S, Abe Y. Dietary troglitazone decreases oxidative stress in early stage type II diabetic rats. Life Sci 2000;66:2043–2049.
106. Gumieniczek A. Effects of pioglitazone on hyperglycemia-induced alterations in antioxidative system in tissues of alloxan-treated diabetic animals. Exp Toxicol Pathol 2005;56:321–326.
107. Gumieniczek A. Effect of the new thiazolidinedione-pioglitazone on the development of oxidative stress in liver and kidney of diabetic rabbits. Life Sci 2003;74:553–562.
108. Dobrian AD, Schriver SD, Khraibi AA, Prewitt RL. Pioglitazone prevents hypertension and reduces oxidative stress in diet-induced obesity. Hypertension 2004;43:48–56.
109. Furuta T, Saito T, Ootaka T, et al. The role of macrophages in diabetic glomerulosclerosis. Am J Kidney Dis 1993;21:480–485.
110. Shikata K, Makino H. Role of macrophages in the pathogenesis of diabetic nephropathy. Contrib Nephrol 2001;134:46–54.
111. Jiang C, Ting AT, Seed B. PPAR-gamma agonists inhibit production of monocyte inflammatory cytokines. Nature 1998;391:82–86.
112. Ricote M, Li AC, Willson TM, Kelly CJ, Glass CK. The peroxisome proliferator-activated receptor-gamma is a negative regulator of macrophage activation. Nature 1998;391:79–82.
113. Dinarello CA. Biologic basis for interleukin-1 in disease. Blood 1996;87:2095–2147.
114. Pfeilschifter J, Pignat W, Vosbeck K, Marki F. Interleukin 1 and tumor necrosis factor synergistically stimulate prostaglandin synthesis and phospholipase A2 release from rat renal mesangial cells. Biochem Biophys Res Commun 1989;159:385–394.
115. Pfeilschifter J, Rob P, Mulsch A, Fandrey J, Vosbeck K, Busse R. Interleukin 1 beta and tumour necrosis factor alpha induce a macrophage-type of nitric oxide synthase in rat renal mesangial cells. Eur J Biochem 1992;203:251–255.
116. Martin M, Neumann D, Hoff T, Resch K, DeWitt DL, Goppelt-Struebe M. Interleukin-1-induced cyclooxygenase 2 expression is suppressed by cyclosporin A in rat mesangial cells. Kidney Int 1994;45:150–158.
117. Rzymkiewicz D, Leingang K, Baird N, Morrison AR. Regulation of prostaglandin endoperoxide synthase gene expression in rat mesangial cells by interleukin-1 beta. Am J Physiol 1994;266: F39–F45.
118. Colville-Nash PR, Gilroy DW. COX-2 and the cyclopentenone prostaglandins–a new chapter in the book of inflammation? Prostaglandins Other Lipid Mediat 2000;62:33–43.
119. Inoue H, Tanabe T, Umesono K. Feedback control of cyclooxygenase-2 expression through PPARgamma. J Biol Chem 2000;275:28,028–28,032.
120. Chawla A, Barak Y, Nagy L, Liao D, Tontonoz P, Evans RM. PPAR-gamma dependent and independent effects on macrophage-gene expression in lipid metabolism and inflammation. Nat Med 2001;7:48–52.

121. Vaidya S, Somers EP, Wright SD, Detmers PA, Bansal VS. 15-Deoxy-Delta12,1412,14-prostaglandin J2 inhibits the beta2 integrin-dependent oxidative burst: involvement of a mechanism distinct from peroxisome proliferator-activated receptor gamma ligation. J Immunol 1999;163: 6187–6192.
122. Petrova TV, Akama KT, Van Eldik LJ. Cyclopentenone prostaglandins suppress activation of microglia: down-regulation of inducible nitric-oxide synthase by 15-deoxy-Delta12,14-prostaglandin J2. Proc Natl Acad Sci USA 1999;96:4668–4673.
123. Straus DS, Pascual G, Li M, et al. 15-deoxy-delta 12,14-prostaglandin J2 inhibits multiple steps in the NF-kappa B signaling pathway. Proc Natl Acad Sci USA 2000;97:4844–4849.
124. Rossi A, Kapahi P, Natoli G, et al. Anti-inflammatory cyclopentenone prostaglandins are direct inhibitors of IkappaB kinase. Nature 2000;403:103–108.
125. Sawano H, Haneda M, Sugimoto T, Inoki K, Koya D, Kikkawa R. 15-Deoxy-Delta12,14-prostaglandin J2 inhibits IL-1beta-induced cyclooxygenase-2 expression in mesangial cells. Kidney Int 2002;61:1957–1967.
126. Ghosh SS, Gehr TW, Ghosh S, et al. PPARgamma ligand attenuates PDGF-induced mesangial cell proliferation: role of MAP kinase. Kidney Int 2003;64:52–62.
127. Yoshimura R, Matsuyama M, Segawa Y, et al. Study of peroxisome proliferator-activated receptor (PPAR)-gamma in renal ischemia-reperfusion injury. Transplant Proc 2004;36:1946–1948.
128. Sivarajah A, Chatterjee PK, Patel NS, et al. Agonists of peroxisome-proliferator activated receptor-gamma reduce renal ischemia/reperfusion injury. Am J Nephrol 2003;23:267–276.
129. Naito Y, Takagi T, Uchiyama K, et al. Suppression of intestinal ischemia-reperfusion injury by a specific peroxisome proliferator-activated receptor-gamma ligand, pioglitazone, in rats. Redox Rep 2002;7:294–299.
130. Crook ED. The role of hypertension, obesity, and diabetes in causing renal vascular disease. Am J Med Sci 1999;317:183–188.
131. van Jaarsveld BC, Krijnen P, Pieterman H, et al. The effect of balloon angioplasty on hypertension in atherosclerotic renal-artery stenosis. Dutch Renal Artery Stenosis Intervention Cooperative Study Group. N Engl J Med 2000;342:1007–1014.
132. Sawamura T, Kume N, Aoyama T, et al. An endothelial receptor for oxidized low-density lipoprotein. Nature 1997;386:73–77.
133. Chinetti G, Griglio S, Antonucci M, et al. Activation of proliferator-activated receptors alpha and gamma induces apoptosis of human monocyte-derived macrophages. J Biol Chem 1998;273: 25,573–25,580.
134. Law RE, Meehan WP, Xi XP, et al. Troglitazone inhibits vascular smooth muscle cell growth and intimal hyperplasia. J Clin Invest 1996;98:1897–905.
135. Murakami K, Tobe K, Ide T, et al. A novel insulin sensitizer acts as a coligand for peroxisome proliferator-activated receptor-alpha (PPAR-alpha) and PPAR-gamma: effect of PPAR-alpha activation on abnormal lipid metabolism in liver of Zucker fatty rats. Diabetes 1998;47:1841–1847.
136. Arici M, Chana R, Lewington A, Brown J, Brunskill NJ. Stimulation of proximal tubular cell apoptosis by albumin-bound fatty acids mediated by peroxisome proliferator activated receptor-gamma. J Am Soc Nephrol 2003;14:17–27.
137. Zafiriou S, Stanners SR, Polhill TS, Poronnik P, Pollock CA. Pioglitazone increases renal tubular cell albumin uptake but limits proinflammatory and fibrotic responses. Kidney Int 2004;65: 1647–1653.
138. Ma LJ, Marcantoni C, Linton MF, Fazio S, Fogo AB. Peroxisome proliferator-activated receptor-gamma agonist troglitazone protects against nondiabetic glomerulosclerosis in rats. Kidney Int 2001;59:1899–1910.
139. Guo B, Koya D, Isono M, Sugimoto T, Kashiwagi A, Haneda M. Peroxisome proliferator-activated receptor-gamma ligands inhibit TGF-beta 1-induced fibronectin expression in glomerular mesangial cells. Diabetes 2004;53:200–208.
140. Portilla D. Energy metabolism and cytotoxicity. Semin Nephrol 2003;23:432–438.
141. Ouali F, Djouadi F, Merlet-Benichou C, Bastin J. Dietary lipids regulate beta-oxidation enzyme gene expression in the developing rat kidney. Am J Physiol 1998;275:F777–F784.
142. Fried LF, Orchard TJ, Kasiske BL. Effect of lipid reduction on the progression of renal disease: a meta-analysis. Kidney Int 2001;59:260–269.
143. Smulders YM, van Eeden AE, Stehouwer CD, Weijers RN, Slaats EH, Silberbusch J. Can reduction in hypertriglyceridaemia slow progression of microalbuminuria in patients with non-insulin-dependent diabetes mellitus? Eur J Clin Invest 1997;27:997–1002.

144. Park CW, Zhang Y, Fan XF, et al. A PPAR alpha agonist improves diabetic nephropathy in db/db mice. J Am Soc Nephrol 2003;14:393A.
145. Wilmer WA, Dixon CL, Hebert C, Lu L, Rovin BH. PPAR-alpha ligands inhibit H_2O_2-mediated activation of transforming growth factor-beta1 in human mesangial cells. Antioxid Redox Signal 2002;4:877–884.
146. Hao CM, Redha R, Morrow J, Guan YF, Bailey MD. Hypertonic stress induces COX2 dependent prostacyclin synthesis in renal medullary interstitial cells (RMICs) and down-stream activation of PPAR delta dependent survival mechanism. J Am Soc Nephrol 2001;12:49A.

17 α-Endosulfine in Diabetic Nephropathy

Jerry Yee, MD, *and Balazs Szamosfalvi,* MD

CONTENTS

EFFECTS OF SULFONYLUREAS ON CULTURED MESANGIAL CELLS

The sulfonylureas (SULF) have long been utilized as oral agents in the treatment of type 2 diabetes mellitus *(1)*. The primary effect of SULF is the stimulation of insulin secretion following binding to specific SULF receptors (SUR) on pancreatic β-cells. However, SUR have extensive representation in a multitude of extrapancreatic tissues. Therefore, it is not unanticipated that SULF may induce metabolic changes aside from that of insulin secretion. These drugs have been shown to increase glucose uptake and glucose transporter (GLUT) expression in myocytes, adipocytes, and skeletal muscle cells *(2–5)*. Moreover, we have documented significant SULF-induced metabolic effects in cultured rat mesangial cells (MCs), including alterations in mesangial matrix metabolism and MC contractility, independent of their effect on the ambient level of glycemia. The latter effect mimicked that provided by other known MC effectors of contractility, for example, atrial natriuretic peptide and angiotensin II.

In short-term (acute) experiments of rat MC, the exposure to a first-generation SULF, tolazamide (1.5 m*M*), augmented mesangial glucose uptake. This effect was attributed to an elevated rate of cytosol-to-membrane translocation of GLUT1. This direct effect subsequently stimulated MC extracellular matrix (ECM) synthesis, driven by transforming growth factor (TGF)-β_1, which was demonstrated to accumulate in the conditioned

From: *Contemporary Diabetes: The Diabetic Kidney*
Edited by: P. Cortes and C. E. Mogensen © Humana Press Inc., Totowa, NJ

media *(6)*. By contrast, chronic exposure of MC to glibenclamide (10 n*M*), a more potent, second-generation SULF, did not enhance MC glucose uptake, yet produced an intense inhibition of high glucose concentration-induced ECM accumulation *(7)*. Taken collectively, SULF, in addition to their action as insulin secretagogues, exert important metabolic changes through affecting MC matrix metabolism to the extent that the development and evolution of diabetic glomerulosclerosis may be altered by them. Furthermore, it is highly probable that the aforementioned effects are mediated via membrane-bound and/or intracellular SUR.

SULFONYLUREA AGENTS REGULATE MESANGIAL ATP-SENSITIVE K CHANNELS

Several SUR have been identified and cloned from diverse species and tissues *(8–10)*. SUR provide the regulatory subunits of adenosine triphosphate (ATP)-sensitive K channels (K_{ATP}). Classical K_{ATP} consist of two subunits, a potassium ion pore and a SUR. These structurally unrelated subunits complex as four heterodimers to comprise a single functional K_{ATP}. The ion pore belongs to the Kir6.*x* subfamily of weak inwardly rectifying K^+ channels and is represented as either Kir6.1 or Kir6.2. SUR are members of the cystic fibrosis transmembrane regulator/multidrug resistance protein subfamily of the ATP-binding cassette protein (ABC) superfamily *(11,12)*. The pancreatic β-cell SUR is a high-affinity receptor and is designated SUR1. This SUR is encoded by the gene *ABCC8*, whereas SUR2, the lower affinity receptor, is encoded by the gene *ABCC9*.

The heterogeneous properties and functional diversity of K_{ATP} are based on differing complexations of Kir6.*x* and SUR isoforms and cellular distribution. Nearly 90% of K_{ATP} are not localized to the plasmalemma, but to endoplasmic reticulum, mitochondria, and secretory granules *(13–16)*. Consequently, nearly 70% of all SULF binding is cytosolic *(17)*, and this intracellular site of action for K_{ATP} represents an important determinant of SULF action. For example, in β-cells, chronic glibenclamide exposure induces translocation of membranous SUR to the cytoplasm, thereby reducing insulin secretion *(18)*. Consistent with the above, the SULF binding site of the β-cell K_{ATP} is on its cytosolic aspect *(19)*. These observations reconcile the greater potency of the more highly lipophilic SULF compounds: they more easily permeate the plasma membrane and have greater affinity for SUR *(20,21)*. Overall, regardless of their location, all SUR ligands act intracellularly, consequently, candidate endogenous SUR ligands would be anticipated to exert their effects intracellularly as well.

Although K_{ATP} were first described in cardiac myocytes, the membrane-bound pancreatic β-cell K_{ATP}, a tetradimer of SUR1/Kir6.2, represents the most extensively studied of these channels, and it is regarded as the "classical" K_{ATP} *(22,23)*. In the functional channel, Kir6.2 confers K_{ATP} inhibition by ATP, whereas SUR increases pore sensitivity to ATP and regulates channel activation by magnesium-bound adenosine diphosphate (MgADP) and closure by SULF *(24,25)*. Finally, SUR respond variably to K_{ATP} channel openers (KCO), for example, diazoxide, cromakalim, or pinacidil.

The prevailing axiom defines K_{ATP} as molecular switches that link the cell's metabolic state to calcium-dependent signaling *(26)*. In the β-cell, SULF and/or elevations of the cytosolic ATP/adenosine diphosphate (ADP) ratio inhibit K_{ATP} leading to a chain of events: channel closure, membrane depolarization, Ca^{2+} influx, and insulin secretion *(25)*. The opposite series of events are observed with declines in the cytosolic ATP/ADP ratio or after exposure to KCO. Currently, the roles of K_{ATP} are broadening with recent evidence reinforcing the diversity of K_{ATP} and the void of knowledge regarding their functions *(9,10,27)*.

SUR2 is the more ubiquitous extrapancreatic K_{ATP} subunit, and it is found as two major low-affinity splice variants, SUR2A and SUR2B. These isoforms respectively reconstitute the cardiac-type K_{ATP} (SUR2A/Kir6.2), predominantly found in heart and skeletal muscle, and the more ubiquitous vascular smooth muscle-type K_{ATP} (SUR2B/Kir6.1 or Kir6.2) found in brain, heart, liver, kidney, intestine, bladder, vascular smooth muscle, and uterus *(9,10,28–30)*. K_{ATP}, in these tissues regulate a myriad functions, including cell survival, differentiation, and responses to ischemic injury, neurotransmitter release, and vascular smooth muscle cell contraction. The latter has been extensively studied in coronary vessels where K_{ATP} control arteriolar tone *(31,32)*. Not unexpectedly, pharmacological evaluations have also documented the diversity of K_{ATP} among various tissues, with respect to their SULF affinities and sensitivity to KCO *(33)*.

Finally, an intact system of actin filaments is critical to extrapancreatic K_{ATP} activity *(34–37)*. Disruption of filamentous actin reduces the sensitivity of cardiac and smooth muscle K_{ATP} for ATP, SULF, and presumably, for any endogenous SUR ligand(s). In the context of diabetic kidney disease, the dependence of K_{ATP} on normal actin assembly becomes highly relevant because high-glucose concentrations induce MC actin fiber disassembly *(38)*. Finally, the discrete localization and control of protein kinase A (PKA) requires actin cytoskeleton targeting by specific proteins, for example, gravin and Wiskott-Aldrich syndrome protein (WAVE), that dually anchor actin and PKA *(39)*.

KIDNEY SUR

The SUR2B splice variant is widely expressed in the kidney, including the distal nephron where it presumably mediates, in part, potassium transport *(40)*. However, in the proximal tubule, the combination of Kir6.1 with SUR2A and/or SUR2B forms a taurine-sensitive K_{ATP} *(41)*. SUR2B may also couple to murine ROMK2, a Kir that resides in the cortical ascending limb and cortical collecting duct of the distal nephron *(42)*. We hypothesized that the observed MC effects of SULF agents were mediated by specific MC K_{ATP} channels. Subsequently, using membrane preparations from rat MC, we demonstrated specific [^{3}H]glibenclamide binding to low-affinity SUR *(8)*. A functional K_{ATP} was subsequently demonstrated in MC. Cultured cells, following a single exposure to glibenclamide (5 μ*M*), initiated prolonged cycles of oscillatory cytoplasmic Ca^{2+} transients that were coupled to the enhancement of MC contractility *(8)*. These observations were in alignment with results of other investigators who demonstrated similar Ca^{2+} oscillations in MC exposed to angiotensin II.

We subsequently cloned two SUR2 cDNAs from rat MC, a 6.7 kbp smooth muscle-type rSUR2B that had been previously described and a unique 4.8 kbp serum-regulatable MC-specific splice variant, mcSUR2B. This variant was homologous, in large part, with the larger splice variant, rSUR2B. Our findings additionally revealed expression of Kir 6.1 but not of Kir6.2 in MC *(43)*. These studies suggest that the K_{ATP} of MC and also of isolated glomeruli are comprised of $(rSUR2B/Kir6.1)_4$ and possibly, $(mcSUR2B/Kir6.1)_4$ *(8,43)*.

In this context, the marked inhibition of established high-glucose concentration-fostered ECM accumulation by glibenclamide at 10 n*M* is a highly relevant observation because the experimental concentrations are within the clinically relevant range for this compound (peak plasma concentration: 50–60 n*M* after a 5-mg dose) *(44)*. In addition, the K_D of 6 n*M* for glibenclamide, as determined by complexation of SUR2B to Kir6.1 in intact cells, is consonant with this hypothesis *(45)*. Finally, immunoreactivity for rSUR2B and mcSUR2 in primary and cloned MC ($16KC_2$) lines as delineated by a specific antibody directed against the common C-terminal epitope of SUR2A and SUR2B further substantiates this argument *(43)*. Thus, it is plausible that the metabolic actions of low-concentration glibenclamide on MC are mediated through K_{ATP} comprised of SUR2B/Kir6.1.

ENDOGENOUS K_{ATP} LIGANDS

The central role that pancreatic β-cell K_{ATP} $(SUR1/Kir6.2)_4$ plays in regulating insulin secretion and the ubiquitous nature of the SUR2-based K_{ATP} led to a search for endogenous ligand(s) of these channels. Subsequently, a putative endogenous polypeptide ligand of K_{ATP}, α-endosulfine was isolated from ovine and porcine brain. Purified α-endosulfine displaced prebound glibenclamide from these K_{ATP}-rich substrates. Because of this initial characterization, human α-endosulfine (*ARPP-19e*) has been cloned and proposed as an endogenous ligand for pancreatic K_{ATP} *(46)*. Consonant with this hypothesis are electrophysiological observations that demonstrate K_{ATP} inhibition by recombinant α-endosulfine in Syrian hamster insulinoma tumor cells and the induction of insulin secretion from MIN6 and RINm5F pancreatic β-cells via a Ca^{2+}-dependent mechanism.

α-Endosulfine and its splice variant β-endosulfine reveal similarity to a group of mammalian neuronal phosphoproteins, which are phosphorylated by PKA. Of these cyclic AMP-regulated phosphoproteins (ARPPs), two closely related isoforms have been characterized by apparent molecular mass, ARPP-16 and ARPP-19. The former is only detected in brain, with enrichment in the neostriatum, whereas the latter is ubiquitously expressed in neurons and non-neuronal tissues, including fibroblasts and renal tubular epithelial cells *(47)*. In vertebrates, the ARPP protein family is characterized by a core of 82 identical amino acids that encompasses an absolutely conserved serine residue, which is phosphorylated, by the catalytic subunit of PKA *(47)*. The conservation of this amino acid contends that ARPP regulation via PKA-dependent phosphorylation represents a fundamental biological process. Although ARPP are without known enzymatic activity, they possess characteristics common to intracellular regulatory proteins that alter the activities of enzymes involved in signal transduction, for example, calmodulin and the PKA inhibitor (Walsh inhibitor, PKI) *(47)*. Presently, little is known regarding the physiological roles of ARPP 16/19, but ARPP-19 mediates nerve growth factor signaling through posttranscriptional control of gene expression via binding to and stabilizing GAP-43 mRNA, which results in amplified protein expression *(48)*.

The human gene encoding α-endosulfine, *ENSA*, had initially been reported on chromosome 14 and colocalized with a known insulin-dependent diabetes mellitus (IDDM) susceptibility locus *(49)*. Subsequently, based on the results derived from the human genome project, *ENSA* was remapped to locus 1q23.1, relegating the previously reported locus to the status of a pseudogene. In functional experiments, recombinant α-endosulfine at micromolar concentrations competitively inhibits [^{3}H]glibenclamide binding to SUR. Moreover, there is also diminution of K_{ATP} conductance in oocytes transduced to express the recombinant channel. The inhibition of current is most evident when α-endosulfine is delivered intracellularly where it can rapidly appose itself to its cytoplasmic locus of action *(50)*.

Although α-endosulfine is expressed in a large number of tissues, including heart, lung, spleen, skeletal muscle, pancreatic somatostatin δ-cells, liver, and kidney *(51)*, its various tissue-specific roles remain at present undetermined. However, it has been recently shown that brain α-endosulfine from Alzheimer's disease patients was greatly reduced *(52)*. Recently, it was posited that α-endosulfine did not mediate its actions in an autocrine or paracrine manner *(51)*. This assumption appears likely given that treatment of pancreatic α cells with somatostatin secretagogues fails to induce α-endosulfine release, K_{ATP} inhibition only occurs in high extracellular α-endosulfine concentrations, plasma α-endosulfine levels are in the picomolar range, and because α-endosulfine is a cytosolic protein that associates with the particulate fraction. In the aggregate, these data favor α-endosulfine as an intracellular regulator *(51)*.

α-ENDOSULFINE REGULATION OF K_{ATP}

As α-endosulfine represents a putative ligand of K_{ATP} and K_{ATP} are present in MC, we postulated that α-endosulfine was expressed in the rat kidney in vivo and in cultured rat MC in vitro. We determined that *ENSA* was expressed abundantly in rat kidney by *in situ* hybridization. Further observations, utilizing Northern blotting and RT-PCR, established α-endosulfine message in cultured MC in vitro and in whole rat kidney in vivo, with expression predominantly localized to the glomeruli. Further studies of α-endosulfine expression by immunoblotting and confocal microscopy confirmed its presence in vitro and in vivo.

ENSA gene and protein expression in MC is altered in response to a hyperglycemic milieu. Cultured cells increased *ENSA* gene expression by twofold following exposure to 30 m*M* glucose within 24–48 h, and this effect persisted for at least 10 d, even after withdrawal of the inciting stimulus *(53)*. Thus, MC expression of SUR2B, Kir 6.1 and α-endosulfine lays the foundation for the existence of a regulatable intracellular K_{ATP}/endosulfine receptor/ligand system, which could influence MC contractility and matrix metabolism *(54)*.

GLOMERULAR EFFECTS OF SULF IN INSULIN-DEFICIENT DIABETES MELLITUS

SULF have been extensively used in the treatment of type 2 diabetes. However, the renal effects of SULF in diabetes have not been determined. A study of complications in patients with type 2 diabetes investigated the effects of intensive glycemic control with insulin or SULF (UK Prospective Diabetes Study) *(55)*. These results revealed a reduction in proteinuria and renal failure, in association with improved glycemic control. However, owing to either the relatively few number of patients who developed renal disease or the confounding effects of combinations of sequential therapies in individual patients, no conclusive differences were detected between insulin- and SULF-treated groups. Since this trial, other studies have proven inconclusive *(56,57)*. Therefore, the current status of clinical knowledge does not render definitive conclusions regarding any beneficial or deleterious renal effects by exogenous SULF or an endogenous SULF-like ligand.

In an attempt to extend prior observations of altered matrix metabolism and increased cellular contractility in MCs after SULF exposure, the effect of chronic administration of various SULF on the progression of diabetic nephropathy was evaluated in animal models of types 1 and 2 diabetes mellitus. Our observations revealed an attenuation of proteinuria

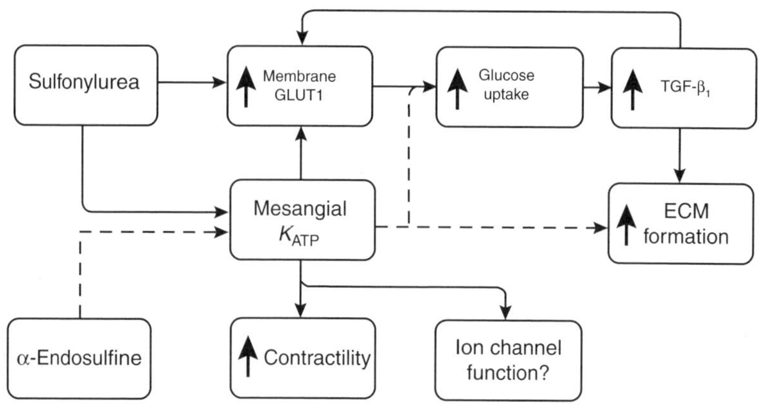

Fig. 1. Mesangial K_{ATP} are formed as tetradimers of Kir6.1 and SUR2B. K_{ATP} mediate changes in extracellular matrix (ECM) metabolism following binding of either sulfonylurea (SULF) or α-endosulfine. Low-concentration SULF inhibits α-endosulfine action at the K_{ATP} site and limits ECM formation. However, high concentrations of SULF increase ECM accumulation as a consequence of the increased expression of GLUT1 and enhanced GLUT1-mediated intracellular glucose transport with the consequent upregulation of TGF-β_1. This growth factor, in turn upregulates membrane-associated GLUT1 expression. Heightened mesangial contractility represents a Ca^{2+}-mediated event in response to exposure to SULF and possibly to α-endosulfine.

and morphological glomerular alterations after glibenclamide or tolazamide administration to streptozotocin-treated rats *(58)*. Notably, these salutary effects proceeded in the absence of changes in glycemia or (as studied in the case of glibenclamide) in glomerular filtration rate or renal hypertrophy. In separate experiments with insulin-resistant db/db mice, SULF treatment did not impact the course of glomerulosclerosis in functional or morphological assays. In toto, these observations imply that the direct glomerular effects of SULF at low concentrations (and by extrapolation, of their endogenous counterpart, α-endosulfine) may suppress or retard the TGF-β_1-mediated accrual of glomerular extracellular matrix (ECM), the hallmark of diabetic glomerulosclerosis and may significantly alter the course of insulin-deficient diabetic kidney disease.

α-ENDOSULFINE EXPRESSION ALTERS MATRIX METABOLISM

To more fully understand the role of *ENSA* expression in MCs with regard to ECM formation, a stably overexpressing α-endosulfine cell line was produced by retroviral transduction. The resulting cell line reliably upregulated *ENSA* by eightfold. In cells, exposed to a high-glucose environment (25 m*M*) for 2 wk, there was increased accumulation of collagen type I in the conditioned medium, compared with control cells transduced by a nonvirus-containing empty vector. A similar finding was noted for type-4 collagen. Contrastingly, *ENSA* downregulation by RNA interference during transient transfection experiments with three different siRNAs led to decrements of types I and IV collagen accumulation in the conditioned media of cells incubated for 2 wk in 5 m*M* glucose. We conclude that, although modifications of ECM gene expression via *ENSA* may not be translated directly to changes in ECM protein expression, these results imply that α-endosulfine enhances ECM accumulation, an effect that is particularly invoked by a high-glucose environment. In addition, in other preliminary data, these effects occur downstream of the perinuclear and nuclear translocation of α-endosulfine in MCs following their cAMP-mediated PKA phosphorylation.

CONCLUSIONS

Heterodimeric expression of SUR2B and Kir6.1 produces functional mesangial K_{ATP} (*see* Fig. 1.). The documentation of a functional α-endosulfine expression system in MC promotes the notion of a regulatable intracellular K_{ATP}/endosulfine receptor/ligand system. Subsequent genomic changes of *ENSA,* particularly in a high-glucose environment, likely regulate ECM protein metabolism via PKA-mediated phosphorylation events. The effects of SULF on mesangial contractility and matrix metabolism in vitro and their partial abrogation of proteinuria and glomerulosclerosis in a rodent model of insulin-deficient diabetes in vivo, may argue for a unique therapeutic role of these agents, in possible opposition to α-endosulfine.

REFERENCES

1. Lebovitz HE, Feinglos MN. Sulfonylurea drugs: mechanism of antidiabetic action and therapeutic usefulness. Diabetes Care 1978;1:189–198.
2. Jacobs DB, Hayes GR, Lockwood DH. In vitro effects of sulfonylurea on glucose transport and translocation of glucose transporters in adipocytes from streptozotocin-induced diabetic rats. Diabetes 1989;38:205–211.
3. Wang PH, Moller D, Flier JR, Nayak RC, Smith RJ. Coordinate regulation of glucose transporter function, number, and gene expression by insulin and sulfonylureas in L6 rat skeletal muscle cells. J Clin Invest 1989;84:62–67.
4. Müller G, Wied S. The sulfonylurea drug glimepiride stimulates glucose transport, glucose transporter translocation, and dephosphorylation in insulin-resistant rat adipocytes in vitro. Diabetes 1993;42:1852–1867.
5. Rogers BJ, Standaert ML, Pollet RJ. Direct effects of sulfonylurea agents on glucose transport in the BC3H-1 myocyte. Diabetes 1987;36:1292–1296.
6. Cortes P, Riser BL, Asano K, Rodrígez-Barbero A, Narins RG, Yee J. Effects of oral antihyperglycemic agents on extracellular matrix synthesis by mesangial cells. Kidney Int 1998;54:1985–1998.
7. Giannico G, Biederman J, Hasset C, Yee J, Cortes P. Amelioration of glucose-induced extracellular matrix formation (ECM) by the sulfonylurea glibenclamide (GLIB) in cultured mesangial cells (MC). J Am Soc Nephrol 2002;13:318A.
8. Asano K, Cortes P, Garvin JL, et al. Characterization of the rat mesangial cell type 2 sulfonylurea receptor. Kid Int 1999;55:2289–2298.
9. Inagaki N, Gonoi T, Clement IV JP, et al. A family of sulfonylurea receptors determines the pharmacological properties of ATP-sensitive K^+ channels. Neuron 1996;16:1011–1017.
10. Chutkow WA, Simon MC, Le Beau MM, Burant CF. Cloning, tissue expression, and chromosomal localization of SUR2, the putative drug-binding subunit of cardiac, skeletal muscle, and vascular K_{ATP} channels. Diabetes 1996;45:1439–1445.
11. Higgins CF. The ABC of Channel Regulation. Cell 1995;82:693–696.
12. Philipson LH, Steiner DF. Pas de deux or more: The sulfonylurea receptor and K^+ channels. Science 1995;268:372, 373.
13. Garlid KD, Paucek P, Yarov-Yarovoy P, Sun X, Schindler PA. The mitochondrial K_{ATP} channel as a receptor for potassium channel openers. J Biol Chem 1996;271:8796–8799.
14. Suzuki M, Kotake K, Fujikura K, et al. Kir6.1: A possible subunit of ATP-sensitive K^+ channels in mitochondria. Biochem Biophys Res Comm 1997;241:693–697.
15. Geng X, Li L, Watkins S, Robbins PD, Drain P. The insulin secretory granule is the major site of K_{ATP} channels of the endocrine pancreas. Diabetes 2003;52:767–776.
16. Suzuki M, Sasaki N, Miki T, et al. Role of sarcolemmal K_{ATP} channels in cardioprotection against ischemia/reperfusion injury in mice. J Clin Invest 2002;109:509–516.
17. Carpentier J-L, Sawano F, Ravazzola M, Malisse WJ. Internalization of ^{3}H-glibenclamide in pancreatic islet cells. Diabetologia 1996;29:259–261.
18. Kawaki J, Nagashima K, Tanaka J, et al. Unresponsiveness to glibenclamide during chronic treatment induced by reduction of ATP-sensitive K^+ channel activity. Diabetes 1999;48:2001–2006.
19. Schwanstecher M, Schwanstecher C, Dickel C, Chudziak F, Moshiri A, Panten U. Location of the sulfonylurea receptor at the cytoplasmic face of the beta-cell membrane. Brit J Pharmacol 1994;113:903–911.

20. Zunkler BJ, Trube G, Panten U. How do sulfonylureas approach their receptor in the β-cell plasma membrane? Naunyn-Schmiedeberg's Arch Pharmacol 1989;340:328–332.
21. Ashcroft SJH, Ashcroft FM. The sulfonylurea receptor. Biochem Biophys Acta 1992;1175:45–59.
22. Dukes ID, Philipson LH. K^+ channels: generating excitement in pancreatic β-cells. Diabetes 1996;45: 845–853.
23. Suzuki M, Fujikura K, Inagaki N, Seino S, Takata K. Localization of the ATP-sensitive K^+ channel subunit Kir6.2 in mouse pancreas. Diabetes 1997;46:1440–1444.
24. Brian J, Aguilar-Brian L. The ABCs of ATP-sensitive potassium channels- more pieces of the puzzle. Curr Opin Cell Biol 1997;9:553–559.
25. Babenko AP, Aguilar-Bryan L, Bryan J. A View of SUR/K_{IR}6.X, K_{ATP} channels. Annu Rev Physiol 1998;60:667–687.
26. Ashcroft FM. Adenosine 5′-triphosphate-sensitive potassium channels. Ann Rev Neurosci 1988;11: 97–118.
27. Seino S, Iwanaga T, Nagashima K, Miki T. Diverse roles in K_{ATP} channels learned from Kir6.2 genetically engineered mice. Diabetes 2000;49:311–318.
28. Lorenz E, Terzic A. Physical association between recombinant cardiac ATP-sensitive K^+ channel subunits Kir6.2 and SUR2A. J Mol Cell Cardiol 1999;31:425–434.
29. Ashcroft SJ, Ashcroft FM. Properties and function of ATP-sensitive K^+ channels. Cell Signal 1990;2:197–214.
30. Gopalakrishnan M, Whitaker KL, Molinari EJ, et al. Characterization of the ATP-Sensitive Potassium Channels (K_{ATP}) Expressed in Guinea Pig Bladder Smooth Muscle Cells. J Pharmacol Exper Therap 1998;289:551–558.
31. Tune JD, Yeh C, Setty S, Downey F. ATP-dependent K^+ channels contribute to local metabolic coronary vasodilatation in experimental diabetes. Diabetes 2002;51:1201–1207.
32. Duncker DJ, van Zon NS, Ishibashi Y, Bache RJ. Role of K_{ATP} channels and adenosine in the regulation of coronary blood flow during exercise with normal and restricted coronary blood flow. J Clin Invest 1996;97:996–1009.
33. Edwards G, Weston AH. The pharmacology of ATP-sensitive potassium channels. Ann Rev Pharmacol Toxicol 1993;33:597–637.
34. Yokoshiki H, Katsube Y, Sunagawa M, Seki T, Sperelakis N. Disruption of actin cytoskeleton attenuates sulfonylurea inhibition of cardiac ATP-sensitive K^+ channels. Eur J Physiol 1997;434:203–205.
35. Song DK, Ashcroft FM. ATP modulation of ATP-sensitive potassium channel ATP sensitivity varies with the type of SUR subunit. J Biol Chem 2001;276:7143–7149.
36. Loffler-Waltz C, Quast U. Disruption of the actin cytoskeleton abolishes high affinity ^3H glibenclamide binding in rat aortic rings. Naunyn-Schmiedebergs Arch Pharmacol 1998;357:183–185.
37. Brady PA, Alekseev AE, Alesandrova LA, Gomez LA, Terzic A. A disrupter of actin filaments impairs sulfonylurea-inhibitory gating of cardiac K_{ATP} channels. Am J Physiol 1996;271:H2710–H2716.
38. Dlugosz JA, Munk S, Ispanovic E, Goldberg HJ, Whiteside C. Mesangial cell filamentous actin disassembly and hypocontractility in high glucose are mediated by PKC-ζ. Am J Physiol Renal Physiol 2002;282:F151–F163.
39. Alto N, Michel JJC, Dodge KL, Langeberg LK, Scott JD. Intracellular targeting of protein kinases and phosphatases. Diabetes 2002;51(3):S385–S388.
40. Beesley AH, Qureshi IZ, Giesberts AN, Parker AJ, J White SJ. Expression of sulfonylurea receptor protein in mouse kidney. Pflugers Arch-Eur J Physiol 1999;438:1–7.
41. Brochiero E, Wallendorf B, Gagnon D, Laprade R, LaPointe JY. Cloning of rabbit Kir6.1, SUR2A, and SUR2B: possible candidates for a renal K_{ATP} channel. Am J Physiol Renal Physiol 2002;282:F289–F300.
42. Tanemoto M, Vanoye CG, Dong K, et al. Rat homolog of sulfonylurea receptor 2B determines glibenclamide sensitivity of ROMK2 in *Xenopus laevis* oocyte. Am J Physiol Renal Physiol 2000;278: F659–F666.
43. Szamosfalvi B, Cortes P, Alviani R, et al. Putative subunits of the rat mesangial K_{ATP}: A type 2B sulfonylurea receptor and an inwardly rectifying K^+ channel. Kid Int 2002;61:1739–1749.
44. Pendergast BD. Glyburide and glipizide, second generation oral sulfonylurea hypoglycemic agents. Clin Pharm 1984;3:473–485.
45. Russ U, HambrockA, Artunc F, et al. Coexpression with the inward rectifier K^+ channel Kir6.1 increases the affinity of the vascular sulfonylurea receptor SUR2B for glibenclamide. Mol Pharmacol 1999;56:955–961.
46. Peyrollier K, Heron Virsolvy-Vergine A, LeCam A, Bataille D. Alpha endosulfine is a novel molecule, structurally related to a family of phosphoproteins. Biochem Biophys Res Commun 1996;223:583–586.

47. Dulubova I, Horiuchi A, Snyder GL, et al. ARPP-16/ARPP-19: a highly conserved family of cAMP-regulated phosphoproteins. J Neurochem 2001;77:229–238.
48. Irwin N, Chao S, Gorichenko L, et al. Nerve growth factor controls GAP-43 mRNA stability via the phosphoprotein ARPP-19. Proc Natl Acad Sci 2002;99:12,427–12,431.
49. Heron L, Virsolvy A, Apiou F, Le Cam A, Bataille D. Isolation, characterization, and chromosomal localization of the human ENSA gene that encodes alpha-endosulfine, a regulator of beta-cell K_{ATP} channels. Diabetes 1999;48:1873–1876.
50. Bataille D, Heron L, Virsolvy A, et al. α-Endosulfine, a new entity in the control of insulin secretion. Cell Mol Life Sci 1999;56:78–84.
51. Gros L, Breant B, Duchene B, et al. Localization of α-endosulfine in pancreatic somatostatin δ-cells and expression during rat pancreas development. Diabetologia 2002;45:703–710.
52. Kim SH Lubec G. Brain α-endosulfine is manifold decreased in brains from patients with Alzheimer's disease: a tentative marker and drug target? Neurosci Lett 2001;310:77–80.
53. Yee J, Cortes P, Barnes JL, Alviani R, Biederman JI, Szamosfalvi B. Rat mesangial α-endosulfine. Kid Int 2004;65:1731–1739.
54. Yee J, Szamosfalvi B. A New Mesangial Triumvirate: Sulfonylureas, Their Receptors and Endosulfines Exp Neph 2002;10:1–6.
55. UK Prospective Diabetes Study (UKPDS) Group. Intensive blood glucose control with sulfonylureas or insulin compared with conventional treatment and risk of complications in patients with type 2 diabetes (UKPDS 33). Lancet 1998;352:837–853.
56. Klein R, Klein BEK, Moss SE, Cruickshanks K. Ten-year incidence of gross proteinuria in people with diabetes. Diabetes 1995;44:916–923.
57. Carpenter A-M, Goetz FC, LeCompte PM, Williamson JR. Glomerulosclerosis in type 2 (non-insulin-dependent) diabetes mellitus: relationship to glycemia in the University Group Diabetes Program (UGDP). Diabetologia 1993;36:1057–1063.
58. Biederman J, Vera E, Pankhaniya R, et al. Effects of sulfonylureas, α-endosulfine counterparts, on glomerulosclerosis in type 1 and type 2 models of diabetes. Kid Int 2005;67:554–565.

18 The Prospect of a Novel Therapeutic, Bone Morphogenetic Protein-7, in Diabetic Nephropathy

Keith A. Hruska, MD, *Laura De Petris,* MD,
Tingting Li, MD, *Song Wang,* MD,
Theresa Geurs, BS, *Frank Strebeck,* BS,
Qing Chen, MD, *and Helen Liapis,* MD

CONTENTS

INTRODUCTION

We are in the midst of a worldwide epidemic of diabetes and hypertension. In the United States, the overall incidence of end-stage kidney disease (ESKD) is increasing at an alarming rate due to this epidemic. Recently, the incidence of ESKD was estimated at 336 per million per year *(1)*, such that the number of patients with ESKD may approach 2.24 million by 2030. Moreover, approx 11% of the population is estimated to have chronic kidney disease (CKD), with nearly half the patients with a glomerular filtration rate (GFR) less than 60 mL/min/1.73 m^2 *(2)*. Similar estimates for other countries have been described in Europe *(3)*, Japan *(4)*, and Australia *(5)*. The most common form of CKD in all of these countries is diabetic nephropathy (DN), accounting for approx 40% of the new cases of ESKD in developed countries.

Despite significant advances in the understanding of the mechanistic pathways mediating the progression of DN to ESKD, options for effective therapy are limited

From: *Contemporary Diabetes: The Diabetic Kidney*
Edited by: P. Cortes and C. E. Mogensen

to treating conventional risk factors including hypertension control, particularly with angiotensin-converting enzyme inhibitors or angiotensin receptor blockers *(6–9)*, tight control of glucose in diabetics *(10,11)*, control of proteinuria *(12,13)*, control of dyslipidemia, and cessation of tobacco use. The prospect of new therapies for CKD and DN are therefore extremely important. Although the primary pathology leading to most forms of CKD differs significantly, all progressive renal diseases, including glomerulonephritis, chronic interstitial nephritis, and DN, exhibit interstitial fibrosis *(14,15)*. Despite the strong correlation between tubulo-interstitial fibrosis and the loss of renal function, the molecular mechanisms underlying fibrosis have remained elusive. However, evidence pointing to the transforming growth factor (TGF)-β superfamily of proteins as primary regulators of fibrosis is accumulating. Indeed, TGF-β1 may be the major stimulator of fibrosis in the kidney, whereas bone morphogenetic protein (BMP)-7 is thought to counteract the profibrotic activity of TGF-β1. Despite recent therapeutic trials in murine and rodent models of acute and chronic renal failure demonstrating the efficacy of BMP-7 in preventing the progression of glomerular injury and renal fibrosis and in some cases reversing glomerulosclerosis and renal fibrosis, questions regarding the molecular mechanisms and clinical relevance of TGF-β and BMP-7 remain.

TGF-β SUPERFAMILY AND SIGNAL TRANSDUCTION

The TGF-β family encodes several secreted factors that regulate a wide variety of cellular processes. The members include TGF-β 1–3, activins, inhibins, BMPs, and growth and differentiation factors (GDFs) *(16,17)*. These secreted proteins bind to type-I and type-II receptors expressed on the cell surface (Fig. 1). There are seven type I, also termed activin receptor-like kinases (Alk), and five type-II receptors, with specific ligand-binding specificity *(16)*. The receptors contain intracellular serine-threonine kinase domains. On binding of ligand, the constitutively active type-II receptor activates the type-I receptor by phosphorylation. This activated receptor then phosphorylates downstream signaling effectors, called Smad proteins (Fig. 1). BMP-mediated signaling activates receptor Smads 1, 5, and 8, whereas activin and TGF-β activate Smads 2 and 3. These activated Smads interact with the common Smad 4, and this complex translocates to the nucleus to regulate target gene transcription. Two inhibitory Smad proteins, Smads 6 and 7, negatively regulate BMP and TGF-β-mediated signaling, respectively. Smad-mediated signaling can be terminated by ubiquitin-mediated degradation. Smurf 1 targets Smads 1 and 5 for destruction *(18)*, Smurf 2 targets Smad 2 *(19)*, and the SCF/Roc1 complex mediates degradation of Smad 3 *(20)*. Moreover, interaction of these ubiquitin-regulatory factors with inhibitory Smads is involved in degradation of the type-I receptor. Interaction of Smurf 1 with Smad 7 targets the TGF-β type-I receptor for degradation *(21)* and Smurf 1 and Smad 6 target the BMP type-I receptor for degradation *(22)*.

The steps leading to receptor activation are regulated at multiple levels. Outside of the cell, the access of TGF-β superfamily ligands to their receptors is controlled by proteins that function to sequester ligands from their respective receptors. Processing of the TGF-β proprotein in the Golgi results in the formation of a latent complex *(23,24)*. The latency-associated protein LAP1, which is the cleaved amino terminus of the TGF-β proprotein, together with latent TGF-β-binding protein 1 and the active TGF-β homodimer, constitute the large latent complex, which associates with the extracellular matrix and can be released and activated by proteolytic cleavage.

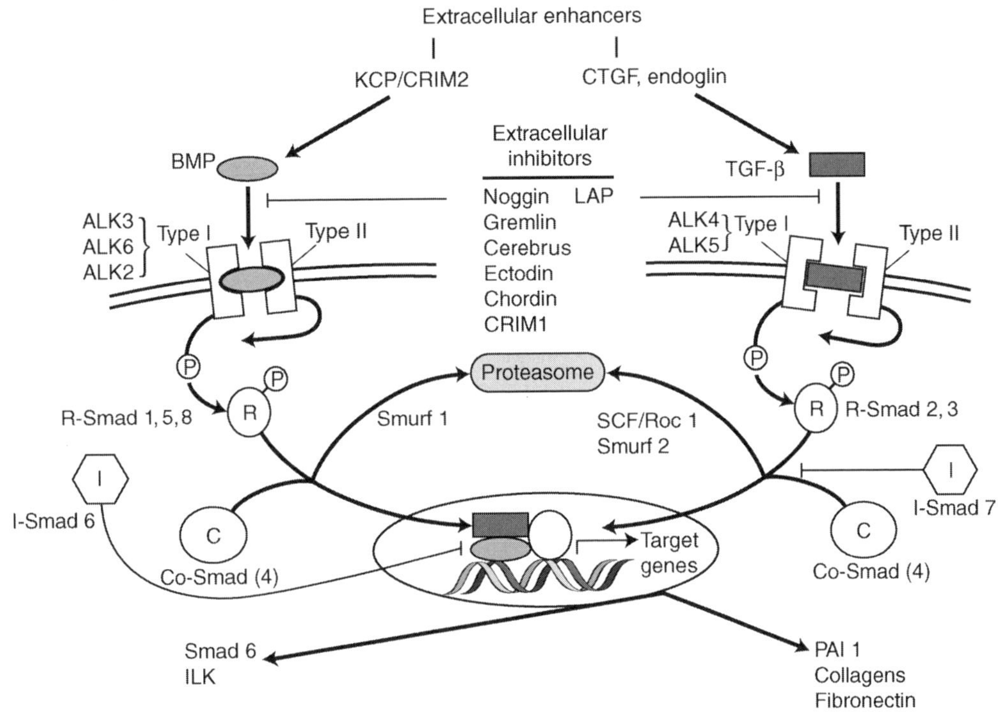

Fig. 1. Schematic BMP and TGF-β signaling (*see* text for details). Ligands bind to type-I and type-II transmembrane receptors. Access of ligands is enhanced or suppressed by extracellular interacting proteins. Type-I receptors phosphorylated by type-II receptors phosphorylate regulatory Smad proteins at serine residues to promote interactions with the ubiquitous co-Smad 4 or with inhibitory Smads 6 and 7. The activated Smad–co-Smad complex translocates to the nucleus to regulate gene expression. Unique ubiquitin ligases, Smurfs, regulate Smad degradation. PAI-1, plasminogen activator inhibitor-1; ILK, integrin-linked kinase stimulated in the medullary collecting duct by BMP-7 *(71)*.

Extracellular inhibitors of BMP signaling include vertebrate chordin, which binds directly to BMPs through the cysteine-rich (CR) domains containing CXXCXC and CCXXC motifs *(25)*, and CR transmembrane (CRIM1), which can regulate secretion and receptor binding of BMPs *(26)*. Signaling by the activin family of ligands is inhibited by follistatins. BMPs can also be bound by Noggin, DAN/Cerebrus, Gremlin, and Ectodin to suppress signaling *(27–29)*. Resolution of the crystal structure of the BMP-7/Noggin complex reveals that Noggin inhibits BMP-7 by blocking surfaces that are required to interact with both type-I and type-II BMP receptors *(30)*. Whereas chordin blocks BMP/receptor interactions, the CR domain protein KCP/CRIM2 enhances BMP/receptor interactions to increase the efficacy of signaling *(31)*. Similarly, the CR domain protein CTGF enhances TGF-β-mediated signaling, whereas suppressing the BMP-dependent pathway *(32)*. Endoglin, a type-III TGF-β receptor, associates with TGF-β and the type-I and type-II receptor complex increasing TGF-β signaling. Interestingly, BMP-2, but not BMP-7, also binds with endoglin and enhances TGF-β signaling *(33)*.

BMP-7 SIGNALING IN KIDNEY DEVELOPMENT

Multiple BMPs have been identified in the developing kidney *(34)*, of which BMP-7 and BMP-4 are the most abundant. BMP-7 is expressed in the ureteric duct at embryonic day 11 postcoitum, and is maintained throughout development in the collecting tubule derivatives of the ureteric duct. BMP-7 is also expressed transiently in the induced mesenchyme, but not the uninduced mesenchyme, and its derivatives. BMP-7 is essential for kidney development as homozygous-null mice have arrested kidney development, possess dysplastic kidneys, and die soon after birth *(35,36)*. Kidney development is normal in the BMP-7-null mice until embryonic day 14.5. Then branching of the ureteric duct, condensation of the metanephric mesenchyme around the ureteric duct, and differentiation of epithelial structures all cease and uninduced mutant mesenchymal cells suffer apoptosis. BMP-7 appears to act as a survival factor for undifferentiated mesenchyme, opposing apoptotic signals. Thus, with additional factors, such as basic fibroblast growth factor 2, BMP-7 expands the stromal progenitor cell population adjacent to the nephrogenic mesenchyme and ensures that the cells are competent to respond to inductive signals *(37)*. The BMP type-I receptors Alk3 and Alk6 are also expressed in the tips and body of the branching ureter, mesenchymal condensates, developing vesicles and comma-shaped bodies *(38)*. All seven Smad proteins are expressed during murine kidney development *(39)*. Expression begins at embryonic day 12 and continues until the end of nephrogenesis at postnatal day 15. The BMP-responsive Smads are mainly expressed in the nephrogenic zone, whereas the TGF-β-responsive Smads are noted in the medullary interstitium. Inhibitory Smad 6 and Smad 7 expression is also evident in mesenchymal cells and in the interstitium.

Extracellular BMP-binding proteins also function in kidney development. The secreted BMP antagonist protein gremlin binds to BMP-2, BMP-4, and BMP-7 in the extracellular compartment and prevents binding to the cognate receptor *(40,41)*. Gremlin-mediated BMP antagonism is essential to induce metanephric kidney development as initiation of ureter growth and branching are disrupted in gremlin-null embryos *(42)*, and the null mice are essentially anephric. Given the potential for BMP-4 to suppress ureteric bud outgrowth *(43)*, it is likely that gremlin suppresses BMP-4 along the posterior nephric duct. The recently identified BMP agonist, KCP protein (also known as CRIM2), is expressed in tubular epithelial cells during development. However, kidney development in KCP-null mice is normal *(31)*.

BMP-7 SIGNALING IN THE ADULT KIDNEY

The role of BMP-7 in the adult kidney is still unresolved. Expression remains high in the collecting tubule, podocytes, glomerular parietal epithelial cells, and renal-artery adventitial cells *(44,45)*. By analyzing the expression pattern of a BMP-7 promoter driving β-galactosidase in transgenic mice, Gould et al. *(46)* demonstrated reporter gene expression in the thick ascending limb, distal convoluted tubule, collecting duct, and podocytes. In proximal tubular cells, BMP-7 expression appears to be weak, though this remains controversial *(47)*. BMP-7 type-II receptors have been described within glomeruli, proximal convoluted tubules, and medullary collecting tubules *(48)*. There is limited information regarding tissue distribution and binding characteristics of the type-I receptor, although Alk 2, 3, and 6 appear to be expressed in the adult kidney. Preliminary studies of Smad 1, Smad 5, and Smad 8 expression in the adult kidney suggest that both Smad 1 and Smad 5 are important mediators of BMP-7 signaling in the adult kidney *(31,49,50)*.

BMP-7 FUNCTION IN ANIMAL MODELS OF ACUTE AND CHRONIC RENAL INJURY

The role of BMP-7 has been evaluated in several models of renal injury, including acute renal failure, chronic renal failure, DN, genetic models of renal disease, and glomerulonephritis. In a mouse model of ischemic acute renal failure *(44,45)*, BMP-7 mRNA is significantly reduced 6 h after injury and remains reduced for up to 4 d after the initial insult, most significantly in the outer medulla and cortex. Administration of recombinant human (rh) BMP-7 protected rats from acute injury, in which tubular necrosis and apoptosis are reduced, and proinflammatory adhesion molecules are reduced. The functional recovery of ischemic kidneys was enhanced. The decrease in BMP-7 expression was reciprocal to TGF-β expression. In the unilateral urinary obstruction (UUO) model, renal BMP-7 expression declines markedly in the obstructed kidney *(51)*. Administration of rhBMP-7 at the time of UUO and every other day thereafter preserved renal function and enhanced recovery of renal function when the UUO was released at day 5. Interstitial inflammation, fibrogenesis, apoptosis, and tubular atrophy was reduced *(51)*. Urine flow and return of GFR to 50% of normal by day 10 was observed with BMP-7 treatment. The effects of BMP-7 on restoration of urine flow and GFR were not seen with enalapril treatment in this model. In a similar study, BMP-7 accelerated the *de novo* recovery of renal function when UUO was removed after 3 d to a GFR of 75% normal at day 10, whereas enalapril restored urine flow but only to a GFR of 25% normal *(52)*.

In a model of glomerulonephritis induced by nephrotoxic serum administration, interstitial fibrosis and epithelial-to-mesenchymal transition is associated with increased TGF-β signaling, resulting in phosphorylation and translocation of Smad 2 and Smad 3 into nuclei *(53)*. The E-cadherin expression is attenuated in tubular epithelial cells, suggesting the conversion of tubular epithelial cells to mesenchymal cells; rhBMP-7 administration improved renal function, prevented tubulo-interstitial fibrosis, and prevented the loss of epithelial E-cadherin expression in a Smad 1-dependent manner. Overall mortality was reduced in the group of animals treated with BMP-7. Mice deficient in the α3 chain of type-IV collagen and RL/MpJlpr/lpr lupus mice are genetic models of chronic renal injury and fibrosis. Decreased tubular expression of BMP-7 was seen during the progression of renal disease in both models. Treatment with rhBMP-7 lead to improved renal function and prevented interstitial fibrosis and tubular atrophy. Decreased type-I collagen and fibronectin expression and increased matrix metalloproteinase (MMP)2 expression were noted in the treated groups *(54)*. Thus, administration of BMP-7 in various models of acute and chronic renal injury appears to attenuate tubulo-interstitial fibrosis and preserve renal function. This also applies to models of DN.

BMP-7 FUNCTION IN ANIMAL MODELS OF DIABETIC NEPHROPATHY

A long-term model of streptozotocin-induced DN was developed in order to study the influence of the BMP family on TGF-β and hyperglycemia-mediated injury (Fig. 2) *(55)*. In Sprague-Dawley rats receiving a single injection of streptozotocin, blood sugars were maintained in the 400–500 mL/dL range with long-acting insulin. In this model, there is a progressive renal hypertrophy that is near maximally established at 16 wk associated with marked increased in GFR and the development of proteinuria (Fig. 2).

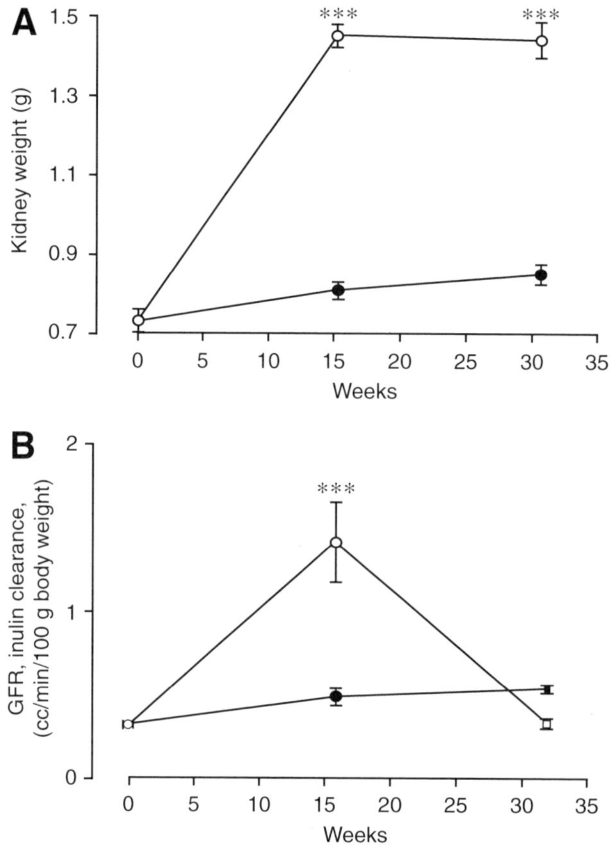

Fig. 2. The long-term streptozotocin (STZ) rodent model of diabetic nephorpathy. A single intravenous dose of STZ is followed by hyperglycemia controlled in the 400–500 mg/dL range by long-acting insulin. At 16 wk, renal hypertrophy and increased GFR is established. From 16 to 32 wk, GFR declines toward normal and glomerulosclerosis develops. Proteinuria is established past the microalbuminuric stage at 16 wk and progresses to the nephrotic range in some rats at 32 wk.

By 16 wk, microalbuminuria has progressed to the stage of frank proteinuria (Fig. 3). The proteinuria is thereafter progressive, reaching nephrotic grade levels between 16 and 32 wk in some animals. The GFRs decreased from the hypertrophic levels toward normal between 16 and 32 wk associated with the onset of focal segmental glomerulosclerosis *(55)* (Fig. 2).

In this model of type 1 DN, BMP-7 levels in the glomerulus and the medulla are reduced by 50–70% at 15–16 wk after injection and continued to decline further to less than 10% of normal by 30–32 wk *(47,55)*. Institution of rhBMP-7 therapy at 16 wk dose-dependently ameliorated proteinuria (Fig. 3) inhibited the development of focal segmental glomerulosclerosis and tubulo-interstitial fibrosis *(55)*. In addition, renal hypertrophy was partially reversed and GFR was preserved compared to diabetic animals receiving vehicle *(55)*.

In another model of DN, the db/db mouse, preliminary studies suggest that BMP-7 was not protective. Dunn et al. suggest there was a high dose-dependent increase in the proteinuria of the db/db mouse *(56)*. Additionally, in protein-overload nephropathy, BMP-7 was not shown to be renoprotective. Therefore, there is more to be learned of the efficacy and mechanism of action of BMP-7 in renal disease.

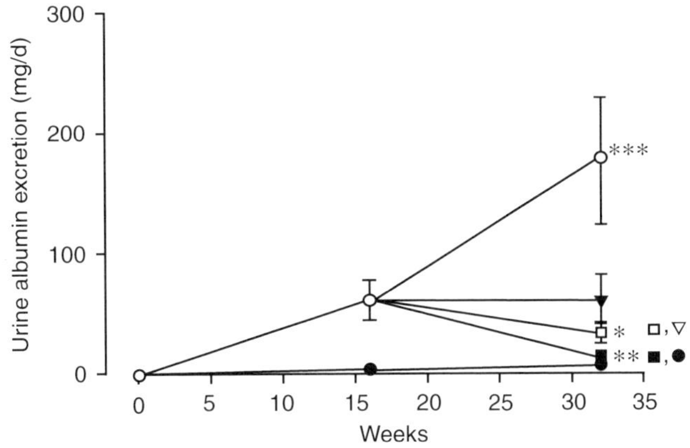

Fig. 3. Proteinuria in our rodent STZ DN model. Frank proteinuria is established at 16 wk and progresses to the nephrotic range in some rats. BMP-7, 10 (▲), 30 (△), and 100 (■) μg/kg injected intravenously twice-weekly dose-dependently reversed proteinuria. ***$p < 0.001$, vehicle treated (○) vs normal (●); **$p < 0.01$, vehicle treated vs BMP-7 100 μg; *$p < 0.05$, vehicle treated vs 30-μg BMP-7 and 20-mg/kg enalapril (□) daily.

MECHANISMS OF BMP-7 ACTION IN CKD

The Role of TGF-β in Renal Disease

Although the primary etiology of renal disease is quite varied, the underlying pathology remains common. One of the most prominent features is the deposition of extracellular matrix (ECM) in the glomerulus, mesangium, and interstitium, as a result of several factors, increased matrix synthesis by accumulating fibroblasts and decreased degradation of this matrix. The role of TGF-β has been studied extensively in models of progressive renal injury. Upregulated expression of TGF-β is a feature of virtually all human and experimental models of renal fibrosis *(57)*. Direct evidence comes from the observation that transgenic mice over expressing TGF-β develop glomerular and interstitial fibrosis *(58)*, as do mice treated with recombinant TGF-β_2 *(59)*. Treatment of rats with replication-defective adenoviral vectors that express soluble TGF-β type-II receptor, a suppressor of signaling, significantly attenuates interstitial collagen deposition in experimental models of kidney injury. Similarly, inhibition of TGF-β by neutralizing antibodies appears to ameliorate injury in the db/db mouse model of DN *(60)*. In addition, TGF-β-mediated epithelial-to-mesenchymal transdifferentiation (EMT) is thought to be a potential source for the large numbers of fibroblasts and myofibroblasts in the fibrotic kidney *(53,61)*. The intracellular signaling molecule Smad 3 mediates TGF-β-stimulated ECM deposition in several cultured systems. In response to TGF-β, Smad 3 stimulates collagen-I promoter expression in cultured human mesangial cells *(62)*. In this system, the TGF-β pathway also stimulated the PI3-kinase-Akt pathway to phosphorylate Smad 3 and enhanced transcriptional activation, leading to increased collagen-I expression *(63)*. The importance of Smad 3 is clear in models of chronic renal disease using Smad 3 knockout mice *(64)*.

In a model for type 1 diabetes mellitus, loss of Smad 3 attenuated the markers of DN. Thickening of the glomerular basement membrane, albuminuria, and upregulation of fibronectin and collagen-IV α3 expression were attenuated, suggesting that local inhibition of Smad 3 may be beneficial in the prevention or treatment of DN *(64)*. Smad 3 is also involved in renal interstitial fibrosis induced by UUO. Following UUO, Smad 3-null mice were protected from tubulo-interstitial fibrosis as manifested by decreased monocyte infiltration and collagen deposition *(65)*.

In Vitro Models of BMP-7 Function

Several studies suggest that BMP-7 may have anti-inflammatory and cytoprotective effects on renal tubular epithelial cells. Gould et al. *(46)* employed a commercial cDNA array to identify genes regulated by exposure of cultured human proximal tubular epithelial cells to BMP-7, tumor necrosis factor (TNF)-α, or the combination of both cytokines. In the same studies, the authors used real-time RT-PCR to confirm that BMP-7 suppresses several TNF-α-stimulated proinflammatory cytokines: interleukins (IL)-6 and -8, chemokines, and monocyte chemoattractant protein-1. BMP-7 also reduced proximal tubular expression of endothelin-2 and the adenosine A1 receptor, but increased endothelin-1. The net effect of these transcriptional changes may be increased blood flow in peritubular capillaries. Neutralization of endogenous BMP-7 in proximal tubular epithelial cells induces the expression of ECM molecules (fibronectin and collagen-III) and the extracellular BMP-binding protein gremlin *(47)*. These studies suggest that loss of endogenous BMP-7 is associated with profibrotic effects.

However, there is also evidence that a broad range of effects of BMP-7 in other cell types reduce TGF-β-mediated fibrosis programs. In vitro, BMP-7 reduces the increased expression of several ECM proteins and matrix accumulation—promoting regulatory molecules that are induced by TGF-β via Smad 2/3 pathways in cultured mesangial cells *(66,67)*. Whereas TGF-β increased collagen type IV, fibronectin, thrombospondin, and CTGF, BMP-7 reduced the expression of these ECM molecules and CTGF. BMP-7 reduced TGF-β-induced ECM protein accumulation primarily by maintaining levels and activity of MMP2, the major metalloproteinase secreted by mesangial cells. Mechanistically, BMP-7 antagonizes TGF-β-dependent upregulation of plasminogen-activated inhibitor-1, an inhibitor of MMP2. In addition, BMP-7 reduces the nuclear accumulation of Smad 3 via a Smad 5-mediated process. BMP-7 signaling via Smad 5 upregulates Smad 6, which blocks the nuclear translocation of phosphorylated Smad 2/3 and therefore counteracts TGF-β-stimulated, plasminogen activator inhibitor-1 expression in mesangial cells *(49)*. The opposing interactions of BMP-7-dependent Smads (1/5) to the TGF-β-induced Smads (2/3) may thus block TGF-β-induced epithelial–mesenchymal transformation *(53)*. Thus, BMP-7 and TGF-β may be taken as opposing forces that can alter the state of the renal epithelia. In recent experimental studies, Zhang et al. *(68)* provide in vitro evidence to support a model of competition between two avenues of direct cell–cell interactions between tubular cells and macrophages, one resulting in profibrogenic activation of tubular cells and another geared toward preventing this profibrogenic cell–cell contact *(69,70)*. In this model, engagement of leukocyte function antigen-1 on the surface of macrophages with tubular cell intercellular adhesion molecule-1 leads to TGF-β mediated activation of a fibrogenic program in tubular cells, whereas binding of macrophage CD44 to tubular cell membrane hyaluronic acid extensions ("cables") prevents this physical association via ICAM-1 and suppresses profibrogenic tubular cell activation. Moreover, these authors described that the hyaluronic acid cables on tubular cell surfaces are regulated by BMP-7 *(68)*. Increased hyaluronic acid cables reduce engagement of ICAM-1 by macrophages perhaps by sterically preventing close contacts between macrophages and the basolateral membrane of tubular cells. These findings elucidate a novel mechanism by which macrophage infiltrates may directly engage tubular cells and, in addition, describe a novel mechanism of antifibrogenic action of BMP-7.

EXTRACELLULAR MODULATION OF BMP-7 FUNCTION

Lin et al. *(31)* recently identified the KCP protein as the first extracellular protein described to enhance BMP function. KCP functions in a paracrine manner and enhances BMP-7 binding to its type-I receptor to increase intracellular concentrations of phosphorylated Smad 1, enhancing Smad 1-mediated transcription. The authors generated KCP-null mice, which were viable, fertile, and had no observable renal pathology *(31)*. In two different models of renal injury, UUO and acute renal failure after folic acid administration, KCP-null mice showed increased susceptibility to developing renal interstitial fibrosis. Surprisingly, the null mice showed signs of interstitial fibrosis in the contralateral "normal" kidney as well. This suggests a possible role of circulating BMP-7 which was lost from the UUO kidney. In the acute renal failure model, 23% mortality was noted within 2 d of administration of folic acid to null mice. Of the surviving mice, increased deposition of ECM was noted, beginning as early as 7 d after injury compared with wild-type mice. KCP expression is not detected in adult kidneys, but is upregulated by renal injury. The time-course of upregulation correlates with the decline in levels of BMP-7 in the UUO and ischemic injury models' renal injury. KCP may augment BMP-7 signaling by increasing association with the BMP type-I receptor.

CONCLUSIONS

BMP-7 is a renal morphogen necessary for normal kidney development. BMP-7 in the adult kidney stimulates differentiation and resists injury to epithelial cells. It prevents myofibroblast transition. In cell-based models and in vivo models of renal injury, BMP-7 antagonizes the fibrogenic actions of TGF-β and serves a cytoprotective role. In several rodent models of renal injury, administration of rhBMP-7 has ameliorated injury and attenuated or reversed tubulo-interstitial fibrosis. These data suggest that BMP-7, its agonists, its receptors, and its effectors may be clinically important targets for developing novel therapies.

REFERENCES

1. USRDS: The United States renal data system. Am J Kidney Dis 2003;42(6 Suppl 5):1–230.
2. Coresh J, Astor BC, Greene T, Eknoyan G, Levey AS. Prevalence of chronic kidney disease and decreased kidney function in the adult US population: third national health and nutrition examination survey. Am J Kidney Dis 2003;41:1–15.
3. Hillege HL, Janssen WMT, Bak AAA, et al. Microalbuminuria is common, also in a nondiabetic, nonhypertensive population, and an independent indicator of cardiovascular risk factors and cardiovascular morbidity. J Int Med 2001;249:519–526.
4. Iseki K. The Okinawa screening program. J Am Soc Neph 2003;14(7 Suppl 2):S127–S130.
5. Chadban SJ, Briganti EM, Kerr PG, et al. Prevalence of kidney damage in Australian adults: the AusDiab kidney study. J Am Soc Neph 2003;14:S131–S138.
6. Berl T, Hunsicker LG, Lewis JB, et al. Cardiovascular outcomes in the Irbesartan diabetic nephropathy trial of patients with type 2 diabetes and overt nephropathy. Ann Intern Med 2003;138:542–549.
7. Lewis EJ, Hunsicker LG, Bain RP, Rohde RD. The effect of angiotensin-converting-enzyme inhibition on diabetic nephropathy. NEJM 1993;329:1456–1462.
8. Jafar TH, Stark PC, Schmid CH, et al. Progression of chronic kidney disease: the role of blood pressure control, proteinuria, and angiotensin-converting enzyme inhibition: a patient-level meta-analysis. Ann Int Med 2003;139:244–252.

9. K/DOQI clinical practice guidelines on hypertension and antihypertensive agents in chronic kidney disease. Am J Kidney Dis 2004;43(5 Suppl 1):1–290.
10. The diabetes control and complications trial (DCCT) research group. Effect of intensive therapy on the development and progression of diabetic nephropathy in the diabetes control and complications trial. Kidney Int 1995;47:1703–1720.
11. Adler AI, Stevens RJ, Manley SE, et al. Development and progression of nephropathy in type 2 diabetes: The United Kingdom prospective diabetes study (UKPDS 64). Kidney Int 2003;63:225–232.
12. Schieppati A, Remuzzi G. Proteinuria and its consequences in renal disease. Acta Paediatr Suppl 2003;443:9–13.
13. Remuzzi G, Ruggenenti P, Perico N. Chronic renal diseases: Renoprotective benefits of renin-angiotensin system inhibition. Ann Intern Med 2002;136:604–615.
14. Eddy AA. Molecular insights into renal interstitial fibrosis. J Am Soc Nephrol 1996;7:2495–2508.
15. Fogo AB. Pathology of progressive nephropathies. Curr Opin Nephrol Hypertens 2000;9:241–246.
16. Shi Y, Massague J. Mechanisms of TGF-β signaling from cell membrane to the nucleus. Cell 2003;113:685–700.
17. Miyazono K, Kusanagi K, Inoue H. Divergence and convergence of TGF-β/BMP signaling. J Cell Physiol 2001;187:265–276.
18. Zhu H, Kavsak P, Abdollah S, Wrana JL, Thomsen GH. A SMAD ubiquitin ligase targets the BMP pathway and affects embryonic pattern formation. Nature 1999;400:687–693.
19. Lo RS, Massagué J. Ubiquitin-dependent degradation of TGF-β-activated Smad2. Nat Cell Biol 1999;1:472–478.
20. Fukuchi M, Imamura T, Chiba T, et al. Ligand-dependent degradation of Smad3 by a ubiquitin ligase complex of ROC1 and associated proteins. Mol Biol Cell 2001;12:1431–1443.
21. Ebisawa T, Fukuchi M, Murakami G, et al. Smurf1 interacts with transforming growth factor-beta type I receptor through Smad7 and induces receptor degradation. J Biol Chem 2001;276: 12,477–12,480.
22. Murakami G, Watabe T, Takaoka K, Miyazono K, Imamura T. Cooperative inhibition of bone morphogenetic protein signaling by Smurf1 and inhibitory Smads. Mol Biol Cell 2003;14:2809–2817.
23. Annes JP, Munger JS, Rifkin DB. Making sense of latent TGFβ activation. J Cell Sci 2003; 116:217–224.
24. Gumienny TL, Padgett RW. The other side of TGF-β superfamily signal regulation: thinking outside the cell. Trends Endo Metab 2002;13:295–299.
25. Garcia Abreu J, Coffinier C, Larrain J, Oelgeschlager M, De Robertis EM. Chordin-like CR domains and the regulation of evolutionarily conserved extracellular signaling systems. Gene 2002;287:39–47.
26. Wilkinson L, Kolle G, Wen D, Piper M, Scott J, Little M. CRIM1 regulates the rate of processing and delivery of bone morphogenetic proteins to the cell surface. J Biol Chem 2003;278:34,181–34,188.
27. Balemans W, Van Hul W. Extracellular regulation of BMP signaling in vertebrates: a cocktail of modulators. Dev Biol 2002;250:231–250.
28. Laurikkala J, Kassai Y, Pakkasjarvi L, Thesleff I, Itoh N. Identification of a secreted BMP antagonist, ectodin, integrating BMP, FGF, and SHH signals from the tooth enamel knot. Dev Biol 2003;264: 91–105.
29. Ohukubo T, Ozawa M. The transcription factor Snail down-regulates the tight junction components independently of E-cadherin down-regulation. J Cell Sci 2004;117(Pt 9):1675–1685.
30. Groppe J, Greenwald J, Wiater E, et al. Structural basis of BMP signalling inhibition by the cystine knot protein Noggin. Nature 2002;420:636–642.
31. Lin J, Patel SR, Cheng X, et al. Kielin/chordin-like protein, a novel enhancer of BMP signaling, attenuates renal fibrotic disease. Nat Med 2005;11:387–393.
32. Abreu JG, Ketpura NI, Reversade B, De Robertis EM. Connective-tissue growth factor (CTGF) modulates cell signalling by BMP and TGF-β. Nat Cell Biol 2002;4:599–604.
33. Chen S, Lechleider RJ. Transforming growth factor-β-induced differentiation of smooth muscle from a neural crest stem cell line. Circ Res 2004;94:1195–1202.
34. Dudley AT, Robertson EJ. Overlapping expression domains of bone morphogenetic protein family members potentially account for limited tissue defects in BMP7 deficient embryos. Develop Dynamics 1997;208:349–362.
35. Dudley AT, Lyons KM, Robertson EJ. A requirement for bone morphogenetic protein-7 during development of the mammalian kidney and eye. Genes Dev 1995;9:2795–2807.
36. Luo G, Hofmann C, Bronckers AL, Sohocki M, Bradley A, Karsenty G. BMP-7 is an inducer of nephrogenesis, and is also required for eye development and skeletal patterning. Genes Dev 1995; 9:2808–2820.

37. Dudley AT, Godin RE, Robertson EJ. Interaction between FGF and BMP signaling pathways regulates development of metanephric mesenchyme. Genes Dev 1999;13:1601–1613.
38. Martinez G, Loveland KL, Clark AT, Dziadek M, Bertram JF. Expression of bone morphogenetic protein receptors in the developing mouse metanephros. Exp Nephrol 2001;9:372–379.
39. Vrljicak P, Myburgh D, Ryan AK, van Rooijen MA, Mummery CL, Gupta IR. Smad expression during kidney development. AJP—Ren Physiol 2004;286:F625–F633.
40. Hsu DR, Economides AN, Wang X, Eimon PM, Harland RM. The Xenopus dorsalizing factor Gremlin identifies a novel family of secreted proteins that antagonize BMP activities. Mol Cell 1998;1:673–683.
41. Khokha MK, Hsu D, Brunet LJ, Dionne MS, Harland RM. Gremlin is the BMP antagonist required for maintenance of Shh and Fgf signals during limb patterning. Nat Genet 2003;34:303–307.
42. Michos O, Panman L, Vintersten K, Beier K, Zeller R, Zuniga A. Gremlin-mediated BMP antagonism induces the epithelial-mesenchymal feedback signaling controlling metanephric kidney and limb organogenesis . Development 2004;131:3401–3410.
43. Miyazaki Y, Oshima K, Fogo A, Hogan BLM, Ichikawa I. Bone morphogenetic protein 4 regulates the budding site and elongation of the mouse ureter. J Clin Invest 2000;105:863–873.
44. Vukicevic S, Basic V, Rogic D, et al. Osteogenic protein-1 (bone morphogenetic protein-7) reduces severity of injury after ischemic acute renal failure in rat. J Clin Invest 1998;102:202–214.
45. Simon M, Maresh JG, Harris SE, et al. Expression of bone morphogenetic protein-7 mRNA in normal and ischemic adult rat kidney. Am J Physiol 1999;276:F382–F389.
46. Gould SE, Day M, Jones S, Dorai H. BMP-7 regulates chemokine, cytokine, and hemodynamic gene expression in proximal tubule cells. Kidney Int 2002;61:51–60.
47. Wang SN, Lapage J, Hirschberg R. Loss of tubular bone morphogenetic protein-7 in diabetic nephropathy. J Am Soc Nephrol 2001;12:2392–2399.
48. Bosukonda D, Shis MS, Sampath KT, Vukicevic S. Characterization of receptors for osteogenic protein-1/bone morphogenetic protein-7 (OP-1/BMP-7) in rat kidneys. Kidney Int 2000;5:1902–1911.
49. Wang S, Hirschberg R. Bone morphogenetic protein-7 signals opposing transforming growth factor β in mesangial cells. J Biol Chem 2004;279:23,200–23,206.
50. Surendran K, Austin PF, Farrell F, Hruska KA. Renal protection in a model of obstructive uropathy by bone morphogenetic protein-7 (BMP-7). J Urology 2005; submitted.
51. Hruska K, Guo G, Wozniak M, et al. Osteogenic protein-1 prevents renal fibrogenesis associated with ureteral obstruction. Am J Phys (Renal) 2000;279:F130–F143.
52. Morrissey J, Hruska K, Guo G, Wang S, Chen Q, Klahr S. Bone morphogenetic protein-7 improves renal fibrosis and accelerates the return of renal function. J Am Soc Nephrol 2002;13:S14–S21.
53. Zeisberg M, Hanai J, Sugimoto H, et al. BMP-7 counteracts TGFβ1-induced epithelial-to-mesenchymal transition and reverses chronic renal injury. Nat Med 2003;9(7):964–968.
54. Zeisberg M, Bottiglio C, Kumar N, et al. Bone morphogenic protein-7 inhibits progresion of chronic renal fibrosis associated with two genetic mouse models. Am J Phys (Renal) 2003;285:F1060–F1067.
55. Wang S, Chen Q, Simon TC, et al. Bone morphogenetic protein-7 (BMP-7), a novel therapy for diabetic nephropathy. Kidney Int 2003;63:2037–2049.
56. Dunn SR, Zhu Y, Qiu G, McCue P, Sharma K. Bone morphogenic protein (BMP-7) increases albuminuria in the dh/db mouse. J Am Soc Neph 2004;15:724A.
57. Bottinger EP, Bitzer M. TGF-β signaling in renal disease. J Am Soc Neph 2002; 13:2600–2610.
58. Kopp JB, Factor VM, Mozes M, et al. Transgenic mice with increased plasma levels of TGF-β1 develop progressive renal disease. Lab Invest 1996;74:991–1033.
59. Ledbetter S, Kurtzberg L, Doyle S, Pratt BM. Renal fibrosis in mice treated with human recombinant transforming growth factor-β2. Kidney Int 2000;58:2367–2376.
60. Ziyadeh FN, Hoffman BB, Han DC, et al. Long-term prevention of renal insufficiency, excess matrix gene expression, and glomerular mesangial matrix expansion by treatment with monoclonal antitransforming growth factor-beta antibody in db/db diabetic mice. Proc Natl Acad Sci 2000;97: 8015–8020.
61. Kalluri R, Neilson EG. Epithelial-mesenchymal transition and its implications for fibrosis. J Clin Invest 2003;112:1776–1784.
62. Poncelet AC, Schnaper HW. Sp1 and Smad proteins cooperate to mediate transforming growth factor-beta 1-induced alpha 2(I) collagen expression in human glomerular mesangial cells. J Biol Chem 2001;276:6983–6992.
63. Runyan CE, Schnaper HW, Poncelet AC. The phosphatidylinositol 3-kinase/Akt pathway enhances Smad3-stimulated mesangial cell collagen I expression in response to transforming growth factor-β1. J Biol Chem 2004;279:2632–2639.

64. Fujimoto M, Maezawa Y, Yokote K, et al. Mice lacking Smad3 are protected against streptozotocin-induced diabetic glomerulopathy. Biochem Biophys Res Com 2003;305:1002–1007.
65. Sato M, Muragaki Y, Saika S, Roberts AB, Ooshima A. Targeted disruption of TGF-β1/Smad3 signaling protects against renal tubulointerstitial fibrosis induced by unilateral ureteral obstruction. J Clin Invest 2003;112:1486–1494.
66. Wang S, Hirschberg R. BMP7 antagonizes TGF-beta-dependent fibrogenesis in mesangial cells. Am J Phys (Renal) 2003;284:F1006–F1013.
67. Zawaideh MA, Surendran K, Hruska KA. BMP-7 inhibits high glucose induced renal glomerular mesangial cell phenotype. J Am Soc Neph 2003;14:62A.
68. Zhang XL, Selbi W, de la Motte C, Hascall V, Phillips A. Renal proximal tubular epithelial cell transforming growth factor-β1 generation and monocyte binding. Am J Pathol 2004;165:763–773.
69. Ito T, Williams JD, Fraser D, Phillips AO. Hyaluronan attenuates transforming growth factor-β1-mediated signaling in renal proximal tubular epithelial cells. Am J Pathol 2004;164:1979–1988.
70. Selbi W, de la Motte C, Hascall V, Phillips A. BMP-7 modulates hyaluronan-mediated proximal tubular cell-monocyte interaction. J Am Soc Neph 2004;15:1199–1211.
71. Leung-Hagesteijn C, Hu MC, Mahendra AS, et al. Integrin-linked kinase mediates bone morphogenetic protein 7-dependent renal epithelial cell morphogenesis. Mol Cell Biol 2005;25:3648–3657.

II Clinical Aspects of Diabetic Nephropathy

A. Genetics and Risks

19 Genetic Determinants of Diabetic Nephropathy in Type 2 Diabetes

Grzegorz Placha, MD, PhD
and Andrzej S. Krolewski, MD, PhD

CONTENTS

INTRODUCTION

Diabetic nephropathy (DN) contributes significantly to morbidity and premature mortality in diabetes mellitus *(1,2)*. Whereas the identification of specific environmental factors involved in the development of proteinuria and progressively declining kidney function have led to clinical measures that modify the natural history of the disease *(3,4)*, available interventions (primarily blood glucose control and treatment with renoprotective and antihypertensive drugs) fall short of the ultimate goal of eradicating this complication. The severity of this deficiency is highlighted best by the fact that an epidemic of end-stage renal disease (ESRD) has developed over the past 20 yr, particularly in patients with type 2 diabetes mellitus (T2DM) in the United States, without any signs of leveling off *(5)*. With T2DM becoming more common among young adults and in pediatric populations *(6)*, one may infer that the burden of ESRD in the US population will increase even further unless more effective clinical measures are found.

Potentially, such measures may result from investigations into the genetic basis underlying susceptibility to the development of DN *(7)*. Knowledge of which genes predispose to DN, and specifically (1) the development of proteinuria and (2) declining kidney function leading to ESRD, will give us a better understanding of the pathogenesis

Parts of this chapter were published previously in the article by Placha G, Canani L, Warram JH, and Krolewski AS, Evidence for Different Susceptibility Genes for Proteinuria and ESRD in Type 2 Diabetes, in Advances in Chronic Kidney Disease, 2005;12:155–169.

From: *Contemporary Diabetes: The Diabetic Kidney*
Edited by: P. Cortes and C. E. Mogensen © Humana Press Inc., Totowa, NJ

of this complication. In a clinical setting, this knowledge may permit us to identify those patients at high risk for DN. Also, new targets for drug development may emerge, especially if the genes found are novel and have not been previously implicated in the pathogenesis of DN.

In this chapter, we review current knowledge of the genetic basis of DN in T2DM. The focus on T2DM is motivated by two reasons

1. T2DM is the major contributor to the ESRD in all populations around the world.
2. In families with T2DM it is possible to dissect the genetic factors contributing to the development of abnormalities in urinary albumin excretion and genetic factors contributing to declining kidney function.

Such a two-disease model for the etiology of DN is assumed in this chapter. This model postulates that a disease process in the glomerulus underlies the development of proteinuria, whereas a separate disease process most likely in the tubules and interstitium underlies declining kidney function. In support of this model in this review, we provide evidence that different genes determine the development of proteinuria and declining kidney function/ESRD.

FAMILIAL AGGREGATION OF PHENOTYPES OF DIABETIC NEPHROPATHY

Proteinuria and kidney function impairment are two phenotypes that are the major hallmarks of DN. Several studies demonstrated that both aggregate in families of diabetic as well as nondiabetic individuals as heritable traits. Before we discuss these results, a few comments are necessary about the ways the studies were designed.

Two different but complementary study designs are used to examine familial aggregation of complex diseases such as DN. Usually, conventional epidemiological designs and methods are used to explore first whether the disease in question clusters in families *(8)*. More formally, the notion of familial clustering or aggregation implies a higher prevalence of disease in family members of cases (index cases) than in the general population or in family members of unaffected individuals (index controls). It should be noted that a disease having no genetic etiology may aggregate or cluster in families owing to a shared environment, such as an infectious agent or a culturally transmitted risk factor such as smoking or dietary preferences.

The relative contributions of heredity and shared environment to the familial aggregation of a disease have been tested historically by comparing the occurrence of the disease in monozygotic and dizygotic twin pairs *(9)*, an impractical approach in T2DM patients with nephropathy. Alternatively, the hereditary and environmental components of familial aggregation can be partitioned on the basis of the pattern of covariance between pairs of relatives within families. Recent developments in statistical genetic analysis now enable the assessment of heritability (h^2) (the proportion of total phenotypic variance owing to additive genetic effects) and the genetic correlation between traits in extended families, taking into account the presence of environmental covariates *(10)*. The proportion of total phenotypic variance owing to additive genetic effects may vary between $h^2 = 0$, i.e., no genetic effect and $h^2 = 1$, i.e., all variance is as a result of genetic effect. This approach has been employed to assess the genetic contributions to variation in urinary albumin excretion (UAE) and glomerular filtration rate (GFR) and has been extended to the mapping of genes for these traits.

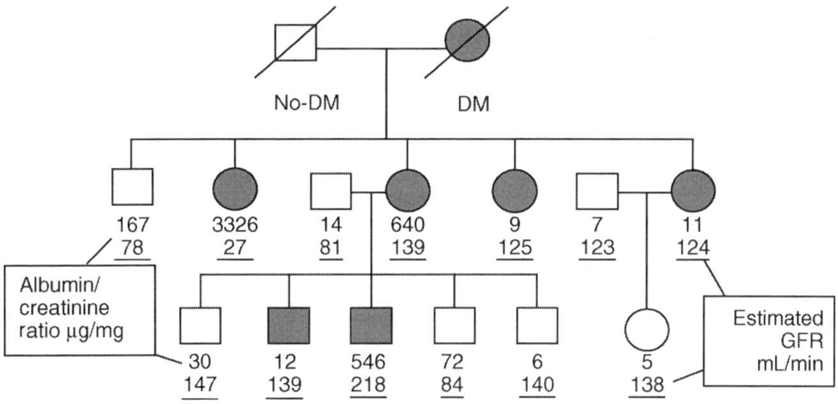

Fig. 1. Example of an extended family from the Joslin Collection of Families with T2DM. Circles indicate women and squares indicate men. Empty symbols indicate the absence of diabetes and filled ones indicate diabetes. Values in italics are the urinary albumin to creatinine ratio (ACR). Underlined values are the GFR estimated from serum cystatin C concentration. (Adapted from ref. *18*.)

Familial Aggregation of Proteinuria and Heritability of Variation in UAE

Familial aggregation of DN was demonstrated first in sibling pairs with type 1 diabetes mellitus (T1DM) *(11–14)* and subsequently in sibling pairs with T2DM. Studies by Faronatto et al. *(15)*, and Canani et al. *(16)* demonstrated that diabetic siblings of diabetic index cases with proteinuria or ESRD had a risk of elevated UAE several times higher than diabetic siblings of diabetic index controls with normoalbuminuria.

The finding of familial aggregation of DN, a discrete outcome, was corroborated in studies of the heritability of UAE, a quantitative trait, in nuclear and extended families *(17–21)*. For example, in a study from our laboratory, Fogarty et al. *(18,19)* examined familial aggregation and estimated the heritability of UAE, measured as the urinary albumin to creatinine ratio (ACR), in 96 extended Caucasian families ascertained for T2DM. An example of a typical family included in the Joslin collection is shown in Fig. 1. In total in these families there were 630 individuals with T2DM and 639 individuals without diabetes, all of whom had measurements of their urinary ACR. The distribution of log-transformed ACR values (logACR) in diabetic and nondiabetic relatives is shown in Fig. 2A. In relatives without diabetes, the distribution of logACR was unimodal (median 6 μg/mg) with a small proportion, about 9%, having abnormal ACR values in the range of microalbuminuria or proteinuria (logACR > 1.5, i.e., ACR > 30 μg of albumin/mg of urinary creatinine). In those with diabetes, the logACR distribution was significantly different. In individuals with diabetes, only 28% had logACR values below the median for relatives without diabetes, another 33% had values between the median and the upper limit of normal, and 39% had values in the range of microalbuminuria or proteinuria. In thinking about the diabetic individuals with an abnormal ACR, one wondered in which the ACR values of their nondiabetic relatives fell in the ACR distribution for nondiabetic individuals. Might they also be in the upper part of that distribution, that is, in the upper range of normoalbuminuria or in the microalbuminuria range?

To test this hypothesis, Fogarty et al. *(19)* examined the relationship between the ACR values in nondiabetic and diabetic individuals in the same family. Median values of logACR were determined separately for the diabetic and nondiabetic members

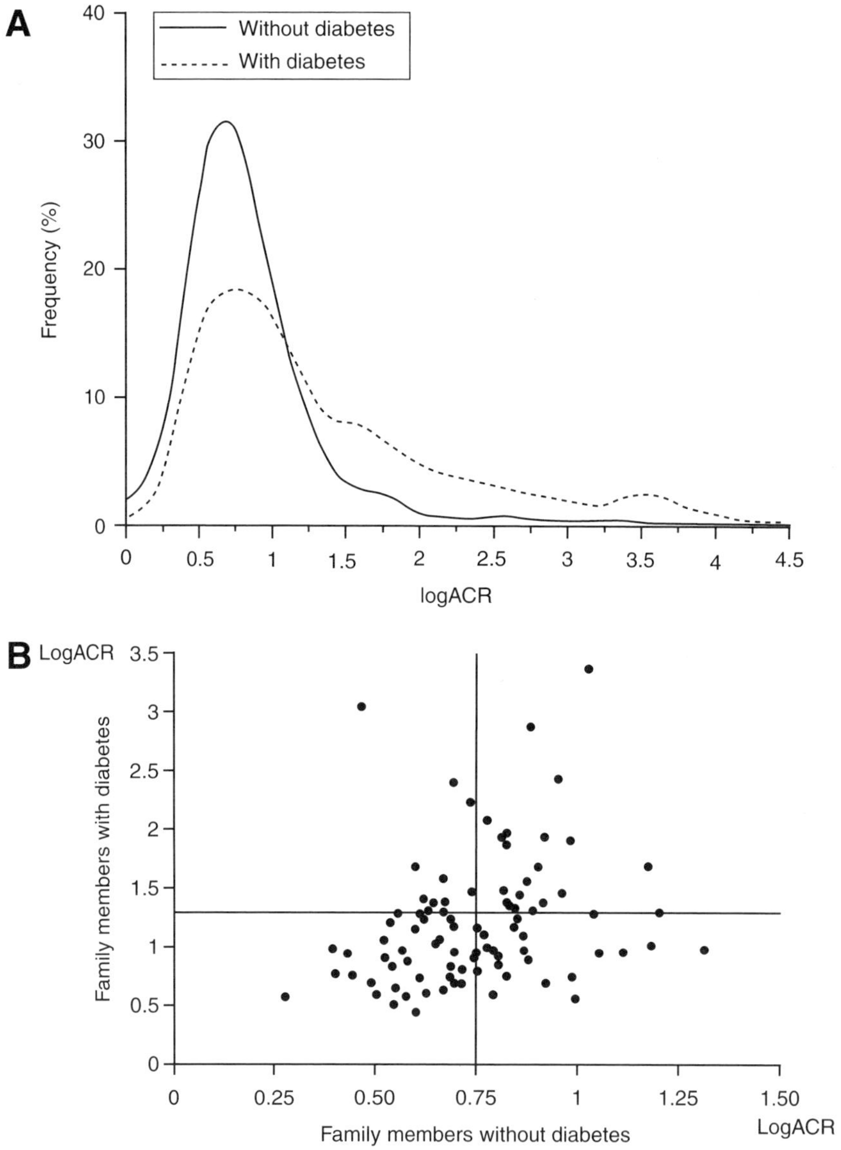

Fig. 2. Distributions of urinary albumin excretion measured as the urinary albumin to creatinine ratio (ACR) in diabetic and nondiabetic members of extended families with type 2 diabetes. (Reproduced with permission from ref. *19*.) **(A)** Comparison of distribution of logACR (ACR transformed to the logarithm base 10) in diabetic (n = 630) and nondiabetic (n = 639) members of the examined families. **(B)** Plot of median logACR in diabetic vs nondiabetic relatives in each of the 96 extended families with type 2 diabetes.

of each family, and the families plotted in Fig. 2B according to the two medians. For the nondiabetic members of the families, the distribution was quite symmetric and none was above the normoalbuminuria range (logACR < 1.5). However, the distribution for the diabetic members was strikingly different, depending on whether their nondiabetic relatives were in the lower or upper half of the range for normoalbuminuria. If the median for the nondiabetic members was in the lower range of normoalbuminuria, very few families had an elevated median value for their diabetic members. This can be

Table 1
Summary of Studies on Familial Clustering of Proteinuria and Heritability of Variation in UAE

Authors	*Population*	*Results of the study*
Faronatto et al., 1997 *(15)*	Caucasians, Italy	Diabetic siblings of index cases with proteinuria had a risk of proteinuria 3.9 times that of diabetic siblings of index cases with normoalbuminuria.
Canani et al., 1999 *(16)*	Caucasians, Southern Brazil	Diabetic siblings of index cases with proteinuria had a risk of proteinuria 3.3 times that of diabetic siblings of index cases with normoalbuminuria.
Forsblom et al., 1999 *(17)*	Caucasians, Finland	In nuclear families ascertained for type 2 diabetes, heritiability of UAE was significant ($h^2 = 0.30$).
Fogarty et al., 2000 *(18)*	Caucasians, New England	In extended families ascertained for type 2 diabetes, heritability of UAE was significant in relatives with diabetes ($h^2 = 0.31$) and those without ($h^2 = 0.20$).
Freedman et al., 2003 *(20)*	Caucasians, USA	In nondiabetic families consisting of sibling pairs concordant for hypertension, heritability of UAE was significant ($h^2 = 0.49$).
Langefeld et al., 2004 *(21)*	Caucasians, North Carolina	In nuclear families consisting of at least two siblings with type 2 diabetes, heritability of UAE was significant ($h^2 = 0.44$).

interpreted as evidence that these families lack susceptibility to DN. In contrast, if the median for the nondiabetic family members was in the upper range of normoalbuminuria, the median for their diabetic relatives was frequently elevated in the range of microalbuminuria or proteinuria. This can be interpreted as evidence that these families were susceptible to DN. Thus, although the median UAE in diabetic relatives was of an order of magnitude higher than that in their nondiabetic relatives, the medians were significantly correlated (Spearman correlation = 0.34, $p < 0.001$). When these data were reanalyzed using variance components analysis and taking into account relevant covariates, a very strong genetic correlation between logACR levels in diabetic and nondiabetic relatives was found *(22)*. This finding strongly supports a hypothesis that the same genes control variation of UAE in diabetic as well as in nondiabetic individuals.

To study further the familial aggregation of UAE variation, a variance components approach was utilized to estimate the heritability for urinary ACR after adjustment for relevant covariates. In the total collection of 6481 pairs of relatives, heritability for UAE ($h^2 = 0.27$, $p < 0.001$) was similar to that for systolic blood pressure (SBP) ($h^2 = 0.24$, $p < 0.001$) *(18)*. Among diabetic family members, the heritability was slightly higher for ACR ($h^2 = 0.31$, $p < 0.001$) and SBP ($h^2 = 0.33$, $p < 0.001$). This finding provided very strong evidence that UAE, as measured by ACR, is a heritable trait in Caucasians with and without diabetes *(18,19)*. Recently, Langefeld et al. *(21)* reported a somewhat higher heritability ($h^2 = 0.44$, $p < 0.001$) of UAE in a large collection of nuclear families with T2DM. Similarly, Freedman et al. *(20)* found higher heritability ($h^2 = 0.49$, $p < 0.001$) of UAE in nuclear families of nondiabetic individuals with hypertension. Summary of the familial aggregation of UAE is shown in Table 1.

To examine the finding of heritability of ACR further, Fogarty et al. *(19)* performed a complex segregation analysis on the members of the 96 families. Likelihood ratio tests were performed to test hypotheses related to genetic transmission. The Mendelian model with multifactorial inheritance was supported more strongly than Mendelian inheritance alone. These analyses suggested that the best model for variation of ACR was multifactorial, with evidence for a common major gene. When the analyses were repeated for diabetic subjects only, the evidence for Mendelian inheritance was improved, and the model with a single major locus with additional multifactorial effects was more strongly supported. The results of this study suggest that variation in ACR is determined by a mixture of genes with large and small effects, as well as other measured covariates such as diabetes and its duration. These findings are consistent with the results of studies of DN in Pima Indians *(19)*.

In summary, the earlier findings have important implications for the design of studies to search for the genes controlling susceptibility to DN. Because UAE can be measured in individuals regardless of diabetes status, it is well suited for analysis as a quantitative trait, with elevated levels being considered a surrogate for nephropathy. The search for nephropathy genes linked to UAE will be more effective because the power of the available pedigrees will be greater for a heritable quantitative trait (UAE) than for a discrete outcome, the presence or absence of proteinuria.

Familial Aggregation of ESRD and Heritability of Variation in GFR

Familial aggregation of ESRD and the heritability of a variation in GFR have been examined in the same fashion as proteinuria and a variation in UAE; the summary of the studies is shown in Table 2.

The first study was by Pettitt et al. *(23)* who described the familial aggregation of impaired kidney function among diabetic parents and their diabetic offspring in Pima Indians with T2DM. Subsequently, Freedman et al. *(24)* reported that in families selected through an index case with ESRD caused by DN, there was an excess of relatives with ESRD in comparison with the risk of ESRD in the general population.

The heritability of GFR was examined in four studies conducted in families ascertained through an individual without diabetes. One analysis was performed in 539 monozygotic and 1208 dizygotic sets of female twins, all of them nondiabetics. The h^2 of serum creatinine was 0.37 and the calculated creatinine clearance using the Cockcroft-Gault formula was 0.63 *(9)*. The heritability of kidney function was computed in multigenerational families in Utah, enriched for the presence of premature cardiovascular disease *(25)*. The examinations were performed three times during a 10-yr follow-up study. The h^2 for serum creatinine varied between 0.25 and 0.31. For GFR estimated using the Modification of Diet in Renal Disease (MDRD) formula, the h^2 ranged from 0.37 to 0.42. Recently, similar data were reported from the Framingham Heart Study, which included 1200 individuals from 330 nuclear families. In this study, the h^2 for various estimates of GFR varied between 0.29 and 0.46 *(26)*. In a more recent report, Langefeld et al. *(21)* examined the h^2 of GFR estimated by the modified MDRD formula in 662 Caucasian individuals with T2DM from 310 families. The h^2 of GFR was 0.75, the highest value in the literature.

In a recent study, we demonstrated that the concentration of serum cystatin C is an accurate estimate of renal function in individuals with T2DM *(27)*. This method provides a more accurate estimate of GFR than other methods (including the MDRD equation), particularly in individuals with normal or elevated values of GFR. By measuring

Table 2
Summary of Studies on Familial Clustering of ESRD and Heritability of Variation of GFR

Authors	*Population*	*Results of the study*
Pettit et al., 1990 *(23)*	Pima Indians, Arizona,	Diabetic siblings and offspring of diabetic index cases with impaired kidney function had elevated serum creatinine.
Freedman et al., 1995 *(24)*	African-Americans, Southern US	Relatives of index cases with type 2 diabetes and ESRD had a risk of ESRD 8.1 times that of relatives of index cases with type 2 diabetes and without DN.
Hunter et al., 2002 *(9)*	Caucasians, UK	In a twin study of adult women, heritabilities of serum creatinine (h^2 = 0.37), and calculated creatinine clearance (h^2 = 0.63) were both significant.
Hunt et al., 2004 *(25)*	Caucasians, Utah	In extended nondiabetic families ascertained for early cardiovascular disease, heritabilities of serum creatinine (h^2 from 0.25 to 0.31) and estimated GFR[a] (h^2 from 0.37 to 0.42) were significant.
Fox et al., 2004 *(26)*	Caucasians, Framingham, MA	In mainly nondiabetic families in the Framingham Heart Study, heritabilities of serum creatinine (h^2 = 0.29), estimated GFR[a] (h^2 = 0.31) and calculated creatinine clearance (h^2 = 0.56) were all significant.
Langefeld et al., 2004 *(21)*	Caucasians, North Carolina	In nuclear families consisting of at least two siblings with type 2 diabetes, heritability of GFR[a] (h^2 = 0.75) was significant.
Placha et al., 2005 *(28)*	Caucasians, New England	In extended families ascertained for type 2 diabetes, heritability of GFR[b] was significant in relatives with diabetes (h^2 = 0.45) and in those without (h^2 = 0.35).

[a]GFR was estimated using serum creatinine levels and the MDRD formula.
[b]GFR was estimated as the reciprocal of serum cystatin C concentration × 100.

families, 63 families out of 104 were included with typical T2DM diagnosed after age 35 yr. The example of the typical family with values of GFR estimated from serum cystatin C is shown in Fig. 1.

To study familial aggregation of variation in renal function, a variance components analysis was used to estimate the heritability for estimated GFR after adjustment for covariates such as sex and age. In our multigenerational families, the heritability (h^2) of GFR estimated by serum cystatin C levels was 0.45 in diabetic relatives and 0.35 in nondiabetic relatives *(28)*. Interestingly, when ACR was included in the variance components analysis as a covariate (in addition to sex and age), the heritability estimates in diabetics and nondiabetics increased slightly to 0.47 and 0.39, respectively. These findings provide very strong evidence that variation in renal function, as measured by estimated GFR, is controlled by genetic factors in individuals with and without diabetes, and they suggest that genes controlling variation in GFR are different from genes controlling ACR.

Table 3
Genetic and Environmental Correlations Between ACR and GFR in Diabetic and Nondiabetic Relatives in the Joslin Collection of Families With T2DM

	Genetic correlation (r_G)	*Environmental correlation* (r_E)
Diabetic relatives	–0.08 (n.s.)	–0.47 ($p < 0.001$)
Nondiabetic relatives	–0.04 (n.s)	–0.31 ($p < 0.005$)

Unpublished data from ref. *28*.

To study further the nature of the relationship between variation in GFR and variation in ACR, we estimated genetic and environmental correlations between these two traits, separately in diabetic and nondiabetic relatives. The results are shown in Table 3. Variation in GFR was not genetically correlated with variation in ACR in diabetic or nondiabetic relatives *(28)*. However, the environmental correlation between these two traits in diabetic and nondiabetic relatives was highly significant statistically, confirming that exposure to elevated levels of ACR is a risk factor for renal function impairment, a conclusion drawn previously from clinical trials on effectiveness of ACE inhibition.

In summary, this pattern of correlations supports further our hypothesis that the genetic factors determining variation in GFR do not overlap with the genetic factors determining variation in ACR. Therefore, our findings provide strong evidence that the search for loci determining variation in GFR must be carried out independently of the search for loci determining variation in ACR.

GENOME SCANS FOR GENES FOR DIABETIC NEPHROPATHY

A promising strategy for identifying genes with major or moderate effects on the development of DN is genotyping suitable families for a large number of genetic markers evenly spread throughout the entire human genome (specifically the 22 autosomes) at 7–15 cM intervals, a strategy referred to as a genome scan. With parametric or non-parametric analytical approaches, one can identify chromosomal regions that harbor genes with major or moderate effects. The evidence for linkage is mapped across the genome in terms of the logarithm of the odds (LOD) favoring linkage vs no linkage at each locus, and the strength of the evidence is assessed as follows. An LOD > 1.15 ($p < 0.01$) indicates potential evidence; an LOD > 1.9 ($p < 0.001$) indicates suggestive evidence; and an LOD > 3.0 ($p < 0.0001$) indicates strong evidence of linkage. With recent improvements in technology, the task of performing a genome scan is well within the capacity of present-day molecular genetics laboratories. The main impediment to the use of this approach is the shortage of DNA from families suitable for genetic studies of DN. Two types of families can be used. One consists of nuclear families with at least two diabetic siblings, at least one of whom is also affected with DN. The other type consists of multigenerational, extended families that include multiple members with T2DM, some of whom are affected with DN and others not. Nondiabetic members may or may not be included. An example of the latter type of families is shown in Fig. 1.

Genome Scans for Genes for Proteinuria or Variation in UAE

A summary of genome scan linkage studies for DN measured as abnormalities in UAE is presented in Table 4.

Table 4
Summary of Results of Genome Scans for Linkage With Proteinuria or Variation in UAE in Families With Type 2 Diabetes

Authors	*Population*	*Results of multipoint linkage analysis*
Imperatore et al., 1998 *(29)*	Pima Indians, Arizona	In a full genome scan of 98 sibling pairs concordant for type 2 diabetes and proteinuria, evidence for linkage with proteinuria was found on chromosomes 3q (LOD = 1.5), 7q (LOD = 2), and 20p (LOD = 1.8).
Vardarli et al., 2002 *(31)*	Caucasians, Turkey	In a partial genome scan of 18 extended families ascertained for early-onset type 2 diabetes (115 relatives with diabetes), evidence for linkage with proteinuria was found on chromosome 18q (LOD = 6.1).
Krolewski et al., 2005 *(22)*	Caucasians, New England	In a full genome scan of 63 extended families ascertained for type 2 diabetes (comprising 5656 relative pairs), evidence for linkage with variation of UAE was found on chromosomes 5q (LOD = 3.4), 7q (LOD = 3.1), and 22q (LOD = 3.7).

A full genome scan for the genes for DN has been carried out in Pima Indian families with T2DM *(29)*. The authors genotyped 98 sibling pairs concordant for T2DM and DN with a 6.4 cM scan. Nephropathy was defined as the presence of overt proteinuria (protein-to-creatinine ratio ≥500 mg/g or a urinary ACR ≥300 mg/g). Three chromosomal regions were identified with at least potential evidence of linkage with nephropathy. However, suggestive evidence for linkage was obtained only on chromosome 7q (multipoint LOD = 2). The other genetic regions potentially linked to nephropathy were on chromosome 3q (multipoint LOD = 1.5), and on chromosome 20p (multipoint LOD = 1.8). Because this study was based on sibling pairs concordant for both T2DM and DN, the positive signals may have been for linkage with either nephropathy or T2DM. However, none of these three regions showed any evidence of linkage with T2DM in a subsequent genome-wide scan for T2DM in Pima Indian families *(30)*.

A partial genome scan for linkage with overt proteinuria was performed in 18 extended Turkish families with 115 members with T2DM *(31)*. Among diabetic family members, there were 61 individuals with normoalbuminuria, 26 with microalbuminuria, and 28 with overt proteinuria. Using parametric linkage analysis, strong evidence of linkage with an elevated UAE (proteinuria only or proteinuria together with microalbuminuria) was found on chromosome 18q. If a dominant mode of inheritance was assumed, the multipoint LOD was 6.6, and if a recessive mode of inheritance was assumed, the multipoint LOD was only 2.2. A reanalysis of the Pima Indian data found weak evidence for linkage with this genetic region (multipoint LOD = 0.7).

We performed a full genome scan for chromosomal regions harboring genes for variation in ACR in 63 extended Caucasian families *(22)*, a subset of the Joslin collection of families with T2DM previously described by Fogarty et al. and Klupa et al. *(18,19,32)*. We measured ACR as a quantitative trait in 426 individuals with and 431 individuals without diabetes. All were genotyped for 381 microsatellite markers spaced

9 cM apart on the 22 autosomes and the results were analyzed using pedigree-based variance-components analysis as implemented in SOLAR *(22)*.

Because the main focus of the study was to identify genes controlling variation in ACR in individuals with diabetes, multipoint variance component linkage analyses were conducted first in the 1332 pairs of relatives with diabetes, and then in all 5656 pairs of all relatives (including diabetic, nondiabetic, and discordant relative pairs). Comparisons of support for linkage from these two analyses at chromosomal regions of interest are measures of the specificity of the effect of that region on variation in ACR. Three possibilities were considered:

1. The effect may be specific to relatives with diabetes if linkage is supported in diabetic pairs and decreases or remains constant in all pairs.
2. The effect may be independent of diabetes status if linkage support is present in pairs of relatives with diabetes and increases significantly in the total sample.
3. The effect may be specific to nondiabetic relatives if there is no linkage support in diabetic pairs but it is present in all pairs of relatives.

In our study we found four chromosomal regions that showed significant or strong support for linkage with ACR. The summary of the findings is shown in Fig. 3. The locations of the linkage peaks are very similar in diabetic as well as in all relative pairs. The support for linkage in genetic regions in all relatives on 22q (multipoint LOD = 3.7), 5q (multipoint LOD = 3.4), and 7q (multipoint LOD = 3.1) was much stronger in all relative pairs than in the subset that included only diabetic relative pairs. The findings are consistent with a hypothesis that these regions harbor genes that determine variation in ACR, in diabetic as well as in nondiabetic relatives *(22)*. In contrast, the linkage support for ACR with chromosome 21p in diabetic relatives only (multipoint LOD = 2.5) is weaker in the group of all relatives (multipoint LOD = 2.1), despite the larger number of relative pairs included in the analysis, a finding consistent with a hypothesis that this genetic region harbors a gene that controls variation of ACR in the presence of diabetes only.

Figure 3 shows also the LOD-1 support intervals for the four chromosomal regions. These intervals vary between 4.7 and 14 million base pairs (Mb) on physical maps and they approximate the locations of the putative susceptibility genes. It is estimated that in each region there are 50–80 genes located, which can be considered as positional candidate genes *(22)*.

The results of our study support a hypothesis that genetic predisposition to diabetic kidney disease may be reflected in the level of urinary albumin excretion, which is controlled by (at least) four genes. In the absence of diabetes, three of these loci may determine the low and the high-normal levels of UAE. With exposure to diabetes, individuals with low levels of UAE remain free of diabetic kidney disease, whereas those with the high-normal levels of UAE may be at risk of worsening to microalbuminuria and overt proteinuria. The risk of the latter may be influenced also by other loci specific for diabetes exposure, for example on chromosome 21p. The nature of the abnormalities in the kidney that determines the level of UAE and is impacted by the genes is unknown.

Genome Scans for Genes for ESRD or Variation in GFR

The summary of the results of the genome-wide scan linkage studies carried out to identify chromosomal regions harboring genes for ESRD or variation in GFR is shown in Table 5.

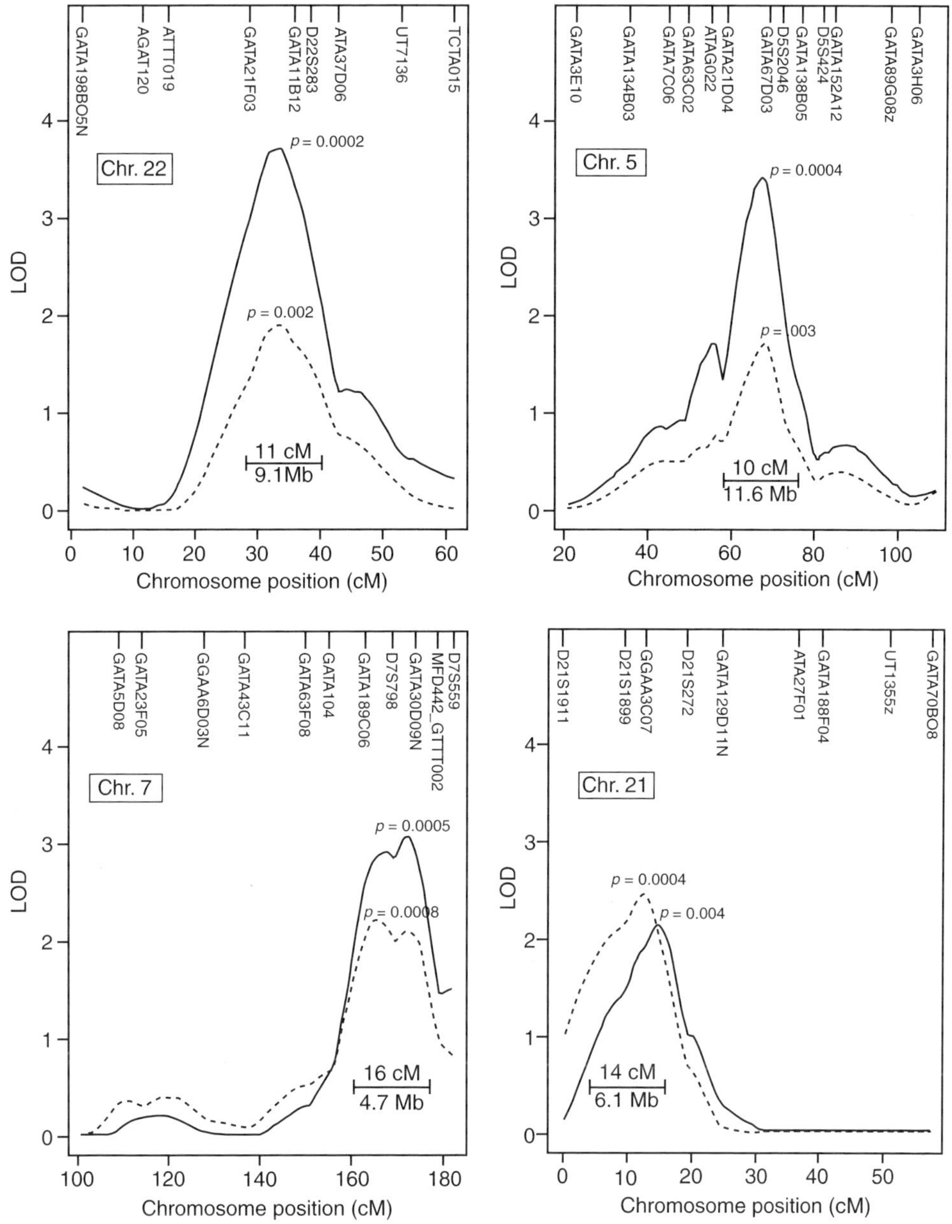

Fig. 3. LOD score plots for ACR on chromosome 22, 5, 7, and 21 for diabetic relative pairs only (broken line) and for all relative pairs (solid line). Empirical *p* values and LOD-1 unit support intervals are shown. Chromosomal positions correspond to the Marshfield map. (Reproduced with permission from ref. *22.*)

A targeted genome scan of a region on human chromosome 10 that is syntenic with the region of the rodent kidney failure-1 gene (*Rf1*) was conducted in two different studies. In the first, 356 African-American sibling pairs affected with ESRD were genotyped for 30 polymorphic markers spaced about 6.6 cM apart on chromosome 10 *(33)*. Strong evidence was found for linkage to a genetic region centromeric from the *Rf1* locus (multipoint LOD = 3.4). The evidence for linkage was similar in the sibling pairs

Table 5
Summary of Results of Genome Scans for Linkage With ESRD or Variation in GFR in Families With Type 2 Diabetes

Authors	*Population*	*Results of multipoint linkage analysis*
Bowden et al., 2004 *(35)*	African Americans, southern US	In a full genome scan of 206 affected sibling pairs with type 2 diabetes and ESRD, evidence for linkage with ESRD was found on chromosomes 3q (LOD = 1.3), 7p (LOD = 1.4), and 18q (LOD = 1.3). The evidence increased for all these regions in ordered subsets analysis.
Placha et al., 2005 *(27)*	Caucasians, New England	In a full genome scan of 63 extended families ascertained for type 2 diabetes (comprising 5656 relative pairs), evidence for linkage with variation in GFR was found on chromosomes 6q (LOD = 2.3) and 7p (LOD = 4.1).

with ESRD owing to diabetes (n = 157) as well as in those with ESRD owing to nondiabetic etiologies (n = 199). The other study, consisting of only 106 diabetic sibling pairs affected with various combinations of proteinuria and ESRD, obtained suggestive evidence of linkage to genetic regions on both the short and long arms of chromosome 10 *(34)*. Neither region, however, overlapped with the region identified in the first study.

A full genome scan for genes controlling the risk for ESRD has been performed in African-American families with T2DM *(35)*. From a collection of 166 nuclear families, 206 sibling pairs affected with both T2DM and ESRD were formed and genotyped for 392 markers with an average spacing of 8.9 cM. In the initial nonparametric linkage analysis, there was evidence for potential linkage on three chromosomes: 3q (multipoint LOD = 1.3), 7p (multipoint LOD = 1.5), and 18q (multipoint LOD = 1.6). However, in the ordered subsets analyses, evidence for linkage for ESRD increased significantly: on 3q to LOD = 4.6 in the optimal subset (estimated to be 29% of the families); on 7p to LOD = 3.6 in the optimal subset (estimated to be 37% of the families); and on 18q to LOD = 3.7 in the optimal subset (estimated to be 64% of the families). Because all sibling pairs also had T2DM, the linkage reported in this study may have been with either ESRD or T2DM. However, the authors preferred the first interpretation for the regions on 3q and 18q because evidence of linkage with proteinuria had been found previously by us on the 3q region in sibling pairs with T1DM discordant for DN *(36)* and on the 18q region in the extended Turkish families with T2DM *(31)*. The authors attributed the evidence of linkage on the 7p region to a T2DM susceptibility locus.

We carried out a full genome scan linkage analysis for chromosomal regions harboring genes for the variation in GFR using the same 63 extended Caucasian families with T2DM as described earlier for the genome scan for variation in ACR *(22,28)*. We estimated GFR by measuring serum levels of cystatin C in 426 individuals with diabetes and 431 individuals without diabetes (*see also* Fig. 1). Relatives in these families formed 5656 relative pairs and were analyzed using pedigree-based variance-component analysis as implemented in SOLAR. After adjustment for covariates such as age, sex, diabetes, diabetes duration, ACR, and mean arterial pressure (MAP), we found evidence for a linkage with the variation in GFR on chromosome 6q (multipoint LOD = 2.3), and on chromosome 7p (multipoint LOD = 4.1). Evidence for linkage was found in both diabetic and nondiabetic relatives. These findings, taken together with the observation that the variation in UAE did not have any genetic correlation with the variation in GFR, suggest that these two chromosomal regions harbor genes specifically controlling variation in GFR and impaired kidney function regardless of diabetes status. Interestingly, the evidence for linkage with variation in GFR on 7p in our study overlaps with the linkage results for ESRD on 7p in the African-American families with T2DM *(35)*. The agreement between these two studies allows us to infer that the evidence obtained in the latter study supports linkage with ESRD rather than with T2DM. This also implies that the genetic region on chromosome 7p harbors genes controlling the risk of declining kidney function in Caucasians as well as in African Americans.

Genome Scans for Genes for Variation in Blood Pressure

Hypertension is a risk factor for elevated ACR as well as diminished GFR, so we carried out multipoint linkage analysis in our 63 families to detect genes that contribute to variation in blood pressure (SBP, diastolic BP [DBP], MAP, or hypertension) in diabetic relative pairs or in all pairs. The goal was to determine whether genes controlling blood pressure would overlap with genes controlling ACR or GFR. In the analyses, after accounting for the effects of significant covariates (such as age, sex, and diabetes status), we found only one chromosomal region with potential evidence (LOD > 1.2) supporting linkage for variation in SBP, DBP, and MAP (Krolewski et al., unpublished data). This region was on chromosome 14p. In diabetic relative pairs, there was potential evidence for linkage with SBP (multipoint LOD = 1.6) and DBP (multipoint LOD = 1.7), and strong evidence for linkage with MAP (multipoint LOD = 3). In all relatives, the LOD scores were similar or smaller then those among diabetic relative pairs (SBP, LOD = 2; DBP, LOD = 1.6; MAP, LOD = 2.6) but at a position 5-11 cM closer to 14pter. These analyses suggest that the region on 14p contains a locus determining variation of blood pressure specifically in diabetic relatives.

There was no evidence supporting linkage for any of the blood pressure measurements on chromosomal regions found to be linked with variation in ACR (shown in Fig. 3) or with variation in GFR. These results provide the first empirical evidence that the frequently observed association between hypertension and elevated ACR and reduced GFR is not the result of pleiotropic effects of a common underlying gene, but is most likely the result of hypertension being a risk factor for both of these nephropathy-related phenotypes.

Positional Cloning of Gene(s) Controlling Risk of Proteinuria and ESRD

Although there is promising evidence of linkage between the variation in UAE and GFR and several chromosomal regions in families with T2DM, the findings need to be replicated in different family collections. However, some investigators have already begun developing physical and transcript maps of these regions to narrow them further, and to identify relevant genes in those smaller critical intervals. Examples of such critical regions are indicated in Fig. 3. This map/location-based approach relies on a comparison of the frequencies of DNA sequence differences (DNA polymorphisms) between properly selected group of cases (either with proteinuria or ESRD) and controls (usually with normoalbuminuric and long duration of diabetes). A large number of polymorphisms in the critical region, in the range of 3000–5000/10,000,000 bp (10 Mb) of the critical region, is required to narrow that region further to less than 1 Mb. Accurate physical and transcript maps of such smaller intervals help to advance the search for a specific susceptibility gene located there that is making individuals susceptible to the development of abnormal urinary excretion or declining renal function.

EXAMINATION OF CANDIDATE GENES FOR DIABETIC NEPHROPATHY

Besides linkage studies for chromosomal regions harboring susceptibility genes for DN and subsequent positional cloning of the putative genes in those regions, an alternative strategy currently employed by many investigators is the "candidate gene" approach *(7,37)*. Unlike genome scans that do not require prior knowledge of the biology of the susceptibility gene, this approach is hypothesis-driven because it focuses on proteins suspected of involvement in the pathogenesis of DN. A gene encoding for one of these proteins is screened for the presence of DNA polymorphisms (single-nucleotide polymorphisms [SNPs], insertion/deletions, or microsatellite markers). Then the distributions of alleles and genotypes of these polymorphisms are examined in unrelated diabetic patients with nephropathy (cases) and unrelated diabetic patients who have remained free of DN despite a long duration of diabetes (controls) to determine whether there are differences. If the groups of cases and controls are inadvertently drawn from populations having different admixtures of subpopulations (population stratification), the case–control study design will return false positive results. Therefore, to confirm positive results from case–control observations, some investigators have turned to the family-based study design, the so-called transmission disequilibrium testing (TDT), which is free of biases owing to the population stratification *(38)*. The selection of "candidate genes" for examination is based on the current understanding of the pathways whereby the hyperglycemia of diabetes is translated into the manifestation of DN. Although the mechanisms have not been fully elucidated, several interrelated pathways can be hypothesized to control the risk of proteinuria and ESRD in patients with diabetes *(39–41)*. In Table 6, four pathways are described, together with a selective list of genes encoding proteins important to each. Sequence differences in any of those genes that result in an abnormal structure or expression of these proteins may contribute to the development of proteinuria and ESRD. Candidate genes located in genetic regions for which there is evidence for linkage with proteinuria (Table 4 and Fig. 3) or ESRD (Table 5) are, for obvious reasons, the primary candidates for examination.

So far, almost 100 different genes have been postulated as candidate genes for DN. These genes were examined mainly in case–control studies. Unfortunately, owing to various methodological deficiencies the results of these studies are difficult to reproduce. In the following sections we describe the results of the examinations of two candidate genes that showed some consistent findings to illustrate the nature of candidate gene studies.

Examination of the Gene Encoding for Apolipoprotein E

Lipid abnormalities have an impact on the progression of DN *(42,43)*. Gene Encoding for apolipoprotein E *(apoE)* is a 299 amino acid glycoprotein that plays an important role in lipid metabolism. It has three common isoforms (E2, E3, and E4), encoded by three alleles (ε2, ε3, and ε4) in exon 4 of the gene encoding apoE *(apoE)* that impact lipid profiles and other cellular functions *(44)*. *apoE* is located on the long arm of chromosome 19, a genetic region for which there is no evidence of linkage with proteinuria or ESRD.

Table 6
Candidate Genes[a] for Susceptibility to the Development of Proteinuria or Declining Kidney Function According to the Presumed Pathway Involved in the Development of DN *(39–41)*

A. Intracellular hyperglycemia: increased level of glucose in endothelial and mesangial cells causes cellular dysfunction. Candidate genes encoding for glucose transporters,[a] aldose reductase,[a] diacylglycerol (DAG) kinase, PKC,[a] nitric oxide synthetases[a]

B. Nonenzymatic glycation: advanced glycation endproducts alter protein function inside as well as outside cells. Candidate genes encoding for glyoxalase I, RAGE[a]

C. Renin–angiotensin system: diabetic milieu causes abnormal kidney hemodynamics. Candidate genes encoding for renin,[a] angiotensinogen,[a] ACE,[a] angiotensin II type 1 receptor[a]

D. Epithelial mesenchymal transdifferentiation: leakage of serum proteins, growth factors, and cytokines into the urinary space initiates and promotes a disease process in tubular cells and interstitium leading to kidney fibrosis. Candidate genes encoding for TGF-β_1,[a] TGF-β_1 receptor, CTGF, CCR2,[a] CCR5[a]

[a]The gene has been examined and reported in the literature.

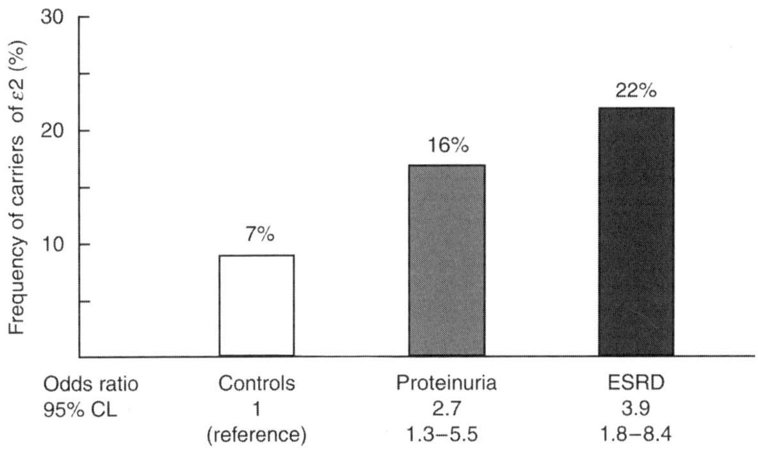

Fig. 4. The frequency of carriers of the ε2 allele according to study groups. (Adapted from ref. *53*.)

Several case–control studies found association between *apoE* polymorphisms and DN in T1 and T2DM, but others did not *(45–52)*. To clarify these controversial findings, Araki et al. *(53)* in our laboratory conducted a large case–control study in T1DM that yielded positive findings. These results were examined further in a TDT family study.

The ε2 allele of *apoE* was significantly more frequent in cases with DN than in diabetic controls with normoalbuminuria despite 15 yr or more duration of T1DM. The frequency of carriers of the ε2 allele is shown in Fig. 4 according to study group, with cases divided into those with proteinuria only and those with ESRD. In comparison with the frequency of ε2 allele carriers in controls (6.6%), the frequencies in cases with proteinuria (16%) and in cases with ESRD (22%) were significantly higher. In comparison with noncarriers, carriers of the ε2 allele had a 2.7-fold higher odds of proteinuria and a 3.9-fold higher odds of having ESRD. Because the odds ratios for proteinuria and ESRD were not significantly different, one may hypothesize that the ε2 allele increases primarily the risk of proteinuria but not ESRD.

Table 7
Transmission Frequencies of the ε2 Allele of the *apoE* Polymorphism From Heterozygous Parents to Offspring According to the Phenotype of the Offspring

DN Status in offspring	*Parental genotype*	*Heterozygous parents*	*ε2 transmitted*		p^a
			Yes	*No*	
With DN					
	ε2/ε3	51	32	19	–
	ε2/ε4	8	6	2	–
	Total	59	38 (64)	21 (36)	0.03
Without DN					
	ε2/ε3	15	5	10	–
	ε2/ε4	5	2	3	–
	Total	20	7 (35)	13 (65)	0.18

[a]Determined by McNemar's test.
Data are *n* or *n*(%). Heterogeneity test: $\chi^2 = 5.3$, p = 0.02. (Reproduced with permission from ref. *53*.)

To exclude the possibility that the association of DN with the ε2 allele of *apoE* in the case–control study was a spurious finding owing to unrecognized population stratification, the association was examined further in a TDT study. Transmission frequencies from parents heterozygous for the ε2 allele to offspring with or without nephropathy are shown in Table 7. As expected for a risk allele, the ε2 allele was preferentially transmitted (in 64%) to offspring with DN and transmitted less than expected (in 35%) to offspring without DN (significance for different patterns of transmission $p = 0.02$). This symmetrically distorted pattern of transmission from the expected 50% strongly supports the association of the ε2 allele of *apoE* with an increased risk of DN.

To exclude the possibility that the association with the ε2 allele might be caused by linkage disequilibrium with another DNA sequence difference in the same region, Araki et al. *(53)* examined the distribution of four additional SNPs flanking *apoE*. He found that the allele frequencies of these SNPs were similar in cases and controls, and the alleles were equally transmitted and not transmitted from heterozygous parents to offspring with and without DN. This negative finding provides support for the conclusion of the study that the *APOE* E2 isoform, which is encoded by the ε2 allele, is causally related to the risk of DN *(53)*.

Recently Araki et al. *(54)* published results of a 4.4 yr follow-up of 429 Japanese subjects with T2DM. Carriers of the ε2 allele had a 2.7 times higher risk of the development of microalbuminuria than noncarriers. Also among patients with microalbuminuria at baseline, carriers of the ε2 allele had a 3.2 times higher risk of progressing to proteinuria than noncarriers. Interestingly, in a multiple logistic regression analysis, the risk of the development of microalbuminuria or progression from microalbuminuria to proteinuria was not changed by adjustment for the levels of total serum cholesterol and triglycerides. This finding indicates that the effect of the *apoE* ε2 isoform on the risk of DN is not mediated through abnormalities in serum lipids levels.

In conclusion, case–control, family-based studies, and follow-up studies provide strong evidence that the ε2 isoform of *apoE*, itself, increases risk of DN in T1 and T2DM, but the impact is primarily on the development of elevated UAE (microalbuminuria and proteinuria) and to lesser degree on ESRD. Furthermore, although the

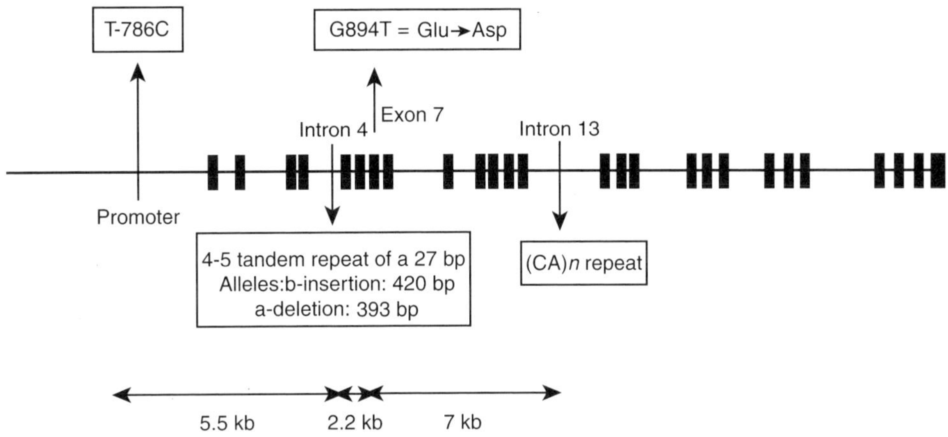

Fig. 5. Organization of eNOS and location of the examined polymorphisms. eNOS is located on chromosome 7q35–36 and is comprised of 26 exons (dark rectangles) and introns (sequences between exons). The protein has 1203 amino acids. The examined polymorphisms are indicated by arrows. Kb is kilobase and bp is base pair. (Reproduced with permission from ref. *65*.)

evidence for the role of the ε2 isoform of *apoE* in the development of DN is becoming clearer, this isoform accounts for only a small proportion of cases with DN and the mechanisms through which this apoE variant causes DN remain to be established *(53)*.

Examination of Gene Encoding for Endothelial Nitric Oxide Synthase

Endothelial dysfunction may be a contributory factor to the variation in UAE and possibly the development of ESRD. This abnormality is prevalent in patients with diabetes and this defect may be owing to decreased availability of nitric oxide (NO) *(55–58)*. This is probably related to the inactivation of NO by a reactive oxygen species generated during nonenzymatic glycation as a consequence of poor glycemic control *(59)*. In addition, the endothelial dysfunction owing to limited availability of NO can be modulated further by the variable production of NO by endothelial nitric oxide synthase (eNOS). In turn, this seems to be associated with polymorphisms in the gene encoding for endothelial nitric oxide synthase *(NOS3) (60,61)*.

NOS3 is a large gene located on the long arm of chromosome 7q35–36. Its organization, including the most frequently examined polymorphisms, is shown in Fig. 5 *(62)*. In early studies, polymorphisms in *NOS3* were associated with an increased risk of myocardial infarction and an elevated risk of ESRD *(63,64)*. To extend the initial observation of an increased risk of ESRD associated with certain polymorphisms in *NOS3*, Zanchi et al. *(65)* in our laboratory carried out a large case–control study in patients with T1DM to examine the risk of proteinuria and ESRD according to the polymorphism shown in Fig. 5. Whereas, an amino acid change in exon 7 and a (CA)n repeat were not associated with DN, the nucleotide change, T-786C, in the promoter of *NOS3* and an insertion/deletion in intron 4 were associated with it. The C allele and a-deletion allele were more frequent in cases suffering from ESRD than in cases with proteinuria or control subjects free of DN. Homozygotes for the C allele of T-786C (OR = 2.8, 95% CI: 1.4–5.6) and carriers of the a-deletion (OR = 2.3, 95% CI: 1.4–4.0) had twice the risk of developing ESRD relative to their comparison groups. In a family-based TDT analysis, the haplotypes defined by these two polymorphisms were determined, and transmission of haplotypes from heterozygous parents to three different groups of offspring was examined. Transmission of the risk haplotype (C/a-deletion) was significantly increased to offspring with ESRD (74%, $p = 0.004$); was insignificantly different from the expected 50% to offspring with proteinuria; and significantly deficient to offspring with normoalbuminuria (35%, $p = 0.04$). Overall, in both case–control and family studies, carriers of the C/a-deletion haplotype had significantly higher risk of ESRD than noncarriers. However, this haplotype did not increase the risk of developing proteinuria.

Several authors reported findings in T2DM, as well as in nondiabetics, that are consistent with the results described earlier *(66–68)*. However, some authors who did not distinguish between cases with proteinuria and cases with ESRD could not replicate our findings *(69)*. Further research is required to examine the molecular as well as physiological mechanisms through which polymorphisms in *NOS3* cause increased risk of ESRD. One must also account for very obvious discrepancies between the association studies summarized earlier and the linkage results summarized in Tables 4 and 5 and Fig. 3. Whereas the association studies point to a role for *NOS3* in the development of ESRD, the evidence for linkage to the genetic region in which *NOS3* is located is with a variation in UAE, not with a variation in GFR.

Considerations Regarding Examination of Other Candidate Genes

We have selectively reviewed recent findings regarding two candidate genes for DN. It is fair to state that the findings for many other candidate genes are far less consistent in most cases and are even conflicting in some. Although the cause of these discrepancies has not been precisely determined, certain explanations should be mentioned to help in the interpretation of these results as well to guide future studies. These explanations relate to the possibility that the "candidate genes" have only a minor impact on DN. Conceivably, the "detectability" of the contributions of these genes may depend on many additional factors such as study designs, the ethnicity of the study population, or the modulating effect of various environmental conditions (e.g., tobacco smoking, glycemic control, or hypertension control).

If an association is found in case–control studies, and is supported by family studies, it may be inferred that the DNA polymorphism is a marker of genetic susceptibility to DN. However, the biological interpretation of the association is not always clear. It may be owing to the polymorphism itself, including a disease-causing allele that directly affects the expression or function of a gene or gene product (e.g., by an amino acid change, frameshift mutation, or premature termination), or the association may result from linkage disequilibrium between the marker polymorphism and a causative polymorphism. This phenomenon is owing to the fact that particular alleles of polymorphisms lying in close genetic proximity to each other have a tendency to segregate together over successive generations *(70)*. Therefore, whereas association between a polymorphism and DN may be demonstrated, confirmation that the polymorphism is actually the cause of genetic susceptibility can only be obtained from functional in vitro and in vivo studies that evaluate the impact of the polymorphism on the pathogenesis of DN.

CONCLUSIONS

Proteinuria and impaired renal function are two clinical phenotypes of DN that aggregate (are heritable) in families with T2DM. Although both are heritable, they are not genetically correlated. These findings support the hypothesis that the development of DN consists of two distinct disease processes, i.e., increasing UAE (proteinuria) and declining renal function. They also strongly justify searches for the putative genes that separately determine variation in these disease processes. These searches have used both genome-wide linkage studies, to map the location of the susceptibility genes for each disease process, and candidate gene investigations, to identify specific genes/proteins involved in these processes.

Using genome scan linkage studies, several research groups have identified genetic regions on chromosomes 5q, 7q, 18q, and 22q that may harbor genes determining either variation in UAE or susceptibility to proteinuria. Although it needs to be investigated further, the linkage data provide strong evidence that the same genes control variation in UAE in individuals with T2DM as in those without. Two genome linkage studies performed in families with T2DM identified genetic regions on chromosome 3q, 6q, 7p, and 18q that harbor susceptibility genes determining variation in GFR or susceptibility to the development of ESRD. Optimism is growing that a positional cloning approach applied to these putative genetic regions will lead to the identification of the susceptibility genes that contribute to abnormalities in UAE as well as declining renal function.

Using the candidate gene approach, several groups are searching for the susceptibility genes for DN. Unfortunately, positive findings can account only for minor genetic effects, pointing out that the major susceptibility genes for each of the two phenotypes are unknown genes, or known genes but their involvement in DN has not been implicated by the current etiological hypotheses.

ACKNOWLEDGMENTS

Support was provided by NIH Grants: DK-58549 and DK-67638. G.P. is a recipient of a fellowship from the Juvenile Diabetes Research Foundation (JDRF # 3-2004-82).

REFERENCES

1. Valmadrid CT, Klein R, Moss SE, Klein BE. The risk of cardiovascular disease mortality associated with microalbuminuria and gross proteinuria in persons with older-onset diabetes mellitus. Arch Intern Med 2000;160:1093–1100.
2. Gerstein HC, Mann JF, Yi Q, et al. Albuminuria and risk of cardiovascular events, death, and heart failure in diabetic and nondiabetic individuals. JAMA 2001;286:421–426.
3. Remuzzi G, Schieppati A, Ruggenenti P. Nephropathy in patients with type 2 diabetes. N Engl J Med 2002;346:1145–1151.
4. Bakris GL. The evolution of treatment guidelines for diabetic nephropathy. Strategies integrate JNC VI, more recent protocols. Postgrad Med 2003;113:35–40.
5. Jones CA, Krolewski AS, Rogus J, Xue JL, Collins A, Warram JH. Epidemic of end stage renal disease in people with diabetes in the US population: Do we know the cause? Kidney Int 2005;67: 1684–1691.
6. Rosenbloom AL, Joe JR, Young RS, Winter WE. Emerging epidemic of type 2 diabetes in youth. Diabetes Care 1999;22:345–354.
7. Krolewski AS. Genetics of diabetic nephropathy: evidence for major and minor gene effects. Kidney Int 1999;55:1582–1596.
8. Liang KY, Beaty TH. Statistical designs for familial aggregation. Stat Method Med Res 2000; 9:543–62.
9. Hunter DJ, Lange M, Snieder H, et al. Genetic contribution to renal function and electrolyte balance: a twin study. Clin Sci 2002;103:259–265.
10. Almasy L, Blangero J. Multipoint quantitative-trait linkage analysis in general pedigrees. Am J Hum Genet 1998;62:1198–1211.
11. Seaquist ER, Goetz FC, Rich S, Barbosa J. Familial clustering of diabetic kidney disease. Evidence for genetic susceptibility to diabetic nephropathy. N Engl J Med 1989;320:1161–1165.

12. Quinn M, Angelico MC, Warram JH, Krolewski AS. Familial factors determine the development of diabetic nephropathy in patients with IDDM. Diabetologia 1996;39:940–945.
13. The Diabetes Control and Complications Trial Research Group. Clustering of long-term complications in families with diabetes in the diabetes control and complications trial. Diabetes 1997;46:1829–1839.
14. Harjutsalo V, Katoh S, Sarti C, Tajima N, Tuomilehto J. Population-based assessment of familial clustering of diabetic nephropathy in type 1 diabetes. Diabetes 204;53:2449–2454.
15. Faronato PP, Maioli M, Tonolo G, Brocco E, Noventa F. Clustering of albumin excretion rate abnormalities in Caucasian patients with NIDDM. The Italian NIDDM Nephropathy Study Group. Diabetologia 1997;40:816–823.
16. Canani LH, Gerchman F, Gross JL. Familial clustering of diabetic nephropathy in Brazilian type 2 diabetic patients. Diabetes 1999;48:909–913.
17. Forsblom CM, Kanninen T, Lehtovitra M, Saloranta C, Groop L. Heritability of albumin excretion rate in families of patients with Type II diabetes. Diabetologia 1999;42:1359–1366.
18. Fogarty DG, Rich SS, Hanna LS, Warram JH, Krolewski AS. Urinary albumin excretion in families with type 2 diabetes is heritable and genetically correlated to blood pressure. Kidney Int 2000;57:250–257.
19. Fogarty DG, Hanna LS, Wantman M, Warram JH, Krolewski AS, Rich SS. Segregation analysis of urinary albumin excretion in families with type 2 diabetes. Diabetes 2000;49:1057–1063.
20. Freedman BI, Beck SR, Rich SS, et al. A genome-wide scan for urinary albumin excretion in hypertensive families. Hypertension 42:291–296.
21. Langefeld CD, Beck SR, Bowden DW, Rich SS, Wagenknecht LE, Freedman BI. Heritability of GFR and albumin in Caucasians with type 2 diabetes mellitus. Am J Kidney Dis 2004;43:796–800.
22. Krolewski AS, Poznik D, Placha G, et al. A genome-wide linkage scan for genes controlling variation in urinary albumin excretion in type 2 diabetes. Kidney Int, in press.
23. Pettitt DJ, Saad MF, Bennett PH, Nelson RG, Knowler WC. Familial predisposition to renal disease in two generations of Pima Indians with type 2 (non-insulin-dependent) diabetes mellitus. Diabetologia 1990;33:438–443.
24. Freedman BI, Tuttle AB, Spray BJ. Familial predisposition to nephropathy in African-Americans with non-insulin-dependent diabetes mellitus. Am J Kidney Dis 1995;25:710–713.
25. Hunt SC, Coon H, Hasstedt SJ, et al. Linkage of serum creatinine and glomerular filtration rate to chromosome 2 in Utah pedigrees. Am J Hypert 2004;17:511–515.
26. Fox CS, Yang Q, Cupples LA, et al. Genome wide linkage analysis to serum creatinine, GFR and creatinine clearance in a community-based population: The Framingham Heart Study. J Am Soc Nephrol 2004;15:2457–2461.
27. Perkins BA, Nelson RG, Ostrander BEP, et al. Detection of renal function decline in patients with diabetes and normal or elevated GFR by serial measurements of serum cystatin C concentration: results of a 4-year follow-up study. J Am Soc nephrol 2005;16:1404–1412.
28. Placha G, Poznik D, Warram JH, Rich SS, Krolewski AS. Genome scan findings in families with type 2 diabetes point to different genetic predispositions to elevated urinary albumin excretion and to impaired renal function. Diabetes 2005;54(Suppl):A199.
29. Imperatore G, Hanson RL, Pettitt DF, Kobes S, Bennett PH, Hanson RL. Sib-pair linkage analysis for susceptibility genes for microvascular complications among Pima Indians with type 2 diabetes. Pima Diabetes Genes Group. Diabetes 1998;47:821–830.
30. Hanson RL, Ehm MG, Pettitt DJ, et al. An autosomal genomic scan for loci linked to type II diabetes mellitus and body-mass index in Pima Indians. Am J Hum Genet 1998;63:1130–1138.
31. Vardali I, Baier LJ, Hanson RL, et al. Gene for susceptibility to diabetic nephropathy in type 2 diabetes maps to 18q22.3-23. Kidney Int 2002;62:2176–2183.
32. Klupa T, Warram JH, Antonellis A, et al. Determinants of the development of diabetes (Maturity-onset diabetes of the young-3) in carriers of HNF-1a mutations. Diabetes Care 2002;25:2292–2301.
33. Freedman BI, Rich SS, Yu H, Roh BH, Bowden DW. Linkage heterogeneity of end-stage renal disease on human chromosome 10. Kidney Int 2002;62:770–774.
34. Iyengar SK, Fox KA, Schachere M, et al. Linkage analysis of candidate loci for end-stage renal disease due to diabetic nephropathy. J Am Soc Nephrol 2003;14:S195–S201.
35. Bowden DW, Colicigno CJ, Langefeld CD, et al. A genome scan for diabetic nephropathy in African Americans. Kidney Int 2004;66:1517–1526.
36. Moczulski DK, Rogus JJ, Antonellis, Warram JH, Krolewski AS. Major susceptibility locus for nephropathy in type 1 diabetes on chromosome 3q: results of novel discordant sib-pair analysis. Diabetes 1998;47:1164–1169.
37. Clark GA. The role of haplotypes in candidate gene studies. Gent Epid 27:321–333.

38. Spielman RS, McGinnis RE, Ewens WJ. Transmission test for linkage disequilibrium: the insulin gene region and insulin-dependent diabetes mellitus (IDDM). Am J Hum Genet 52:506–516.
39. Brownlee M. Biochemistry and molecular cell biology of diabetic complications. Nature 414:813–829.
40. Jerums G, Panagiotopoulos S, Forbs J, Osicka T, Cooper M. Evolving concepts in advanced glycation, diabetic nephropathy, and diabetic vascular disease. Arch Biochem Bioph 419:55–62.
41. He Z, King GI. Microvascular complications of diabetes. Endocrinol Metab Clin North Am 33:215–238.
42. Watts GF, Powrie JK, O'Brien SF, Shaw KM. Apolipoprotein B independently predicts progression of very-low-level albuminuria in insulin-dependent diabetes mellitus. Metabolism 45:1101–1107.
43. Krolewski AS, Warram JH, Christlieb AR. Hypercholesterolemia—a determinant of renal function loss and deaths in IDDM patients with nephropathy. Kidney Int Suppl 1994;45:S125–S131.
44. Mahley RW, Apolipoprotein E. Cholesterol transport protein with expanding role in cell biology. Science 1988;240:622–630.
45. Chowdhury TA, Dyer PH, Kumar S, et al. Association of apolipoprotein epsilon2 allele with diabetic nephropathy in Caucasian subjects with IDDM. Diabetes 1998;47:278–280.
46. Hadjadj S, Gallois Y, Simard G, et al. Lack of relationship in long-term type 1 diabetic patients between diabetic nephropathy and polymorphisms in apolipoprotein varepsilon, lipoprotein lipase and cholesterol ester transfer protein. Nephrol Dial Transplant 2000;15:1971–1976.
47. Tarnow L, Stehouwer CD, Emeis JJ, et al. Plasminogen activator inhibitor-1 and apolipoprotein E gene polymorphisms and diabetic angiopathy. Nephrol Dial Transplant 2000;15:625–630.
48. Eto M, Horita K, Morikawa A, et al. Increased frequency of apolipoprotein epsilon 2 allele in non-insulin dependent diabetic (NIDDM) patients with nephropathy. Clin Genet 1995;10:288–292.
49. Kimura H, Suzuki Y, Gejyo F, et al. Apolipoprotein E4 reduces risk of diabetic nephropathy in patients with NIDDM. Am J Kidney Dis 1998;31:666–673.
50. Ukkola O, Kervinen K, Salmela PI, von Dickhoff K, Laakso M, Kesaniemi YA. Apolipoprotein E phenotype is related to macro- and microangiopathy in patients with non-insulin-dependent diabetes mellitus. Atherosclerosis 1993;101:915–967.
51. Boizel R, Benhamou PY, Corticelli K, et al. ApoE polymorphism and albuminuria in diabetes mellitus: a role for LDL in the development of nephropathy in NIDDM. Nephrol Dial Transplant 1998;13:72–75.
52. Vauhkonen I, Niskanen L, Ryynanen M, et al. Divergent association of apolipoprotein E polymorphism with vascular disease in patients with NIDDM and control subjects. Diabet Med 1997;14:748–756.
53. Araki S, Moczulski DK, Hanna LS, Scott LJ, Warram JH, Krolewski AS. APOE polymorphisms and the development of diabetic nephropathy in Type 1 diabetes. Diabetes 2000;49:2190–2195.
54. Araki S, Koya D, Makiishi T, et al. APOE polymorphism and the progression of diabetic nephropathy in Japanese subject with type 2 diabetes. Diabetes Care 2003;26:2416–2420.
55. Calver A, Collier J, Vallance P. Inhibition and stimulation of nitric oxide synthesis in the human forearm arterial bed of patients with insulin-dependent diabetes. J Clin Invest 1992;90:2548–2554.
56. Elliot TG, Cockcroff JR, Groop PH, Viberti GC, Ritter JM. Inhibition of nitric oxide synthesis in forearm vasculature of insulin-dependent diabetic patients. Blunted vasoconstriction in patients with microalbuminuria. Clin Sci 1993;85:687–693.
57. Zenere B, Arcaro G, Saggiani F, Rossi L, Muggeo M, Lechi A. Noninvasive detection of functional alterations of the arterial wall in IDDM patients with and without microalbuminuria. Diabetes Care 1995;18:975–982.
58. Lekakis J, Papamichael C, Anastatsiou H, et al. Endothelial dysfunction of conduit arteries in insulin-dependent diabetes mellitus without microalbuminuria. Cardiovasc Res 1997;34:164–168.
59. Bucala R, Tracey KJ, Cerami A. Advanced glycosylation products quench nitric oxide and mediate defective endothelium-dependent vasodilatation in experimental diabetes. J Clin Invest 1991;87: 432–438.
60. Tsukada T, Yokoyama K, Arai T, et al. Evidence of association of the ecNOS gene polymorphism with plasma NO metabolite levels in humans. Bioch Bioph Res Comm 245:190–193.
61. Komatsu M, Kawagishi T, Emoto M, et al. eNOS gene polymorphism is associated with endothelium-dependent vasodilatation in type 2 diabetes. Am J Physiol 2002;283:H557–H561.
62. Marsden PA, Heng HH, Scherer SW, et al. Structure and chromosomal localization of the human constitutive endothelial nitric oxide synthase gene. J Biol Chem 1993;268(23):17,478–17,488.
63. Wang XL, Sim AS, Badenhop RF, McCredie M, Wilcken DEL. A smoking dependent risk of coronary artery disease associated with a polymorphism of the endothelial nitric oxide synthase gene. Nature Med 1996;2:41–45.

64. Wang Y, Kikuchi S, Suzuki H, Nagase S, Koyama A. Endothelial nitric oxide synthase gene polymorphism in intron 4 affects the progression of renal failure in non-diabetic renal diseases. Nephrol Dial Transplant 1999;14:2898–2902.
65. Zanchi A, Moczulski DK, Hanna LS, Wantman M, Warram JH, Krolewski AS. Risk of advanced diabetic nephropathy in type 1 diabetes is associated with endothelial nitric oxide synthase gene polymorphism. Kidney Int 2000;57:405–413.
66. Neugebauer S, Baba T, Watanabe T. Association of the nitric oxide synthase gene polymorphism with an increased risk for progression to diabetic nephropathy in type 2 diabetes. Diabetes 2000;49:500–503.
67. Asakimori Y, Yorioka N, Taniguchi Y, et al. T(-786)->C polymorphism of the endothelial nitric oxide synthase gene influences the progression of renal disease. Nephron 2002;91:747–751.
68. Buraczynska M, Ksiazek P, Zaluska W, Nowizka T, Ksiasek A. Endothelial nitric oxide synthase gene intron 4 polymorphism in patients with end-stage renal disease. Nephrol Dial Transplant 2004;19: 2302–2306.
69. Rippin JD, Patel A, Belyaev ND, Gill GV, Barnett AH, Bain SC. Nitric oxide synthase gene polymorphisms and diabetic nephropathy. Diabetologia 2003;46:426–428.
70. Pericak-Vance MA. Linkage disequilibrium and allelic association. In: Haines JL, Pericak-Vance MA, eds. Approaches to gene mapping in complex human diseases. Wiley-Liss, New York, 1998, pp. 323–333.

20 Major Risks Indicators for Diabetic Kidney Disease

Katherine R. Tuttle, MD

CONTENTS

INTRODUCTION

Risks for diabetic kidney disease have traditionally focused on those associated with loss of renal function, particularly glomerular filtration rate (GFR). The ultimate consequence of GFR loss, end-stage renal disease (ESRD), has long been the primary domain for many nephrologists. However, loss of renal function also encompasses many aspects other than GFR. A number of comorbidities result from, or are exacerbated by, damage to the kidney: hypertension, anemia, disordered bone and mineral metabolism, dyslipidemia, and inflammation, among others. Many of these disturbances are more prevalent, occur earlier, and are more severe in diabetes than in other forms of chronic kidney disease (CKD) *(1–4)*. Furthermore, they may contribute to further kidney damage, as well as to cardiovascular disease (CVD). The latter issue is of particular concern because most people with diabetes who develop CKD will die of CVD rather than reach ESRD *(5)*. Therefore, kidney damage and associated comorbidities can be viewed as fundamental participants in a self-perpetuating, positive feedback cycle that produces widespread injury to the circulation with multiple target organ consequences. Because diabetes and CKD pose such a high risk of mortality and major adverse events, the purpose of this chapter is to review major risks indicators. Identification of risks allows for development of improved strategies for detection, intervention, and novel therapeutic approaches.

PREDICTORS OF KIDNEY DISEASE IN EARLY DIABETES

Renal Hemodynamics

Genetic predisposition undoubtedly contributes to the development of kidney disease in diabetes, as discussed in the chapter by Placha and Krolewski. In addition, early renal

From: *Contemporary Diabetes: The Diabetic Kidney*
Edited by: P. Cortes and C. E. Mogensen © Humana Press Inc., Totowa, NJ

functional changes have also been associated with subsequent kidney disease. Glomerular hyperfiltration, a higher than normal GFR, has long been recognized in recent-onset type-1 or -2 diabetes *(6–11)*. In observational studies of persons with type-1 diabetes, those with higher GFR levels have been described as being more likely to develop micro- or macroalbuminuria many years later *(12,13)*. However, these studies are limited by lack of very long-term follow-up (>30 yr) necessary to potentially associate early glomerular hyperfiltration with late loss of kidney function.

Animal models have provided a great deal of insight into the early renal hemodynamic disturbances in diabetes. In classic physiologic studies, diabetic rats studied with micropuncture techniques were found to have high GFR owing to increased glomerular perfusion and pressure *(14)*. Intraglomerular hypertension was shown to play a key role in hyperfiltration and subsequent renal injury in diabetes or with high-protein diets in other experimental models *(14,15)*. Furthermore, feeding diabetic rats a high-protein diet greatly exacerbated renal injury and loss of function *(16)*. Conversely, a low-protein diet protected the kidney even in the setting of continued hyperglycemia *(16)*. Another important observation from this study was that the diabetic rats exhibited greater sensitivity to the renal hemodynamic effects of dietary protein than the normal rats *(16)*. These data suggested that interactions between the defining feature of diabetes, hyperglycemia, and dietary protein produce an augmented glomerular hyperfiltration response and, consequently, kidney damage.

In human physiologic studies, we aimed to further investigate how hyperglycemia and dietary protein interact in diabetes. Persons with diabetes were studied after an overnight fast with the plasma glucose level clamped at an ambient level of approx 200 mg/dL *(17,18)*. In studies of both type-1 and -2 diabetes, GFR and renal plasma flow were normal in the fasting state. However, when a mixed amino acid (AA) solution designed to resemble a protein meal was infused intravenously, the renal hemodynamic responses diverged sharply between the diabetic participants and normal controls. Those with either type-1 or -2 diabetes had an augmented glomerular hyperfiltration response that was greatly increased beyond that of nondiabetic individuals. Filtration fraction, an indirect indicator of glomerular hypertension, was also increased in diabetes. Acute (36 h) control of hyperglycemia did not correct this augmented response, but after 3 wk of strict glycemic control, renal hemodynamics were normal in both the fasting and AA-stimulated states. These data suggested that hyperglycemia was necessary but not sufficient to produce glomerular hyperfiltration in diabetes. Moreover, sensitivity to the AA stimulus to raise GFR was enhanced by chronic hyperglycemia. Thus, human studies were consistent with the animal models in demonstrating greater sensitivity to renal hemodynamic effects of dietary protein, acting through increased AA levels, in diabetes.

Hormonal responses to protein feeding or an AA infusion could be responsible for increasing renal perfusion and GFR. Glucagon levels are increased after a protein meal, and infusion of glucagon has been reported to cause glomerular hyperfiltration in diabetic and normal subjects *(19–22)*. Renal vasodilatory prostaglandins have also been implicated in producing glomerular hyperfiltration induced by diabetes and/or AAs *(23–26)*. Therefore, we studied a group of individuals with type-1 diabetes by blocking either glucagon secretion (octreotide) or prostaglandin production (indomethacin) during AA infusion *(27)*. Neither of these inhibitors prevented the augmented glomerular hyperfiltration response to AAs in the diabetic participants. We also evaluated the renal hemodynamic response to a glucagon infusion in the same participants. Those with diabetes also had an augmented response to the glucagon stimulus, suggesting that the enhanced renal hemodynamic sensitivity was not specific for AAs. The increases in GFR and renal plasma flow during glucagon infusion were blocked by indomethacin, indicating that prostaglandins were responsible for this response. In summary, individuals with diabetes have enhanced sensitivity to AAs as well as to glucagon, another stimulus that raises GFR. Although glucagon and prostaglandins do not appear to be primary causes of AA-induced renal hemodynamic changes in diabetes, they could produce glomerular hyperfiltration under other conditions, such as more severe hyperglycemia.

Cellular Mechanisms

More recently, we have explored the kidney's response to AAs at the cellular level. We hypothesized that AAs could directly injure cells and participate in processes induced by high levels of glucose. In other words, interactions between AAs and glucose that exacerbate kidney damage could occur at the cellular level. The mesangial cell culture model was chosen because it is a key cell involved in regulation of renal hemodynamics, as well as the profibrotic and proliferative response to injury in diabetes. The model utilizes four main experimental conditions: increased AA, high glucose (30.5 m*M*; HG), the combination of both AA and HG (AA/HG), and control *(28)*. The mixture of AAs used in the cell culture studies is derived from the same solution (Travasol 10%, Baxter, Deerfield, IL, USA) that was infused in the human studies previously described *(17,18,27)*. This mixture is designed to resemble a protein meal, and the levels are increased 1.5–sixfold above control, depending on the AA. We first demonstrated that increased AAs, alone or in combination with a high glucose level, induced mesangial cell proliferation and fibrosis *(28)*. In addition, the profibrotic response was mediated by increased expression and activation of transforming growth factor-β. The matrix protein, thrombospondin-1, was responsible for increased transforming growth factor-β activation under these circumstances. These responses to the AA and AA/HG conditions were remarkably similar to those of the HG condition. For the mesangial cell proliferation response, the combination condition of AA/HG produced an even greater response than either HG or AA alone.

Because of the remarkable similarities between effects of glucose and AAs on mesangial cells, we hypothesized that a common metabolic pathway could be responsible. Advanced glycation end products (AGEs) are formed by nonenzymatic glycation of free amino groups, followed by a complex series of sequential glycation and oxidation reactions. Although previous research has focused on hyperglycemia as the main causal factor, increased availability of free amino groups could also initiate these reactions. If so, then cell signaling pathways associated with AGEs should also be activated and participate in the injury responses. In a series of experiments, we found that AGE formation was increased by the AA condition, and that the combination condition of AA/HG appeared to produce an even greater amount of AGEs *(29)*. Preventing AGE formation with aminoguanidine blocked the profibrotic mesangial cell response. We also found that cell signaling pathways associated with AGEs, oxidative stress, and activation of protein kinase C and mitogen-activated protein kinases extracellular signal-related kinases 1,2, were increased by the AA, HG, and AA/HG conditions. Their causal roles in the profibrotic response were confirmed by specific inhibition of these processes. To our knowledge, this was the first demonstration that AAs induce AGE formation in mesangial cells, and that they appear to enhance such an effect of glucose. These observations provide insight into cellular mechanisms of injury induced by AAs and a potential explanation for increased sensitivity of the diabetic kidney to damage resulting from high dietary protein. Furthermore, AGEs are associated with widespread vascular damage and consumption of foods with increased amounts of AGE-modified proteins increase circulating AGEs and inflammatory markers in diabetic subjects *(30)*. We speculate that AA-induced injury could be produced at sites other than the kidney, and that the arterial circulation may be particularly vulnerable. In support of this notion, a recent study of persons with type-1 diabetes and early CKD (on average stage 2) showed that a modest reduction of dietary protein decreased the combined end point of death and ESRD *(31)*. Deaths were predominantly owing to CVD and were decreased as much, or more, than cases of ESRD. Thus, limiting exposure to dietary protein and, consequently, increased levels of AAs, may protect against CVD as well as CKD. Our data provide insight into a potential underlying mechanism.

KIDNEY DISEASE AS A WINDOW TO THE CIRCULATION

Development of kidney disease in diabetes reflects processes operative at distant sites that have a major impact on risks of adverse outcomes. In the chapters by Sowers et al. and Stehouwer et al., hypertension, CVD, and endothelial dysfunction in diabetes are reviewed in depth. This section will address how early and late indicators of CKD provide insight into global circulatory dysfunction. Albuminuria is the earliest clinical indicator of CKD in diabetes. However, albuminuria also increases risk of CVD events and death independent of traditional risk factors *(32,33)*. Although this relationship is particularly apparent in diabetes, albuminuria also appears to increase CVD risk in other groups, including those with essential hypertension and the general population *(34,35)*. In a study of persons undergoing elective coronary angiography, we found a direct correlation between albuminuria levels and severity of coronary artery disease *(36)*. This relationship was most pronounced in the subset of individuals with type-2 diabetes. Importantly, the levels of albuminuria that correlated with coronary artery disease were largely below the traditional threshold for defining microalbuminuria (albumin-to-creatinine ratio <30 mg/g). This concept is also supported by data from the Heart Outcomes Prevention Evaluation (HOPE) study that showed that risk of major CVD events in high-risk patients, with and without diabetes, increases at levels of albuminuria far below the traditional threshold for microalbuminuria *(37)*. Therefore, elevated levels of albuminuria defined by predicting progression of kidney disease may be higher than those that predict clinically important CVD.

As for most CVD risk factors, the relationship to CKD appears to be continuous. Risk of major CVD events increases even further as albuminuria progresses to clinical albuminuria (albumin-to-creatinine ratio > 300 mg/g) or overt proteinuria (dipstick-positive, protein-to-creatinine ratio >500 mg/g). Risks for strokes and coronary events are amplified as proteinuria increases *(38)*. Once GFR begins to fall, the risk of CVD continues to escalate *(39)*. In fact, most people with CKD will die of CVD and not reach ESRD *(5)*. People with both diabetes and decreased GFR are at especially high risk of cardiac death *(5,40)*.

The strong influence of kidney disease on CVD is likely to be multifactorial. There are several possible explanations: vascular disease expressed at the level of the kidney reflects greater severity; persons with CKD have a greater burden of traditional risk factors including diabetes; CKD produces nontraditional risk factors *(41)*. It is important to recognize that these possibilities are not mutually exclusive. Endothelial injury, a key component of the atherosclerotic process, occurs in the glomerular microcirculation and in the circulation at large. Albuminuria is believed to be an excellent marker of this process. In persons with known coronary heart disease, defined by a previous myocardial infarction, albuminuria correlated directly with the transvascular escape rate of albumin *(42)*. Even in apparently healthy persons, increased levels of albuminuria are associated with endothelial dysfunction, as determined by impaired flow-associated dilation of the brachial artery *(43)*. Thus, albuminuria can be considered an indicator of endothelial injury in the kidney as well as at distant sites in the circulation.

Persons with type-2 diabetes and albuminuria have a particularly high risk of CVD *(32,33)*. Albuminuria is highly prevalent in this group, approx 40% overall, with a range of 10–80%, depending on the population studied *(44)*. A seminal question is whether or not reduction of albuminuria predicts improved risk status. In secondary analyses of the Reduction in Endpoints in Noninsulin-dependent diabetes mellitus with the Angiotensin II Antagonist Losartan (RENAAL) trial, lowering albuminuria was associated with reduced risk of renal and cardiovascular events *(45,46)*. This has been interpreted to mean that albuminuria should be a therapeutic target in type 2 diabetes. However, a limitation of this interpretation is that those who were responsive to treatment with the angiotensin receptor blocker may have had less severe disease. Nevertheless, the hypothesis that albuminuria should be a therapeutic target is an important one worthy of prospective testing. Other important questions are embedded in this hypothesis: Do albuminuria-reducing treatments other than angiotensin receptor blockers improve outcomes? Do treatments without an effect on albuminuria improve outcomes?

In summary, indicators of CKD in diabetes, albuminuria, and decreased GFR, reflect damage to the kidney that predicts a broad spectrum of adverse outcomes in multiple vascular target organs.

CONCLUSIONS

Risks for diabetic kidney disease have traditionally focused on those associated with loss of renal function, particularly GFR. Loss of renal function also encompasses many aspects other than GFR: hypertension, anemia, disordered bone, and mineral metabolism, dyslipidemia, and inflammation, among others. Many of these disturbances are more prevalent, occur earlier, and are more severe in diabetes than in other forms of CKD. Furthermore, they may contribute to further kidney damage, as well as to CVD. The latter issue is of particular concern because most people with diabetes who develop CKD will die of CVD rather than reach ESRD. Predictors of early kidney disease, focusing on renal hemodynamic disturbances produced by diabetes and nutritional influences (excess dietary protein), were discussed. Evidence for a direct effect of dietary protein, acting through increased AAs, to induce mesangial cell injury was also presented. Finally, the concept that indicators of CKD, albuminuria, and decreased GFR, reflect widespread circulatory disease was reviewed.

Development of kidney disease in diabetes heralds a number of adverse outcomes. An understanding of major risks indicators should facilitate future research designed to elucidate basic mechanisms of disease at one end of the spectrum, whereas improving design of clinical trials on the other. Indeed, identification of major risks indicators is a critical component of translational research, the bench-to-bedside paradigm.

REFERENCES

1. Tarnow L, Rossing P, Gall MA, Nielsen FS, Parving HH. Prevalence of arterial hypertension in diabetic patients before and after the JNC-V. Diabetes Care 1994;17:1247–1251.

2. Deray G, Heurtier A, Grimaldi A, Vacher VL, Bagnis CI. Anemia and diabetes. Am J Nephrol 2004;24:522–526.
3. Hörl WH. The clinical consequences of secondary hyperparathyroidism: focus on clinical outcomes. Nephrol Dial Transplant 2004;19:v2–v8.
4. Kaysen GA, Eiserich JP. The role of oxidative stress-altered lipoprotein structure and function and microinflammation on cardiovascular risk in patients with minor renal dysfunction. J Am Soc Nephrol 2004;15:538–548.
5. Foley RN, Murray AM, Li S, et al. Chronic kidney disease and the risk for cardiovascular disease, renal replacement, and death in the United States Medicare population, 1998 to 1999. J Am Soc Nephrol 2005;16:489–495.
6. Stalder G, Schmid R. Severe functional disorders of glomerular capillaries and renal hemodynamics in treated diabetes mellitus during childhood. Ann Peadiatr (Basel) 1959;193:129–138.
7. Mogensen CE, Andersen MJ. Increased kidney size and glomerular filtration rate in early juvenile diabetes. Diabetes 1973;22:706–712.
8. Christiansen JS, Gammelgaard J, Frandsen M, Parving HH. Increased kidney size, glomerular filtration rate, and renal plasma flow in short-term insulin-dependent diabetics. Diabetologia 1981;20:451–456.
9. Nelson RG, Tan M, Beck GJ, et al. Changing glomerular filtration with progression from impaired glucose tolerance to type II diabetes mellitus. Diabetologia 1999;42:90–93.
10. Keller CK, Bergis KH, Fliser D, Ritz E. Renal findings in patients with short-term type 2 diabetes. J Am Soc Nephrol 1996;7:2627–2635.
11. Lee KU, Park JY, Hwang IR, et al. Glomerular hyperfiltration in Koreans with non-insulin-dependent diabetes mellitus. Am J Kidney Dis 1995;26:722–726.
12. Dahlquist G, Stattin EL, Rudberg S. Urinary albumin excretion rate and glomerular filtration rate in the prediction of diabetic nephropathy; a long-term follow-up study of childhood onset type-1 diabetic patients. Nephrol Dial Transplant 2001;16:1382–1386.
13. Chiarelli F, Verrotti A, Morgese G. Glomerular hyperfiltration increases the risk of developing microalbuminuria in diabetic children. Pediatr Nephrol 1995;9:154–158.
14. Hostetter TH, Troy JL, Brenner BM. Glomerular hemodynamics in experimental diabetes mellitus. Kidney Int 1981;19:410–415.
15. Brenner BM, Meyer TW, Hostetter TH. Dietary protein intake and the progressive nature of kidney disease: the role of hemodynamically mediated glomerular injury in the pathogenesis of progressive glomerular sclerosis in aging, renal ablation, and intrinsic renal disease. N Engl J Med 1982;307: 652–659.
16. Zatz R, Meyer TW, Rennke HG, Brenner BM. Predominance of hemodynamic rather than metabolic factors in the pathogenesis of diabetic glomerulopathy. Proc Natl Acad Sci USA 1985;82:5863–5867.
17. Tuttle KR, Bruton JL, Perusek MC, Lancaster JL, Kopp DT, DeFronzo RA. Effect of strick glycemic control on renal hemodynamic response to amino acids and renal enlargement in insulin-dependent diabetes mellitus. N Engl J Med 1991;324:1626–1632.
18. Tuttle KR, Bruton JL. Effect of insulin therapy on renal hemodynamic response to amino acids and renal hypertrophy in non-insulin-dependent diabetes. Kidney Int 1992;42:167–173.
19. Giordano M, Castellino P, McConnell EL, DeFronzo RA. Effect of amino acid infusion on renal hemodynamics in humans: a dose-response study. Am J Physiol Renal Fluid Electrolyte Physiol 1994;267:F703–F708.
20. Wada L, Don BR, Schambelan M. Hormonal mediators of amino acid-induced glomerular hyperfiltration in humans. Am J Physiol Renal Fluid Electrolyte Physiol 1991;260:F787–F792.
21. Parving HH, Christiansen JS, Noer I, Tronier B, Mogensen CE. The effect of glucagon on kidney function in short-term insulin-dependent juvenile diabetes. Diabetologia 1980;19:350–354.
22. Parving HH, Noer J, Kehlet H, Mogensen CE, Svendsen PA, Heding L. The effect of short-term glucagon infusion on kidney function in normal man. Diabetologia 1977;13:323–325.
23. Fioretto P, Trevisan R, Valerio A, et al. Impaired renal response to a meat meal in insulin-dependent diabetics: role of glucagon and prostaglandins. Am J Physiol Renal Fluid Electrolyte Physiol 1990;258: F675–F683.
24. Hirschberg RR, Zipser RD, Slomowitz LA, Kopple JD. Glucagon and prostaglandins are mediators of amino acid-induced rise in renal hemodynamics. Kidney Int 1988;33:1147–1155.
25. Krishna GG, Newell G, Miller E, et al. Protein-induced glomerular hyperfiltration: role of hormonal factors. Kidney Int 1988;33:578–583.
26. Vanrenterghem YF, Verberckmoes RK, Roels LM, Michielsen PJ. Role of prostaglandins in protein-induced glomerular hyperfiltration in normal humans. Am J Physiol Renal Fluid Electrolyte Physiol 1988;254:F463–F469.

27. Tuttle KR, Puhlman ME, Cooney SK, Short RA. Effects of amino acids and glucagon on renal hemodynamics in type 1 diabetes. Am J Physiol Renal Physiol 2002;282:F103–F112.
28. Meek RL, Cooney SK, Flynn SD, et al. Amino acids induce indicators of response to injury in glomerular mesangial cells. Am J Physiol Renal Physiol 2003;285:F79–F86.
29. Tuttle KR, Johnson EC, Cooney SK, et al. Amino acids injure mesangial cells by advanced glycation end products, oxidative stress, and protein kinase C. Kidney Int 2005;67:953–968.
30. Vlassara H, Cai W, Crandall J, et al. Inflammatory mediators are induced by dietary glycotoxins, a major risk factor for diabetic angiopathy. Proc Natl Acad Sci USA 2002;99:15,596–15,601.
31. Hanson HP, Tauber-Lassen E, Jensen BR, Parving HH. Effect of dietary protein restriction on prognosis in patients with diabetic nephropathy. Kidney Int 2002;62:220–228.
32. Mogensen CE. Microalbuminuria predicts clinical proteinuria and early mortality in maturity-onset diabetes. N Engl J Med 1984;310:356–360.
33. Dineen SF, Gerstein HC. The association of microalbuminuria and mortality in non-insulin-dependent diabetes mellitus. Arch Intern Med 1997;157:1413–1418.
34. Jensen JS, Feldt-Rasmussen B, Strandgaard S, Schroll M, Borch-Johnsen K. Arterial hypertension, microalbuminuria, and risk of ischemic heart disease. Hypertension 2000;35:898–903.
35. Hillege HL, Fidler V, Diercks GF, et al. Prevention of Renal and Vascular End Stage Disease (PREVEND) Study Group. Urinary albumin excretion predicts cardiovascular and noncardiovascular mortality in general population. Circulation 2002;106:1777–1782.
36. Tuttle KR, Puhlman ME, Cooney SK, Short RA. Urinary albumin and insulin as predictors of coronary artery disease: An angiographic study. Am J Kidney Dis 1999;34:918–925.
37. Gerstein HC, Mann JF, Yi Q, Zinman B, et al. Albuminuria and risk of cardiovascular events, death, and heart failure in diabetic and nondiabetic individuals. JAMA 2001;286:421–426.
38. Miettinen H, Haffner SM, Lehto S, Ronnemaa T, Pyorala K, Laakso M. Proteinuria predicts stroke and other atherosclerotic vascular events in nondiabetic and non-insulin-dependent diabetic subjects. Stroke 1996;27:2033–2039.
39. Valmadrid CT, Klein R, Moss SE, Klein BE. The risk of cardiovascular disease mortality associated with microalbuminuria and gross proteinuria in persons with older-onset diabetes mellitus. Arch Int Med 2000;160:1093–1100.
40. Szczech LA, Best PJ, Crowley E, et al. Brooks MM, Berger PB, Bittner V, Gersh BJ, Jones R, Califf RM, Ting HH, Whitlow PJ, Detre KM, Holmes D, for the Bypass Angioplasty Revascularization Investigation (BARI) Investigators. Outcomes of patients with chronic renal insufficiency in the bypass angioplasty revascularization investigation. Circulation 2002;105:2253–2258.
41. Hostetter TH. Chronic kidney disease predicts cardiovascular disease. N Engl J Med 2004;351: 1344–1345.
42. Jensen JS. Renal and systemic transvascular albumin leakage in severe atherosclerosis. Arterioscler Throm Vasc Biol 1995;15:1324–1329.
43. Clausen P, Jensen JS, Jensen G, Borch-Johnsen, Feldt-Rasmussen B. Elevated urinary albumin excretion is associated with impaired arterial dilatory capacity in clinically healthy subjects. Circulation 2001;103:1869–1874.
44. Tuttle KR. Cardiovascular implications of albuminuria. J Clin Hypertens 2004;6:13–17.
45. de Zeeuw D, Remuzzi G, Parving HH, et al. Albuminuria, a therapeutic target for cardiovascular protection in type 2 diabetic patients with nephropathy. Circulation 2004;110:921–927.
46. de Zeeuw D, Remuzzi G, Parving HH, et al. Proteinuria, a target for renoprotection in patients with type 2 diabetic nephropathy: lessons from RENAAL. Kidney Int 2004;65:2309–2320.

II Clinical Aspects of Diabetic Nephropathy

B. Histopathology and Special Populations

21 The Structure of Human Diabetic Nephropathy

Michael Mauer, MD *and Behzad Najafian,* MD

CONTENTS

INTRODUCTION

This chapter outlines the histopathology of human diabetic nephropathy (DN). The classical structural changes of DN have been well described and demonstrated in general renal and renal pathology textbooks. The emphasis here is on current and evolving studies and concepts in this field. As renal lesions in type 1 diabetes are believed to be more unique to DN and more uniform and as lesions in type 2 diabetes are more heterogeneous and, perhaps, more frequently complicated by renal diseases other than diabetes, this chapter primarily focuses on the structural changes in type 1 diabetes. We will, however, discuss nephropathy of type 2 diabetes and its differences from type 1 diabetes at the end of this chapter.

EVOLUTION OF THE STRUCTURAL CHANGES OF DIABETIC NEPHROPATHY

The sequence of structural changes in DN can be considered along either chronological or functional time scales. The functional alterations are expressed as the evolution of events related to clinical findings such as progression from normoalbuminuria to

From: *Contemporary Diabetes: The Diabetic Kidney*
Edited by: P. Cortes and C. E. Mogensen © Humana Press Inc., Totowa, NJ

microalbuminuria and to proteinuria or from hyperfiltration to progressive glomerular filtration rate (GFR) decline and end-stage renal disease (ESRD). The functional sequence is not always progressive and studies show that patients can regress from microalbuminuria to normoalbuminuria *(1)*. Thus, the consideration of structural changes could be more meaningful if evaluated along with functional alterations. The first structural change that can be quantified by stereological methods is thickening of glomerular basement membrane (GBM) *(2)*. Tubular basement membrane (TBM) thickening develops in parallel to GBM thickening (*see* below) *(3,4)*. Exudative lesions of DN include arteriolar hyalinosis, glomerular capillary subendothelial hyaline accumulation (hyaline caps), and capsular drops (hyaline material between the parietal epithelium and Bowman's capsule). Arteriolar hyalinosis can be seen within 3–5 yr after onset of diabetes or following transplantation of a normal kidney into the diabetic patient *(5)*. Experimental and human studies suggest these lesions may trigger inflammatory cascades through complement fixation *(6)*. Increases in the fractional volume of mesangium per glomerulus [Vv(Mes/glom)] can be documented 4–5 yr after the onset of type 1 diabetes *(2)*. Increased fractional volume of mesangial matrix per glomerulus [Vv(MM/glom)] precedes increased Vv(Mes/glom) and represents the main component of glomerular mesangial expansion in diabetic glomerulopathy *(7)*. The relative contribution of cell number vs cell size to the expansion of the cellular component of the mesangium is currently unknown. Late finding of increased Vv(Mes/glom) compared with GBM thickening can be the result of more interglomerular variability of this parameter among normal subjects *(8)* or nonlinearity of the relationship of mesangial expansion to diabetes duration, with more rapid development after 15 yr of diabetes *(9)*. The fractional volume of interstitium per renal cortex [Vv(Int/cortex)] initially decreases *(10)*. This, perhaps, is owing to hypertrophy of tubules, which make up to 85% or more of the renal cortex and are the main contributor to kidney enlargement in early diabetes, reducing the relative volume of interstitium to the volume of the renal cortex. Initial expansion of cortical interstitium is primarily owing to an increase in its cellular component *(11)*, whereas increased fractional volume of interstitium occupied by extracellular matrix (ECM) fibrillar collagen is measurable only in later stages when GFR has already declined *(11)*. Diffuse diabetic glomerulosclerosis is defined as widespread mesangial expansion within and among glomeruli, whereas nodular glomerulosclerosis (Kimmelstiel-Wilson [K-W] nodules) represents marked segmental expansion of mesangium appearing as round fibrillar nodules, with palisading of mesangial nuclei around the periphery often surrounded by compressed appearing capillary loops. Glomerular capillary wall detachment from mesangial anchoring points (mesangiolysis), leading to microaneurysm formation *(12,13)* (*see* also glomerulotubular junction abnormalities) has been proposed as underlying mechanism of these lesions. Generally, K-W nodules are primarily restricted to proteinuric patients with established diabetic glomerulopathy. However, occasional findings of nodular lesions in some patients with little or no diffuse mesangial expansion or albuminuria suggests that these two forms of diabetic mesangial expansion may, at least in part, have different pathogenesis.

The accumulation of different ECM components of mesangium, GBM, and TBM in DN does not occur proportionally. For instance, densities of α_3 and α_4 chains of type-IV collagen increase in the GBM, whereas those of α_1 and α_2 chains decrease in the mesangium and the subendothelial space of patients with DN *(14,15)*. Quantitative immunogold electron microscopic studies have shown that densities of types-IV *(15)* and -VI collagen *(16)* were decreased in the mesangial matrix of patients with advanced mesangial expansion. However, given the marked increased amount of Vv(MM/glom), the absolute amount of these components per glomerulus was increased. Progression of DN toward renal insufficiency is accompanied by progressive global glomerulosclerosis. Expression of scar collagen can be found in globally sclerosed glomeruli or in advanced nodular glomerulosclerosis *(14,17)*. Globally sclerosed glomeruli are more often than by chance oriented in the plane vertical to the renal capsule in diabetic patients, suggesting a vaso-occlusive pathophysiology *(18)*. Moreover, more severe arteriolar hyalinosis is associated with increased number of globally sclerosed glomeruli *(19)*. Mesangial expansion and global glomerular sclerosis are correlated in type 1 diabetic patients *(19,20)*, whereas heterogeneity of renal lesions in type 2 diabetes may disturb this correlation.

PODOCYTE CHANGES IN DIABETIC NEPHROPATHY

Podocyte injury is putatively the main culprit in many progressive glomerulopathies *(21)* including DN. Using conventional methods, perhaps, the first recognizable podocyte alteration in DN is foot process effacement.

It is known that foot process effacement is accompanied by excess filtration of protein in ultrafiltrate. However, this may not be detectable in the terminal urine until the capacity of tubular protein reabsorption is surpassed. Foot processes are interconnected by slit diaphragm complexes, creating a zipper-like structure, which is thought to act as a sieve restricting the loss of large molecules into the urinary space. Nephrinuria can be detected in 30% of normoalbuminuric type 1 diabetic patients, suggesting early damage to the slit diaphragm *(22)*. Foot process effacement is equivalent to reduced length density of slit diaphragms per GBM surface [Lv(SD/GBM)]. Consequently, reduced density of profiles of slit diaphragms would be seen on two-dimensional images of transmission electron microscope along the cross-section of GBM whenever foot process width is increased. This observation by many investigators has been expressed as reduced number of slits per GBM length, ignoring the fact that GBM is a complex three-dimensional structure, which is better characterized as a surface than a length. More disconcerting, a reduction in slit diaphragm length has been interpreted as reduced expression of components within the slit diaphragm rather than a decrease in the availability of the structure where these components reside. This critique is particularly applicable to reduced immunostainings for these molecules unless their quantitation is expressed in relationship to the available slit diaphragm structure.

Podocyte Number vs Number Density

Podocyte damage, if severe enough, leads to podocyte loss. Increased urinary excretion of podocytes has been detected in microalbuminuric and proteinuric type 2 diabetic patients *(23)*. There has been a debate concerning whether reduction in podocyte number or reduction in podocyte number density is a better correlate or predictor of renal dysfunction in DN *(24–27)*. Studies of Pima Indian patients with type 2 diabetes showed marked reduction in both the number [N(PC/glom)] and the number density of podocytes per glomerulus [Nv(PC/glom)] in patients with clinical proteinuria compared with normal controls and subjects with early diabetes *(24)*. These studies used the Weibel-Gomez method for enumerating podocytes *(28)*, which necessarily makes assumptions regarding podocyte nuclear shape, size and distribution, rendering the method vulnerable to bias. Steffes et al. *(29)*, using the same method, obtained comparable results in type 1 diabetic patients. Dalla Vestra et al. *(27)* (same method) showed both N(PC/glom) and Nv(PC/glom) decreased in type 2 diabetic patients with microalbuminuria or proteinuria *(27)*. However, only Nv(PC/glom) correlated with albumin excretion rate (AER), suggesting that this parameter was of greater functional importance. White et al. *(30)* obtained comparable results in type 2 diabetic patients using the disector/fractionator method, which is an unbiased method with no size or shape assumptions *(30)*. Both N(PC/glom) and Nv(PC/glom) correlated with proteinuria in their study. On the other hand, the same group found no difference in N(PC/glom) in type 1 diabetic patients with clinical proteinuria compared with normal controls and in N(PC/glom) in baseline compared with 3-yr follow-up biopsies *(26)*. However, Nv(PC/glom) was less in diabetic patients (secondary to increased glomerular volume) compared with control subjects and negatively correlated with AER in proteinuric patients. No difference was found in GBM surface area between proteinuric diabetic patients and normal subjects, implying that decreased Nv(PC/glom) was not accompanied by increased surface to be covered by podocytes. Uncovering changes in N(PC/glom) and Nv(PC/glom) in diabetes in longitudinal studies is presumably more difficult than comparison of normal subjects with diabetic patients. In the former, the differences among the groups may not be large enough to be demonstrated by any reasonably practical methodology. In other words, more precise and standardized methods may be required to obtain reproducible results. In this regard, we prefer the disector/fractionator method. However, another potentially confounding variable is that precise cell identification by location becomes increasingly difficult as diabetic glomerulopathy advances, especially when examined by light microscopy. Electron microscopy or immunohistochemistry may be needed in those situations. Obviously, more studies are required to illuminate numerical podocyte changes during the natural history of diabetic nephropathy.

Podocyte Detachment From GBM

Detachment of podocytes has been reported in glomerulopathies with severe podocyte damage. We have documented obvious and substantial podocyte foot process detachment from GBM in proteinuric type 1 diabetic patients *(31)*. We also found that a small but measurable fraction of GBM is denuded of podocyte foot processes in normoalbuminuric and microalbuminuric longstanding type 1 diabetic patients. Podocyte foot process detachment correlates inversely with GFR and directly with AER. Podocyte detachment is known to be associated with tuft to Bowman's capsule adhesions (TBCA) *(32)*, a finding that is frequent in proteinuric type 1 diabetic patients *(33)*. Also, denuded areas of GBM may explain nonselective (shunt) permeability defects in proteinuric diabetic patients *(34)*. However, this detachment process was not seen in a small cohort of patients with steroid resistant nephrotic syndrome who later developed focal segmental glomerulosclerosis (Lee HS et al., unpublished observations), thus ruling out proteinuria *per se* as a sufficient cause of this phenomenon.

GLOMERULAR ARTERIOLES AND THE JUXTAGLOMERULAR APPARATUS

Hyalinosis of both afferent and efferent arterioles, defined by the replacement of the smooth muscle cells of arteriolar walls by homogeneous, transluscent appearing periodic acid-Shiff positive material consisting of immunoglobins, complement, fibrinogen, albumin, and other plasma proteins *(35,36)* is fairly specific for DN. Exceptions include cyanotic congenital heart disease and cystic fibrosis (CF), conditions not readily confused with diabetes, except for CF patients with both conditions. This finding must be differentiated from hypertensive arteriolosclerosis, in which hyalinosis only affects the afferent arteriole. Arteriolar hyalinosis secondary to calcineurin inhibitors may also be indistinguishable from diabetic changes *(37)*. Østerby et al. *(38)* showed that matrix volume fraction is increased in afferent and efferent arterioles of microalbuminuric type 1 diabetic patients and this increase correlates with the extent of glomerulopathy, suggesting a common pathophysiology. Østerby also demonstrated enlargement of the glomerular vascular pole area and the presence of more than one efferent arteriole also were shown in type 1 diabetic patients *(39)*. The pathophysiology and significance of these findings are unclear.

Paulsen et al. found that the juxtaglomerular apparatus (JGA) may manifest different abnormalities such as hypertrophy or sclerosis independent of the severity of glomerulopathy in type 1 diabetic patients *(40)*. The same study reported the frequent finding of T-lymphocytes in JGA of diabetic patients, suggestive of a process representing the polyendocrinopathy often seen in type 1 diabetic patients. The latter finding was confirmed in our laboratory and was shown to occur primarily in the earlier years of type 1 diabetes and was associated with larger glomeruli and greater filtration surface, this perhaps supporting Paulsen's hypothesis that autoimmune JGA injury could be protective of DN *(41)*.

STRUCTURAL–FUNCTIONAL RELATIONSHIPS IN DIABETIC NEPHROPATHY

Mesangial expansion is the major hallmark of nephropathy in type 1 diabetic patients *(42)* and is, more or less, related to all other renal structural or functional alterations of the disease. Increased Vv(Mes/glom) closely correlates with a decrease in peripheral GBM filtration surface density [Sv(PGBM/glom)]. On the other hand, total filtration surface per glomerulus [S(PGBM/glom)] is highly correlated with GFR across the spectrum from hyperfiltration to renal insufficiency in type 1 diabetes *(42–45)*. Vv(Mes/glom) is also related to the AER *(42,46)* and high blood pressure *(20,42)*. Similarly, but less strongly than for Vv(Mes/glom), GBM width is directly correlated with blood pressure and AER and inversely correlated with GFR *(42,46)*. In fact, the rate of development of mesangial expansion and GBM thickening varies among patients *(42,46)*. For example, relatively marked GBM thickening can be seen without remarkable mesangial expansion and vice versa, preventing a precise correlation between these parameters *(42,47)*. Considering both Vv(Mes/glom) and GBM width as predictor variables, and using multiple regression analyses these structural variables explain 59% of the variability in AER in type 1 diabetic patients, with AER ranging from normoalbuminuria to proteinuria *(46)*.

Percent global glomerulosclerosis *(19)* and interstitial expansion *(48)* along with glomerular structural changes are correlated with deterioration of renal function in type 1 diabetic patients with a wide spectrum of AER and GFR. However, sequential renal biopsies of normoalbuminuric and microalbuminuric patients showed that the increase in AER correlated with the increase in Vv(Mes/glom), whereas the Vv(Int/cortex) did not change during the 5-yr interval of the study *(49)*. This suggests that the correlation of Vv(Int/cortex) with renal function may be in great part driven by the more advanced cases. In general, it appears that during most of the natural history of DN glomerular structural parameters are more important determinants of renal dysfunction, whereas Vv(Int/cortex) is a stronger determinant of the rate of progression from moderate to severe renal insufficiency *(50)*.

The average GBM width and Vv(Mes/glom) is increased in normoalbuminuric patients with long-standing (20 yr) type 1 diabetes *(46,51)*. However, individual values of these parameter within this group vary from the normal range to increased values that overlap those of patients with microalbuminuria and proteinuria *(46,51)*. Although GBM width and Vv(Mes/glom) in patients with microalbuminuria are rarely in the normal range, overlap with values observed in normoalbuminuric (and proteinuric) patients exists *(46,51)*. Studies of identical twin pairs discordant for type 1 diabetes showed, in every pair studied, that the diabetic twin had higher values for GBM and TBM width and Vv(Mes/glom) than the nondiabetic sibling, even if values for GBM width and Vv(Mes/glom) of the diabetic twin were within the normal range *(3)*.These studies suggested that the metabolic abnormalities of diabetes are necessary for the development of glomerular abnormalities and that all type 1 diabetic patients develop diabetic glomerulopathy changes, albeit, some so slowly that their structural measures remain in the normal range despite many years of diabetes. Unpublished analyses of data from these same studies showed that glomerular structural parameters of the nondiabetic twins did not predict the rate of development of diabetic glomerulopathy lesions in the diabetic twins, indicating that genetic or environmental determinants of variability in these structural parameters before the onset of diabetes do not represent risk factors for DN.

Volume and number of glomeruli are shown to be related to nephropathy risk. Mean glomerular volumes were higher in type 1 diabetic patients developing DN after 25 yr of diabetes compared with a group that developed nephropathy after only 15 yr *(52)*. This study suggested that glomerular size or the capacity for glomerular expansion may determine the rate of progressive deterioration of renal function in patients who develop DN. The number of glomeruli per kidney varies widely among normal individuals *(53)*. The number of glomeruli were reportedly not different among type 1 and 2 diabetic patients with proteinuria but without advanced renal insufficiency and nondiabetic patients *(54)*. This study showed that a subgroup of type 1 diabetic patients with severe renal dysfunction had less glomeruli compared with patients with mild or no glomerulopathy. This could be owing either to resorption of sclerotic glomeruli *(54)* or to greater susceptibility to glomerulopathy in patients with fewer glomeruli. However, the proteinuric type 1 diabetic patients in this study without advanced renal insufficiency had glomerular number no different from normal. This is concordant with the former hypothesis. Moreover, the rate of development of diabetic glomerulopathy lesions in type 1 diabetic patients with a single transplanted kidney is not different from native (two) kidneys of type 1 diabetic patients with duration of diabetes matched with the time after transplantation in the one kidney patients (Chang S, personal communication). These studies imply that reduced number of glomeruli does not accelerate the early lesions of diabetic glomerulopathy. Reduced number of glomeruli, however, could speed the rate of progression to ESRD in established DN.

TUFT TO BOWMAN'S CAPSULE ADHESIONS

TBCA are rare findings in normoalbuminuric and microalbuminuric type 1 diabetic patients *(55)*. TBCA are frequent in proteinuric patients, and show marked predilection for the area of the glomerulotubular junction *(56)*, (equivalent to tip lesions). These

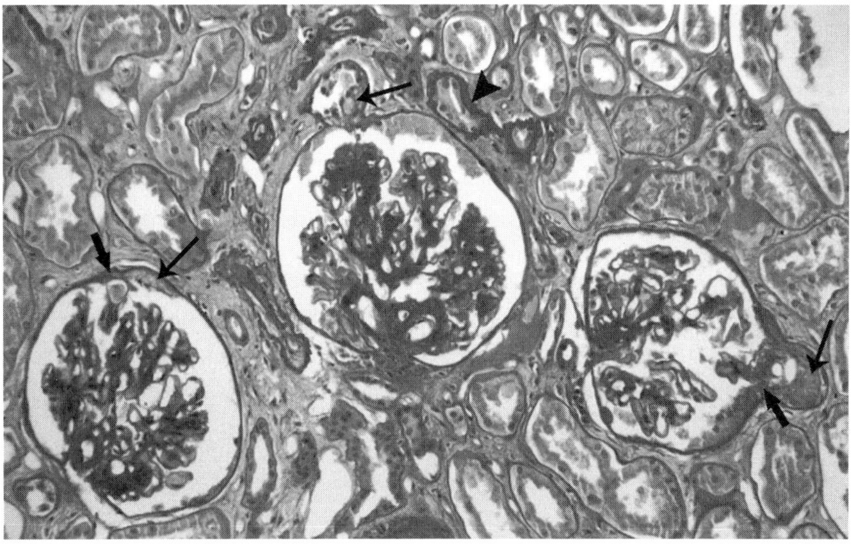

Fig. 1. Three glomeruli with tuft to Bowman's capsule adhesions (bold arrows) and glomerulotubular junction abnormalities (the middle and right glomeruli) from a proteinuric type 1 diabetic patient. Presumed paraglomerular filtration (thin arrows) resulting in reduplicated Bowman's capsule and tubular basement membranes. An atrophic tubule with flat epithelial cells is connected to the middle glomerulus. Atrophic tubular profiles with thick, wrinkled basement membranes (arrowhead) surrounding this glomerulus may be cross-sections of the same atrophic tubule, thus representing nephrocentric tubular atrophy.

lesions are composed of TBCA and dilated capillary loops, frequently filled with foam cells and, often, tuft collapse. Advanced lesions are associated with segmental sclerosis and the dilated capillary loops may be replaced by K-W nodules. The association of both microaneurysms and K-W nodules with tip lesions in type 1 diabetic patients is in accordance with the hypothesis that mesangiolysis is a precursor lesion of K-W nodules *(16)*. However, the absence of K-W nodules in nondiabetic renal diseases with either tip lesions or microaneurysms suggests that additional specifically diabetic pathogenetic variables are necessary for K-W nodules to develop. Glomerular tuft prolapse into the very proximal segment of the proximal tubule was suggested as a precursor of tip lesions *(57)*. However, this phenomenon is rarely, if ever, present in DN. Moreover, most adhesions in type 1 diabetic patients were shown to be localized in a zone comprising the one-sixth of the Bowman's capsule inner surface that is adjacent to (rather than at) the glomerulotubular junction, or prolapsing into the proximal tubular lumen *(56)*. Our observations show that tip lesions in DN are associated with proximal tubular atrophy and contribute to renal function impairment in proteinuric patients. Hence, the suggestion of a less dire prognosis in patients with tip lesions and focal segmental glomerulosclerosis may not be applicable to DN. Diffuse podocyte damage, perhaps as a prerequisite for TBCA is present in established DN (*see* "Podocyte Changes in Diabetic Nephropathy" section). Once TBCA develops, the aberrant filtration through Bowman's capsule (paraglomerular filtration) is thought to advance around the Bowman's capsule, toward the proximal portion of the proximal tubule leading to progressive nephrocentric tubular atrophy and nephron loss (Fig. 1) *(58)*. TBCA in DN is, in fact, frequently accompanied by Bowman's capsule thickening and/or reduplication at the adhesion site. The space formed between the two layers of Bowman's capsule basement membrane extends toward and beyond the glomerulotubular junction, mimicking a progressive dissecting process with a sharp cut-off point. The normal proximal tubular epithelial cells of the segment proximal to this cut-off point are invariably associated with flat epithelial cells. There is usually a sharp transition from flat cells to normal appearing proximal tubular epithelial cells with brush borders (distal to the cut-off point). However, some glomeruli with tip lesions are attached to long atrophic tubules covered with cuboidal cells with no discernible brush borders and thickened but not reduplicated TBMs. The surface of glomerular capillary loops of tip lesions is frequently populated with flat cells with dark nuclei and small cytoplasm with no resemblance to podocytes. These cells are continuous with the flat cells covering Bowman's capsule basement membrane and the atrophic segment of the proximal tubule. To our knowledge, there is no study revealing the origin of these cells. Howie et al. *(59)* showed that the flat cells covering the atrophic segment of the proximal tubules are epithelial membrane antigen (EMA)-positive, suggestive of a possible origin from the EMA-positive cells normally present as a necklace at the glomerulotubular junction. The frequent finding of Bowman's capsule reduplication and TBCA at the opposite side of the vascular pole of atubular glomeruli in proteinuric type 1 diabetic patients is in accordance with the hypothesis that TBCA, and specially tip lesions, can lead to progressive tubular atrophy and atubular glomeruli. Our studies show that only 32% of glomeruli in proteinuric type 1 diabetic patients have normal glomerulotubular junctions and 17% of these glomeruli are atubular *(33)*. We hypothesize that appearance of TBCA with the advent of proteinuria in type 1 diabetic patients reflects the beginning of a new phase in the natural history of DN, characterized by accentuation of glomerulosclerosis, tubular atrophy, interstitial expansion leading, ultimately, to progressive renal function loss and chronic renal failure. This association with overt proteinuria could explain why proteinuria typically ushers in a phase of progressive GFR loss in diabetes and why therapies that reduce proteinuria could slow this decline toward ESRD.

TUBULES

TBM thickening is an early abnormality in type 1 diabetes that parallels GBM thickening and can be detected in normoalbuminuric patients using stereological methods *(4)*. TBM width correlates with GBM width and Vv(Mes/glom) and more specifically with Vv(MM/glom), consistent with the idea that the TBM changes are part of a broad accumulation of basement membrane ECM material in the diabetic kidney *(8)* and arguing against the hypothesis that glomerular hemodynamic abnormalities are causally related to the development of the early lesions of diabetic glomerulopathy *(60)*. This accumulation of ECM material can be owing to increased matrix production, decreased matrix removal (suggested by increased expression of Plasminogen active inhibitor-1 [PAI-1] in glomeruli of diabetic patients *[61]* or both). Both nephrocenteric and diffuse tubular atrophy can be seen in DN. Nephrocentric tubular atrophy usually precedes appearance of diffuse tubular atrophy. As mentioned above, nephrocentric tubular atrophy is initiated by TBCA, mostly involves proximal tubules and manifests as focal profiles of atrophic tubules around segmentally or globally sclerosed glomeruli (Fig. 1). Interstitial expansion is accentuated around these atrophic tubules and is often accompanied by lymphocytic infiltration. Our observations, based on serial sectioning studies of atrophic tubules attached to glomeruli with glomerulotubular junction abnormalities, indicates that the atrophic segment of these tubules is covered by flat cells, overlying a basement membrane that is detached from an outer TBM. The space between these two layers of TBM is filled with an amorphous material, which proximally is continuous with the space between the layers of reduplicated Bowman's capsule associated with TBCA *(33)*. Transition of this atrophic segment to a normal-appearing tubule is usually abrupt and happens at the point where the two layers of reduplicated TBM fuse together. We hypothesize that paraglomerular filtration originating from TBCA infiltrates into the Bowman's capsule and TBM and dissects them into two layers or results in the production of a second layer. This process, if it progresses distally, could lead to progressive nephrocentric tubular atrophy and/or detachment of the atrophic tubule from glomerulotubular junction and development of atubular glomeruli, and thus contributes to GFR loss in proteinuric patients.

COMPARISON OF TYPE 1 AND 2 DIABETES

Although more than 80% of diabetic ESRD patients have type 2 diabetes, renal pathology and structural–functional relationships have been less well studied in type 2 diabetic patients. Although, several reports indicate a high incidence of nondiabetic renal lesions in type 2 diabetic patients, this may represent selection bias toward biopsy of atypical cases, as the frequency of finding other diseases, in substantial measure, reflects local institutional biopsy policies and criteria *(62)*. In fact, when biopsies in type 2 diabetic patients are done only for research purposes, the frequency of changes diagnostic of other conditions is low (Fioretto P, personal communication). Moreover, an autopsy study of type 2 diabetic patients did not confirm a high incidence of nondiabetic glomerulopathies in proteinuric cases, arguing against the findings of aforementioned studies *(63)*. Most studies of type 2 diabetic patients show that renal lesions are more heterogeneous in comparison with those in type 1 diabetes *(64)*. A study of microalbuminuric type 2 diabetic patients showed that only one-third of patients had changes typical of DN in type 1 diabetes, including glomerular hypertrophy, mesangial expansion, and arteriolar hyalinosis. Despite persistent microalbuminuria, 30% of patients had normal or near normal renal structures and the remaining 40% showed atypical patterns of renal injury with absent or mild diabetic glomerulopathy, associated with severe tubulo-interstitial lesions and/or arteriolar hyalinosis and global glomerulosclerosis, whereas nonsclerosed glomeruli showed only mild diabetic changes *(65)*. Østerby et al. *(66)* found that in Caucasian type 2 diabetic patients with proteinuria, all the glomerular structural parameters were on average abnormal, although some patients had glomerular structure within the normal range. In contrast, these parameters were always severely altered in type 1 diabetic patients with overt nephropathy. In general, it appears that in type 1 diabetes the most dominant structural changes are those of diabetic glomerulopathy, whereas a substantial proportion of type 2 diabetic patients have global glomerulosclerosis, and tubulo-interstitial and vascular injury out of proportion to diabetic glomerulopathy.

PREVENTION AND REVERSAL OF DIABETIC NEPHROPATHY LESIONS

Although prevention of DN lesions in animal models with insulin treatment or reversal of lesions with islet transplantation was known from earlier studies *(67–69)*, reversibility of lesions in human had been more challenging to document. Diabetic patients who have received renal allografts develop DN lesions at rates similar to those in diabetic patients with native kidneys *(58,70)*. On the other hand, intensive treatment of hyperglycemia not only reduces incidence of microalbuminuria in type 1 diabetic patients *(71)*, but also reduces GBM thickening *(72)*, and, in patients who have renal allografts, results in less accumulation of mesangial matrix *(73)*. Pancreas transplantation 2–4 yr after renal transplantation is associated 4–6 yr later with less mesangial expansion than after kidney transplantation alone *(74)*. Simultaneous kidney/pancreas transplantation prevents DN lesions *(75)*. We documented that although DN lesions do not change 5 yr after pancreas transplantation *(76)*, significant improvement or preventing diabetic glomerulopathy lesions including reduction in the thickness of GBM and TBM and mesangial matrix, disappearance of K-W nodular lesions representing substantial remodeling of the glomerular architecture, was seen 10 yr after pancreas transplantation alone *(77)*. Possible explanations for this delayed healing could be relative insusceptibility of heavily glycosylated and cross-linked ECM molecules to degradation *(78)* or phenotypical alterations in renal cells that persists despite the return of normoglycemia (cellular memory) *(79)*. The rate of development of DN in transplanted kidneys is highly variable and is only partially explained by differences in glycemic control in the postransplant period. This argues for the importance of genetic variability in tissue responses on exposure to hyperglycemia *(70)*. Our preliminary observations that the in vitro behavior of skin fibroblasts of kidney transplant donors is predictive of the rate of development of GBM thickening in type 1 diabetic kidney transplant recipients is in accordance with this hypothesis (unpublished data).

KIDNEY BIOPSY AND NEW DIRECTIONS OF TECHNOLOGY

Animal models have expanded our understanding of DN. However, undeniable differences between the natural history and characteristics of human and animal DN make it difficult to simply extrapolate this knowledge to humans. On the other hand, a major limitation for studying human diabetic renal disease is that current clinical practice usually does not require biopsy for diagnosis or as a guide for management except for atypical situations, in which DN is often complicated by another condition and therefore, the sample would not be representative of the disease. Thanks to advancing technologies the yield of information obtainable from a kidney biopsy can be far beyond the traditional routine examinations. Immunohistochemical stainings either on paraffin embedded or frozen tissues, immunogold electron microscopy and *in situ* hibridization techniques have provided valuable information about expression and trafficking of molecules. Unbiased stereological methods, using reproducible nonsubjective methods, have been answering questions on structural alterations from GBM width changes to number of podocytes and glomeruli. Availability of high throughput molecular diagnostics, such as DNA, protein and tissue microarrays on specimens obtained by kidney biopsy could allow monitoring of thousands of genes or proteins in a single experiment *(80)*. However, interpretation of these tests may be difficult owing to pathology related tissue heterogeneity in the cellular makeup of biopsy materials. Thus, established DN is often associated with altered cellular composition of the renal cortex. For example, increased number of lymphocytes in interstitium or fibroblasts populating sclerosed glomeruli, are common findings. Interpretation of gene–protein expressions without considering these compositional changes could be rather misleading. Laser capture microdissection may provide more precise sampling of structural components, and is applicable to archived materials. Yet, exact isolation of components of complex structures such as gloemruli is currently not possible. Moreover, the quality and quantity of mRNA obtained in fixed tissues might be less than adequate. Viable cells obtained from renal biopsies can be cultured and used for in vitro studies. One advantage of these in vitro studies is that activities of cells with different genomic contents can be evaluated in a well-controlled in vitro environment. On the other hand, living in a different environment (high glucose concentration in diabetic patients) for a long time may impose long-lasting effects on cells even if they are cultured through several in vitro passages (memory phenomenon). Analysis of cell turnover, cell–ECM interactions, cellular metabolism, and signal transduction pathways in diabetic milieu, cell–cell interaction and cellular response to mechanical forces are other possibilities of in vitro studies. Having said all this, and despite the inherent challenges of every method, there is enormous potential for studies that can be generated by using the material obtained through kidney biopsies. Moreover, as we have argued above, the processes of DN genesis and progression may be markedly different. Studying the kidney at the early preclinical stages necessitates research biopsies. Efforts to correlate these early structural findings with potential predictive biomarkers of pathobiological significances are clearly important. Studies of serum, plasma, renal and other cells, urine, DNA, and so on, together with careful renal structural measures at various stages in the evolution of nephropathy in type 1 and 2 diabetes will undoubtedly yield clinical and basic research advances. Finally, the goal of studies of primary prevention of diabetic renal disease, given the extremely long time from normoalbuminuria to currently accepted hard renal disease end points, could be met by using renal structural progression as important study end point. Otherwise primary prevention trial would be of impractical length, or forced to use end points, which may be imprecise surrogates of serious risk. It is not unreasonable to assume that therapies that substantially slow the earliest lesions of DN will delay or prevent the ultimate clinical expression of the disease, making renal structure, alone or combined with early functional changes, a useful marker of progression. Renal biopsy clinical trials, coupled with the application of the new tools for tissue studies outlined above, could facilitate progress in this field.

CONCLUSIONS

Accumulation of extracellular basement membrane matrix material is the hallmark of structural changes in DN. Glomerular and TBM thickenings, increased glomerular mesangium, decreased glomerular filtration surface density, glomerular and arteriolar exudative lesions, and K-W nodules are classical structural findings of DN. Podocyte damage and loss may also contribute to renal functional impairment. TBCAs, glomerulotubular junction abnormalities and atubular glomeruli are frequent findings in proteinuric type 1 diabetic patients and are rare or absent in normoalbuminuric and microalbuminuric patients. Progression of human diabetic nephropathy lesions is, at least partially, preventable with strict control of glycemia and reversible with long-term normoglycemia induced by pancreas transplantation. Structural changes of nephropathy in type 2 diabetic patients are more heterogeneous and arteriolosclerosis, global glomerulosclerosis, interstitial fibrosis, and tubular atrophy may be found in the absence of significant diabetic glomerulopathy.

REFERENCES

1. Perkins BA, Ficociello LH, Silva KH, Finkelstein DM, Warram JH, Krolewski AS. Regression of microalbuminuria in type 1 diabetes. N Engl J Med 2003;348:2285–2293.
2. Østerby R. Early phases in the development of diabetic glomerulopathy. Acta Med Scand Suppl 1974;574:3–82.

3. Steffes MW, Sutherland DE, Goetz FC, Rich SS, Mauer SM. Studies of kidney and muscle biopsy specimens from identical twins discordant for type I diabetes mellitus. N Engl J Med 1985;312: 1282–1287.
4. Brito PL, Fioretto P, Drummond K, et al. Proximal tubular basement membrane width in insulin-dependent diabetes mellitus. Kidney Int 1998;53:754–761.
5. Mauer SM, Barbosa J, Vernier RL, et al. Development of diabetic vascular lesions in normal kidneys transplanted into patients with diabetes mellitus. N Engl J Med 1976;295:916–920.
6. Burkholder PM. Immunohistopathologic study of localized plasma proteins and fixation of guinea pig complement in renal lesions of diabetic glomerulosclerosis. Diabetes 1965;14:755–770.
7. Steffes MW, Bilous RW, Sutherland DE, Mauer SM. Cell and matrix components of the glomerular mesangium in type I diabetes. Diabetes 1992;41:679–684.
8. Steffes MW, Barbosa J, Basgen JM, Sutherland DE, Najarian JS, Mauer SM. Quantitative glomerular morphology of the normal human kidney. Lab Invest 1983;49:82–86.
9. Drummond KN, Kramer MS, Suissa S, et al. International diabetic nephropathy study group. Effects of duration and age at onset of type 1 diabetes on preclinical manifestations of nephropathy. Diabetes 2003;52:1818–1824.
10. Drummond K, Mauer M. International diabetic nephropathy study group. The early natural history of nephropathy in type 1 diabetes: II. Early renal structural changes in type 1 diabetes. Diabetes 2002;51:1580–1587.
11. Katz A, Caramori ML, Sisson-Ross S, Groppoli T, Basgen JM, Mauer M. An increase in the cell component of the cortical interstitium antedates interstitial fibrosis in type 1 diabetic patients. Kidney Int 2002;61:2058–2066.
12. Stout LC, Kumar S, Whorton EB. Focal mesangiolysis and the pathogenesis of the Kimmelstiel-Wilson nodule. Hum Pathol 1993;24:77–89.
13. Saito Y, Kida H, Takeda S, et al. Mesangiolysis in diabetic glomeruli: its role in the formation of nodular lesions. Kidney Int 1988;34:389–396.
14. Kim Y, Kleppel MM, Butkowski R, Mauer SM, Wieslander J, Michael AF. Differential expression of basement membrane collagen chains in diabetic nephropathy. Am J Pathol 1991;138:413–420.
15. Zhu D, Kim Y, Steffes MW, Groppoli TJ, Butkowski RJ, Mauer SM. Glomerular distribution of type IV collagen in diabetes by high resolution quantitative immunochemistry. Kidney Int 1994;45:425–433.
16. Moriya T, Groppoli TJ, Kim Y, Mauer M. Quantitative immunoelectron microscopy of type VI collagen in glomeruli in type I diabetic patients. Kidney Int 2001;59:317–323.
17. Falk RJ, Scheinman JI, Mauer SM, Michael AF. Polyantigenic expansion of basement membrane constituents in diabetic nephropathy. Diabetes 1983;32(2):34–39.
18. Hørlyck A, Gundersen HJ, Østerby R. The cortical distribution pattern of diabetic glomerulopathy. Diabetologia 1986;29:146–150.
19. Harris RD, Steffes MW, Bilous RW, Sutherland DE, Mauer SM. Global glomerular sclerosis and glomerular arteriolar hyalinosis in insulin dependent diabetes. Kidney Int 1991;40:107–114.
20. Mauer SM, Sutherland DE, Steffes MW. Relationship of systemic blood pressure to nephropathology in insulin-dependent diabetes mellitus. Kidney Int 1992;41:736–740.
21. Kriz W, Gretz N, Lemley KV. Progression of glomerular diseases: is the podocyte the culprit? Kidney Int 1998;54:687–697.
22. Pätäri A, Forsblom C, Havana M, Taipale H, Groop PH, Holthofer H. Nephrinuria in diabetic nephropathy of type 1 diabetes. Diabetes 2003;52:2969–2974.
23. Nakamura T, Ushiyama C, Suzuki S, et al. Urinary excretion of podocytes in patients with diabetic nephropathy. Nephrol Dial Transplant 2000;15:1379–1383.
24. Pagtalunan ME, Miller PL, Jumping-Eagle S, et al. Podocyte loss and progressive glomerular injury in type II diabetes. J Clin Invest 1997;99:342–348.
25. Meyer TW, Bennett PH, Nelson RG. Podocyte number predicts long-term urinary albumin excretion in Pima Indians with type II diabetes and microalbuminuria. Diabetologia 1999;42:1341–1344.
26. White KE, Bilous RW, Marshall SM, et al. Podocyte number in normotensive type 1 diabetic patients with albuminuria. Diabetes 2002;51:3083–3089.
27. Dalla Vestra M, Masiero A, Roiter AM, Saller A, Crepaldi G, Fioretto P. Is podocyte injury relevant in diabetic nephropathy? Studies in patients with type 2 diabetes. Diabetes 2003;52:1031–1035.
28. Weibel ER, Gomez DM. A principle for counting tissue structures on random sections. J Appl Physiol 1962;17:343–348.
29. Steffes MW, Schmidt D, McCrery R, Basgen JM. International diabetic nephropathy study group. Glomerular cell number in normal subjects and in type 1 diabetic patients. Kidney Int 2001;59: 2104–2113.

30. White KE, Bilous RW. Diabiopsies study group. Structural alterations to the podocyte are related to proteinuria in type 2 diabetic patients. Nephrol Dial Transplant 2004;19:1437–1440.
31. Toyoda M, Najafian B, Groppoli T, Basgen J, Kim Y, Mauer M. Problems in the measurement of podocyte structural parameters in proteinuric type 1 diabetic patients. J Am Soc Nephrol 2003;14:597A.
32. Kriz W, LeHir M. Pathways to nephron loss starting from glomerular diseases-insights from animal models. Kidney Int 2005;67:404–419.
33. Najafian B, Kim Y, Crosson JT, Mauer M. Atubular glomeruli and glomerulotubular junction abnormalities in diabetic nephropathy. J Am Soc Nephrol 2003;14:908–917.
34. Tomlanovich S, Deen WM, Jones HW 3rd, Schwartz HC, Myers BD. Functional nature of glomerular injury in progressive diabetic glomerulopathy. Diabetes 1987;36:556–565.
35. Brown DM, Mauer SM. Diabetes Mellitus. In: Pediatric Nephrology. Holliday M, Barrat M, Vernier RL (eds.), Baltimore: Williams & Wilkins, 1987, pp. 513–519.
36. Mauer SM, Miller K, Goetz FC, et al. Immunopathology of renal extracellular membranes in kidneys transplanted into patients with diabetes mellitus. Diabetes 1976;25:709–712.
37. Fioretto P, Steffes MW, Mihatsch MJ, Strom EH, Sutherland DE, Mauer M. Cyclosporine associated lesions in native kidneys of diabetic pancreas transplant recipients. Kidney Int 1995;48:489–495.
38. Østerby R, Hartmann A, Bangstad HJ. Structural changes in renal arterioles in Type I diabetic patients. Diabetologia 2002;45:542–549.
39. Østerby R, Hartmann A, Nyengaard JR, Bangstad HJ. Development of renal structural lesions in type 1 diabetic patients with microalbuminuria. Observations by light microscopy in 8-year follow-up biopsies. Virchows Arch 2002;440:94–101.
40. Paulsen EP, Burke BA, Vernier RL, Mallare MJ, Innes DJ Jr, Sturgill BC. Juxtaglomerular body abnormalities in youth-onset diabetic subjects. Kidney Int 1994;45:1132–1139.
41. Moriya R, Manivel JC, Mauer M. Juxtaglomerular apparatus T-cell infiltration affects glomerular structure in Type 1 diabetic patients. Diabetologia 2004;47:82–88.
42. Mauer SM, Steffes MW, Ellis EN, Sutherland DE, Brown DM, Goetz FC. Structural-functional relationships in diabetic nephropathy. J Clin Invest 1984;74:1143–1155.
43. Ellis EN, Steffes MW, Goetz FC, Sutherland DE, Mauer SM. Glomerular filtration surface in type I diabetes mellitus. Kidney Int 1986;29:889–894.
44. Østerby R, Gundersen HJ, Nyberg G, Aurell M. Advanced diabetic glomerulopathy. Quantitative structural characterization of nonoccluded glomeruli. Diabetes 1987;36:612–619.
45. Hirose K, Tsuchida H, Østerby R, Gundersen HJ. A strong correlation between glomerular filtration rate and filtration surface in diabetic kidney hyperfunction. Lab Invest 1980;43:434–437.
46. Caramori ML, Kim Y, Huang C, et al. Cellular basis of diabetic nephropathy: 1. Study design and renal structural-functional relationships in patients with long-standing type 1 diabetes. Diabetes 2002;51:506–513. Erratum in: Diabetes 2002;51:1294.
47. Mauer SM. Structural-functional correlations of diabetic nephropathy. Kidney Int 1994;45:612–622. Erratum in: Kidney Int 1994;46:285.
48. Lane PH, Steffes MW, Fioretto P, Mauer SM. Renal interstitial expansion in insulin-dependent diabetes mellitus. Kidney Int 1993;43:661–667.
49. Fioretto P, Steffes MW, Sutherland DE, Mauer M. Sequential renal biopsies in insulin-dependent diabetic patients: structural factors associated with clinical progression. Kidney Int 1995;48:1929–1935.
50. Taft JL, Nolan CJ, Yeung SP, Hewitson TD, Martin FI. Clinical and histological correlations of decline in renal function in diabetic patients with proteinuria. Diabetes 1994;43:1046–1051.
51. Fioretto P, Steffes MW, Mauer M. Glomerular structure in nonproteinuric IDDM patients with various levels of albuminuria. Diabetes 1994;43:1358–1364.
52. Bilous RW, Mauer SM, Sutherland DE, Steffes MW. Mean glomerular volume and rate of development of diabetic nephropathy. Diabetes 1989;38:1142–1147.
53. Nyengaard JR, Bendtsen TF. Glomerular number and size in relation to age, kidney weight, and body surface in normal man. Anat Rec 1992;232:194–201.
54. Bendtsen TF, Nyengaard JR. Glomerutubular junction abnormalities are associated with proteinuria in type 1 diabetes. J Am Soc Nephrol, in press.
55. Najafian B, Crosson JT, Kim Y, Mauer M. The frequency of glomerulotubular junction abnormalities and atubular glomeruli in relation to albumin excretion rtae in type 1 diabetic patients. J Am Soc Nephrol 2003;14:597A.
56. Najafian B, Crosson JT, Kim Y, Mauer M. Predilection of tuft to Bowman's capsule adhesions for glomerulotubular junction area in type 1 diabetes mellitus. J Am Soc Nephrol 2004;15:729A.
57. Howie AJ, Ferreira MA, Majumdar A, Lipkin GW. Glomerular prolapse as precursor of one type of segmental sclerosing lesions. J Pathol 2000;190:478–483.

58. Kriz W, Elger M, Hosser H, et al. How does podocyte damage result in tubular damage? Kidney Blood Press Res 1999;22:26–36.
59. Howie AJ. Epithelial membrane antigen in normal and proteinuric glomeruli and in damaged proximal tubules. J Pathol 1986;148:55–60.
60. Brenner BM, Hostetter TH, Olson JL, Rennke HG, Venkatachalam MA. The role of glomerular hyperfiltration in the initiation and progression of diabetic nephropathy. Acta Endocrinol Suppl (Copenh) 1981;242:7–10.
61. Paueksakon P, Revelo MP, Ma LJ, Marcantoni C, Fogo AB. Microangiopathic injury and augmented PAI-1 in human diabetic nephropathy. Kidney Int 2002;61:2142–2148.
62. Mazzucco G, Bertani T, Fortunato M, et al. Different patterns of renal damage in type 2 diabetes mellitus: a multicentric study on 393 biopsies. Am J Kidney Dis 2002;39:713–720.
63. Carpenter AM, Goetz FC, LeCompte PM, Williamson JR. Glomerulosclerosis in type 2 (non-insulin-dependent) diabetes mellitus: relationship to glycaemia in the University Group Diabetes Program (UGDP). Diabetologia 1993;36:1057–1063.
64. Fioretto P, Stehouwer CD, Mauer M, et al. Heterogeneous nature of microalbuminuria in NIDDM: studies of endothelial function and renal structure. Diabetologia 1998;41:233–236.
65. Fioretto P, Mauer M, Brocco E, et al. Patterns of renal injury in NIDDM patients with microalbuminuria. Diabetologia 1996;39:1569–1576.
66. Østerby R, Gall MA, Schmitz A, Nielsen FS, Nyberg G, Parving HH. Glomerular structure and function in proteinuric type 2 (non-insulin-dependent) diabetic patients. Diabetologia 1993;36:1064–1070.
67. Rasch R. Prevention of diabetic glomerulopathy in streptozotocin diabetic rats by insulin treatment. The mesangial regions. Diabetologia 1979;17:243–248.
68. Rasch R. Prevention of diabetic glomerulopathy in streptozotocin diabetic rats by insulin treatment. Diabetologia 1979;16:319–324.
69. Steffes MW, Brown DM, Basgen JM, Mauer SM. Amelioration of mesangial volume and surface alterations following islet transplantation in diabetic rats. Diabetes 1980;29:509–515.
70. Mauer SM, Goetz FC, McHugh LE, et al. Long-term study of normal kidneys transplanted into patients with type I diabetes. Diabetes 1989;38:516–523.
71. Writing Team for the Diabetes Control and Complications Trial/Epidemiology of Diabetes Interventions and Complications Research Group. Sustained effect of intensive treatment of type 1 diabetes mellitus on development and progression of diabetic nephropathy: the Epidemiology of Diabetes Interventions and Complications (EDIC) study. JAMA 2003;290:2159–2167.
72. Bangstad HJ, Østerby R, Dahl-Jorgensen K, Berg KJ, Hartmann A, Hanssen KF. Improvement of blood glucose control in IDDM patients retards the progression of morphological changes in early diabetic nephropathy. Diabetologia 1994;37:483–490.
73. Barbosa J, Steffes MW, Sutherland DE, Connett JE, Rao KV, Mauer SM. Effect of glycemic control on early diabetic renal lesions. A 5-year randomized controlled clinical trial of insulin-dependent diabetic kidney transplant recipients. JAMA 1994;272:600–606.
74. Bilous RW, Mauer SM, Sutherland DE, Najarian JS, Goetz FC, Steffes MW. The effects of pancreas transplantation on the glomerular structure of renal allografts in patients with insulin-dependent diabetes. N Engl J Med 1989;321:80–85.
75. Bohman SO, Wilczek H, Tyden G, Jaremko G, Lundgren G, Groth CG. Recurrent diabetic nephropathy in renal allografts placed in diabetic patients and protective effect of simultaneous pancreatic transplantation. Transplant Proc 1987;19:2290–2293.
76. Fioretto P, Mauer SM, Bilous RW, Goetz FC, Sutherland DE, Steffes MW. Effects of pancreas transplantation on glomerular structure in insulin-dependent diabetic patients with their own kidneys. Lancet 1993;342:1193–1196.
77. Fioretto P, Steffes MW, Sutherland DE, Goetz FC, Mauer M. Reversal of lesions of diabetic nephropathy after pancreas transplantation. N Engl J Med 1998;339:69–75.
78. Lubec G, Pollak A. Reduced susceptibility of nonenzymatically glucosylated glomerular basement membrane to proteases: is thickening of diabetic glomerular basement membranes due to reduced proteolytic degradation? Ren Physiol 1980;3:4–8.
79. Roy S, Sala R, Cagliero E, Lorenzi M. Overexpression of fibronectin induced by diabetes or high glucose: phenomenon with a memory. Proc Natl Acad Sci USA 1990;87:404–408.
80. Susztak K, Sharma K, Schiffer M, McCue P, Ciccone E, Bottinger EP. Genomic strategies for diabetic nephropathy. J Am Soc Nephrol 2003;14:S271–S278.

22 Diabetic Kidney Disease in Transitional and Disadvantaged Populations

E. Jennifer Weil, MD
and Robert G. Nelson, MD, PhD

Contents

INTRODUCTION

The International Diabetes Federation estimates that the number of people with diabetes worldwide is 171 million and projects that number will increase to 334 million by the year 2030 *(1)*. Most of the increase will be the result of type 2 diabetes (T2DM) and disadvantaged people and those from transitional populations—people undergoing rapid change in their economies, lifestyles, and health—will be affected disproportionately (Fig. 1). Transitional and disadvantaged populations may include people of any race or ethnicity, but those most at risk for T2DM are Asians, Pacific Islanders, Australian Aborigines, African Americans, Hispanics, and Native Americans. These particular populations are also at higher risk for developing diabetic nephropathy (DN). Factors contributing to the high rate of DN in these transitional and disadvantaged populations may include differences in access to health care, genetic susceptibility, and environmental exposures.

From: *Contemporary Diabetes: The Diabetic Kidney*
Edited by: P. Cortes and C. E. Mogensen © Humana Press Inc., Totowa, NJ

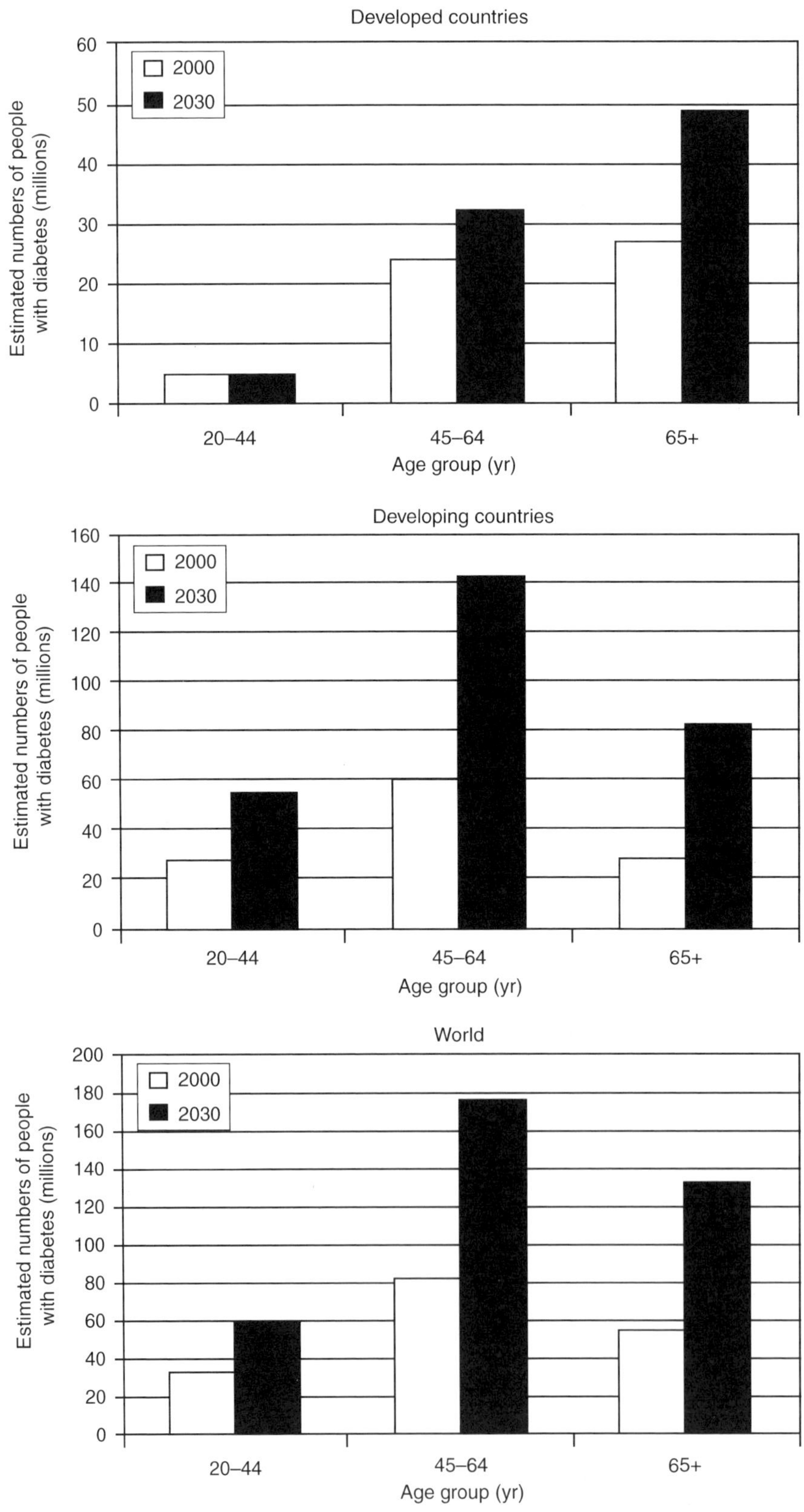
Developed countries
2000
2030
Estimated numbers of people with diabetes (millions)
60
50
40
30
20
10
0
20–44
45–64
65+
Age group (yr)
Developing countries
2000
2030
Estimated numbers of people with diabetes (millions)
160
140
120
100
80
60
40
20
0
20–44
45–64
65+
Age group (yr)
World
2000
2030
Estimated numbers of people with diabetes (millions)
200
180
160
140
120
100
80
60
40
20
0
20–44
45–64
65+
Age group (yr)

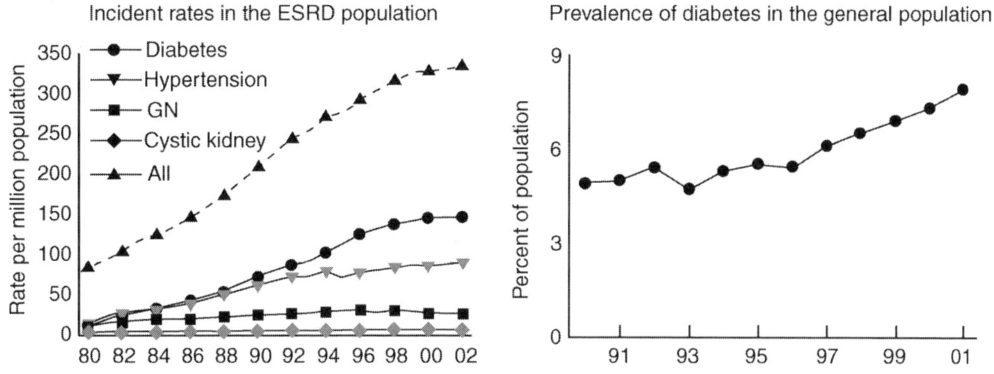

Fig. 2. Adjusted end-stage renal disease (ESRD) incident rates, by primary diagnosis, and diabetes in the general population. Incident ESRD patients; rates adjusted for age, gender, and race. Data on the prevalence of diabetes in the general population obtained from the CDC's behavioral risk factor surveillance system. The data reported here have been supplied by the US Renal Data System. The interpretation and reporting of these data are the responsibility of the author(s) and in no way should be seen as an official policy or interpretation of the US government *(8)*.

The pace of transition from agricultural to industrial economies has accelerated throughout the world in recent years. As developing countries undergo economic expansion, farmers switch from planting diverse crops for home consumption to cultivating high-yield crops to be sold at market. With the increased efficiency of mechanized agriculture, fewer people are required to grow the crops, prompting many to move from rural communities to seek economic opportunity in cities *(2)*. In 1900, just 10% of the world's population inhabited cities. Today, that figure is nearly 50% *(3)*.

The profound changes in economy, physical activity, and diet *(4)*, associated with the transition to an urban lifestyle, lead to changing patterns of disease, with increased frequencies of obesity, hypertension, the metabolic syndrome, and T2DM. This review will focus on the epidemic of DN in transitional and disadvantaged populations. Our goal is to describe the frequency of DN in these vulnerable populations, to identify risks for DN of particular relevance and importance to these populations, and to describe efforts to reduce these risks. We will also consider the management of DN in countries where limited resources influence the standard of care patients receive.

EPIDEMIOLOGICAL OVERVIEW

Diabetic kidney disease progresses from early stages, marked by hyperfiltration and microalbuminuria (30–300 mg/g albumin:creatinine), to later stages characterized by macroalbuminuria (>300 mg/g albumin:creatinine), declining glomerular filtration rate (GFR), and finally, end-stage renal disease (ESRD). Diabetes is the most common cause of ESRD in the United States (Fig. 2) and other developed nations. Many years are often required to progress through these stages, providing opportunities for prevention and early intervention.

The prevalence of early DN (pre-ESRD) depends on a number of factors including glycemic control, diabetes duration, and blood pressure *(5)*. The effect of race and/or

Fig. 1. Estimated number of adults with diabetes by age-group, year, and countries for the developed and developing categories and for the world. (© 2004, American Diabetes Association.) Reprinted with permission from the American Diabetes Association *(1)*.

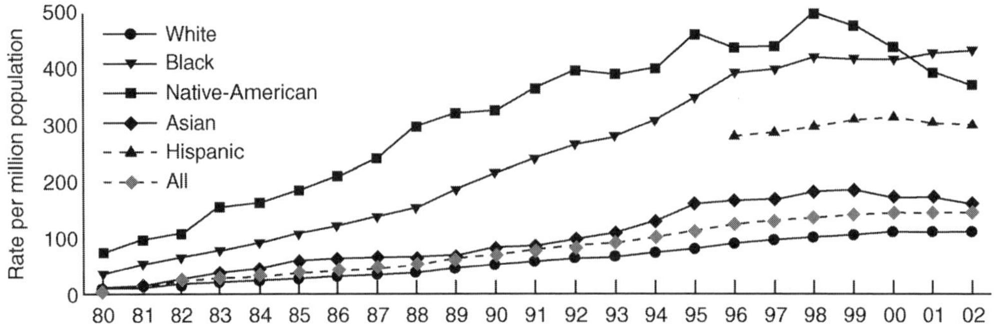

Fig. 3. Adjusted incident rates of end-stage renal disease (ESRD) owing to diabetes by race/ethnicity. Incident ESRD patients; adjusted for age and gender. For Hispanic patients, we present data beginning in 1996, the first full year after the April 1995 introduction of the revised Medical Evidence form, which contains more specific questions on race and ethnicity. The data reported here have been supplied by the US Renal Data System. The interpretation and reporting of these data are the responsibility of the author(s) and in no way should be seen as an official policy or interpretation of the US government *(8)*.

ethnicity on the prevalence of early DN may be confounded by these factors. For example, no ethnic differences in the prevalence of microalbuminuria were found among newly diagnosed diabetic participants in the UK Prospective Diabetes Study (UKPDS), which included Afro-Caribbean and Asian patients as well as whites *(6)*. Similarly, a US study of patients with variable duration of T2DM found a similar prevalence of microalbuminuria among various ethnic and racial groups *(7)*. However, that same study found the odds of microalbuminuria to be greater among hypertensive Hispanics than among hypertensive whites. Furthermore, among patients without hypertension, the odds of microalbuminuria was highest among Asians.

Transitional and disadvantaged populations are disproportionately represented among patients with diabetic ESRD. In the United States, the US Renal Data System (USRDS) reports that the incidence rate of diabetic ESRD among transitional and disadvantaged populations is much greater than the rate in the majority white population (Fig. 3) *(8)*. In Europe, several centers have reported disproportionate representation of transitional and minority populations among patients with ESRD *(9–11)*.

In 2004, the USRDS began collecting information, on a voluntary basis, from nations other than the United States *(8)*. Many European countries participated, but specific incidence estimates for transitional or disadvantaged dialysis patients within those countries were not reported. The USRDS also received data from several developing nations. Of these, Malaysia had the highest proportion of diabetic ESRD (Fig. 4). Malaysia has undergone rapid economic transition, and the high incidence of ESRD attributed to DN presumably reflects the growing prevalence of T2DM. In 1984, the prevalence of diabetes was 4% among the residents of three villages in Kuala Selangor province *(12)*. By 1996, the national prevalence of diabetes in Malaysia was 7%—a 75% increase from the estimates in Kuala Selangor province—and an additional 5% of the population had impaired glucose tolerance *(13)*.

Because many studies that examine the epidemiology of DN in T2DM rely on data collected at the time of initiation of dialysis, the quality of epidemiological information is best from developed countries where dialysis is offered. The burden of DN, however, may be greatest in developing countries, where patients with early DN are likely to be underdiagnosed and patients with kidney failure from diabetes are unlikely to receive

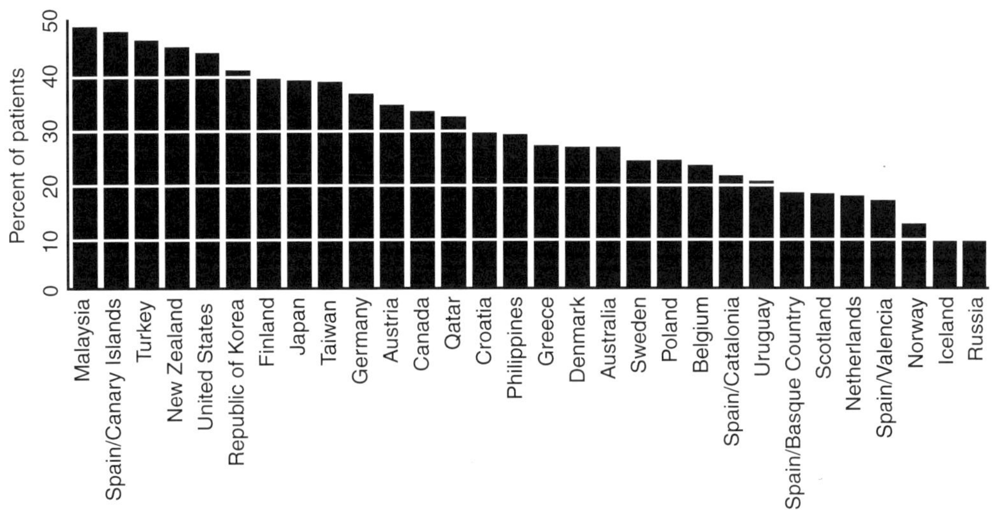

Fig. 4. Percent of incident end-stage renal disease (ESRD) patients with diabetes in 2002. Data presented only for those countries from which relevant information was available. All rates are unadjusted. Data from Israel, Japan, Luxembourg, and Taiwan represent dialysis only. The data reported here have been supplied by the US Renal Data System. The interpretation and reporting of these data are the responsibility of the author(s) and in no way should be seen as an official policy or interpretation of the US government *(8)*.

dialysis. Under these circumstances, accurate data on the frequency of DN in developing countries are sparse or nonexistent. Nevertheless, data about the frequency of DN and diabetic ESRD are available from some developing countries and from emigrants to the developed countries. These data reflect the different methods and definitions of the authors who report them and different ages of those who were examined. Accordingly, they are neither exhaustive nor definitive, but they reflect the scope of the problem of DN in transitional and disadvantaged populations and they are reviewed next.

Asians

A large, recent cross-sectional study of early DN from 103 centers in 10 Asian countries (Singapore, Hong Kong, Philippines, People's Republic of China, Taiwan, Thailand, Malaysia, Indonesia, Pakistan, and South Korea) reported a prevalence of microalbuminuria among patients with T2DM of 39.8% *(14)*. By contrast, a national survey of microalbuminuria among diabetic patients in the United States reported a prevalence of 28.8% *(15)*. The authors speculate that the reason for higher prevalence of microalbuminuria among the Asian patients is poor blood pressure control, with only 10.6% of patients with microalbuminuria achieving a blood pressure goal of 130/80 mmHg or below *(14)*.

Asians are also at high risk for diabetic ESRD. In Asian countries where dialysis is not widely available, the prevalence of diabetic ESRD is uncertain. On the other hand, Asians living in Australia and the United States are disproportionately represented among those receiving ESRD care for DN *(8,16)*. In Australia, the incidence rate of diabetic ESRD among Asian immigrants is up to 10 times that of nonindigenous Australians *(16)*. In the United States, the incidence rate of diabetic ESRD among Asians is less than that of whites, but since 1992 Asians have had the greatest increase in ESRD incidence from DN among the various ethnic groups tracked by the USRDS *(8)*.

Moreover, in Hawaii, the most common cause of ESRD among people of Japanese and Filipino ancestry is DN *(17)*.

Indo-Asians

The prevalence of microalbuminuria in patients with T2DM from one center in India was 36.3% *(18)*. Because the prevalence of T2DM is rising throughout India *(19)*, the frequency of DN is likely to increase further.

DN is the leading cause of ESRD in Chennai, India *(20)* (*vide infra*). Similarly, Indo-Asians treated at two centers in the United Kingdom have an age-adjusted annual incidence of ESRD that is three to five times that of whites and most of the ESRD in the Indo-Asians is attributable to DN *(10,21)*. In the Netherlands, the relative risk for dialysis among Indo-Asian patients with diabetes is 40 times that of the white population. This risk is much higher than expected, because the prevalence of T2DM among the Netherlands Indo-Asian population is only eight times that of the white population *(11)*.

Pacific Islanders

Early diabetic kidney disease is prevalent among Pacific Islanders with T2DM. The prevalence of microalbuminuria among diabetic subjects in Nauru is 41% *(22)* and in one ethnic group in New Guinea is 26% *(23)*. In South Auckland, the prevalence of microalbuminuria among diabetic Pacific Islanders is 33.3% *(24)*.

In New Zealand, immigrants from the Pacific Islands have the highest rates of ESRD attributable to T2DM; more than 10 times that of nonindigenous people *(16)*. Likewise, DN is the overwhelming cause of ESRD among Native Hawaiians—68.6% of ESRD is caused by DN *(17)*. In Micronesia, 75% of the incidence of ESRD among the indigenous populations of Guam (Safa S, personal communication) and the Commonwealth of the Northern Mariana Islands *(25)* is attributed to DN.

Indigenous Australians and New Zealanders

The prevalence of microalbuminuria is high among Australian Aborigines, regardless of whether or not they have diabetes *(26)*. Indeed, among those with microalbuminuria, only 21.5% meet diagnostic criteria for T2DM. In Aboriginal patients with diagnosed T2DM, the odds of microalbuminuria was 1.8 times that of white Australians *(27)*. Similarly, in South Auckland, New Zealand, the prevalence of microalbuminuria among diabetic Maori was 1.2 times that of whites with diabetes *(24)*.

ESRD disproportionately affects the indigenous peoples of Australia and New Zealand. Aboriginal Australians constitute less than 2% of the Australian population but represent 10% of new patients starting dialysis *(28)*. From 1992 to 2001, the incidence rate of ESRD attributed to DN among Australian Aboriginals was 50–100 times that of nonindigenous Australians and the rate among Maoris was 23 times that of nonindigenous people *(29)*.

African Americans and Afro-Caribbeans

One study of African-American patients with newly diagnosed T2DM reported a prevalence of microalbuminuria of 23.4% *(30)*. In another small study, African-American patients with T2DM of longer duration had a prevalence of microalbuminuria of 36% *(31)*. A large study of US veterans found that after adjustment for age, sex, and economic status, African-American veterans were 1.3 times more likely to have early DN than Caucasians *(32)*. In the United Kingdom, elevated urinary albumin excretion was found in 37% of Africans and Afro-Caribbeans with T2DM *(33)*.

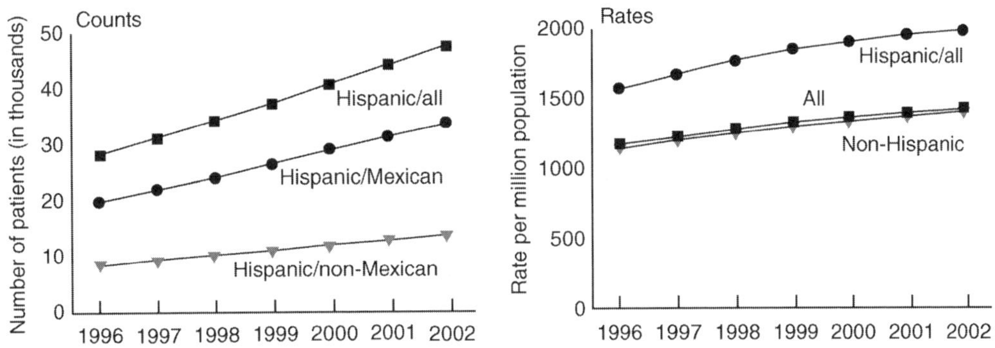

Fig. 5. Prevalence counts and adjusted rates, by ethnicity. December 31 point-prevalent end-stage renal disease patients. Rates adjusted for age and gender. For Hispanic patients, we present data beginning in 1996, the first full year after the April 1995 introduction of the revised Medical Evidence form, which contains more specific questions on race and ethnicity. The data reported here have been supplied by the US Renal Data System. The interpretation and reporting of these data are the responsibility of the author(s) and in no way should be seen as an official policy or interpretation of the US government *(8)*.

In the study of US veterans *(32)*, diabetic ESRD was 1.9 times more likely to be present in African Americans than whites. The USRDS reported that in 1996, DN surpassed hypertension as the most common cause of ESRD among African Americans *(8)*. In the United Kingdom, Afro-Caribbeans have a relative risk of diabetic ESRD that is 1.76 times that of whites of *(9,33)*.

Hispanics and Latin Americans

The term "Hispanic" refers to Spanish-speaking people in the United States and includes Mexican Americans, Puerto Rican Americans, and Cuban Americans, as well as other immigrants from Latin America and their descendants. The risk of DN among Hispanics in the United States varies with the prevalence of T2DM; Mexican Americans and Puerto Rican Americans have much higher prevalence of T2DM than Cuban Americans *(34)*. Mexican Americans with T2DM are more likely to have diabetic complications than are diabetic non-Hispanic whites of a similar age *(35)* and Hispanics are more likely to have microalbuminuria (but not macroalbuminuria) than African-Americans or Asians *(31)*. Outside the United States, Latin Americans also have high rates of DN. Of 304 Mexican patients with T2DM from the Mexico City, 84.4% of men and 63.8% of women had microalbuminuria *(36)*. Almost nothing is known about the frequency of early DN in Latin America.

The USRDS began to collect data on Hispanic patients in 1995 and found that Hispanics are disproportionately represented among patients with diabetic ESRD *(8)*. However, the USRDS distinguishes only between Mexican-Americans and non-Mexican Hispanic. Thus, incidence and prevalence of ESRD is known only for Hispanics as a whole and for Mexican Americans. Nevertheless, the USRDS data suggest that incidence rates of ESRD for Hispanics are 1.5 times those of non-Hispanic whites (Fig. 5) *(8)*.

Native Americans

Elevated protein excretion is present in 33% of Native Americans with diabetes, of whom 10% have microalbuminuria and 23% have overt proteinuria *(37)*. A longitudinal study of Pima Indians found that the incidence rate of proteinuria is increasing despite better control of blood glucose and blood pressure, and that increasing average duration of diabetes is largely responsible for this finding *(38)*.

Native Americans and Alaskan Natives experience high rates of ESRD attributable to DN. In 1999, 68% of Native Americans and Alaskan Natives who initiated ESRD treatment in the United States had DN as the underlying cause of kidney failure. By contrast, only 25% of whites and 42% of African Americans had diabetic ESRD *(37)*. However, since 1992 the overall trend of diabetic ESRD incidence among Native Americans aged 40–59 yr has declined *(8)*. This may reflect improvements in the medical treatment of early kidney disease *(39)*.

ENVIRONMENTAL FACTORS

Environmental factors that affect the development of DN may be divided into those present before birth, for example, maternal malnutrition, diabetes during pregnancy, and maternal vitamin A deficiency; those present before the development of diabetes that affect the risk of diabetes and its progression, for example, diet, exercise, access to medical care, compliance with medicines; and those that add to the risk of progressive kidney disease in people with established diabetes, for example, infections and environmental toxins. All of these factors are important in transitional and disadvantaged populations and are deeply intertwined with socioeconomic factors. Diabetes and diabetes control will be discussed in the section on socioeconomic factors (*vide infra*). Here we shall focus on maternal malnutrition and diabetes during prenatal life, infections, and environmental toxins because these are environmental factors that may disproportionately affect transitional and disadvantaged populations.

Intrauterine Exposures

Maternal malnutrition often causes intrauterine growth retardation (IUGR) in offspring. Low birthweight, a manifestation of IUGR, may then increase the risk of both T2DM *(40–42)* and DN *(43,44)*. IUGR affects 25% of live births in developing countries annually *(45)* and represents a major potential cause of kidney disease in these populations. The mechanism for increased susceptibility to kidney disease among individuals with low birthweight is thought to be impaired nephron development. With fewer nephrons and a correspondingly reduced filtration surface area, the resulting hyperfiltration may accelerate damage to the glomeruli initiated by diabetes *(46)*. Elevated urinary albumin is more prevalent among diabetic Pima Indians with low birthweight (Fig. 6). Another manifestation of low nephron mass may be hypertension, which was found more frequently in persons of low birthweight, including indigenous Australians *(47)*.

Glomerulomegaly has been reported in two transitional populations at high risk for diabetic kidney disease, Aboriginals *(48,49)* and Pima Indians *(50,51)*, and it may reflect an attempt by the kidneys to maintain adequate filtration surface area through expansion of existing glomeruli in people with reduced nephron mass.

Exposure to maternal diabetes *in utero* may also greatly increase the risk of DN. Animal experiments demonstrate that maternal diabetes during pregnancy reduces the number of nephrons in offspring *(52)*. In Pima-Indians, the odds of elevated urinary albumin excretion was nearly four times as high in subjects exposed to diabetes *in utero* than in those exposed to a normal uterine environment (Fig. 7) *(53)*. Hence, the increasing frequency of exposure to maternal diabetes in Pima-Indians *(54)* may, in part, explain

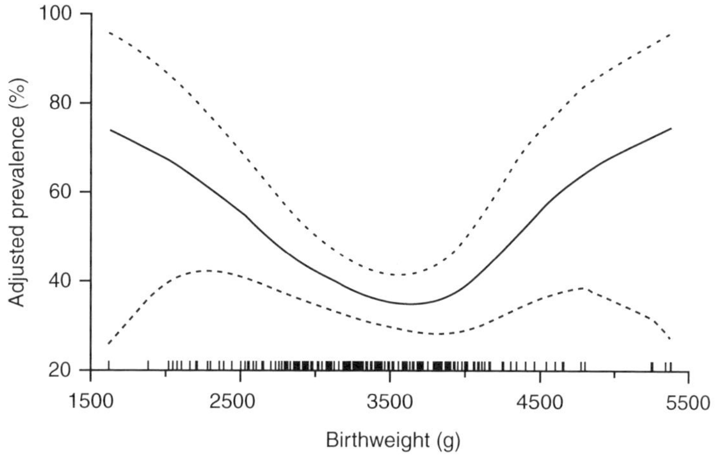

Fig. 6. Prevalence of elevated urinary albumin excretion (albumin-to-creatinine ratio ≥30 mg/g) in diabetic Pima Indians by birthweight, adjusted for age, sex, duration of diabetes, HbA1C, and mean arterial pressure. Dashed lines represent twice the pointwise asymptotic standard errors of the estimated curve, and the vertical tics on the *x*-axis are a frequency plot of birthweights. Values of the covariates were set to their sample means. Reprinted with the permission of Oxford University Press *(53)*.

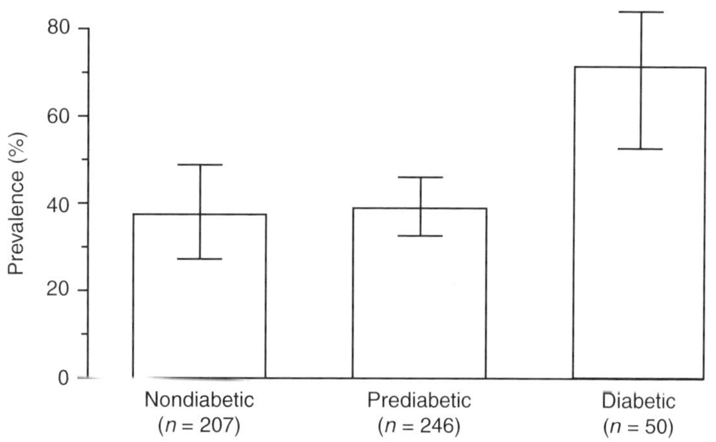

Fig. 7. Predicted prevalence (95% CIs) of elevated UAE (albumin-to-creatinine ratio ≥30 mg/g), in diabetic Pima Indians, by maternal diabetes status, adjusted for age, sex, duration of diabetes, HbA1C, and MAP. Values of the covariates were set to their sample means. © 1998 American Diabetes Association; reprinted with permission from the American Diabetes Association *(1)*.

the secular increase in incidence of proteinuria in this population, as each successive generation has a higher rate of diabetes and diabetic kidney disease as a result of this exposure *(54)*. Given that the largest increase in the prevalence of diabetes during the childbearing years over the next several decades will occur in the developing world, populations in these countries will be disproportionately affected by the impact of this exposure *(1)*.

Vitamin A (retinol) and its main derivative, retinoic acid, are involved in nephrogenesis, and rats exhibit a dose-dependent effect of vitamin A on nephron number *(55)*. Both retinal and retinoic acid are potent stimulators of nephrogenesis, with a single injection of retinoic acid given to a pregnant rat at midgestation inducing supernumerary nephrons. Although human data on the relationship between vitamin A and nephron mass are not available, the existing animal data suggest that a mild vitamin A deficiency during pregnancy could lead to a nephron deficit in the offspring that enhances the risk of kidney disease. Although vitamin A deficiency is not a major health problem in developed countries, it is frequently encountered in developing countries, particularly in pregnant women, in whom intake of vitamin A may be inadequate to meet the increased demands encountered during pregnancy. Accordingly, fetal vitamin A deficiency may disproportionately affect minority and disadvantaged populations and contribute to their increasing incidence rate of kidney disease.

Infections

Once diabetes is established, the risk of DN may be increased by chronic or repeated infections. Australian researchers have documented a high prevalence of parasitic and bacterial infections among Aboriginals who later developed DN *(56)*. The highest risk appears to result from repeated bacterial infections of the eyes, ears, nose, chest, skin, and gut. Although infections with *streptococci* are known to cause poststreptococcal glomerulonephritis (PSGN), a condition that is relatively common among Aboriginals *(57)*, infections with other organisms may also contribute to progressive kidney disease in DN through immune activation and mesangial proliferation *(58)*. Close living quarters and poor hygiene are largely responsible for the repeated bacterial and parasitic infections in the Aboriginal community.

Environmental Toxins

Exposure to environmental toxins may not increase the risk of DN *per se*, but may well accelerate its progression by adding to the burden of interstitial kidney disease *(59)*. Transitional and disadvantaged populations may experience high levels of toxic exposure at work, because access to types of employment in which such exposures are less may be limited by language and educational attainment. Those who live and work in rural environments may be exposed more frequently to nephrotoxins used in industrial agriculture including fertilizers, herbicides, and insecticides containing heavy metals like arsenic. Urban workers may be exposed to hydrocarbons and heavy metals used in manufacturing, including cadmium, mercury, and lead.

Toxic exposures may also occur at home. As recent immigrants to cities, members of transitional and disadvantaged populations may be less likely to own land or have influence over land use and more likely to live in neighborhoods where they are exposed to toxic chemicals at unhealthy levels. Cultural practices that arise in response to economic forces and social disruption may also lead to toxic exposures that harm the kidney. Moonshine, for example, is an alcoholic beverage made cheaply by distilling ethanol in radiators typically lined with lead and using copper pipe soldered with lead. Drinking moonshine distilled in such containers may result in lead nephropathy, which could hasten progression of DN as well *(60)*.

Exposure to Tobacco

In patients with T2DM, tobacco is an independent risk factor for onset and progression of DN *(61,62)*, and smoking also increases the risk of diabetic ESRD *(63)*. Unfortunately, the prevalence of smoking is often high in developing countries. In Latin America, for example, the prevalence of smoking is variable, from 24.1% in Paraguay to

66.3% in the Dominican Republic *(64)*. In African Americans, exposure to cigaret smoke increases the risk of DN *(65)*, but this finding has not been confirmed in other transitional and disadvantaged populations. Nevertheless, in the United States, members of transitional and disadvantaged populations are disproportionately inclined to substance abuse, including tobacco *(66)*. Economic transition appears to increase the prevalence of cigaret smoking among Australian Aboriginals *(67)*, and migration from rural to urban areas is associated with increased prevalence of tobacco abuse in China *(68)*. Why economic transition is associated with increased prevalence of smoking is unclear. Tobacco abuse may cause smokers to feel more relaxed and in control *(68)* or may result from increased disposable income and increased access to cigarets in urban areas *(72)*.

SOCIOECONOMIC FACTORS

Economic transition can have different effects on socioeconomic status (SES) and on the risk of developing T2DM. People who successfully undergo economic transition—those who migrate to cities and take industrial jobs that pay well—experience an increase in SES and greater access to food. In India, higher SES increases the risk of diabetes *(69)* and in the United States, the risk of T2DM is highest among Hispanics of highest SES *(70)*. On the other hand, higher SES is generally associated with better education and with the resources to make healthier food choices. In the United States, for example, the risk of T2DM among African Americans is lowest in those of higher SES *(71)*. Different levels of acculturation may, in part, explain the differential effects of SES on the risk of T2DM in different populations *(72)*.

SES also has an effect on the risk of diabetic complications. Once T2DM is diagnosed, diabetes duration, glycemic control, blood pressure, and microalbuminuria all predict future kidney disease. Control of glycemia is dependent on a host of factors and poor glycemic control disproportionately affects many members of transitional and disadvantaged populations. In the Third National Health and Nutrition Examination Survey, glycemic control was poorer among Blacks and Mexican Americans than in non-Hispanic whites *(73)*. In India, urban patients of lower SES were more likely than those of higher status to develop complications of T2DM *(69)*. Poor glycemic control may be exacerbated by a number of socioeconomic factors. Economic realities may make proper diet, diabetes testing equipment, and medicines unaffordable. Furthermore, transitional and disadvantaged populations may have limited access to education, including health education. The benefits of medicines prescribed to control blood sugar and blood pressure may not be as clear to poorly educated patients, and the side effects of these medicines may discourage compliance. Noncompliance, however, has very real consequences in DN. Thirty-six percent of Mexican-American subjects 65 yr or older with self-reported diabetes said that they took their prescribed diabetes medicines inconsistently. Those who took their medicines inconsistently increased their odds of kidney disease by 1.6 compared with those with good consistency over a 7-yr period, after controlling for age, sex, diabetes duration, education, income, marital status, language of interview, insurance status, medication type, cognitive function, presence of depressive symptoms, and activities of daily living *(74)*.

SES is correlated with progression of kidney disease in a number of transitional and disadvantaged populations. Among Native Americans living in Minnesota, family income and educational attainment are inversely associated with increased urine albumin excretion *(75)*. African Americans with early decline in kidney function are more likely to be of low SES and have suboptimal health behaviors and suboptimal control of glucose and blood pressure *(76)*. Similarly, socioeconomic factors are strongly associated with the incidence of ESRD among indigenous Australians. Leaving school before the age of 15 yr, unemployment, low household income, and overcrowding in the home were all found to correlate with increased risk of ESRD *(30)*.

BARRIERS TO CARE

There are many obstacles to the prevention, timely diagnosis, and treatment of T2DM and DN in transitional and disadvantaged populations. Most important of these are the same lifestyle changes that increase the risk of T2DM and DN. Changes in caloric balance that accompany the transition from a subsistence lifestyle (hunting, gathering, or intensive agriculture) to an industrial lifestyle are not easily reversed once a diagnosis of T2DM is made. Hence, a dietary prescription may be difficult to implement and sustain for some members of transitional and disadvantaged populations *(77)*. The poverty that is associated with obesity and poor diet also limits the funds available to pay for healthy foods, exercise, access to a health care professional, and medicine once diabetes develops.

"Functional health literacy" is a measure of a patient's ability to perform basic reading and numerical tasks required to function in the health care environment. It is distinct from educational level or language ability *(78)*. Poor functional health literacy limits effective communication between the patient and their health care provider, so patients are often confused about their disease and the process of care required to successfully manage their disease, and the practitioner is frustrated by their patient's lack of understanding and inability to implement treatment plans *(79,80)*.

Intertwined with impaired functional health literacy are complex patterns of health beliefs, motivations, and behaviors that also act as barriers to care of people with T2DM. These include lack of perception of the seriousness of their illness, denial of illness, lack of trust in the health care provider or system, shame, discomfort with the gender of the practitioner, faith in God, and bad experiences either on the part of the patient or the patient's family and friends *(81)*. Members of transitional and disadvantaged populations often feel more comfortable using home remedies or seeking the help of a traditional healer and, as a result, may seek the help of Western medicine only as a last resort. By the time such a patient comes to the attention of a practitioner of Western medicine, it is often too late to prevent DN and the only therapy that remains is dialysis *(81)*.

Inadequate transportation may limit access to health care among transitional and disadvantaged populations. For example, in small villages near Chennai, India, there are two physicians for every 25,000 people. Although care and medicines are free, the patient must travel to the health care center without assistance. There are often no roads and no bus. If there is a bus, the patient must pay the fare. Once on the bus, it may take half a day to get to the health center and half a day to return. This means the loss of 1 d wage. As a result, few patients will seek the care of a physician unless they are completely incapacitated and will not seek care for chronic diseases, such as T2DM, that may have no symptoms *(20)*.

Other barriers related to transportation include bureaucracy, time, and child care. Government or private organizations may provide programs with various benefits, but the process of registering for these programs may be so complicated that benefits are largely unused. Moreover, patients may be too busy because of long work hours to

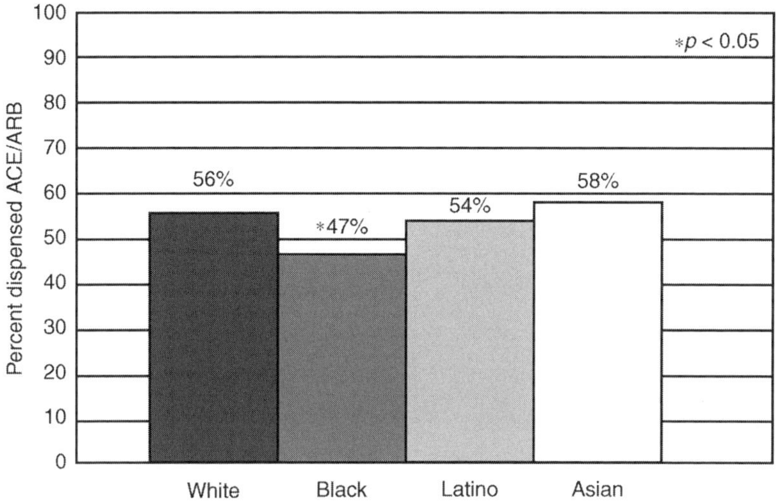

Fig. 8. Angiotensin-converting enzyme (ACE)/angiotensin receptor blocker (ARB) use among ethnic groups with albuminuria. The asterisk indicates a significant ($p < 0.05$) difference in rates of ACE/ARB use compared with rates of use in whites with albuminuria in the absence of hypertension. Reprinted with the permission from Blackwell *(88)*.

schedule frequent visits or providers may not have enough hours in their schedules to see all the patients who seek their care. Women especially may not seek medical assistance if they cannot find someone else to care for their families.

Even when barriers to care are removed, the risk of DN may still remain elevated if standards of care are not met by the providers. Kaiser Permanente of Northern California maintains a longitudinal registry of patients with diabetes and monitors outcomes in these patients. All patients have unfettered access to providers and to pharmacy benefits. Among 38,887 diabetic patients who were at high risk for DN because of hypertension and/or elevated albuminuria, 61% received angiotensin-converting enzyme (ACE) inhibitors or angiotensin receptor blockers (ARBs). Although there was no statistically significant difference in overall prescription rate for ACE inhibitors or ARBs among the racial and ethnic groups in the study, African Americans with albuminuria as a sole indication for therapy with these agents were less likely to have ACE inhibitors or ARBs prescribed (Fig. 8) *(82)*. Among the Kaiser patients, Asians, African-Americans, and Hispanics had higher incidence rates of ESRD than non-Hispanic whites, despite equal access to care *(83)*. The persistence of ethnic disparities after removal of barriers to care suggests that other genetic, socioeconomic, and environmental factors may still have profound effects on outcomes of diabetes *(83)*.

RATE OF PROGRESSION

A subanalysis of the Modification of Diet in Renal Disease study *(84)*, a study that largely excluded patients with diabetes, suggested that African Americans have a more rapid progression of kidney disease than whites. This observation was ascribed to difficulty in achieving blood pressure control in African Americans. Similarly, Pima Indians with DN also experience rapid progression of kidney disease relative to whites *(46)*. The rate of decline of GFR in Pima Indians was 13.8 mL/min/1.73m^2/yr, or roughly four times the rate of decline in whites from Italy *(85)* and differences in glycemic and blood pressure control may account, at least in part, for these differences. On the other hand, a small, retrospective study in London found that Indo-Asians with DN had a significantly higher rate of doubling of serum creatinine than whites or Afro-Caribbeans despite similarities in blood pressure, glycemic control, smoking behavior, baseline proteinuria, and use of ACE inhibitors *(86)*, again suggesting that other genetic, socioeconomic, and environmental factors must be involved in the more rapid progression of DN in transitional and disadvantaged populations.

COMORBIDITIES

T2DM and DN often coexist with other medical problems in patients from transitional and disadvantaged populations. These comorbidities are often other health manifestations of the same economic and lifestyle transition that led to T2DM and they include obesity and its complications (e.g., obstructive sleep apnea, degenerative joint disease), hyperlipidemia and its complications (stroke, angina, myocardial infarction, peripheral vascular disease), and hypertension and its complications (vascular disease, kidney failure). Other diabetic complications, including retinopathy, neuropathy, and vascular disease, also occur more frequently in people with DN.

A relationship between DN and heart disease has been noted in many studies. Microalbuminuria confers a risk of myocardial infarction that equals or exceeds that of hypertension. This is true among members of transitional and disadvantaged populations as well as in nonminority groups *(87–89)*. The Strong Heart Study, for example, reported an association of diabetic microalbuminuria with left ventricular hypertrophy and with serum markers of systemic inflammation suggestive of atherosclerosis among Native Americans *(90)*.

Several infectious diseases, including HIV, PSGN, and hepatitis C, are associated with kidney complications. None of these infectious diseases have a direct relationship with obesity, the metabolic syndrome, or T2DM, but they may confuse the diagnosis of DN or complicate its course.

The HIV appears to cause kidney disease by direct infection of glomerular endothelial and mesangial cells. In the United States, African Americans are disproportionately infected with HIV *(91)* and they have a higher risk of the HIV-associated nephropathy than whites *(92)*.

PSGN results after a throat or skin infection with specific nephritogenic strains of group A streptococcus (such as type 12 and type 49) and usually occurs sporadically. However, PSGN may also occur in epidemic form and is spread among people with close contact. Skin infections with streptococcal organisms are implicated in the high rates of ESRD seen in the Aboriginal population in Australia *(93,94)* and in other transitional and disadvantaged populations who often live in crowded conditions that favor transmission of streptococcus or staphylococcus organisms. Perhaps a postinfectious glomerulonephritis following either one of these common skin infections complicates DN and results in an accelerated decline in kidney function *(95)*. Alternatively, skin infections may hasten progression of DN by immune activation and mesangial proliferation *(94)*.

Hepatitis C is a blood-borne viral infection that is associated with an increased risk of T2DM *(96–98)*. Hepatitis C is quite prevalent among certain racial and ethnic minorities within the United States and is newly emerging as a comorbidity among Afro-Caribbeans *(99)* and Native Americans with T2DM *(100)*. The kidney disease associated with hepatitis C is immune-mediated and may be found in patients with microalbuminuria and coexisting DN *(101,102)*.

PREVENTION OF DN IN TRANSITIONAL AND DISADVANTAGED POPULATIONS

Prevention of T2DM

A recent large clinical trial demonstrates that T2DM can be prevented in certain transitional and disadvantaged populations. The Diabetes Prevention Program included African Americans, Hispanics, and Native Americans *(103)* as well as non-Hispanic whites. By using either a strategy of lifestyle modification to encourage increased exercise and promote weight loss or the drug metformin, diabetes was significantly delayed; more so in subjects receiving the lifestyle modification than in those receiving metformin. The effect of intervention was equivalent in all racial and ethnic groups.

Community-based efforts to prevent T2DM, however, have been less successful than the more intensive clinical trials. A program among elementary school children in the Mohawk community in Canada that encouraged healthy eating and more physical activity reported no effect of intervention on body mass index, physical activity, fitness, or diet. The investigators concluded that although early results showed some successes in reducing risk factors for T2DM, these benefits were not maintained long-term *(104,105)*.

Although there are no published reports of success in community-based primary prevention of T2DM, expert opinion suggests that gaining community support is critical to the success of interventions in transitional and disadvantaged populations *(106)*. Unless diabetes prevention is seen as a goal by the members and leadership of a community, success may be difficult or impossible. Moreover, integration of members of the community into the diabetes prevention team is one way to provide sustainable leadership *(107–109)*.

A central paradox of T2DM among members of many transitional and disadvantaged populations is that economic transition often increases the risk of diabetes and the SES as well. The challenge in diabetes prevention is to find ways to encourage economic growth although decreasing the risk of T2DM.

Prevention of DN

Early detection of DN may reduce the progression of kidney disease and widespread screening for T2DM and DN is available at low cost to high-risk transitional and disadvantaged populations *(110,111)*. In the United States, for example, the National Kidney Foundation's Kidney Early Evaluation Program (KEEP) is a traveling screening program that targets high-risk populations and raises awareness of kidney disease in these groups. KEEP provides free screening and educational information, and the message it provides is that kidney disease and its complications can be prevented or delayed *(112)*.

Another model program was implemented in the Tiwi Islands for members of an Australian Aboriginal community that has extraordinarily high rates of T2DM, DN, and ESRD. Patients are screened systematically for hypertension, diabetes, and elevated albuminuria. Once identified, they are given aggressive blood pressure management with the ACE inhibitor perindopril. Additional antihypertensive medicines are added as needed to control blood pressure. Those receiving the intervention had a marked decline in blood pressure and a slowing of the progression of albuminuria and the loss of GFR in comparison with the historical controls. A drop in all-cause mortality was also noted in the treatment group *(113–115)*.

A third model for the early detection of T2DM and DN in a transitional and disadvantaged population is that of Mani and the Kidney Help Trust of Chennai, India. By training young women as preventive social health workers and providing them with bicycles and simple screening tools, population screening was successfully carried out in this region. Eleven percent of the screened population had T2DM, and DN was the leading cause of ESRD. Once patients were diagnosed with either diabetes or hypertension, medicines were dispensed and the patients were followed by a preventive social health worker as well as by a physician. Metformin was prescribed for patients with diabetes and reserpine was used to treat blood pressure, because ACE inhibitors and ARBs were too expensive. Although tight glycemic control was rarely achieved, blood pressure was reportedly reduced to the target of 140/90 mmHg or below in more than 95% of the subjects. Whether this approach to care in rural, underserved areas will translate to a reduction in the frequency of kidney failure from diabetic kidney disease, however, remains to be determined *(20)*.

Slowing Progression, Delaying ESRD, and Preventing Cardiovascular Mortality

Once DN is established, therapeutic efforts should focus on slowing the rate of progression of kidney disease and delaying ESRD. Although early referral to a nephrologist may be an ideal way to care for patients with established DN *(116,117)*, economic reality suggests that primary care providers are often the sole providers of care for members of transitional and disadvantaged populations. Fortunately, therapy may be simplified so that nurses *(125)* or even low-skilled workers can implement it *(61,112,113,122)*.

Among the antihypertensive medications, ARBs have been shown in large clinical trials to slow the progression of established DN in T2DM in a number of racial and ethnic groups (Fig. 9). The Reduction of Endpoints in NIDDM with the Angiontensin II Antagonist Losartan (RENAAL) study included 252 Asian patients, 230 African-American patients, and 176 Hispanic patients, and the Irbesartan in Diabetic Nephropathy (IDNT) included 85 Asians, 228 African Americans, and 83 Hispanics *(119,120)*. A subgroup analysis of the Asian patients enrolled in RENAAL found that losartan was effective in reducing the endpoints of doubling of serum creatinine, ESRD, and all-cause mortality. Moreover, Asians had the lowest rate of discontinuation of any subgroup in RENAAL, suggesting that losartan is associated with fewer side effects in Asians than in other populations *(121)*.

Another goal of prevention is reduction of mortality from cardiovascular disease in patients with established DN. Heart disease is common in developing countries and the frequency of heart disease is likely to worsen as populations undergo economic and lifestyle transition and the prevalence of diabetes increases *(122)*. Although multifactorial intervention to prevent cardiovascular mortality in patients with T2DM may be ideal *(130)*, the cost of such therapy is prohibitive in many parts of the developing world. Hence, efforts to delay or prevent the onset of diabetes may be the most cost-effective way to reduce the frequency of diabetic kidney disease.

TREATMENT OF ESRD

No Therapy At All

Once DN progresses to ESRD, options for therapy are limited to dialysis, transplantation, or no therapy at all. Although dialysis is widely available in most developed countries, the same is not true in the developing world. Indeed, whereas dialysis is

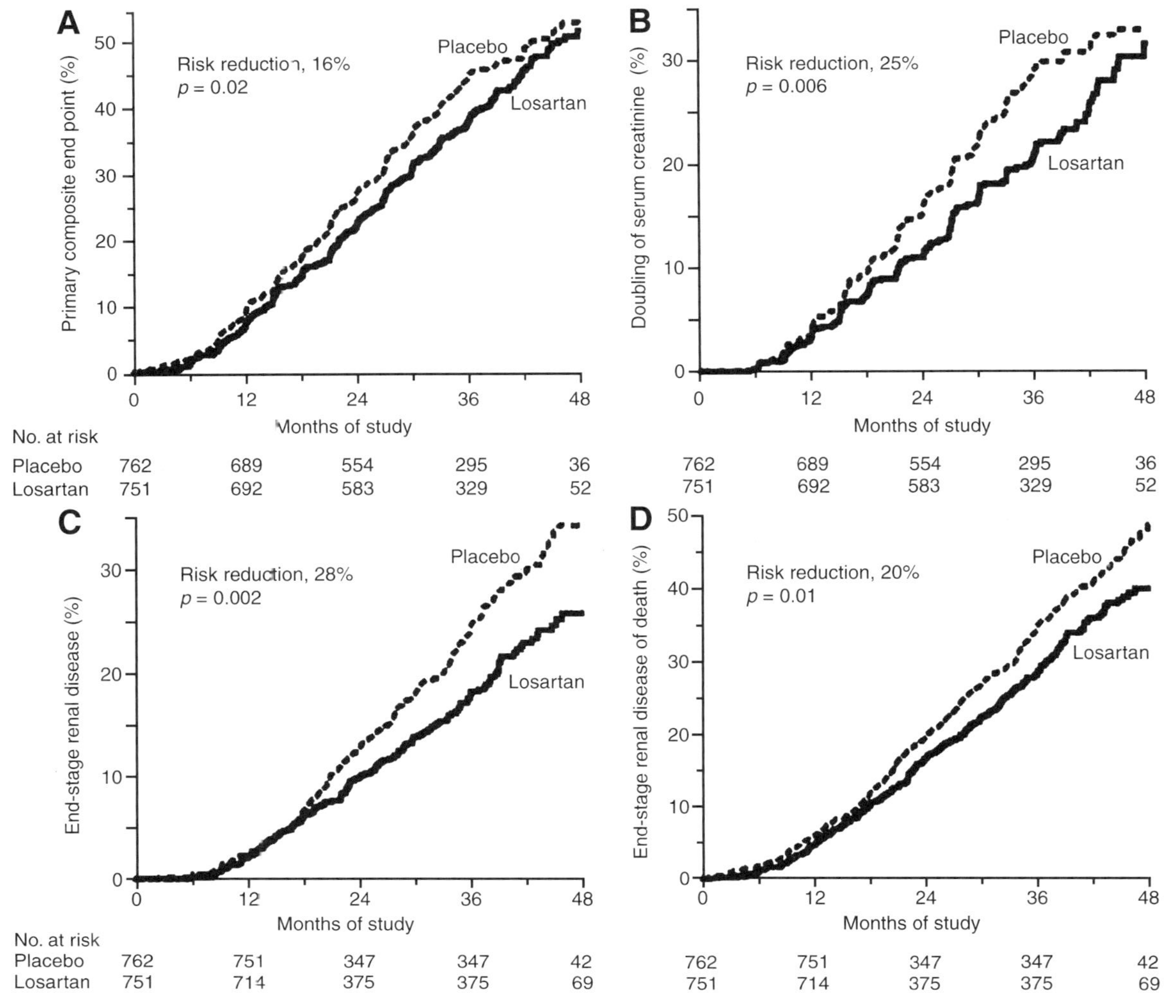

Fig. 9. Kaplan-Meier Curves of the percentage of patients with the primary composite end point (**A**) and its individual components, a doubling of the serum creatinine concentration (**B**), end-stage renal disease (**C**), and the combined end point of end-stage renal disease or death (**D**). The mean follow-up time was 3.4 yr (42 mo). (*[119]*.)

available to all who need it in Brazil, many of the world's other transitional and disadvantaged populations with DN are more like those in Nigeria, where there is no government funding for dialysis or it is reserved for people with acute renal failure *(124,125)*. In South Africa, dialysis is provided only as a bridge to transplantation when a living donor is available *(126)*. Technology itself is not the restricting factor, as dialysis is available in large cities within developing nations and used by wealthy people who can pay for each treatment *(127)*. Rather, the prohibitive cost of dialysis is the problem, and most people with irreversible kidney failure secondary to DN cannot afford dialysis and therefore die.

Dialysis in Remote Locations

The difficulties of providing dialysis to patients who live in remote locations are considerable *(128)*. The Australian Remote Area Dialysis Program was established in 1989 by the Royal Perth Hospital and oversees many patients on home hemodialysis. Because nearly half of indigenous patients with ESRD come from regions without dialysis facilities *(129)*, practitioners have had to develop other novel approaches to dialysis. "Community hemodialysis" is used in some areas—a dialysis machine is located at a community center in a small village and shared by two or more patients. Patients use the dialysis machine with the assistance of a paid caregiver who has undergone basic training in its set-up and use *(130)*. Continuous ambulatory peritoneal dialysis is another dialysis modality that can be used in remote locations *(131)*. However, long-term continuous ambulatory peritoneal dialysis is limited in both indigenous Australians and indigenous Canadians by high rates of infection *(132,133)*.

Disparities in Dialysis

Within developed nations, members of transitional and disadvantaged populations are disproportionately represented among dialysis patients *(134)*. Limited access to care in the early and middle stages of kidney disease may be responsible, in part, for this disparity. Limited access to expert care may also result in "late" referral to a nephrologist. When patients start dialysis within 3 or 4 mo of their first visit with a nephrologist, the window of opportunity to slow the kidney disease has long passed. Data from the USRDS suggest that African Americans, Hispanics, and Asians are disproportionately represented among patients with late referral *(135,136)*. Once started on dialysis, ethnic minorities may receive an inadequate dose of dialysis relative to whites *(137)*. Patients who receive lower doses of dialysis have higher mortality rates *(138)*.

Nonetheless, members of transitional and disadvantaged populations who receive dialysis often have lower mortality rates than their white counterparts, both in the United States *(139)* and in the United Kingdom *(140)*. Higher cardiovascular mortality among whites treated with dialysis may be responsible for this finding *(141)*. Among diabetic dialysis patients, Hispanics have lower mortality than non-Hispanics *(142)* and Pima Indians have substantially lower mortality rates than diabetic blacks and whites of similar age *(143)*. Asian Americans have intermediate outcomes that are superior to both white and African Americans *(144)*. On the other hand, survival among dialysis patients was similar for indigenous (Native American) Canadians and white patients after adjustment for comorbidity *(145)* and in Australia, overall mortality rates for patients receiving renal replacement therapy (RRT) were higher among Maori and Aboriginals (but not Pacific Islanders) than among whites, even when adjusted for comorbidities *(146)*.

Kidney Transplantation

Kidney transplantation is considered the most desirable form of RRT, but rates of kidney transplant are limited worldwide by organ availability. Many studies find that transitional and disadvantaged populations have less access to kidney transplantation than the majority population *(147,148)*.

In the United States, African Americans undergo renal transplantation less often than whites, in part because they are less likely to want a kidney transplant, but also because African Americans who do want a kidney transplant are less likely to be referred to transplant centers, even after adjusting for coexisting morbidity *(149)*. Moreover, once referred, African Americans are less likely than whites to complete the evaluation necessary before being listed for transplant *(150,151)*. Barriers to completion include limited access to transportation, child-care responsibilities, and lack of available time away from work; factors that affect transitional and disadvantaged populations disproportionately. After receiving a kidney transplant, African Americans have shorter graft survival than whites *(152)*.

In Australia and New Zealand, the proportion of indigenous patients, including Pacific Islanders, who are referred for kidney transplantation is lower than among non-indigenous patients. Furthermore, once accepted for transplantation, indigenous people are less likely to receive a graft. This finding is due, in part, to lower rates of living donation among Aboriginal patients, but among the Maori rates of living donation are equal to those of non-indigenous donation and Pacific Islanders are actually more likely to participate in living donation than non-indigenous families. Among those who received cadaveric grafts, indigenous people receive fewer well-matched grafts *(146)*.

In the United Kingdom, Indo-Asian patients are slightly less likely to be referred for transplant than whites, their rates of transplantation are lower, and they are more likely to receive grafts with less human leukocyte antigen matches. Transplant survival is also lower among Indo-Asians than whites in the United Kingdom *(153)*.

In Pakistan, kidney transplantation offers the best hope for survival for many patients with kidney failure. Given the absence of governmental funding for dialysis, patients with ESRD and a paid or otherwise willing donor can receive a kidney transplant at a fraction of the cost of dialysis. One program in Pakistan funds kidney transplantation through a community–government partnership. Through this program, more than 100 kidney transplants have been performed each year since 1995 and free immunosuppressive drugs are given to those who receive a transplant *(154)*. Partnerships of this sort may offer hope to people with kidney failure in many parts of the developing world, where the costs of dialysis are beyond reach.

RENOPROTECTION AND FINANCIAL CONSIDERATIONS

The bulk of the cost of treating DN is the cost of providing RRT to patients who develop ESRD. Worldwide, the total population of patients with diabetic ESRD is expected to double *(155)* and the worldwide cost is expected to exceed US $1 trillion by the year 2010 *(156)*. Of the million-plus people in the world who are currently receiving dialysis, 90% live in the developed world, where the health care budget can accommodate treatments that may cost US $66,000 per patient per year *(157,158)*. But transitional and dis-advantaged patients living in the developing world generally do not receive RRT because the cost is prohibitive. Consequently, treatments directed at preventing DN or slowing its progression are essential to the management of these patients. If the decline in GFR could be slowed by merely 10% in patients with GFR less than 60 mL/min, the cumulative saving from reduced dialysis costs would be approx $18 billion in the United States between 2002 and 2010 *(159)*. Because transitional and disadvantaged patients in developing nations are generally not offered dialysis, the worldwide benefit of early treatment could best be measured in terms of lives saved rather than in dollars spent.

CONCLUSIONS

In conclusion, diabetic kidney failure is a common and growing problem in many transitional and disadvantaged populations throughout the world. Poverty and, paradoxically, the rapid emergence from poverty are, in part, responsible for the growing epidemic because these factors increase the risk of diabetes. Unfortunately, particularly in developing countries, the costs associated with management of diabetic kidney failure already far exceed the available resources. Accordingly, efforts should be directed toward reducing the number of people who reach kidney failure, through diabetes prevention and early screening and intervention in those who already have diabetes.

REFERENCES

1. Wild S, Roglic G, Green A, Sicree R, King H. Global prevalence of diabetes: estimates for the year 2000 and projections for 2030. Diabetes Care 2004;27(5):1047–1053.
2. Caballero B, Rubinstein S. Environmental factors affecting nutritional status in urban areas of developing countries. Arch Latinoam Nutr 1997;47(2 Suppl 1):3–8.
3. http://www.fao.org/FOCUS/E/obesity/obes2.htm. Retrieved April 21, 2005.
4. Kuhnlein HV, Receveur O. Dietary change and traditional food systems of indigenous peoples. Annu Rev Nutr 1996;16:417–442.
5. Gall MA, Hougaard P, Borch-Johnsen K, Parving HH. Risk factors for development of incipient and overt diabetic nephropathy in patients with non-insulin dependent diabetes mellitus: prospective, observational study. BMJ 1997;314:783–788.
6. UK Prospective Diabetes Study Group. UK Prospective Diabetes Study. XII: Differences between Asian, Afro-Caribbean and white Caucasian type 2 diabetic patients at diagnosis of diabetes. Diabet Med 1994;11:670–677.
7. Young BA, Katon WJ, Von Korff M, et al. Racial and ethnic differences in microalbuminuria prevalence in a diabetes population: the pathways study. J Am Soc Nephrol 2005;16:219–228.
8. U.S. Renal Data System. USRDS 2004 Annual Data Report: Atlas of End-Stage Renal Disease in the United States, National Institutes of Health, National Institute of Diabetes and Digestive and Kidney Diseases, Bethesda, MD, 2004.
9. Clark TJ, Richards NT, Adu D, Michael J. Increased prevalence of dialysis dependent renal failure in ethnic minorities in the West Midlands. Nephr Dial Transplant 1993;8:146–148.
10. Lightstone L, Rees AJ, Tomson C, Walls J, Winearls CG, Feehally J. High incidence of end-stage renal disease in Indo-Asians in the UK. QJM 1995;88:191–195.
11. Chandie Shaw PK, Vandenbroucke JP, Tjandra YI, et al. Increased end-stage diabetic nephropathy in Indo-Asian immigrants living in the Netherlands. Diabetologia 2002;45:337–341.
12. Khebir BV, Osman A, Khalid BA. Changing prevalence of diabetes mellitus amongst rural Malays in Kuala Selangor over a 10-year period. Med J Malaysia 1996;51:41–47.
13. Hooi LS, Wong HS, Morad Z. Prevention of renal failure: The Malaysian experience. Kidney Int Suppl 2005;94:S70–S74.
14. Wu AY, Kong NC, de Leon FA, et al. MAPS Investigators. An alarmingly high prevalence of diabetic nephropathy in Asian type 2 diabetic patients: the Microalbuminuria Prevalence (MAP) Study. Diabetologia 2005;48:17–26.
15. Jones CA, Francis ME, Eberhardt MS, et al. Microalbuminuria in the US population: third national health and nutrition examination survey. Am J Kidney Dis 2002;39:445–459.
16. Stewart JH, McCredie MR, McDonald SP. Incidence of end-stage renal disease in overseas-born, compared with Australian-born, non-indigenous Australians. Nephrology (Carlton) 2004;9:247–252.
17. Mau MK, West M, Sugihara J, Kamaka M, Mikami J, Cheng SF. Renal disease disparities in Asian and Pacific-based populations in Hawaii. J Natl Med Assoc 2003;95:955–963.

18. Varghese A, Deepa R, Rema M, Mohan V. Prevalence of microalbuminuria in type 2 diabetes mellitus at a diabetes centre in southern India. Postgrad Med J 2001;77:399–402.
19. Ramachandran A, Snehalatha C, Latha E, Vijay V, Viswanathan M. Rising prevalence of NIDDM in an urban population in India. Diabetologia 1997;40:232–237.
20. Mani MK. Experience with a program for prevention of chronic renal failure in India. Kidney Int Suppl 2005;(94):S75–S78.
21. Ball S, Lloyd J, Cairns T, et al. Why is there so much end-stage renal failure of undetermined cause in UK Indo-Asians? QJM 2001;94:187–193.
22. Collins VR, Dowse GK, Finch CF, Zimmet PZ, Linnane AW. Prevalence and risk factors for micro- and macroalbuminuria in diabetic subjects and entire population of Nauru. Diabetes 1989;38: 1602–1610.
23. Hodge AM, Dowse GK, Zimmet PZ. Microalbuminuria, cardiovascular risk factors, and insulin resistance in two populations with a high risk of type 2 diabetes mellitus. Diabet Med 1996;13:441–449.
24. Simmons D, Shaw LM, Scott DJ, Kenealy T, Scragg RK. Diabetic nephropathy and microalbuminuria in the community. The South Auckland Diabetes Survey. Diabet Care 1994;17:1404–1410.
25. Abidi SM, Negrete HO, Zahid I, Bennett PH, Nelson RG. Diabetic end-stager renal disease in the indigenous population of the Commonwealth of the Northern Mariana islands. Nephrology 2005; 10:291–295.
26. Rowley KG, Iser DM, Best JD, O'Dea K, Leonard D, McDermott R. Albuminuria in Australian Aboriginal people: prevalence and associations with components of the metabolic syndrome. Diabetologia 2000;43:1397–1403.
27. McGill MJ, Donnelly R, Molyneaux L, Yue DK. Ethnic differences in the prevalence of hypertension and proteinuria in NIDDM. Diabetes Res Clin Pract 1996;33(3):173–179.
28. Cass A, Cunningham J, Snelling P, Wang Z, Hoy W. End-stage renal disease in indigenous Australians: a disease of disadvantage. Ethn Dis 2002;12:373–378.
29. Stewart JH, McCredie MR, McDonald SP. The incidence of treated end-stage renal disease in New Zealand Maori and Pacific Island people and in Indigenous Australians. Nephrol Dial Transplant 2004;19:678–685.
30. Kohler KA, McClellan WM, Ziemer DC, Kleinbaum DG, Boring JR. Risk factors for microalbuminuria in black Americans with newly diagnosed type 2 diabetes. Am J Kidney Dis 2000;36: 903–913.
31. Konen JC, Summerson JH, Bell RA. Abnormal urinary protein excretion in African Americans with type 2 diabetes mellitus. Ethn Dis 1999;9(1):3–9.
32. Young BA, Katon WJ, Von Korff M, et al. Racial and ethnic differences in microalbuminuria prevalence in a diabetes population: the pathways study. J Am Soc Nephrol. 2005;16:219–228.
33. Oli JM, Watkins PJ, Wild B, Adegoke OJ. Albuminuria in Afro-Caribbeans with type 2 diabetes mellitus: is the sickle cell trait a risk factor? Diabet Med 2004;21:483–486.
34 Flegal KM, Ezzati TM, Harris MI, et al. Prevalence of diabetes in Mexican Americans, Cubans, and Puerto Ricans from the Hispanic health and nutrition examination survey, 1982–1984. Diabetes Care 1991;14:628–638.
35. Kuo YF, Raji MA, Markides KS, Ray LA, Espino DV, Goodwin JS. Inconsistent use of diabetes medications, diabetes complications, and mortality in older Mexican Americans over a 7-year period: data from the Hispanic established population for the epidemiologic study of the elderly. Diabetes Care 2003;26:3054–3060.
36. Gonzalez Villalpando C, Stern MP, Arredondo Perez B, et al. Nephropathy in low income diabetics: the Mexico City diabetes study. Arch Med Res 1996;27:367–72.
37. Narva AS. Kidney disease in Native Americans. J Natl Med Assoc 2002;94:738–742.
38. Nelson RG, Morgenstern H, Bennett PH. Intrauterine diabetes exposure and the risk of renal disease in diabetic Pima Indians. Diabetes 1998;47:1489–1493.
39. Burrows NR, Narva AS, Geiss LS, Engelgau MM, Acton KJ. End-stage renal disease due to diabetes among southwestern American Indians, 1990-2001. Diabetes Care 2005;28:1041–1044.
40. Phipps K, Barker DJ, Hales CN, Fall CH, Osmond C, Clark PM. Fetal growth and impaired glucose tolerance in men and women. Diabetologia 1993;36:225–228.
41. Hales CN, Barker DJ, Clark PM, et al. Fetal and infant growth and impaired glucose tolerance at age 64. BMJ 1991;303:1019–1022.
42. Barker DJ, Hales CN, Fall CH, Osmond C, Phipps K, Clark PM. Type 2 (non-insulin-dependent) diabetes mellitus, hypertension and hyperlipidaemia (syndrome X): relation to reduced fetal growth. Diabetologia 1993;36:62–67.

43. Lopes AA, Port FK. Differences in the patterns of age-specific black/white comparisons between end-stage renal disease attributed and not attributed to diabetes. Am J Kidney Dis 1995;25: 714–721.
44. Nelson RG, Morgenstern H, Bennett PH. Birth weight and renal disease in Pima Indians with type 2 diabetes mellitus. Am J Epidemiol 1998;148:650–656.
45. de Onis M, Blossner M, Villar J. Levels and patterns of intrauterine growth retardation in developing countries. Eur J Clin Nutr 1998;52 Suppl. (1):S5–S15.
46. Lemley KV. A basis for accelerated progression of diabetic nephropathy in Pima Indians. Kidney Int Suppl 2003;83:S38–S42.
47. Singh GR, Hoy WE. Kidney volume, blood pressure, and albuminuria: findings in an Australian aboriginal community. Am J Kidney Dis 2004;43:254–259.
48. Young RJ, Hoy WE, Kincaid-Smith P, Seymour AE, Bertram JF. Glomerular size and glomerulosclerosis in Australian aborigines. Am J Kidney Dis 2000;36:481–489.
49. Bertram JF, Young RJ, Seymour AE, Kincaid-Smith P, Hoy W. Glomerulomegaly in Australian Aborigines. Nephrology 1998;4:S46–S53.
50. Schmidt K, Pesce C, Liu Q, et al. Large glomerular size in Pima Indians: lack of change with diabetic nephropathy. J Am Soc Nephrol 1992;3:229–235.
51. Pagtalunan ME, Miller PL, Jumping-Eagle S, et al. Podocyte loss and progressive glomerular injury in type II diabetes. J Clin Invest 1997;99:342–348.
52. Amri K, Freund N, Vilar J, Merlet-Benichou C, Lelievre-Pegorier M. Adverse effects of hyperglycemia on kidney development in rats: in vivo and in vitro studies. Diabetes 1999;48: 2240–2245.
53. Dabelea D, Pettitt DJ. Intrauterine diabetic environment confers risks for type 2 diabetes mellitus and obesity in the offspring, in addition to genetic susceptibility. J Pediatr Endocrinol Metab 2001;14:1085–1091.
54. Nelson RG. Intrauterine determinants of diabetic kidney disease in disadvantaged populations. Kidney Int Suppl 2003;83:S13–S16.
55. Merlet-Benichou C. Influence of fetal environment on kidney development. Int J Dev Biol 1999;43: 453–456.
56. Thomas M. Antecedents of renal disease in Aborigines. Nephrology (Carlton) 2004;9(4):S113–S116.
57. Moore L, Lloyd MS, Puglsey D, Seymour AE. Renal disease in the Australian Aboriginal population: a pathological study. Nephrology 1996;2:315–321.
58. Thomas M. Kidney disease in Australian Aboriginals: time for decisive action. MJA 1998;168: 532–533.
59. Yaqoob M, Patrick AW, McClelland P, et al. Occupational hydrocarbon exposure and diabetic nephropathy. Diabet Med 1994;11:789–793.
60. Tsaih SW, Korrick S, Schwartz J, et al. Lead, diabetes, hypertension, and renal function: the normative aging study. Environ Health Perspect 2004;112:1178–1182.
61. Biesenbach G, Grafinger P, Janko O, Zazgornik J. Influence of cigarette-smoking on the progression of clinical diabetic nephropathy in type 2 diabetic patients. Clin Nephrol 1997;48:146–150.
62. Orth SR, Stockmann A, Conradt C, et al. Smoking as a risk factor for end-stage renal failure in men with primary renal disease. Kidney Int 1998;54:926–931.
63. Muhlhauser I. Cigarette smoking and diabetes: an update. Diabet Med 1994;11:336–343.
64. da Costa e Silva VL, Koifman S. Smoking in Latin America: a major public health problem. Cad Saude Publica 1998;14(3):99–108.
65. Kohler KA, McClellan WM, Ziemer DC, Kleinbaum DG, Boring JR. Smoking and microalbuminuria: a case–control study in African-Americans with type 2 diabetes. Diabetes Care 2002;25:243–245.
66. Barbeau EM, Wolin KY, Naumova EN, Balbach E. Tobacco advertising in communities: associations with race and class. Prev Med 2005;40:16–22.
67. Perkins JJ, Sanson-Fisher RW, Blunden S, Lunnay D, Redman S, Hensley MJ. The prevalence of drug use in urban aboriginal communities. Addiction 1994;89:1319–1331.
68. Chen X, Li X, Stanton B, et al. Cigarette smoking among rural-to-urban migrants in Beijing, China. Prev Med 2004;39:666–673.
69. Ramachandran A, Snehalatha C, Vinitha R, et al. Prevalence of overweight in urban Indian adolescent school children. Diabetes Res Clin Pract 2002;57:185–190.
70. Pazmino PA, Pazmino AK. Diabetic renal failure in Texas: influence of ethnicity and household income. Tex Med 2003;99:57–65.
71. Brancati FL, Whelton PK, Kuller LH, Klag MJ. Diabetes mellitus, race, and socioeconomic status. A population-based study. Ann Epidemiol 1996;6:67–73.

72. Hazuda HP, Haffner SM, Stern MP, Eifler CW. Effects of acculturation and socioeconomic status on obesity and diabetes in Mexican Americans. The San Antonio Heart Study. Am J Epidemiol 1988; 128:1289–1301.
73. Harris MI, Flegal KM, Cowie CC, et al. Prevalence of diabetes, impaired fasting glucose, and impaired glucose tolerance in U.S. adults. The third national health and nutrition examination survey, 1988–1994. Diabetes Care 1998;21:518–524.
74. Kuo YF, Raji MA, Markides KS, Ray LA, Espino DV, Goodwin JS. Inconsistent use of diabetes medications, diabetes complications, and mortality in older Mexican Americans over a 7-year period: data from the Hispanic established population for the epidemiologic study of the elderly. Diabetes Care 2003;26:3054–3060.
75. Kasiske BL, Rith-Najarian S, Casper ML, Croft JB. American Indian heritage and risk factors for renal injury. Kidney Int 1998;54:1305–1310.
76. Krop JS, Coresh J, Chambless LE, et al. A community-based study of explanatory factors for the excess risk for early renal function decline in blacks vs whites with diabetes: the Atherosclerosis risk in communities study. Arch Intern Med 1999;159:1777–1783.
77. Shobhana R, Begum R, Snehalatha C, Vijay V, Ramachandran A. Patients' adherence to diabetes treatment. J Assoc Physicians India 1999;47:1173–1175.
78. Ad Hoc Committee on Health Literacy for the Council on Scientific Affairs, American Medical Association. Health Literacy: Report of the council on scientific affairs. JAMA 1999;281:552–557.
79. Georges CA, Bolton LB, Bennett C. Functional health literacy: an issue in African-American and other ethnic and racial communities. J Natl Black Nurses Assoc 2004;15:1–4.
80. Schillinger D, Bindman A, Wang F, Stewart A, Piette J. Functional health literacy and the quality of physician-patient communication among diabetes patients. Patient Educ Couns 2004;52:315–323.
81. Larkey LK, Hecht ML, Miller K, Alatorre C. Hispanic cultural norms for health-seeking behaviors in the face of symptoms. Health Educ Behav 2001;28:65–80.
82. Rosen AB, Karter AJ, Liu JY, Selby JV, Schneider EC. Use of angiotensin-converting enzyme inhibitors and angiotensin receptor blockers in high-risk clinical and ethnic groups with diabetes. J Gen Int Med 2004;19:669–675.
83. Karter AJ, Ferrara A, Liu JY, Moffet HH, Ackerson LM, Selby JV. Ethnic disparities in diabetic complications in an insured population. JAMA 2002;287:2519–2527. Erratum in: JAMA 2002; 288:46.
84. Hebert LA, Kusek JW, Greene T, et al. Effects of blood pressure control on progressive renal disease in blacks and whites. Modification of Diet in Renal Disease Study Group. Hypertension 1997;30 (3 Part 1):428–435.
85. Nosadini R, Velussi M, Brocco E, et al. Course of renal function in type 2 diabetic patients with abnormalities of albumin excretion rate. Diabetes 2000;49:476–484.
86. Earle KK, Porter KA, Ostberg J, Yudkin JS. Variation in the progression of diabetic nephropathy according to racial origin. Nephrol Dial Transplant 2001;16:286–290.
87. Hoy W, McDonald SP. Albuminuria: marker or target in indigenous populations. Kidney Int Suppl 2004;92:S25–S31.
88. Jones CA, Francis ME, Eberhardt MS, et al. Microalbuminuria in the US population: third National Health and Nutrition Examination Survey. Am J Kidney Dis 2002;39:445–459.
89. Gerstein HC, Mann JF, Yi Q, et al. Albuminuria and risk of cardiovascular events, death, and heart failure in diabetic and nondiabetic individuals. JAMA 2001;286:421–426.
90. Palmieri V, Tracy RP, Roman MJ, et al. Strong Heart Study. Relation of left ventricular hypertrophy to inflammation and albuminuria in adults with type 2 diabetes: the strong heart study. Diabetes Care 2003;26:2764–2769.
91. Centers for Disease Control and Prevention (CDC). Health disparities experienced by black or African Americans—United States. MMWR Morb Mortal Wkly Rep 2005;54:1–3.
92. Abbott KC, Hypolite I, Welch PG, Agodoa LY. Human immunodeficiency virus/acquired immunodeficiency syndrome-associated nephropathy at end-stage renal disease in the United States: patient characteristics and survival in the pre highly active antiretroviral therapy era. J Nephrol 2001;14: 377–383.
93. Currie BJ, Carapetis JR. Skin infections and infestations in Aboriginal communities in northern Australia. Australas J Dermatol 2000;41:139–143.
94. Thomas M. Deprivation and dialysis: pathways to kidney failure in Australian Aborigines. Adv Chronic Kidney Dis 2005;12:84–87.
95. Haas M. Postinfectious glomerulonephritis complicating diabetic nephropathy: a frequent association, but how clinically important? Hum Pathol 2003;34:1225–1227.

96. Thuluvath PJ, John PR. Association between hepatitis C, diabetes mellitus, and race. a case–control study. Am J Gastroenterol 2003;98:438–441.
97. el-Zayadi AR, Selim OE, Hamdy H, Dabbous H, Ahdy A, Moniem SA. Association of chronic hepatitis C infection and diabetes mellitus. Trop Gastroenterol 1998;19:141–144.
98. Knobler H, Schattner A. TNF-{alpha}, chronic hepatitis C and diabetes: a novel triad. QJM 2005; 98:1–6.
99. Gray H, Wreghitt T, Stratton IM, Alexander GJ, Turner RC, O'Rahilly S. High prevalence of hepatitis C infection in Afro-Caribbean patients with type 2 diabetes and abnormal liver function tests. Diabet Med 1995;12:244–249.
100. Wilson C. Hepatitis C infection and type 2 diabetes in American-Indian women. Diabetes Care 2004;27:2116–2119.
101. Liangpunsakul S, Chalasani N. Relationship between hepatitis C and microalbuminuria: results from the NHANES III. Kidney Int 2005;67:285–290.
102. Crook ED, Patel SR. Diabetic nephropathy in African-American patients. Curr Diab Rep 2004;4: 455–461.
103. Knowler WC, Barrett-Connor E, Fowler SE, et al. Reduction in the incidence of type 2 diabetes with lifestyle intervention or metformin. N Engl J Med 2002;346:393–403.
104. Macaulay AC, Paradis G, Potvin L, et al. The Kahnawake schools diabetes prevention project: intervention, evaluation, and baseline results of a diabetes primary prevention program with a native community in Canada. Prev Med 1997;26:779–790.
105. Paradis G, Levesque L, Macaulay AC, et al. Impact of a diabetes prevention program on body size, physical activity, and diet among Kanien'keha:ka (Mohawk) children 6 to 11 years old: 8-year results from the Kahnawake schools diabetes prevention project. Pediatrics 2005;115:333–339.
106. Devanesen D, Intersectoral action for Aboriginal primary health care. Paper presented at AAHPP and PHA (HPSIG) Ninth national health promotion conference. People, places and programs: exploring better practice in health promotion for diverse Populations. 18029, The Baufort Hotel, Darwin. Subsequently published at http://www.nt.gov.au/health/pdf/Intersec.%20Action.pdf
107. Irish A, Warr K, Snelling P. Foreword from the organisers. Nephrology (Carlton) 2004;9(Suppl 4): S107,S108.
108. Cass A, Lowell A, Christie M, et al. Sharing the true stories: improving communication between Aboriginal patients and healthcare workers. Med J Aust 2002;176:466–470.
109. O'Hare JP, Raymond NT, Mughal S, et al. Evaluation of delivery of enhanced diabetes care to patients of South Asian ethnicity: the United Kingdom Asian diabetes study (UKADS). Diabet Med 2004;21: 1357–1365.
110. Schieppati A, Perico N, Remuzzi G. Preventing end-stage renal disease: the potential impact of screening and intervention in developing countries. Kidney Int 2003;63:1948–1950.
111. Plata R, Silva C, Yahuita J, Perez L, Schieppati A, Remuzzi G. The first clinical and epidemiological programme on renal disease in Bolivia: a model for prevention and early diagnosis of renal diseases in the developing countries. Nephrol Dial Transplant 1998;13:3034–3036.
112. National Kidney Foundation. Kidney Early Evaluation Program. Am J Kidney Dis 2005;45(2 Suppl 2): S1–S135.
113. Hoy WE, Baker PR, Kelly AM, Wang Z. Reducing premature death and renal failure in Australian aboriginals. A community-based cardiovascular and renal protective program. Med J Aust 2000; 172:473–478.
114. Hoy WE, Wang Z, Baker PR, Kelly AM. Secondary prevention of renal and cardiovascular disease: results of a renal and cardiovascular treatment program in an Australian aboriginal community. J Am Soc Nephrol 2003;14(7 Suppl 2):S178–S185.
115. Hoy WE, Wang Z, Baker PR, Kelly AM. Reduction in natural death and renal failure from a systematic screening and treatment program in an Australian Aboriginal community. Kidney Int Suppl 2003;83:S66–S73.
116. Frimat L, Loos-Ayav C, Panescu V, Cordebar N, Briancon S, Kessler M. Early referral to a nephrologist is associated with better outcomes in type 2 diabetes patients with end-stage renal disease. Diabetes Metab 2004;30:67–74.
117. Ifudu O, Friedman EA. Managing chronic renal insufficiency—intertwined roles of non-nephrologist and nephrologist. J Natl Med Assoc 2003;95:43–54.
118. O'Sullivan C, Brady SJ, Lawton PD, Love CM. Everybody's business. Nephrology (Carlton) 2004;9(Suppl 4):S117–S120.
119. Brenner BM, Cooper ME, de Zeeuw D, et al. Effects of losartan on renal and cardiovascular outcomes in patients with type 2 diabetes and nephropathy. N Engl J Med 2001;345:861–869.

120. Lewis EJ, Hunsicker LG, Clarke WR, et al. Renoprotective effect of the angiotensin-receptor antagonist irbesartan in patients with nephropathy due to type 2 diabetes. N Engl J Med 2001;345:851–860.
121. Chan JC, Wat NM, So WY, et al. Renin angiotensin aldosterone system blockade and renal disease in patients with type 2 diabetes. An Asian perspective from the RENAAL Study. Diabetes Care 2004; 27:874–879.
122. Reddy KS. Cardiovascular diseases in the developing countries: dimensions, determinants, dynamics and directions for public health action. Public Health Nutr 2002;5:231–237.
123. Gaede P, Vedel P, Larsen N, Jensen GV, Parving HH, Pedersen O. Multifactorial intervention and cardiovascular disease in patients with type 2 diabetes. N Engl J Med 2003;348:383–393.
124. Zatz R, Romao JE, Jr, Noronha IL. Nephrology in Latin America, with special emphasis on Brazil. Kidney Int Suppl 2003;83:S131–S134.
125. Bamgboye EL. Hemodialysis: management problems in developing countries, with Nigeria as a surrogate. Kidney Int Suppl 2003;83:S93–S95.
126. Naicker S. End-stage renal disease in sub-Saharan and South Africa. Kidney Int Suppl 2003;83:S119–S122.
127. De Vecchi AF, Dratwa M, Wiedemann ME. Healthcare systems and end-stage renal disease (ESRD) therapies—an international review: costs and reimbursement/funding of ESRD therapies. Nephrol Dial Transplant 1999;14(Suppl 6):31–41.
128. Villarba A, Warr K. Home haemodialysis in remote Australia. Nephrology (Carlton) 2004; 9(Suppl 4):S134–S137.
129. Cass A, Cunningham J, Wang Z, Hoy W. Regional variation in the incidence of end-stage renal disease in Indigenous Australians. Med J Aust 2001;175:24–27.
130. Kneipp E, Murray R, Warr K, Fitzclarence C, Wearne M, Maguire G. Bring me home: renal dialysis in the Kimberley. Nephrology (Carlton) 2004;9(4):S121–S125.
131. Carruthers D, Warr K. Supporting peritoneal dialysis in remote Australia. Nephrology (Carlton) 2004;9(4):S129–S133.
132. Lim WH. Is there a role for peritoneal dialysis in remote aboriginal patients with end-stage renal disease in Australia? Nephrology (Carlton) 2004;9(4):S126–S128.
133. Tonelli M, Hemmelgarn B, Manns B, et al. Use and outcomes of peritoneal dialysis among Aboriginal people in Canada. J Am Soc Nephrol 2005;16:482–488.
134. Feldman HI, Klag MJ, Chiapella AP, Whelton PK. End-stage renal disease in US minority groups. Am J Kidney Dis 1992;19:397–410.
135. Ifudu O, Dawood M, Iofel Y, Valcourt JS, Friedman EA. Delayed referral of black, Hispanic, and older patients with chronic renal failure. Am J Kidney Dis 1999;33:728–733.
136. Kausz AT, Obrador GT, Arora P, Ruthazer R, Levey AS, Pereira BJ. Late initiation of dialysis among women and ethnic minorities in the United States. J Am Soc Nephrol 2000;11:2351–2357.
137. Owen WF, Jr, Chertow GM, Lazarus JM, Lowrie EG. Dose of hemodialysis and survival: differences by race and sex. JAMA 1998;280:1764–1768.
138. Eknoyan G, Beck GJ, Cheung AK, et al. Effect of dialysis dose and membrane flux in maintenance hemodialysis. N Engl J Med 2002;347(25):2010–2019.
139. Mesler DE, Byrne-Logan S, McCarthy EP, Ash AS, Moskowitz MA. How much better can we predict dialysis patient survival using clinical data? Health Serv Res 1999;34(1 Part 2):365–375.
140. Prasad S, Singh S, Duncan N, et al. Ethnicity and survival on dialysis in west London. Kidney Int 2004;66:2416–2421.
141. Parekh RS, Zhang L, Fivush BA, Klag MJ. Incidence of atherosclerosis by race in the dialysis morbidity and mortality study: a sample of the US ESRD population. J Am Soc Nephrol 2005;16:1420–1426
142. Murthy BV, Molony DA, Stack AG. Survival advantage of Hispanic patients initiating dialysis in the United States is modified by race. J Am Soc Nephrol 2005;16:782–790.
143. Nelson RG, Hanson RL, Pettitt DJ, Knowler WC, Bennett PH. Survival during renal replacement therapy for diabetic end-stage renal disease in Pima Indians. Diabetes Care 1996;19:1333–1337.
144. Frankenfield DL, Ramirez SP, McClellan WM, Frederick PR, Rocco MV. Differences in intermediate outcomes for Asian and non-Asian adult hemodialysis patients in the United States. Kidney Int 2003;64:623–631.
145. Dyck RF, Tan L. Rates and outcomes of diabetic end-stage renal disease among registered native people in Saskatchewan. Canadian Med Assoc J 1994;150:203–208.
146. McDonald SP, Russ GR. Current incidence, treatment patterns and outcome of end-stage renal disease among indigenous groups in Australia and New Zealand. Nephrology 2003;8:42–48.
147. Gadegbeku C, Freeman M, Agodoa L. Racial disparities in renal replacement therapy. J Natl Med Assoc 2002;94(8):45S–54S.

148. Sequist TD, Narva AS, Stiles SK, Karp SK, Cass A, Ayanian JZ. Access to renal transplantation among American Indians and Hispanics. Am J Kidney Dis 2004;44:344–352.
149. Ayanian JZ, Cleary PD, Weissman JS, Epstein AM. The effect of patients' preferences on racial differences in access to renal transplantation. N Engl J Med 1999;341:1661–1669.
150. Alexander GC, Sehgal AR. Barriers to cadaveric renal transplantation among blacks, women, and the poor. JAMA 1998;280:1148–1152.
151. Epstein AM, Ayanian JZ, Keogh JH, et al. Racial disparities in access to renal transplantation—clinically appropriate or due to underuse or overuse? N Engl J Med 2000;343:1537–1544.
152. Young CJ, Gaston RS. Renal transplantation in black Americans. N Engl J Med 2000;343: 1545–1552.
153. Jeffrey RF, Woodrow G, Mahler J, Johnson R, Newstead CG. Indo-Asian experience of renal transplantation in Yorkshire: results of a 10-year survey. Transplantation 2002;73:1652–1657.
154. Rizvi SA, Naqvi SA, Hussain Z, et al. Renal transplantation in developing countries. Kidney Int Suppl 2003;83:S96–S100.
155. Mitch WE. Treating diabetic nephropathy—are there only economic issues? N Engl J Med 2004;351: 1934–1936.
156. Dirks JH. The drumbeat of renal failure: symbiosis of prevention and renal replacement therapy. Blood Purif 2004;22:6–8.
157. Schieppati A, Perico N, Remuzzi G. Preventing end-stage renal disease: the potential impact of screening and intervention in developing countries. Nephrol Dial Transplant 2003;18:858–859.
158. Lysaght MJ. Maintenance dialysis population dynamics: current trends and long-term implications. J Am Soc Nephrol 2002;13(1):S37–S40.
159. Trivedi HS, Pang MM, Campbell A, Saab P. Slowing the progression of chronic renal failure: economic benefits and patients' perspectives. Am J Kidney Dis 2002;39:721–729.

II Clinical Aspects of Diabetic Nephropathy

C. Diagnosis and Treatment

23 Screening and Treatment of Early Diabetic Renal Disease in Type 1 and Type 2 Diabetes

Ellie Chuang, MD *and Mark E. Molitch,* MD

Contents

INTRODUCTION

As has been discussed elsewhere in this text, diabetes mellitus is the leading cause of end-stage renal disease (ESRD) and the care of patients with diabetes and ESRD contributes significantly to health care costs. Of patients with type 1 diabetes, approx 20–30% will eventually develop ESRD *(1–5)*, whereas about 10–20% of those with type 2 diabetes will do so *(2,5–8)*. In the past couple of decades, there have been notable advances in our knowledge regarding the early stages of diabetic kidney disease, including the advent of interventions that can significantly slow or even reverse the course of progressive disease. In this chapter, we will review the definition and detection of early diabetic kidney disease, its natural history, current proven therapies, and potential future therapies.

DEFINITION AND NATURAL HISTORY

It is known that diabetic nephropathy (DN) can be detected before the onset of decreased glomerular filtration rate (GFR) in most patients by detecting abnormal amounts of albumin in the urine. Two stages have been designated: microalbuminuria (defined as urine albumin between 30 and 300 mg/24 h, 20–200 μg/min on a timed sample, or spot urine albumin to creatinine ratio 30–300 mg/g) and albuminuria, also termed clinical albuminuria, macroalbuminuria, and overt nephropathy (>300 mg/24 h, >200 μg/min on a timed sample, or spot urine albumin to creatinine [ACR] ratio >300 mg/g). Short-term hyperglycemia, exercise, urinary tract infections, marked hypertension, heart failure, and acute, febrile illness can cause transient elevations *(9)*; there is also marked day-to-day variability in albumin excretion, so that at least two of

From: *Contemporary Diabetes: The Diabetic Kidney*
Edited by: P. Cortes and C. E. Mogensen © Humana Press Inc., Totowa, NJ

three collections done should show elevated levels before a patient is designated as having microalbuminuria.

In type 1 diabetes, microalbuminuria is rarely present at diagnosis, but persistent and untreated microalbuminuria will progress to albuminuria in 30–80% of individuals over 10–15 yr, and of those, 50–78% will progress to ESRD over the next 10–18 yr *(1–5,10)*. Hypertension usually develops as a complication of nephropathy. In type 2 diabetes, microalbuminuria and even albuminuria may be present at or soon after diagnosis, in part due to the fact that diabetes has often already been present for years. Left untreated, 20–40% of such patients will develop overt nephropathy, with only approx 20% of those patients progressing to ESRD over the next 20 yr *(5,7,8,11)*. In fact, more patients with albuminuria and type 2 diabetes will die from cardiovascular disease than progress to ESRD *(12,13)*. Hypertension is frequently already present at the time of diagnosis of diabetes, often as part of the metabolic syndrome. Based on the current evidence that early intervention may slow the progression of diabetic kidney disease, it is now the standard of care to do annual screening for microalbuminuria, in type 1 diabetes starting at puberty or 5 yr after diagnosis, and in type 2 diabetes beginning at diagnosis *(14)*.

However, cross-sectional studies have found decreased GFR in the absence of increased urine albumin excretion (UAE) in a substantial percentage of adults with type 2 diabetes *(15)*. In the Third National Health and Nutrition Examination Survey, which collected demographic and health information from a nationally representative sample of the US population, 13% of adults with type 2 diabetes had a GFR <60 mL/min/1.73 m^2. Among these, an absence of increased UAE (defined in this study as a spot urine ACR ≥17 mg/g in men and ≥25 mg/g in women) was noted in approx 40%, whereas absence of both increased UAE and diabetic retinopathy was noted in 30% *(15)*. Decreased GFR in the absence of increased UAE among adults with both type 1 and 2 diabetes have also been reported in other studies *(16)*. In follow-up, the rates of decline of GFR in those with type 2 diabetes with initial GFR levels <60 mL/min/1.73 m^2 were similar, regardless of the presence or absence of albuminuria *(17)*. Thus, these studies demonstrate that substantial declines in GFR may be noted in adults with type 1 and 2 diabetes in the absence of increased UAE. Because these studies did not perform kidney biopsies, investigators can only speculate on the etiology of decreased GFR in the absence of increased UAE. Pathological evidence of DN has been documented in adults with diabetes even in the absence of increased UAE *(18,19)*. In addition, older patients with type 2 diabetes may also have vascular and tubulo-interstitial changes owing to the presence of comorbid conditions, including long-standing hypertension and renal vascular disease, and potential senescence of glomeruli owing to aging itself *(20,21)*. Conversely, studies have also reported a range of biopsy findings from normal to typical diabetic changes and frequently other kidney diseases in adults with type 2 diabetes and increased UAE *(22–24)*. Therefore, in addition to yearly screening for albuminuria, the yearly measurement of serum creatinine with estimation of GFR using the adjusted Modification Diet in Renal Disease (MDRD) *(25)* or other formulas *(26–28)* should also be carried out.

CURRENT TARGETS FOR INTERVENTION

Glycemic Control

Several large prospective randomized trials have demonstrated the efficacy of improved glycemic control in preventing progression of diabetic kidney disease in persons with type 1 diabetes. A number of observational studies have shown that the development of microalbuminuria is associated with poorer glycemic control *(6,29–34)*. Several small, prospective, interventional studies from the early 1980s showed that improved glycemic control caused a decrease in the development and progression of albuminuria but in most cases, the small sizes of the cohorts precluded statistical significance *(35–41)*. A meta-analysis of these studies concluded that intensive therapy significantly reduced the risk of nephropathy progression (OR 0.34, 95% CI 0.20–0.58, $p < 0.001$) *(42)*. The Diabetes Control and Complications Trial (DCCT) of 1441 subjects with type 1 diabetes showed that an intensive glycemic control regimen compared with a conventional control regimen resulted in a sustained mean hemoglobin (Hb)A_{1c} 2% lower with the intensive regimen *(43)*. After a mean duration of 9 yr, the intensively treated subjects showed significantly lower rates of microalbuminuria compared with the conventionally treated subjects, in both the primary prevention group (risk reduction 34%) and the secondary prevention group (risk reduction 43%) *(43,44)*. In the similarly designed Stockholm study with 102 patients with type-1 diabetes, intensive insulin therapy resulting in a mean HbA_{1c} of 7.1% was associated with albuminuria in only 1 out of 48 patients (2.1%), whereas conventional therapy, resulting in a mean HbA_{1c} of 8.5% was associated with albuminuria in 9 of 54 patients (16.6%) ($p = 0.01$) *(45)*.

In the follow-up Epidemiology of Diabetes Interventions and Complications Study, 1349 of the DCCT subjects were followed. The previous difference in HbA_{1c} between the original intensive and conventional treatment groups disappeared within 2 yr such that both groups then maintained mean HbA_{1c} values around 8% for the subsequent 6 yr. Interestingly, despite closure of the gap in glycemic control, there appeared to be a sustained protective effect of earlier intensive control, with a 59% risk reduction in the development of new microalbuminuria (15.8% in the original conventional group vs 6.8% in the original intensive group) and an 84% risk reduction in development of albuminuria (9.4% in the original conventional group vs 1.4% in the original intensive group) *(46)*, suggesting the presence of a "metabolic memory" effect and emphasizing the importance of early intervention.

Several major intervention studies have also been carried out with type 2 diabetes subjects. Using a similar design as the DCCT, the Kumamoto study separated 110 Japanese subjects with type 2 diabetes into primary prevention and secondary intervention cohorts, randomizing them to intensive (HbA_{1c} 7.1%) or conventional (HbA_{1c} 9.4%) glycemic control with insulin *(47)*. Over 6 yr, intensively treated subjects sustained a significant reduction in both new onset and progression of nephropathy compared with conventionally treated subjects. In the prevention cohort, 7.7% developed microalbuminuria in the intensive group vs 28% in the conventional group ($p = 0.032$). After 8 yr, these percentages were 11.5 and 43.5%. Progression to albuminuria was also reduced (11.5% of intensive vs 32% of conventional) *(48)*. The UK Prospective Diabetes Study (UKPDS) randomly assigned newly diagnosed patients with type 2 diabetes to intensive management using a sulfonylurea or insulin, or to conventional management with diet alone. The average HbA_{1c} for the intensive group was 7% as compared with 7.9% for the conventional group during the study *(49)*. After 9 yr of intensive therapy, the risk reduction for the development of microalbuminuria was 24% *(49)*. The degree of risk reduction was similar whether intensive therapy was achieved with sulfonylurea or insulin. However, when better glycemic control was achieved with metformin in the UKPDS, no effect was found on albuminuria *(50)*. In the Veterans Affairs Cooperative Study on glycemic control and complications in Type 2 Diabetes

Feasibility Trial, 95 males with a mean duration of diabetes of 7.8 yr and no microalbuminuria were randomized to intensive diabetes control (mean HbA1c 7.1% at 2 yr) or conventional control (mean HbA1c 9.2% at 2 yr). In this Veterans Affairs Study, 17% of the intensively treated group developed microalbuminuria vs 35% in the conventionally treated group, whereas 12% intensively treated subjects developed albuminuria vs 36% of conventionally treated subjects *(51)*.

Based on these and other data showing that improving glycemic control reduces the rates of not only nephropathy but also retinopathy and neuropathy, the American Diabetes Association (ADA) recommends for adults with diabetes a goal HbA_{1c} of less than 7% *(14)*, whereas the American Association of Clinical Endocrinologists and the European Noninsulin-Dependent Diabetes Mellitus (NIDDM) Working Group recommend a treatment goal of less than 6.5% *(52,53)*. It should be noted that attempts to attain tighter glycemic control may be complicated by an increased frequency of hypoglycemia, especially in patients treated with insulin.

Hypertension/Renin–Angiotensin–Aldosterone System Blockade

Hypertension frequently coexists with diabetes mellitus in adults. The prevalence is greater than 50% in persons with type 2 diabetes mellitus *(54)*, increasing with age, and approx 25% in those with type 1 diabetes *(55)*. As mentioned previously, the onset of hypertension in type 1 diabetes appears to be primarily a complication of DN, whereas in type 2 the hypertension is frequently present at the time of the diagnosis of diabetes with both being components of the metabolic syndrome. Despite the possible difference in pathophysiology of hypertension in the two types of diabetes, it is clear that uncontrolled hypertension increases the risk for progressive renal damage in patients with either type.

Treatment of hypertension in diabetes clearly decreases the risk of microvascular and macrovascular complications, including nephropathy. Large prospective, randomized trials (UKPDS and the Appropriate Blood Pressure Control in Diabetes trial) have shown decreased rates of progression of nephropathy with lowering of blood pressure *(56,57)*. Based on these and other trials, the Joint National Committee on Prevention, Detection, Evaluation, and Treatment of High Blood Pressure (JNC), the ADA, and the National Kidney Foundation have all redefined the goal blood pressure in individuals with diabetes as <130/80 mmHg *(58–60)*. Although the primary goal is blood pressure lowering, the possible differential class effects above and beyond direct effects on blood pressure have been and are continuing to be addressed in large, prospective, and randomized clinical trials. As has been found in multiple clinical trials, the great majority of subjects with diabetes required at least two, and many, even three or more antihypertensive agents in order to reach target blood pressures *(61)*. Most patients with diabetes on appropriately aggressive therapy, therefore, will ultimately end up taking agents from multiple drug classes.

Antihypertensive agents that block the renin–angiotensin–aldosterone system (RAAS) appear to have beneficial effects on the progression of nephropathy above and beyond their blood pressure-lowering effects. They appear to do this by decreasing intraglomerular pressure and by blocking the vasoconstrictive and trophic effects of the RAAS that are thought to be important factors in the pathogenesis of vascular injury in diabetes *(62–64)*. Studies have shown angiotensin-converting enzyme (ACE) inhibitors to be of superior benefit in comparison with other classes of antihypertensive agents in decreasing the development of microalbuminuria and albuminuria in patients with type 1 diabetes, including those without hypertension *(65,66)*. Currently, there are little data regarding angiotensin receptor blockers (ARBs) in type 1 diabetes and nephropathy, but the efficacy and superiority of ACE inhibitors have generally been extrapolated to ARBs.

Until recently, there has been little data from large prospective trials regarding the effectiveness of ACE inhibitors for nephropathy in patients with type 2 diabetes, but again, there have been a presumed extension of their benefits to such patients. A small study of 156 normotensive, normoalbuminuric patients with type 2 diabetes treated with either enalapril or placebo for 6 yr demonstrated a significant risk reduction of 12.5% in the development of microalbuminuria with enalapril as well as a significant attenuation in decline in GFR (mean decrease of 0.025 mL/s/yr with enalapril vs 0.04 mL/s/yr with placebo, $p = 0.040$) *(67)*. In the Microalbuminuria, Cardiovascular, and Renal Outcomes–Heart Outcomes Prevention Evaluation (MICRO-HOPE) study of 3577 primarily type 2 diabetic subjects, ramipril showed a statistically significant benefit over placebo in preventing the progression from microalbuminuria to overt nephropathy (24% risk reduction), and a nonsignificant decrease in development of new microalbuminuria *(68)*. The more recently published Bergamo Nephrologic Diabetes Complications Trial (BENEDICT) randomized 1204 subjects with type 2 diabetes, hypertension, and no albuminuria to trandolopril, verapamil, both, or placebo. Over more than 3 yr of the study, the primary endpoint of persistent microalbuminuria occurred in 5.7% of subjects receiving trandolapril and verapamil, 6% of those on trandolapril only, 11.9% of those on verapamil only, and 10% of those receiving placebo *(69)*. This study confirmed the efficacy of an ACE inhibitor in type 2 diabetes as well as its superiority to verapamil.

For ARBs, more evidence of benefit in prevention of progression of nephropathy exists for type 2 than for type 1 diabetes. The Reduction of Endpoints in NIDDM with the Angiotensin II Antagonist Losartan (RENAAL) study enrolled 1513 hypertensive patients with type 2 diabetes who had albuminuria and serum creatinine levels of 1.3–3 mg/dL. Patients were randomized to losartan or placebo and the blood pressure was controlled (<140/90) with other non-ACE inhibitor and non-ARB medications. Losartan use resulted in a relative risk reduction of 16% in comparison with placebo in the composite endpoint of a doubling of the serum creatinine, ESRD, or death *(70)*. In a study of 1715 diabetic patients with similar baseline characteristics and a similar study design, the Irbesartan Diabetic Nephropathy Trial (IDNT) found that irbesartan treatment resulted in a 20% risk reduction of the same composite endpoint as was used in RENAAL, whereas no benefit was found with the dihydropyridine calcium channel blocker (CCB) amlodipine *(71)*. In a third study of 590 patients with microalbuminuria and hypertension, irbesartan was found to decrease the rate of progression to albuminuria by 24% using a dose of 150 mg/d and by 38% using a dose of 300 mg/d *(72)*. The Microalbuminuria Reduction with Valsartan Trial of Valsartan vs Amlodipine (MARVAL) demonstrated that valsartan decreased microalbuminuria and macroalbuminuria associated with type 2 diabetes more effectively than other antihypertensive classes *(73)*.

Interestingly, subanalyses from the RENAAL study demonstrated that the degree of albuminuria reduction with losartan in the first 6 mo correlated positively with reduction in the renal events and ESRD; every 50% reduction in albuminuria was associated with a 36% risk reduction in renal endpoint and a 45% risk reduction for ESRD during later follow-up *(74)*. A similar association was found for cardiovascular endpoints *(75)*. It has thus been suggested that reduction of urinary albumin be a specific therapeutic goal, with a suggested target of less than 500 mg/d *(76)*.

Theoretically, the idea of dual blockade of the RAAS with an ACE inhibitor plus an ARB is attractive, as neither ACE inhibition nor angiotensin subtype-1 (AT_1) receptor blockade alone by pharmacological agents leads to complete RAAS blockade, and clinical trials of each drug class alone have demonstrated slowing but not arrest of nephropathy progression. Therefore, ACE inhibitor in addition to ARB therapy, blocking the RAAS at different levels and theoretically more completely, would potentially have additive effects not only on decreasing blood pressure but also vascular complications. This is supported by animal studies *(77)*, but few human clinical studies have been published as yet. A number of small studies have provided evidence that combination therapy may be of more benefit than monotherapy in slowing progression of DN with respect to albuminuria levels *(78–81)*. In the largest, the Candesartan and Lisinopril Microalbuminuria (CALM) study of 199 diabetic subjects, candesartan plus lisinopril therapy for 6 mo led to greater blood pressure reduction than either agent alone, as well as greater reduction in microalbuminuria; however, it was not clear whether the latter effect was owing to the greater blood pressure change or to more complete RAAS blockade *(82)*.

The addition of a nondihydropyridine CCB to an ACE inhibitor has been shown in a small study to decrease proteinuria in patients with DN by a greater degree than either agent alone *(83)*. There are also a couple of small studies suggesting that addition of an aldosterone antagonist to an ACE inhibitor may lead to a greater decrease in proteinuria than either alone *(84,85)*.

A more detailed discussion of the data regarding the relative efficacy of the different antihypertensive classes in slowing the progression of DN is beyond the scope of this review. Here we provide some basic guidelines regarding the therapy of hypertension in early diabetic kidney disease: blockade of the RAAS is clearly paramount, and thus far data support the likely interchangeability of ARBs and ACE inhibitors as first-line agents. Thiazide diuretics are a valuable second-line agent particularly as many patients have a component of volume overload; CCBs and β-blockers are safe and effective in diabetic patients and represent, in most cases, useful third-line add-on therapy. α-Agonists and peripheral vasodilators are best considered as fourth- or fifth-line antihypertensive agents. A full review of contraindications and other considerations regarding the different classes of agents are not discussed here, but may be found elsewhere (e.g., Chuang and Molitch *[86]*). Escalation of dosage and stepwise addition of different pharmacological agents should be done in as timely a manner as possible (barring serious or intolerable side effects) so as to reach goal blood pressure as rapidly as possible. The reduction of urinary albumin to less than 500 mg/d may also be beneficial in slowing progression of nephropathy, and dual ACE inhibitor/ARB therapy or the addition of a nondihydropyridine CCB or aldosterone antagonist to RAAS blockade may assist in attaining this target.

Although management of hypertension in diabetes will often require pharmacological agents, it is important not to neglect lifestyle changes. Weight loss has been shown to decrease blood pressure *(87–89)*. Diet composition appears to affect blood pressure as well. The Dietary Approaches to Stop Hypertension (DASH) trial found that a diet high in fruits, vegetables, and low-fat dairy products; low in red meat, sweets, and saturated fats led to blood pressure reductions, particularly in hypertensive patients (systolic blood pressure [SBP] reduction 11.4, diastolic blood pressure [DBP] reduction 5.5 mmHg) *(90)*. The so-called DASH diet also appeared to enhance blood pressure response to the ARB losartan in a study of 55 hypertensive patients *(91)*. In hypertensive subjects in the DASH-Sodium study, the DASH diet plus a "low" sodium intake (500–1000 mg/d) was

Table 1
Recommendations for Lifestyle Modifications in Patients With Diabetes and Hypertension

Modification type	*Recommendations*	*Potential decrease in BP*
Weight loss	Decrease weight by diet and/or exercise, ideally to BMI <25 kg/m^2	5–20 mm Hg reduction in SBP per 10 kg of weight lost
Dietary	Dietary Approaches to Stop Hypertension (DASH) diet (high in fruits, vegetables, low-fat dairy products; low in red meat, sweets, saturated fats)	8–14 mm Hg reduction in SBP, 5.5 mm reduction in DBP *(90)*
Sodium reduction	Dietary sodium <2.4 g/d	2–8 mm Hg reduction in SBP
Exercise	Aerobic exercise for at least 30 min most days of the week	4–9 mm Hg reduction in SBP, 4–8 mm reduction in DBP[94]
Alcohol use	Men: ≤2 drinks[a] per day Women: ≤1 drink per day	2–3 mm Hg reduction in both SBP and DBP *(98)*
Tobacco use	Complete cessation	Up to 7 mm Hg reduction in SBP, 4 mm in DBP *(97)*

BMI, body massindex; SBP, systolic blood pressure; DBP, diastolic blood pressure.
[a]One drink, 1 oz (30 mL) ethanol: 24 oz beer, 10 oz wine, or 2 oz 100-proof whiskey.
Data in part from JNC VII guidelines *(58)*, except where indicated.

found to lead to a further decrease in SBP of 11.5 mm Hg compared with that seen on the DASH diet and a "high" sodium intake (approx 3600 mg/d) *(92)*. Again, reducing sodium intake appeared to potentiate the blood pressure effects of losartan in a small study of type 2 diabetic patients *(93)*. The JNC VII guidelines recommend daily intake of sodium less than 2.4 g *(58)*. Increasing physical activity also lowers blood pressure *(94,95)*.

It should also be remembered that tobacco and alcohol consumption can increase blood pressure *(96–98)*. It is important to counsel patients about the risks of either habit above and beyond causing hypertension, and about strategies for cessation or reduction. For alcohol consumption, the JNC VII guidelines recommend no more than two drinks a day for men (total of 1 oz [30 mL] ethanol, for example, 24 oz [720 mL] of beer, 10 oz [300 mL] of wine, or 2 oz [60 mL] of 100-proof whiskey), one drink a day for women *(58)*. Reduction in alcohol consumption can lead to a 2–3 mmHg drop in both SBP and DBP *(98)*. Based on the described studies and others, the JNC VII guidelines have published the approximate potential reduction in SBP resulting from each lifestyle change. These approximations are included in Table 1.

Protein Restriction

A rat model of DN has shown that restriction of dietary protein intake also reduces hyperfiltration and intraglomerular pressure and retards the progression of renal disease *(99)*. A 4-yr prospective, blinded, and controlled study of 82 subjects with type 1 diabetes and decreasing GFR showed that a low-protein diet (mean 0.89 g/kg/d) compared with usual-protein diet (1.02 g/kg/d) led to a relative risk reduction in ESRD or death of 23% after adjustment for baseline cardiovascular disease ($p = 0.01$) *(100)*. Several small studies in humans with DN have shown that a protein-restricted diet of 0.6 g/kg/d retards the rate of fall of GFR by approx 25% *(101)*. Although the MDRD, in which only 3% of the patients had non-insulin dependent diabetes mellitus (NIDDM) and none had insulin-dependent diabetes mellitus (IDDM), failed to show a clear benefit of protein restriction in retarding the progression of renal disease *(102)*, a meta-analysis suggested that a low-protein diet of about 0.6 g/kg/d in patients with DN results in a significantly reduced rate of decline of the GFR (relative risk 0.56) *(103)*.

At this point in time, the general consensus is to prescribe a protein intake of approximately the adult recommended dietary allowance of 0.8 g/kg/d (approx 10% of daily calories) in the patient with nephropathy. However, it has been suggested that once the GFR begins to fall, further restriction to 0.6 g/kg/d may prove useful in slowing the decline of GFR in selected patients *(103)*. It is also recommended that patients with diabetes and nephropathy be counseled against utilizing a high-protein diet such as the Atkins diet to attain weight loss or glycemic control.

Lipid-Lowering Agents

More aggressive lipid-lowering in patients with diabetes has recently become the standard of care, with the National Cholesterol Education Program (NCEP) designating persons with diabetes as having a coronary heart disease equivalent and recommending a low-density lipoprotein (LDL) target of less than 100 mg/dL *(104)*. Because of their very high risk for coronary artery disease *(12,13)* it may well be that the recently recommended lower goal of less than 70 mg/dL for LDL cholesterol *(105)* may be more appropriate for patients with established nephropathy. Thus, many patients with diabetes, particularly those with type 2, will require lipid-lowering therapy, frequently with a statin, regardless of their renal status. However, it is interesting to note that animal studies have shown that high-cholesterol diets worsen renal injury, whereas lowering blood lipids by medications ameliorates the renal injury *(106–109)*. A relationship between hyperlipidemia and DN has also been suggested by epidemiological studies *(29)*. A meta-analysis of 12 small, controlled studies in humans concluded that treatment was associated with a lower rate of decline in GFR compared with no treatment– 0.156 mL/min/mo vs – 0.285 mL/min/mo, respectively, $p = 0.008$). This effect did not correlate with either the percent change in cholesterol or with the type of lipid-lowering agent used, although all but two trials utilized statins (the other two, gemfibrozil, and probucol). Seven of the trials included only patients with DN *(110)*.

POSSIBLE TARGETS FOR INTERVENTION

With our increasing knowledge of the pathophysiology of diabetic kidney disease, a number of promising avenues of research for future therapies have opened. We will sketch a brief overview of some of these research areas; more detailed information about a number of them may be found in other chapters of this text.

Reduction of Advanced Glycation Endproducts

Intracellular hyperglycemia leads to the formation of advanced glycation endproducts (AGEs), which have been found in animal models to serve as mediators of glucose-induced damage in various target tissues, including the kidney *(111–113)*. Early glycation products, such as Amadori-modified proteins, have been shown to be associated with nephropathy in patients with type 1 diabetes *(114)*. Several drugs already being used for diabetic complications appear to have an effect on AGE accumulation, including the ARB valsartan, the ACE inhibitors ramipril and enalapril, and the antihyperglycemic medication metformin *(115–118)*. Experiments in animal models with a number of substances found to decrease or inhibit AGEs, including aminoguanidine (pimagedine), pyridoxamine, lipoic acid, vitamin E, benfotiamine, and monoclonal antibodies to Amadori-modified glycated albumin have demonstrated slowing in the progression of diabetic vascular complications *(112,116,119–121)*.

The ACTION I (A Clinical Trial In Overt Nephropathy of Type 1 Diabetics) trial randomized 690 subjects with type 1 diabetes, nephropathy, and retinopathy to placebo, aminoguanidine 150 mg twice a day, or aminoguanidine 300 mg twice a day. Over the approx 3-yr study period, fewer treatment patients (26%) reached the primary endpoint of doubled serum creatinine than did placebo patients, but this was not statistically significant ($p = 0.099$). There was a significant decrease in three-step or greater progression of retinopathy, however (10% treated vs 16% placebo, $p = 0.030$) *(122)*.

Protein Kinase C Inhibition

Intracellular hyperglycemia also leads to tissue damage via activation of protein kinase C (PKC), leading to increased production of cytokines, extracellular matrix (ECM), plasminogen activator inhibitor, and endothelin-1 *(112)*. Inhibition of PKC has been shown to reduce urinary albumin and mesangial expansion in db/db mice *(123)*, and to also be renoprotective in humans *(124)*.

Growth Factors

Transforming growth factor (TGF)-β, vascular endothelial growth factor, and connective tissue growth factor may all be important mediators of DN *(125–127)*. Monoclonal antibodies to TGF-β in a diabetic mouse model are renoprotective *(128)*. Human studies with interventions affecting these growth factors have not yet been reported.

Peroxisome Proliferator-Activated Receptors

The peroxisome proliferator-activated receptors (PPARs)-γ agonists are currently used for glycemic control in diabetes, but studies in animals and humans have suggested they may have a role in therapy and prevention of DN independent of their glucose-lowering effects *(129–132)*. As previously mentioned, PPAR-α agonists such as gemfibrozil may also have renoprotective effects *(110)*. Although long-term human studies with such agents are ongoing, their results with respect to nephropathy have not yet been reported.

Other

Pentoxifylline, currently used to treat peripheral vascular disease, has been shown in animal and cellular studies to have beneficial effects on cell proliferation, inflammation, and ECM accumulation. Some human studies have suggested they may have an additive effect on microalbuminuria reduction when used with ACE inhibitors *(133,134)*.

CONCLUSIONS

Patients with diabetes who are at high risk of developing ESRD can now be identified at a point very early in the course of their development of this complication. A number of therapies (summarized in Table 2) have been identified that can slow progression of this

Table 2
Summary of Therapeutic Interventions in Early Diabetic Kidney Disease

Target	*Goal*	*Therapy*
Hyperglycemia	$HbA_{1c} < 7\%$	Type-1 diabetes: Insulin Type-2 diabetes: Oral antihyperglyemic agents and/or insulin
Hypertension	BP < 130/80 mm Hg (Consider goal urine albumin < 500 mg/d)	• Lifestyle changes (*see* Table 1) • If pharmacological therapy also required, ACE-inhibitor or ARB; additional agents as needed to reach goal
Microalbuminuria/ albuminuria (without hypertension)	Consider goal urine albumin < 500 mg/d	Consider ACE-inhibitor or ARB
Hyperlipidemia	LDL < 100 mg/dL (Consider goal LDL < 70 mg/dL)	• In general, statin, plus other lipid-lowering agents as necessary to reach goal • Consider therapy if albuminuria present, even if LDL <100 mg/dL already
Dietary protein	Normal GFR: 0.8 g/kg/d Decreased GFR: 0.6 g/kg/d	Nutrition consult

complication, which is associated with a great deal of morbidity and mortality, as well as staggering costs. There is no question in the present day and age that aggressive control of hyperglycemia and hypertension is beneficial in this regard, or that drugs inhibiting RAAS activity are beneficial independent of their blood pressure effects. Protein restriction may also be of benefit in selected patients. Lipid-lowering agents should be used as recommended to attain cholesterol and triglyceride targets, and may contribute a renoprotective effect as well. It is less clear at this time whether reduction of UAE should be a specific goal, and it also remains controversial regarding whether normotensive patients with microalbuminuria or albuminuria should be treated. Although most studies show that current therapies can only slow the progression of disease, it is possible that when instituted very early they may actually halt progression in some patients. Furthermore, a number of promising possibilities are on the horizon. Thus, although the number of people in the world with diabetes is steadily increasing, it may well be that the proportion and possibly the absolute numbers who develop ESRD will decrease.

REFERENCES

1. Andersen AR, Christiansen JS, Andersen JK, et al. Diabetic nephropathy in Type 1 (insulin-dependent) diabetes: an epidemiological study. Diabetologia 1983;25:496–501.
2. Krolewski AS, Warram JH, Christlieb AR, et al. The changing natural history of nephropathy in type I diabetes. Am J Med 1985;78:785–794.
3. Rossing P, Rossing K, Jacobsen P, et al. Unchanged incidence of diabetic nephropathy in IDDM patients. Diabetes 1995;44:739–743.
4. Krolewski M, Eggers PW, Warram JH. Magnitude of end-stage renal disease in IDDM: a 35 year follow-up study. Kidney Int 1996;50:2041–2046.
5. DeFronzo RA. Diabetic nephropathy: etiologic and therapeutic considerations. Diabet Rev 1995;3:510–564.

6. Bojestig M, Arnqvist HJ, Karlberg BE, et al. Glycemic control and prognosis in type I diabetic patients with microalbuminuria. Diabetes Care 1996;19:313–317.
7. Humphrey LL, Ballard DJ, Frohnert PP, et al. Chronic renal failure in non-insulin-dependent diabetes mellitus. A population-based study in Rochester, Minnesota. Ann Intern Med 1989;111: 788–796.
8. Ritz E, Stefanski A. Diabetic nephropathy in type II diabetes. Am J Kidney Dis 1996;27:167–194.
9. Mogensen CE, Vestbo E, Poulsen PL, et al. Microalbuminuria and potential confounders. A review and some observations on variability of urinary albumin excretion. Diabetes Care 1995;18:572–581.
10. Caramori M, Fioretto P, Mauer M. The need for early predictors of diabetic nephropathy risk: is albumin excretion rate sufficient? Diabetes 2000;49:1399–1408.
11. Krolewski AS, Warram JH. Natural history of diabetic nephropathy. Diabet Rev 1995;3:446–459.
12. Dinneen SF, Gerstein HC. The association of microalbuminuria and mortality in non-insulin-dependent diabetes mellitus. A systematic overview of the literature. Arch Int Med 1997;157:1413–1418.
13. Adler AI, Stevens RJ, Manley SE, et al. Development and progression of nephropathy in type 2 diabetes: the United Kingdom Prospective Diabetes Study (UKPDS 64). Kidney Int 2003;63:225–232.
14. American Diabetes Association. Standards of medical care in diabetes. Diabetes Care 2005;28(1): S4–S36.
15. Kramer H, Nguyen Q, Curhan G, et al. Renal insufficiency in the absence of albuminuria and retinopathy among adults with type 2 diabetes mellitus. JAMA 2003;289:3273–3277.
16. Tsalamandris C, Allen T, Gilbert RE, et al. Progressive decline in renal function in diabetic patients with and without albuminuria. Diabetes 1994;43:649–655.
17. MacIsaac RJ, Tsalamandris C, Panangiotopoulos S, et al. Nonalbuminuric renal insufficiency in type 2 diabetes. Diabetes Care 2004;27:195–200.
18. Lane P, Steffes M, Mauer S. Glomerular structure in IDDM women with low glomerular filtration rate and normal urinary albumin excretion. Diabetes 1992;41:581–586.
19. Steele D, Yeron R, Abendroth C, et al. Diabetic glomerulosclerosis and chronic renal failure with absent-to-minimal microalbuminuria. Am J Kidney Dis 1992;20:80–83.
20. Ruggenenti P, Remuzzi G. Nephropathy of type 1 and type 2 diabetes: diverse pathophysiology, same treatment? Nephrol Dial Transplant 2000;15:1900–1902.
21. Gambara V, Mecca G, Remuzzi G, et al. Heterogeneous nature of renal lesions in type II diabetes. J Am Soc Nephrol 1993;3:1458–1466.
22. Fioretto P, Mauer M, Brocco E, et al. Patterns of renal injury in NIDDM patients with microalbuminuria. Diabetologia 1996;39:1569–1576.
23. Wirta O, Pasternack A, Mustonen J, et al. Albumin excretion rate and its relation to kidney disease in non-insulin-dependent diabetes mellitus. J Int Med 1995;237:367–373.
24. Bertani T, Gambara V, Remuzzi G. Structural basis of diabetic nephropathy in microalbuminuric NIDDM patients: a light microscopy study. Diabetologia 1996;39:1625–1628.
25. Levey AS, Bosch JP, Lewis JB, et al. A more accurate method to estimate glomerular filtration rate from serum creatinine: a new prediction equation. Modification of Diet in Renal Disease Study Group. Ann Intern Med 1999;130:461–470.
26. Cockcroft DW, Gault MH. Prediction of creatinine clearance from serum creatinine. Nephron 1976;16:31–41.
27. National Kidney Foundation. K/DOQI Clinical Practice Guidelines for Chronic Kidney Disease. Part 5: Evaluation of laboratory measurements for clinical assessment of kidney disease. Am J Kidney Dis 2002;39:S76–S92.
28. Rule AD, Larson TS, Bergstralh EJ, et al. Using serum creatinine to estimate glomerular filtration rate: accuracy in good health and in chronic kidney disease. Ann Intern Med 2004;141:929–937.
29. Coonrod BA, Ellis D, Becker DJ, et al. Predictors of microalbuminuria in individuals with IDDM. Pittsburgh Epidemiology of Diabetes Complications Study. Diabetes Care 1993;16:1376–1383.
30. McCance DR, Hadden DR, Atkinson AB, et al. The relationship between long-term glycaemic control and diabetic nephropathy. Q J Med 1992;82:53–61.
31. Klein R, Klein B, Moss S. The incidence of gross proteinuria in people with insulin-dependent diabetes mellitus. Arch Intern Med 1991;151:1344–1348.
32. Chantelau E, Wichmann P. Pathological proteinuria in patients with insulin-dependent diabetes mellitus: relation to intensive insulin therapy. Exp Clin Endocrinol 1992;99:164–168.
33. Chase HP, Jackson WE, Hoops SL, et al. Glucose control and the renal and retinal complications of insulin-dependent diabetes. JAMA 1989;261:1155–1160.
34. Krolewski AS, Laffel LM, Krolewski M, et al. Glycosylated hemoglobin and the risk of microalbuminuria in patients with insulin-dependent diabetes mellitus. N Engl J Med 1995;332:1251–1255.

35. The Kroc Collaborative Study Group. Blood glucose control and the evolution of diabetic retinopathy and albuminuria. A preliminary multicenter trial. N Engl J Med 1984;311:365–372.
36. Lauritzen T, Frost-Larsen K, Larsen HW, et al. Two-year experience with continuous subcutaneous insulin infusion in relation to retinopathy and neuropathy. Diabetes 1985;3:74–79.
37. Feldt-Rasmussen B, Mathiesen ER, Deckert T. Effect of two years of strict metabolic control on progression of incipient nephropathy in insulin-dependent diabetes. Lancet 1986;2:1300–1304.
38. Feldt-Rasmussen B, Mathiesen ER, Jensen T, et al. Effect of improved metabolic control on loss of kidney function in type 1 (insulin-dependent) diabetic patients: an update of the Steno studies. Diabetologia 1991;34:164–170.
39. Dahl-Jorgensen K, Hanssen KF, Kierulf P, et al. Reduction of urinary albumin excretion after 4 years of continuous subcutaneous insulin infusion in insulin-dependent diabetes mellitus. The Oslo Study. Acta Endocrinol 1988;117:19–25.
40. Dahl-Jorgensen K, Bjoro T, Kierulf P, et al. Long-term glycemic control and kidney function in insulin-dependent diabetes mellitus. Kidney Int 1992;41:920–923.
41. Beck-Nielsen H, Olesen T, Mogensen CE, et al. Effect of near normoglycemia for 5 years on progression of early diabetic retinopathy and renal involvement. Diabetes Res 1990;15:185–190.
42. Wang P, Lau J, Chalmers T. Meta-analysis of effects of intensive blood-glucose control on late complications of type 1 diabetes. Lancet 1993;341:1306–1309.
43. The DCCT Research Group. The effect of intensive treatment of diabetes on the development and progression of long-term complications in insulin-dependent diabetes mellitus. N Engl J Med 1993;329:977–986.
44. The DCCT Research Group. Effect of intensive therapy on the development and progression of diabetic nephropathy in the Diabetes Control and Complications Trial (DCCT). Kidney Int 1995;47:1703–1720.
45. Reichard P, Nilsson BY, Rosenqvist U. The effect of long-term intensified insulin treatment on the development of microvascular complications of diabetes mellitus. N Engl J Med 1993;329:304–309.
46. The Epidemiology of Diabetes Interventions and Complications (EDIC)/Diabetes Control and Complications Trial (DCCT) Study. Sustained effects of intensive treatment of type 1 diabetes mellitus on the development and progression of diabetic nephropathy. JAMA 2003;290:2159–2167.
47. Ohkubo Y, Kishikawa H, Araki E, et al. Intensive insulin therapy prevents the progression of diabetic microvascular complications in Japanese patients with non-insulin-dependent diabetes mellitus: a randomized prospective 6-year study. Diabetes Res Clin Pract 1995;28:103–117.
48. Shichiri M, Kishikawa H, Ohkubo Y, et al. Long-term results of the Kumamoto Study on optimal diabetes control in type 2 diabetic patients. Diabetes Care 2000;23 (Suppl 2):B21–B25.
49. UK Prospective Diabetes Study Group. Intensive blood-glucose control with sulphonylureas or insulin compared with conventional treatment and risk of complications in patients with type 2 diabetes (UKPDS 33). Lancet 1998;252:837–853.
50. UK Prospective Diabetes Study Group. Effect of intensive blood–glucose control with metformin on complications in overweight patients with type 2 diabetes (UKPDS 34). Lancet 1998;352:854–865.
51. Levin SR, Coburn JW, Abraira C, et al. Effect of intensive glycemic control on microalbuminuria in type 2 diabetes. Veterans Affairs Cooperative Study on Glycemic Control and Complications in Type 2 Diabetes Feasibility Trial investigators. Diabetes Care 2000;23:1478–1485.
52. American Association of Clinical Endocrinologists, American College of Endocrinology. Medical guidelines for the management of diabetes mellitus: the AACE system of intensive diabetes self-management—2002 update. Endocr Pract 2002;8(1):40–82.
53. European NIDDM Policy Group. A desktop guide for the management of non-insulin-dependent diabetes mellitus (NIDDM). 2005. Available at http://www.rbh.nthames.nhs.uk/prestige/niddm/niddm.htm. Accessed on May 22, 2005.
54. National Institute of Diabetes and Digestive and Kidney Diseases (NIDDK). National Diabetes Statistics. National Diabetes Information Clearing house Website. 2004. Available at http://diabetes.niddk. nih.gov/dm/pubs/statistics/index.htm. Accessed on August 12, 2004.
55. Collado-Mesa F, Colhoun HM, Stevens LK, et al. Prevalence and management of hypertension in type 1 diabetes mellitus in Europe: the EURODIAB IDDM Complications Study. Diab Med 1999;16:41–48.
56. UK Prospective Diabetes Study Group. Tight blood pressure control and risk of macrovascular and microvascular complications in type 2 diabetes: UKPDS 38. BMJ 1998;317:703–713.
57. Schrier RW, Estacio RO, Esler A, et al. Effects of aggressive blood pressure control in normotensive type 2 diabetic patients on albuminuria, retinopathy and strokes. Kidney Int 2002;61:1086–1097.

58. Chobanian AV, Bakris GL, Black HR, et al. The seventh report of the Joint National Committee on Prevention, Detection, Evaluation, and Treatment of High Blood Pressure: the JNC 7 report. JAMA 2003;289:2560–2572.
59. Arauz-Pacheco C, Parrott MA, Raskin P. Hypertension management in adults with diabetes. Diabetes Care 2004;27(1):S65–S67.
60. NKF-Kidney Disease Outcomes Quality Initiative (K/DOQI). Guideline 8: Pharmacological therapy: Diabetic kidney disease. Am J Kidney Dis 2004;43:S142–S158.
61. Bakris GL. The importance of blood pressure control in the patient with diabetes. Am J Med 2004;116:S30–S38.
62. Zatz R, Anderson S, Meyer TW, et al. Lowering of arterial blood pressure limits glomerular sclerosis in rats with renal ablation and in experimental diabetes. Kidney Int Suppl 1987;20:S123–S129.
63. Zatz R, Dunn BR, Meyer TW, et al. Prevention of diabetic glomerulopathy by pharmacological amelioration of glomerular capillary hypertension. J Clin Invest 1986;77:1925–1930.
64. Goa KL, Haria M, Wilde MI. Lisinopril. A review of its pharmacology and use in the management of the complications of diabetes mellitus. Drugs 1997;53:1081–1105.
65. ACE Inhibitors in Diabetic Nephropathy Trialist Group. Should all patients with type 1 diabetes mellitus and microalbuminuria receive angiotensin-converting enzyme inhibitors? A meta-analysis of individual patient data. Ann Intern Med 2001;134:370–379.
66. Lewis EJ, Hunsicker LG, Bain RP, et al. The effect of angiotensin-converting-enzyme inhibition on diabetic nephropathy. N Engl J Med 1993;329:1456–1462.
67. Ravid M, Brosh D, Levi Z, et al. Use of enalapril to attenuate decline in renal function in normotensive, normoalbuminuric patients with type 2 diabetes mellitus: A randomized, controlled trial. Ann Intern Med 1998;128:982–988.
68. Heart Outcomes Prevention Evaluation Study Investigators. Effects of ramipril on cardiovascular and microvascular outcomes in people with diabetes mellitus: results of the HOPE study and MICRO-HOPE substudy. Lancet 2000;355:253–259.
69. Ruggenenti P, Fassi A, Ilieva AP, et al. Preventing microalbuminuria in type 2 diabetes. N Engl J Med 2004;351:1941–1951.
70. Brenner BM, Cooper ME, de Zeeuw D, et al. Effects of losartan on renal and cardiovascular outcomes in patients with type 2 diabetes and nephropathy. N Engl J Med 2001;345:861–869.
71. Lewis EJ, Hunsicker LG, Clarke WR, et al. Renoprotective effect of the angiotensin-receptor antagonist irbesartan in patients with nephropathy due to type 2 diabetes. N Engl J Med 2001;345:851–860.
72. Parving HH, Lehnert H, Brochner-Mortensen J, et al. The effect of irbesartan on the development of diabetic nephropathy in patients with type 2 diabetes. N Engl J Med 2001;345:870–878.
73. Viberti G, Wheeldon NM, for the MicroAlbuminuria Reduction With VALsartan (MARVAL) Study Investigators. Microalbuminuria reduction with valsartan in patients with type 2 diabetes mellitus: a blood pressure-independent effect. Circulation 2002;106:672–678.
74. de Zeeuw D, Remuzzi G, Parving HH, et al. Proteinuria, a target for renoprotection in patients with type 2 diabetic nephropathy: lessons from RENAAL. Kidney Int 2004;65:2309–2320.
75. de Zeeuw D, Remuzzi G, Parving HH, et al. Albuminuria, a therapeutic target for cardiovascular protection in type 2 diabetic patients with nephropathy. Circulation 2004;110:921–927.
76. de Zeeuw D. Should albuminuria be a therapeutic target in patients with hypertension and diabetes? Am J Hypertension 2004;17:S11–S15.
77. Taal MW, Brenner BM. Renoprotective benefits of RAS inhibition: from ACEI to angiotensin II antagonists. Kidney Int 2000;57:1803–1817.
78. Jacobsen P, Parving HH. Beneficial impact on cardiovascular risk factors by dual blockade of the renin-angiotensin system in diabetic nephropathy. Kidney Int Suppl 2004;66:S108–S110.
79. Rossing K, Jacobsen P, Pietraszek L, et al. Renoprotective effects of adding angiotensin II receptor blocker to maximal recommended doses of ACE inhibitor in diabetic nephropathy: a randomized double-blind crossover trial. Diabetes Care 2003;26:2268–2274.
80. Laverman GD, Navis G, Henning RH, et al. Dual renin-angiotensin system blockade at optimal doses for proteinuria. Kidney Int 2002;62:1020–1025.
81. Hebert LA, Falkenhain ME, Nahman NS Jr, et al. Combination ACE inhibitor and angiotensin II receptor antagonist therapy in diabetic nephropathy. Am J Nephrol 1999;19:1–6.
82. Mogensen CE, Neldam S, Tikkanen I, et al. Randomised controlled trial of dual blockade of renin-angiotensin system in patients with hypertension, microalbuminuria, and non-insulin dependent diabetes: the candesartan and lisinopril microalbuminuria (CALM) study. Brit Med J 2000;321: 1440–1444.

83. Bakris GL, Weir MR, DeQuattro V, et al. Effects of an ACE inhibitor/calcium antagonist combination on proteinuria in diabetic nephropathy. Kidney Int 1998;54:1283–1289.
84. Epstein M, Buckalew VJ, Martinez F, et al. Antiproteinuric efficacy of eplerenone, enalapril and eplerenone/enalapril combination therapy in diabetic hypertensives with microalbuminuria. Am J Hypertens 2002;15:24A.
85. Chrysostomou A, Becker G. Spironolactone in addition to ACE inhibition to reduce proteinuria in patients with chronic renal disease. N Engl J Med 2001;345:925, 926.
86. Chuang E, Molitch ME. Treatment of hypertension in diabetes. In: Fonseca V, ed. Clinical Diabetes. Elsevier Press, Inc., "in press."
87. Reisin E, Frohlich E, Messerli F, et al. Cardiovascular changes after weight reduction in obesity hypertension. Ann Intern Med 1983;98:315–319.
88. Stamler R, Stamler J, Grimm R, et al. Nutritional therapy for high blood pressure: Final report of a four-year randomized controlled trial—the Hypertension Control Program. JAMA 1987;257: 1484–1491.
89. Wassertheil-Smoller S, Blaufox M, Oberman A, et al. The Trial of Antihypertensive Interventions and Management (TAIM) study: Adequate weight loss, alone and combined with drug therapy in the treatment of mild hypertension. Arch Intern Med 1992;152:131–136.
90. Appel LJ, Moore TJ, Obarzanek E, et al. A clinical trial of the effects of dietary patterns on blood pressure. N Engl J Med 1997;336:1117–1124.
91. Conlin P, Erlinger T, Bohannon A, et al. The DASH diet enhances the blood pressure response to losartan in hypertensive patients. Am J Hypertens 2003;16:337–342.
92. Sacks FM, Svetkey LP, Vollmer WM, et al. Effects on blood pressure of reduced dietary sodium and the Dietary Approaches to Stop Hypertension (DASH) diet. N Engl J Med 2001;344:3–10.
93. Houlihan C, Allen T, Baxter A, et al. A low-sodium diet potentiates the effects of losartan in type 2 diabetes. Diabetes Care 2002;25:663–671.
94. Kelley G, McClellan P. Antihypertensive effects of aerobic exercise: a brief mata-analysis of randomized control trials. Am J Hypertension 1994;7:115–119.
95. Kelley G, Kelley K. Progressive resistance exercise and resting blood pressure: a meta-analysis of randomized control trials. Hypertension. 2000;35:838–843.
96. Groppelli A, Giorgi DM, Omboni S, et al. Persistent blood pressure increase induced by heavy smoking. J Hypertens 1992;10:495–499.
97. Verdecchia P, Schillaci G, Borgioni C, et al. Cigarette smoking, ambulatory blood pressure and cardiac hypertrophy in essential hypertension. J Hypertens 1995;13:1209–1215.
98. Xin X, He J, Frontini MG, et al. Effects of alcohol reduction on blood pressure: a meta-analysis of randomized controlled trials. Hypertension 2001;38:1112–1117.
99. Zatz R, Meyer TW, Rennke HG, et al. Predominance of hemodynamic rather than metabolic factors in the pathogenesis of diabetic glomerulopathy. Proc Natl Acad Sci USA 1985;82:5963–5967.
100. Hansen HP, Tauber-Lassen E, Jensen B, et al. Effect of dietary protein restriction on prognosis in patients with diabetic nephropathy. Kidney Int 2002;62:220–228.
101. Zeller K. Low-protein diets in renal disease. Diabetes Care 1991;14:856–866.
102. Klahr S, Levey A, Beck G, et al. The effects of dietary protein restriction and blood-pressure control on the progression of chronic renal disease. N Engl J Med 1994;330:877–884.
103. Pedrini M, Levey A, Lau J, et al. The effect of dietary protein restriction on the progression of diabetic and nondiabetic renal diseases: a meta-analysis. Ann Int Med 1996;124:627–632.
104. National Cholesterol Education Program (NCEP) Expert panel on detection, evaluation, and treatment of high blood cholesterol in adults. Third Report of the National Cholesterol Education Program (NCEP) Expert Panel on Detection, Evaluation, and Treatment of High Blood Cholesterol in Adults (Adult Treatment Panel III). 2002. Available at http://www.nhlbi.nih.gov/guidelines/cholesterol/. Accessed on May 22, 2005.
105. Grundy SM, Cleeman JI, Merz CN, et al. Implications of recent clinical trials for the National Cholesterol Education Program Adult Treatment Panel III Guidelines. J Am Coll Cardiol 2004;44:720–732.
106. Kasiske BL, O'Donnell M, Schmitz P, et al. Renal injury of diet-induced hypercholesterolemia in rats. Kidney Int 1990;37:880–891.
107. Wellman K, Volk B. Renal changes in experimental hypercholesterolemia in normal and subdiabetic rabbits. II. Long-term studies. Lab Invest 1971;24:144–155.
108. Kasiske BL, O'Donnell MP, Cleary MP, et al. Treatment of hyperlipidemia reduces glomerular injury in obese Zucker rats. Kidney Int 1988;33:667–672.
109. Kasiske BL, O'Donnell MP, Garvis WJ, et al. Pharmacologic treatment of hyperlipidemia reduces glomerular injury in rat 5/6 nephrectomy model of chronic renal failure. Circ Res 1988;62:367–374.

110. Fried LF, Orchard TJ, Kasiske BL. Effect of lipid reduction on the progression of renal disease: A meta-analysis. Kidney Int 2001;59:260–269.
111. Hudson B, Schmidt A. RAGE: a novel target for drug intervention in diabetic vascular disease. Pharm Res 2004;21:1079–1086.
112. Nishikawa T, Edelstein D, Brownlee M. The missing link: A single unifying mechanism for diabetic complications. Kidney Int Suppl 2000;77:S26–S30.
113. Soulis T, Cooper ME, Vranes D, et al. Effects of aminoguanidine in preventing experimental diabetic nephropathy are related to the duration of treatment. Kidney Int 1996;50:627–634.
114. Schalkwijk C, Ligtvoet N, Twaalfhoven H, et al. Amadori albumin in type 1 diabetic patients: correlation with markers of endothelial function, association with diabetic nephropathy, and localization in retinal capillaries. Diabetes 1999;48:2446–2453.
115. Forbes JM, Thomas MC, Thorpe SR, et al. The effects of valsartan on the accumulation of circulating and renal advanced glycation end products in experimental diabetes. Kidney Int Suppl 2004;92: S105–S107.
116. Alderson NL, Chachich ME, Frizzell N, et al. Effect of antioxidants and ACE inhibition on chemical modification of proteins and progression of nephropathy in the streptozotocin diabetic rat. Diabetologia 2004;47:1385–1395.
117. Forbes JM, Cooper ME, Thallas V, et al. Reduction of the accumulation of advanced glycation end products by ACE inhibition in experimental diabetic nephropathy. Diabetes 2002;51:3274–3282.
118. Beisswenger P, Ruggiero-Lopez D. Metformin inhibition of glycation processes. Diabetes Metab 2003;29:3274–3282.
119. Metz TO, Alderson NL, Thorpe SR, et al. Pyridoxamine, an inhibitor of advanced glycation and lipoxidation reactions: a novel therapy for treatment of diabetic complications. Arch Biochem Biophys 2003;419:41–49.
120. Hammes HP, Du X, Edelstein D, et al. Benfotiamine blocks three major pathways of hyperglycemic damage and prevents experimental diabetic retinopathy. Nat Med 2003;9:294–299.
121. Cohen M, Sharma K, Jin Y, et al. Prevention of diabetic nephropathy in db/db mice with glycated albumin anatagonists. A novel treatment strategy. J Clin Invest 1995;95:2338–2345.
122. Bolton W, Cattran D, Williams M, et al. Randomized trial of an inhibitor of formation of advanced glycation end products in diabetic nephropathy. Am J Nephrol 2004;24:32–40.
123. Koya D, Haneda M, Nakagawa H, et al. Amelioration of accelerated diabetic mesangial expansion by treatment with a PKC beta inhibitor in diabetic db/db mice, a rodent model for type 2 diabetes. FASEB J 2000;14:439–447.
124. Tuttle K, Bakris GL, Toto R, et al. Effect of ruboxistaurin on type 2 diabetes nephropathy. Diabetes Care 2005;28:7686–7690.
125. Hoffman BB, Sharma K, Ziyadeh FN. Potential role of TGF-beta in diabetic nephropathy. Miner Electrolyte Metab 1998;24:190–196.
126. Aiello LP, Wong JS. Role of vascular endothelial growth factor in diabetic vascular complications. Kidney Int Suppl 2000;77:S113–S119.
127. Twigg SM, Cooper ME. The time has come to target connective tissue growth factor in diabetic complications. Diabetologia 2004;47:965–968.
128. Ziyadeh FN, Hoffman BB, Han DC, et al. Long-term prevention of renal insufficiency, excess matrix gene expression, and glomerular mesangial matrix expansion by treatment with monoclonal antitransforming growth factor-beta antibody in db/db diabetic mice. Proc Natl Acad Sci USA 2000;97:8015–8020.
129. Buckingham R, Al-Barazanji K, Toseland C, et al. Peroxisome proliferator-activated receptor-gamma agonist, rosiglitazone, protects against nephropathy and pancreatic islet abnormalities in Zucker fatty rats. Diabetes 1998;47:1326–1334.
130. Isshiki K, Haneda M, Koya D, et al. Thiazolidinedione compounds ameliorate glomerular dysfunction independent of their insulin-sensitizing action in diabetic rats. Diabetes 2000;49:1022–1032.
131. Bakris GL, Viberti G, Weston W, et al. Rosiglitazone reduces urinary albumin excretion in type 2 diabetes. J Hum Hypertens 2003;17:7–12.
132. Imano E, Kanda T, Nakatani Y, et al. Effect of troglitazone on microalbuminuria in patients with incipient diabetic nephropathy. Diabetes Care 1998;21:2135–2139.
133. Lin SL, Chen YM, Chiang WC, et al. Pentoxifylline: a potential therapy for chronic kidney disease. Nephrology 2004;9:198–204.
134. Ha SW, Bae JS, Yeo HJ, et al. TGF-beta-induced protein beta ig-h3 is upregulated by high glucose in vascular smooth muscle cells. J Cell Biochem 2003;88:774–782.

24 Treatment in Advanced Renal Disease in Type 1 and Type 2 Diabetes

Eberhard Ritz, MD *and Gunter Wolf,* MD

CONTENTS

INTRODUCTION

Not so long ago, terminal renal failure used to be a death sentence for the diabetic patient. In 1972, in a famous paper entitled "The Sad Truth About Hemodialysis in Diabetic Nephropathy," Ghavamian arrived at the conclusion that "dialysis for such patients … carries little likelihood of long-term survival or improvement in quality of life" *(1)*. Although survival of uremic diabetic patients has improved dramatically in recent years, such historical experience underlines the particular susceptibility of the diabetic patient to cardiovascular (CV) complications and infectious episodes.

In the pioneer report on kidney transplantation combined with pancreatic–duodenal allotransplantation, only 2 of 10 patients with juvenile-onset diabetes were alive 7 mo postoperatively *(2)*. Meanwhile, the outcome of combined pancreas–kidney transplantation has improved dramatically and this alternative has become the procedure providing best survival and quality of life *(3)* in the type 1 diabetic patient.

Chronic ambulatory peritoneal dialysis (PD) is a complementary modality that may, in certain situations, particularly as long as residual renal function persists, be superior to hemodialysis (HD) treatment *(4)*.

From: *Contemporary Diabetes: The Diabetic Kidney*
Edited by: P. Cortes and C. E. Mogensen © Humana Press Inc., Totowa, NJ

Table 1
Incidence of Patients Admitted to Renal Replacement Programs With Diabetes as a Comorbid Condition According to National Registries

Country	*Year*	*New patients total (pmp)*	*Diabetes (% of total)*	*Diabetes (pmp)*
Australia	2002	94	26	24.4
Catalonia	2002	146.8	21	30.7
Denmark	2002	128.7	26	34
Germany	2002	174	36	62.6
Heidelberg[a]	2001	183	48.9	101[b]
New Zealand	2002	115	45	51.7
Poland	2002	99.1	23.9	24.1
Russia	2002	14.7	9.1	1.3
United States	2002	326	45.3	148

Data are given as patients per million population (pmp) or percent.
[a]According to Schwenger *(15)*.
[b]Type 1 diabetes, 6 pmp; type 2 diabetes, 92 pmp.

EPIDEMIOLOGY

There has been a secular trend of decreasing prevalence of nephropathy in type 1 diabetic patients *(5)*, presumably because of progressively better management of glycemia and hypertension. Although in type 2 diabetic patients aggressive early multifactorial intervention reduces the frequency of CV and renal end points *(6)*, there is no evidence of a decreasing incidence of advanced nephropathy in patients with type 2 diabetes, presumably because of the dramatic increase of type 2 diabetes in the Western world *(7)* and the high renal risk in type 2 diabetes *(8)*, which at least in young, type 2 diabetics may even be greater than in type 1 diabetics *(9)*. Apart from the increasing prevalence of type 2 diabetes in the population *(7)* and the aging of the population (type 2 diabetes is more frequent at advanced age), better survival of diabetic patients with nephropathy is a major reason for this epidemiological scenario of rising numbers of type 2 diabetics with end-stage renal disease (ESRD) *(10,11)*. Follow-up of the United Kingdom Prospective Diabetes Study concerning type 2 diabetics showed that approx 2–3% of patients per year progress from normo- to microalbuminuria, from micro- to macroalbuminuria and from macroalbuminuria to impaired renal function or terminal renal failure, respectively *(8)*. It is of note that—as in the nondiabetic patient with chronic kidney disease *(8)*—the risk to succumb to cardiovascular disease (CVD) is greater than the chance to live long enough until ESRD has occurred.

As shown in Table 1, according to numerous national registries, ESRD with diabetes as a comorbid condition has become the single most frequent diagnosis for patients entering renal replacement programs. Most of these patients, in our experience of less than 90%, suffer from type 2 diabetes. The incidence continues to increase throughout the Western world; in Europe the incidence has doubled within the last decade *(12)*, and has recently started to increase in developing countries as well.

According to the US Renal Data System (2004; incidence data from 2002) diabetic nephropathy (DN) was the primary diagnosis in 45% of incident patients (i.e., 148 out of 326 patients per million). This was an increase by 221% compared with 1990 *(13,14)*.

Table 2
Most Frequent Causes of Death in Diabetic Hemodialyzed Patients (Rates Per 1000 Patient Years at Risk in the Years 1996–1998)

Cause of death	*Rates per 1000 patient years at risk*
Cardiac arrest	59.4
Septicemia	30.5
Myocardial infarction	26.7
Cardiac arrhythmia	16.0
Stroke	16.8
Others	46.5

After refs. *19* and *20*.

In 2000–2003, the actual proportion of diabetic patients among those admitted for renal replacement therapy (RRT) varied considerably between different countries as illustrated in Table 1. Registry figures, for example, those from Germany, tend to underestimate the renal burden of diabetes: we found that diabetes was present in not less than 48.9% of patients admitted for RRT in Heidelberg *(15)*. However, clinical features of classical Kimmelstiel Wilson's disease were found only in 60%. Atypical presentation consistent with ischemic nephropathy accounted for 13% and known primary renal disease (e.g., polycystic kidney disease, analgesic nephropathy, glomerulo-nephritis) with superimposed diabetes for 27% of the cases. Survival of the diabetic patient on HD is similar *(16)*, however, whether or not diabetic or primary nondiabetic renal disease accounts for end-stage renal failure. In the Heidelberg series, diabetes had not been diagnosed at the time of admission in 11% of the diabetic patients with renal failure, presumably because the patient had lost weight secondary to anorexia, thus self-correcting hyperglycemia.

Survival of diabetic patients on dialysis is considerably worse than in nondiabetic patients. In a prospective study in Germany, the 5-yr survival of type 2 diabetics on dialysis was not more than 5% *(17)* corresponding to the survival of patients with metastasizing gastrointestinal carcinoma; it has somewhat improved recently: in the 4D Trial *(18)* the annual mortality was 13%. The main causes of death in hemodialyzed diabetic patients are CV event and septicemia (Table 2) *(19,20)*.

Survival rates in dialyzed diabetic patients are much better in Eastern countries such as Japan *(21)*. This is presumably related to the generally lower rate of CV death in the background population of Japan.

It is known that 5–10% of patients develop diabetes *de novo* on dialysis, presumably because they had been prediabetic to begin with *(13)*. They had presumably a temporary reversal of hyperglycemia following weight loss from anorexia in the predialytic stage and recurrence after weight gain on dialysis. Recently, it has been found *(22)* that in the United States by the end of the first year of RRT, close to two-thirds of patients have the diagnosis of diabetes. This was particularly the case in patients in whom the diagnosis had been "hypertensive nephropathy" when they entered HD programs.

It is of importance that an increasing proportion of patients present as acute irreversible renal failure, mostly acute on chronic renal failure, usually after cardiac or septic complications with or without administration of radiocontrast or nonsteroidals. This was seen in 27% of the diabetic patients in the Heidelberg series *(15)*. The prognosis is particularly poor in patients admitted as emergencies with acute renal failure *(15,23)*.

Late referral continues to be a problem. In Heidelberg, the median interval between referral and start of dialysis was 17 wk. One-year mortality was 37% in diabetic and 30.6% in nondiabetic patients referred less than 17 wk and only 7.3% and 4.1%, respectively, for those referred more than 17 wk—in other words late referral had a greater impact than diabetes *(24)*. Patients referred late have particularly insufficient control of risk factors and have more frequently no vascular access. The latter is the main factor causing increased morbidity and mortality.

CARDIAC PROBLEMS IN THE DIABETIC PATIENT

Epidemiology

In the diabetic patient on RRT, cardiac problems are the main difficulty faced by the nephrologist. Even before dialysis, heart disease is more frequent in diabetic (46.4%) than nondiabetic patients (32.2%) *(25)*. This includes myocardial infarction (MI), angina pectoris, necessity for coronary artery bypass grafting (CABG) or percutaneous transluminal coronary angioplasty (PTCA), or a pathological coronary angiogram and congestive heart failure (CHF) *(20)*. In preterminal diabetic patients compared with nondiabetic patients, the odds ratio for a new CV event is 5.3 *(26)* and progression (i.e., either new events or worsening of existing pathology) is seen in 20% of the patients over a 23-mo follow-up period. In 433 Canadian patients, 116 of whom were diabetics, the latter had left ventricular hypertrophy (LVH), ischemic heart disease, and CHF more frequently *(27)*. No difference between diabetic and nondiabetic patients was found with respect to *de novo* appearance or progression of LVH and CHF. In contrast, the relative risks to develop ischemic heart disease *de novo* and to die from CV causes were significantly higher in dialyzed diabetic compared with nondiabetic patients, suggesting accelerated atherogenesis. It is noteworthy that although the risk of CV death is reduced, it is not completely abrogated by transplantation. It was recently found that the hazard ratio to develop an acute coronary syndrome after transplantation was still 0.38 and the rate of new events was 0.79 per patient-year compared with 1.67 prior to transplantation *(28)*.

If the diabetic patient on dialysis develops an acute coronary syndrome, his or her chances of survival is very poor *(29)*. Cardiac mortality at 1 yr is 42% and at 5 yr is 75%. Unfortunately, up-to-date interventions including thrombolysis, PTCA, or CABG are not widely used in the high-risk population of renal patients irrespective of the presence or absence of diabetes *(30)*. The risk of an adverse cardiac outcome in the diabetic patient with ischemic heart disease is amplified because of the coexistence of more severe LVH *(27)*, CHF *(31)*, disturbed sympathetic innervation *(32)*, and microvessel disease *(33)*.

Diagnosis

It is particularly difficult to establish the diagnosis of coronary heart disease in the diabetic patient with renal failure. Because of autonomic polyneuropathy, coronary disease is often silent with episodes of silent myocardial ischemia and silent MI. Coronary heart disease is not well predicted by baseline or exercise EKG (the latter is difficult to perform in polyneuropathic patients with muscular atrophy or arterial occlusive disease). Conventional screening tests such as treadmill or exercise EKG are therefore unreliable. Dipyridamol thallium scans predict myocardial ischemia, but are not well correlated to the findings on coronarography (i.e., do not well predict the presence of lesions necessitating intervention). However, it has been recommended as a screening

Table 3
Cardiac Findings in Diabetic Patients on Dialysis

Baseline	*Diabetic patients (n = 116) (%)*	*Nondiabetic patients (n = 317) (%)*	*p*
Concentric LV hypertrophy	50	38	0.04
Ischemic heart disease	32	18	0.003
Cardiac failure	48	24	0.00001
Follow-up	*Adjusted relative risk (diabetic/nondiabetic)*		*p*
Ischemic heart disease		3.2	0.0002
Overall mortality		2.3	0.0001
Cardiovascular mortality		2.6	0.0001

After ref. *27*.

test. The diagnostic value of magnetic resonance tomography angiography is currently under evaluation. Unfortunately, the best approach is still to study the patient directly with coronary angiography if there is a suspicion of coronary heart disease: LV dilatation on echocardiography, regional contraction abnormalities on echocardiography, sudden deterioration of cardiac function with pulmonary edema, and arrhythmia or an increase in troponin T concentration. Troponin T is excreted via the kidney and it has long been controversial whether it is a faithful predictor of myocardial ischemia in the presence of renal failure, but this issue has recently been settled *(34)*. In the renal patient, troponin T concentrations are predictive of cardiac death *(35)* even in the absence of overt coronary heart disease, presumably reflecting diffuse myocardial microvascular ischemia. Nevertheless, an acute major increase is a reliable indicator of MI in the uremic diabetic patient as well (Table 3).

Intervention

Much new information on interventions has become available. There is no doubt that interventional management is superior to conservative management with calcium channel blockers *(36)*. It has remained controversial, however, whether PTCA (± stent) or coronary bypass is the preferred modality of treatment. Although prospective data are not available, very compelling observational information in a large patient sample indicates that CABG has the disadvantage of higher in hospital death rates (12.5% vs 5.4% in PTCA), but the advantage of better long-term survival (56.9 vs 52.9%) *(37)*. The most powerful predictors of cardiac death are old age and diabetes, the relative risk being 1.37 in diabetic compared with nondiabetic patients. Table 4 compares the results of cardiac intervention in diabetic and nondiabetic dialysis patients *(38)*. Compared with PTCA without stent, PTCA plus stent was superior in nondiabetic, but not in diabetic patients. Similar to the result of the Bypass Angioplasty Revascularization Investigation (BARI) study in nonrenal patients CABG was superior in both nondiabetic and diabetic patients. It is important that such benefit was seen only when internal mammary grafts were used and not saphenous bypass grafts.

There is some discussion concerning the use of β-blockers and statines. In the past, we had strongly advocated more liberal use of β-blockers in patients with diabetes *(39)*,

Table 4
Comparison of Cardiac Intervention in Diabetic and Nondiabetic Dialysis Patients

	Relative risk of all-cause death compared with PTCA without stent	
	PTCA+Stent	*Coronary artery bypass surgery*
Nondiabetic	0.9 (0.86–0.97)	0.79 (0.7–0.85)
Diabetic	0.99 (0.91–1.08)[a]	0.81 (0.75–0.86)[b]

After ref. *38*.
[a] p = N.S.
[b] p = 0.0001.

Table 5
Suggested Preventive Maneuvers in Diabetic Patients With Renal Failure and Risk of Cardiovascular Disease

Start intervention in early stage of renal disease
Angiotensin-converting enzyme inhibitors or angiotensin receptor blockers
Low target blood pressure values
Aspirin
Control of hypervolemia (low salt intake, diuretics)
Statines
Treat anemia

based on the observation that only 3% of dialyzed type 2 diabetic patients who died from cardiac causes had been on β-blockers, but no less than 30% of those who survived *(16)*. There had been much concern to use β-blockers because of adverse metabolic side effects. Meanwhile, a prospective trial in dialysis patients with CHF documented functional improvement and better survival with administration of carvedilol compared with placebo *(40)*.

Prevention of Cardiac Disease

Concerning the prevention of cardiac disease, current recommendation suggest that low-density lipoprotein cholesterol should be lowered to values less than 100 mg/dL in diabetic patients. The recent 4D Trial in hemodialyzed type 2 diabetics *(18)* had shown no positive effect of the administration of atorvastatin on a composite CV end point. Table 5 summarizes the recommended measures to prevent coronary heart disease in the diabetic patient.

Several predictors of cardiac death had been identified in diabetic patients, i.e., a history of vascular disease, specifically MI or angina pectoris *(17)*, proliferative retinopathy, and polyneuropathy (presumably inducing unbalanced autonomic cardiac innervation *[16]*) and serum lipid levels *(41)*. The latter observation is remarkable because in nondiabetic patients on HD, an inverse relation is usually found between cholesterol and survival, presumably because low cholesterol is an index of microinflammation/malnutrition *(42)*. In prospective studies, strong predictors of CV death were smoking *(43)* as well as poor glycemic control before dialysis *(44)* or on HD *(45)*.

HYPERTENSION

At any given level of glomerular filtration rate (GFR), blood pressure tends to be higher in diabetic compared with nondiabetic patients with renal failure. Because of their beneficial effect on CV complications *(46)* and progression *(47–49)*, angiotensin-converting enzyme (ACE) inhibitors or angiotensin receptor blockers (ARBs) are obligatory in our view, unless there are contraindications, for example, hyperkalemia resistant to correctice manuvers such as administration of loop diuretics, dietary potassium restriction, or correction of metabolic acidosis. The widespread practice to withdraw ACE inhibitors or ARBs in advanced renal failure in the hope of decreasing the serum creatinine concentration does not make sense, unless there has been an abrupt recent increase in serum creatinine *(50)*. In the Irbesartan Diabetic Nephropathy Trial (IDNT) study, we saw that Irbesartan prolonged the time to dialysis even in the far-advanced stages of renal failure.

Because of their marked propensity to retain salt, patients with DN are prone to develop hypervolemia and edema. Therefore, dietary salt restriction and administration of loop diuretics are usually indicated. In the diabetic patient on dialysis it is important to recommend dietary restriction of salt and to achieve adequate dry weight.

GLYCEMIC CONTROL

On the one hand, renal failure causes insulin resistance, among others, by cumulation of a (hypothetical) circulating factor interfering with the action of insulin. As a result, patients tend to develop impaired glucose tolerance and hyperglycemia. Because the hypothetical low-molecular-weight circulating insulin inhibitor is apparently dialyzable, insulin resistance is improved after the start of dialysis.

On the other hand, the half-life of insulin is prolonged, predisposing to hypoglycemic episodes. This risk is further compounded by anorexia and by cumulation of most sulfonylurea compounds (with the exception of gliquidone or glimerpiride). Glinides and glitazones do not cumulate, but long-term safety data in renal failure are not available.

It follows from the above that the net result of these opposing influences is difficult to predict, so that close monitoring of glycemia is advisable.

In the treatment of these patients there is an increasing tendency to use more liberally short-acting insulins with or without a basis of long-acting insulin. The goal is to prevent catabolism and malnutrition. Insulin administration is obligatory during intercurrent illness, infection, surgery, or MI *(51)*.

MALNUTRITION

Diabetic patients with renal failure are often severely catabolic and tend to develop malnutrition. This risk is particularly high during periods of intercurrent illness or fasting, but may also be the result of ill-advised recommendations to restrict protein intake, particularly when these anorectic patients concomitantly reduce energy intake. Malnutrition is a potent, independent predictor of death *(52)* and its presence justifies an early start of renal replacement treatment.

Anorectic obese patients with type 2 diabetes and advanced renal failure often undergo massive weight loss, leading to normalization of fasting glucose and even of glycemia after a glucose load.

Low muscle mass because of wasting is an important cause why physicians misjudge the severity of renal failure, because at any given level of GFR the serum creatinine concentration will then be spuriously low. Misjudgement of the extent of renal impairment may contribute to dosing errors of drugs that cumulate in renal failure and may also delay the start of RRT. In cases of doubt, it is advised to measure or estimate the creatinine clearance.

ANEMIA

Patients with DN tend to have more severe anemia than nondiabetic patients. In a small series of type 1 diabetic patients in an early stage of DN *(53)*, nearly 50% of the patients were anemic, compared with matched control patients with glomerulonephritis. This observation has recently been confirmed in a large series *(54)*. Ishimura found more severe anemia in type 2 diabetic patients with advanced renal disease compared with matched nondiabetic controls *(55)*. Anemia may be present even at an early stage of renal dysfunction *(54)*. Diabetic patients have inadequately low erythropoietin (EPO) concentrations in relation to the degree of anemia *(56)*. The assumption that treatment of anemia by EPO improves end-organ damage is unproven, but plausible. A positive effect on retinopathy *(57,58)* and polyneuropathy *(59)* is suggested by uncontrolled observations. The role of anemia and its reversal by EPO in patients with peripheral artery disease is unclear. One retrospective study claimed an adverse effect *(60)*, but the relative roles of improving oxygen supply vs increasing viscosity and other potential adverse effects on microrheology have not been worked out. Anemia has also been claimed to either improve *(61)* or aggravate *(62)* insulin resistance, but confounding effects of EPO treatment on appetite and food intake have not been excluded.

Current guidelines suggest work-up for anemia when hemoglobin (Hb) is less than 13.5 g/dL in adult males and 11.5 g/dL in premenopausal females (European Best Practise Guidelines, 2004). Two major studies currently investigate whether prevention of anemia by administration of EPO ameliorates cardiovascular surrogate markers and improves outcome.

CALCIUM PHOSPHATE METABOLISM

Although a detailed description of this complex topic is beyond the scope of this chapter, optimal management of the disturbed calcium phosphate metabolism reduces morbidity and mortality of patients with DN. Recently, the adverse effects of secondary hyperparathyroidism and its management because of its adverse effects on CVD have attracted considerable interest *(63)*. Hyper-parathyroidism tends to be less severe in the diabetic patient with renal failure.

Nevertheless, it causes problems in diabetic patients as well. First, hyperparathyroidism interferes with insulin sensitivity and secretion through various mechanisms *(64)*. Second, the use of calcitriol to suppress parathyroid hormone (PTH) secretion together with the use of calcium-containing oral phosphate binders presumably aggravates vascular calcification. Furthermore, the concentration of 1,25-dihydoxy-vitamin D_3 (calcitriol) is decreased in chronic renal failure and exerts adverse pathophysiological effects on its own. For example, a decrease in calcitriol may contribute to the progression of renal failure by aggravating podocyte injury *(65)*. Diabetic patients have also an increased risk to develop life-threatening calciphylaxis and low bone turnover. The 2003 K-DOQI guidelines recommend to limit the use of calcium-containing phosphate binders and propose an upper limit of 1.5-g calcium salts per day. New noncalcium phosphate binders are already on the market or currently tested in clinical trials (sevelamer, lanthanum, iron compounds). Future approaches to control calcium metabolism will include calcimimetic agents that increase the sensitivity of the calcium-sensing receptor in the parathyroid gland, thus lowering PTH concentrations and at the same time serum calcium and phosphorous concentrations *(66)*.

MANAGEMENT OF TERMINAL RENAL FAILURE

Vascular Access

Timely creation of vascular access is of overriding importance. This should be considered when the GFR is approx 20–25 mL/min. Although venous run-off problems are not unusual because of hypoplastic veins, particularly in elderly female diabetics or patients with venous occlusion after infections or infusions, it is inadequate arterial inflow that is increasingly recognized as a major cause of fistula malfunction *(67)*. If radial arteries are severely sclerotic, anastomosis at a more proximal level may be necessary. Use of native vessels for creation of the fistula is clearly the first choice *(68)* because results of polytetrafluoroethylene grafts are definitely inferior. It is often necessary, however, to create an upper arm of fistula *(68,69)* or use more sophisticated surgical approaches *(70)*. The most common underlying cause of fistula malfunction is the inability of sclerotic radial arteries to undergo vasodilatation and remodeling to permit an increase in blood flow from 10–20 to 1000 mL/min *(67)*. Arteriosclerosis of arm arteries may not only jeopardize fistula flow, but may also predispose to a "steal phenomenon" with finger gangrene *(71)*.

Initiation of Renal Replacement Therapy

Most nephrologists agree that in diabetic compared with nondiabetic patients, RRT should be started earlier at a GFR of approx 15 mL/min. An even earlier start may be justified when hypervolemia and blood pressure become uncontrollable, when the patient is severely anorectic or cachectic, and when the patient vomits as the combined result of uremia and gastroparesis. In this situation, clinical findings are more important than laboratory values.

Hemodialysis

Interdialytic and Intradialytic Blood Pressure

Dialyzed diabetic patients tend to be more hypertensive than dialyzed nondiabetic patients. In diabetic patients, blood pressure is exquisitely volume-dependent. The problem is further compounded by autonomic denervation, more pronounced aortic stiffness, and LVH with reduced LV compliance. As a result, the patients are predisposed to intradialytic hypotension. It is therefore often difficult to reach target "dry weight" by ultrafiltration. Nevertheless, reduced dietary salt intake and ultrafiltration often permit hypertension control without medication, but most patients require antihypertensive drugs.

Disturbed LV compliance causes an abrupt decrease of cardiac output when LV filling pressure decreases during ultrafiltration *(72)*. One or more of the following approaches are useful to avoid intradialytic hypotension: omission of antihypertensive agents immediately before dialysis sessions, long dialysis sessions, lowering of dialysate temperature, controlled ultrafiltration, and correction of anemia by EPO therapy. If nothing works, however, alternative treatment modalities such as continuous ambulatory peritoneal dialysis (CAPD) should be considered. Intradialytic hypotension increases the risk of cardiac death by a factor of 3 *(16)*. It also predisposes to myocardial ischemia, arrhythmia, deterioration of maculopathy, cortical atrophy of the brain and, particularly in the elderly, nonthrombotic mesenteric infarction. Sudden death on dialysis is preceded by a hypotensive episode in up to 30% of patients *(73)*. Pulse pressure and impaired elasticity of central arteries are major predictors of cardiovascular events and of death in non-uremic patients and in nondiabetic dialyzed patients, but for uncertain reasons not so in diabetic patients on dialysis *(73)*.

Metabolic Control on Hemodialysis

Dialysis treatment partially reverses insulin resistance, so that insulin requirements are often less than before dialysis. Even patients with type 1 diabetes may occasionally lose their need for insulin, at least transiently, on institution of HD. In other patients, however, insulin requirements increase, presumably because anorexia is reversed so that appetite and food consumption increase. It is most convenient to use a dialysate that contains usually about 200 mg/dL of glucose. This allows insulin to be administered at the usual times of the day, reduces the risk of hyperglycemic or hypoglycemic episodes during dialysis, and also causes less hypotensive episodes.

Adequate control of glycemia is important because hyperglycemia (and the resulting hyperosmolarity) causes thirst, high fluid intake, and hypervolemia as well as an osmotic shift of water and K^+ from the intracellular to the extracellular space. The consequences are circulatory congestion and hyperkalemia. Diabetics with poor glucose control are also more susceptible to infection. Finally, in dialyzed diabetic patients, poor glycemic control definitely increases the risk of death, mainly from CV causes *(45)*.

Asssessment of glycemic control using HbA1c is confounded by carbamylation of Hb and by altered red blood cell survival *(74)*. HbA1c values above 7.5% cause modest overestimation of hyperglycemia in diabetic patients with ESRD.

Diminished insulin-mediated glucose uptake as evidence of insulin resistance has been noted in the hearts of uremic animals *(75)* and this has been related to reduced ischemia tolerance of the heart *(33)*. Insulin should presumably be administered more generously, which might also be beneficial to control malnutrition and anemia management.

In view of the dramatic results of insulin and glucose administration after MI *(76)*, although recently not confirmed, and of the impressive benefit from intensive insulin therapy in critically ill patients, particularly in those with acute renal failure *(77)*, liberal administration of insulin is advisable in diabetic patients with ischemic heart disease.

Malnutrition on Hemodialysis

Because of anorexia and prolonged habituation to dietary restriction, the dietary intake of diabetic patients on HD often falls short of the required intake of energy (30–35 kcal/kg/d) and protein (1.3 g/kg/d). By X-ray absorptiometry, Okuno documented a decrease in body fat mass in diabetic compared with nondiabetic patients on HD *(78)*. This finding is particularly problematic because malnutrition is a potent predictor of mortality *(52)*. It is also of concern that malnutrition and/or microinflammation tend to be more common in diabetic patients *(79,80)*. Malnutrition is a predictor of mortality in diabetic patients *(81)*.

Peritoneal Dialysis

According to the US Renal Data System (2004), 11.5% of all patients with diabetes receiving RRT are treated with peritoneal dialysis (PD), whereas 68.8% receive maintenance HD and 17.9% undergo transplantation. There are often good *a priori* reasons to offer initially CAPD treatment to diabetic patients. In diabetic patients with ESRD, forearm vessels are often sclerosed, so it is difficult to create a fistula. The alternative of HD via intravenous catheters (instead of using AV fistulas or grafts) is not sufficient in the long run, because blood flow is low and the risk of infection high. Long-term dialysis via catheters was identified as one major predictor of poor survival on HD *(82)*.

There are further reasons to offer PD as the initial mode of RRT to the diabetic patient. During the first 2 yr of treatment, survival is better for patients treated with PD compared with HD *(83)* and this is also true for diabetic patients. The survival advantage was no longer demonstrable beyond the second year (presumably because by then residual renal function has decayed). Moreover, PD provides low and sustained ultrafiltration without rapid fluctuations of fluid volume and electrolyte concentrations (features that are advantageous for blood pressure control and prevention of heart failure).

An interesting concept has been proposed by Van Biesen *(4)*. When patients started PD and were then transferred to HD after residual renal function had decayed, they had better long-term survival compared with patients who started on HD and remained on HD throughout. As a potential explanation, it has been proposed that early start on CAPD prevents cumulative organ damage in the late stages of uremia. Survival of patients who had remained on CAPD for more than 48 mo, however, was inferior when compared with patients on HD, presumably because CAPD is no longer sufficiently effective once residual renal function has gone, at least in heavy patients. These optimistic views have recently been challenged by the result of a national survey in the United States, which showed that even in the initial years of treatment survival on CAPD was worse, particularly in diabetic patients with coronary heart disease *(84)*. Protection of residual renal function in patients on CAPD was recently achieved in patients, including diabetic patients, undergoing CAPD by administering ARBs, which attenuated the rate of loss of residual renal function *(85)*.

It is relevant that CAPD treatment is not a contraindication to renal transplantation. PD catheters should be left in place after transplantation until stable renal function has been attained and should be then removed.

In the past it was felt to be an attractive concept to administer insulin by injection into the CAPD fluid with the goal of providing insulin via the more physiological portal route. Unfortunately, there are many practical problems. Selection of the dose is difficult because since insulin binds to the surface of dialysis bags and tubing and is degraded by insulinases in the peritoneum. Moreover, absorption from the peritoneal cavity shows large interindividual variations. There is no firm evidence that the procedure permits better control of glycemia or dyslipidemia *(86)*. As a result, most nephrologists no longer use this approach.

Although protein is lost across the peritoneal membrane, the main nutritional problem is gain of glucose and calories because high glucose concentrations in the dialysate are necessary for the osmotic removal of excess body fluid. This leads to weight gain and obesity. Daily glucose absorption is 100–150 g and a CAPD patient is exposed to 3–7 t of fluid containing 50–175 kg glucose per year. The use of glucose-containing fluid has another interesting disadvantage. Heat sterilization of glucose under acid conditions creates highly reactive glucose degradation products (GDPs) such as methylglyoxal, glyoxalformaldehyde, deoxyglucosone, and 3,4-dideoxyglucosone-3-ene. GDPs are cytotoxic and also lead to the formation of advanced glycation endproducts (AGEs). Even in nondiabetic patients on CAPD, deposits of AGE are found in the peritoneal membrane and this is accompanied by fibrogenesis and neoangiogenesis with deterioration of peritoneal membrane properties. These observations led to the misleading, term "local diabetes mellitus." Heat sterilization using two-compartment bags circumvents the generation of toxic GDP. In prospective studies, CAPD fluid thus sterilized was much less toxic than conventional CAPD fluids, despite the high glucose concentration *(86)*.

TRANSPLANTATION IN THE DIABETIC PATIENT (KIDNEY ALONE AND PANCREAS PLUS KIDNEY)

Outcome of Kidney Transplantation

There is consensus that medical rehabilitation of the diabetic patient with uremia is best after transplantation *(87)*. Although survival of the diabetic patient with a kidney graft is worse compared with a grafted nondiabetic patient, the gain in life expectancy of the diabetic patient with a graft, compared with the dialyzed diabetic patient on the waiting list, is proportionally much greater than in the nondiabetic patients, because on dialysis survival of the diabetic patient is poor. The higher mortality of the diabetic compared with the nondiabetic patient with a kidney graft is mainly explained by pre-existing vascular disease *(28)*, LVH, and post-transplant hypertension. Woolfe *(87)* calculated the adjusted relative risk of death of transplant recipients as compared with patients on the waiting list. It was 0.27 for diabetic patients compared with 0.39 in nondiabetic patients with glomerulonephritis. Obviously, the perioperative risk is higher in diabetic than in nondiabetic patients, but nevertheless, in diabetic patients the predicted survival on the waiting list was only 8 yr and after transplantation no less than 19 yr. The majority of diabetic patients receiving a transplant are currently C-peptide-negative type 1, although in carefully selected type 2 diabetic patients without vascular disease who had received kidney grafts, graft and patient survival are impressive *(88)*. Diabetic patients must be subjected to rigorous pretransplantation evaluation, among others, to exclude CVD. In most centers, routine coronary angiography is therefore performed. As an alternative, Manske has devised an algorithm to identify the diabetic patient who should receive coronarography *(89)*. Patients should also be examined by X-ray, Doppler sonography, and (if necessary) angiography of pelvic arteries to avoid placement of a renal allograft into an iliac artery with heavy calcification or compromised arterial flow risking ischemia of the extremity and amputation.

Kidney Plus Pancreas Transplantation

Despite great excitement about the seminal double transplantation by Kelly *(90)* in Minneapolis, the results of simultaneous pancreas and kidney transplantation (SPK) had remained disappointing for a long time. The breakthrough came with the introduction of calcineurin inhibitors and low steroid protocols. In an impressivly large single-center experience comprising 335 patients, Becker *(3)* recently showed that survival of patients with SPK approached that of patients transplanted for nondiabetic renal disease and was clearly superior to diabetic recipients of living donor kidney grafts and particularly of cadaver kidney grafts (Fig. 1). The Kaplan-Meier estimate

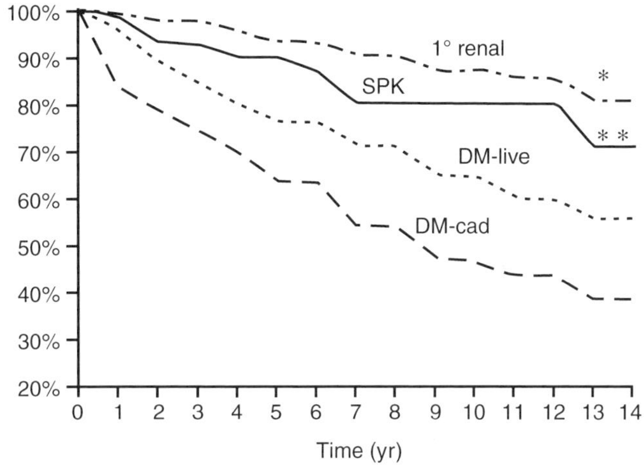

Fig. 1. Kaplan-Meier patient survival estimates in diabetic patients after simultaneous pancreas–kidney (SPK), cadaveric (DM-cad), or live-donor kidney transplantation (DM-live), compared with patients with nondiabetic primary renal disease undergoing cadaveric kidney transplantation (1° renal) (after ref. *3*). $*p = 0.0029 \times 1°$ vs all others. $**p = 0.004$ SPK vs DM-cad and DM-live.

of patient survival in 215 SPK vs 111 live-donor kidney graft recipients after 10 yr was 82% vs 71%. The annual mortality rate was 1.5% for SPK recipients, 3.65% for living donor kidney graft recipients, and 6.27% for cadaver donor kidney graft recipients. Reversibility of established microvascular complications after SPK is minor at best, with the important exception of autonomic polyneuropathy *(91)*, particularly improved cardiorespiratory reflexes, and some improvement in nerve conduction velocity *(92)*. Further benefits include improved gastric and bladder function *(93)* as well as superior quality of life, better metabolic control *(94)*, and improved survival *(3)*. Consequently, today SPK should be the preferred treatment modality for the type 1 diabetic who meets the selection criteria. As of 2003, more than 19,400 pancreas transplants have been performed, the majority in the United States. There is an increasing tendency for early or even pre-emptive SPK. Because graft outcome is progressively more adverse with increasing time spent on HD, this strategy is sensible. In the United States, diabetics younger than 55 yr are usually considered for SPK at a GFR less than 40mL/min, whereas criteria in Europe are more conservative with a GFR below 20mL/min.

Pancreas After Kidney Transplantation

An alternative strategy must be considered in the diabetic patient who has a live kidney donor: to first transplant the living donor kidney, and subsequently, once stable renal function is achieved (GFR >50mL/min), to transplant a cadaver donor pancreas. The outcomes are quite satisfactory *(95)*.

Procedure and Management

Today, the preferred SPK technique is enteric drainage. Bladder drainage has been increasingly abandoned because of irritation of mucosa, development of strictures, bicarbonate wasting with metabolic acidosis, recurrent urinary tract infections, and reflux pancreatitis.

Metabolic Results

Oral glucose tolerance normalizes unless the graft is damaged by ischemia or subclinical rejection related to HLA–DR mismatch. Most investigators find either normalization of insulin sensitivity or some impairment of insulin-stimulated nonoxidated glucose metabolism with hepatic insulin resistance *(96)* possibly related to insulin delivery into the systemic circulation (as opposed to the physiological delivery into the portal circulation). Impressive normalization of lipoprotein lipase activity and of the lipid spectrum pointing to reduced atherogenic risk have also been reported.

Diagnosis of Rejection

An interesting issue is whether rejection affects kidney and pancreatic grafts in parallel. Although this is mostly so (permitting to use the renal function as a surrogate marker of rejection of the pancreas), it is by no means obligatory, but episodes of isolated rejection of the pancreas are rare so that monitoring the kidney graft is the usual procedure. The pancreatic graft can be monitored by duplex sonography, if necessary, or pancreas graft biopsy. Pancreas grafts are usually lost because of alloimmunity reactions, but in rare cases, graft loss resulting from destruction by autoimmune mechanisms (with GAD-antibodies and IA2-antibodies) has been observed *(97)*. Recurrence of autoimmune inflammation with selective loss of insulin-producing β-cells (whereas sparing glucagon, somatostatin, and pancreatic polypeptide-secreting cells) and lymphocytic infiltration have been noted in the pioneer era when segmental pancreatic grafts were performed in monozygotic twins and when insulitis often recurred in the recipient. Today this has become rare, presumably because immunosuppression keeps autoimmunity under control. Rejection of the pancreas responds poorly to steroid treatment. Its treatment should always include T-cell antibodies.

Islet Cell Transplantation

Although more advanced procedures such as transplantation of stem cells or precursor cells, transplantation of encapsulated islet cells, islet xenotransplants, or insulin gene therapy are still beyond the horizon, islet cell transplantation has so far already yielded some interesting, but not yet definitive results. As of November 2004, worldwide more than 800 patients received islet cell transplants. Only eight centers have more than 10 yr experience with this method, although several additional centers have started an islet cell transplantation program since 2000. Patient survival was 79% and 14% of patients were off insulin, but measureable C-peptide greater than 0.5ng/mL as evidence of residual islet function was noted in 45%. Minor intraportal insulin secretion may be relevant because it may normalize hepatic glucose production *(98)*. This area got a major boost by Shapiro *(99)*, who reported on successful islet transplantation achieving insulin independence in seven consecutive patients using a steroid-free immunosuppression regimen consisting of sirolimus, tacrolimus, and taclizumab. The generalizibility of the results is currently evaluated by a multicenter study.

CONCLUSIONS

Diabetes has become the single most frequent comorbid condition in patients entering renal replacement programs, the proportion of incident patients with diabetes ranging from 30% to 50% in all Western countries. The majority suffer from diabetic glomerulosclerosis, but approx 20% suffer from ischemic nephropathy and from another nondiabetic renal disease, respectively. A frequent mode of presentation in ESRD is irreversible acute, mostly acute on chronic, renal failure. The therapeutic options comprise HD, CAPD, and transplantation, either kidney alone or kidney plus pancreas (SPK). An emerging problem is the appearance of diabetes type 2 in nondiabetic patients having undergone renal transplantation. The prognosis of diabetics on RRT is consistently worse than in nondiabetic patients. The main causes of death are cardiac disease and peripheral artery disease. The main clinical problems are difficulties with vascular access, accelerated coronary heart disease and CHF, complications of neuropathic and/or vascular diabetic foot, anemia, malnutrition, and changes in the pharmacokinetics of insulin, and some oral antidiabetic agents.

REFERENCES

1. Ghavamian M, Gutch CF, Kopp KF, Kolff WJ. The sad truth about hemodialysis in diabetic nephropathy. JAMA 1972;222:1386–1389.
2. Lillehei RC, Simmons RL, Najarian JS, et al. Pancreatico-duodenal allotransplantation: experimental and clinical experience. Ann Surg 1970;172:405–436.
3. Becker BN, Brazy PC, Becker YT, et al. Simultaneous pancreas–kidney transplantation reduces excess mortality in type-l diabetic patients with end-stage renal disease. Kidney Int 2000;57: 2129–2135.
4. Van Biesen W, Vanholder RC, Veys N, Dhondt A, Lameire NH. An evaluation of an integrative care approach for end-stage renal disease patients. J Am Soc Nephrol 2000;11:116–125.
5. Bojestig M, Arnqvist HJ, Hermansson G, Karlberg BE, Ludvigsson J. Declining incidence of nephropathy in insulin-dependent diabetes mellitus. N Engl J Med 1994;330:15–18.
6. Gaede P, Vedel P, Larsen N, Jensen GV, Parving HH, Pedersen O. Multifactorial intervention and cardiovascular disease in patients with type-2 diabetes. N Engl J Med 2003;348:383–393.
7. Zimmet P, Alberti KG, Shaw J. Global and societal implications of the diabetes epidemic. Nature 2001;414:782–787.
8. Adler AI, Stevens RJ, Manley SE, Bilous RW, Cull CA, Holman RR. Development and progression of nephropathy in type-2 diabetes: the United Kingdom prospective diabetes study (UKPDS 64). Kidney Int 2003;63:225–232.
9. Yokoyama H, Okudaira M, Otani T, et al. Higher incidence of diabetic nephropathy in type 2 than in type 1 diabetes in early-onset diabetes in Japan. Kidney Int 2000;58:302–311.
10. Ritz E, Orth SR. Nephropathy in patients with type-2 diabetes mellitus. N Engl J Med 1999;341: 1127–1133.
11. McBean AM, Li S, Gilbertson DT, Collins AJ. Differences in diabetes prevalence, incidence, and mortality among the elderly of four racial/ethnic groups: whites, blacks, hispanics, and asians. Diabetes Care 2004;27:2317–2324
12. Stengel B, Billon S, Van Dijk PC, et al. Trends in the incidence of renal replacement therapy for end-stage renal disease in Europe, 1990–1999. Nephrol Dial Transplant 2003;18:1824–1833.
13. Ritz E, Stefanski A. Diabetic nephropathy in type II diabetes. Am J Kidney Dis 1996;27:167–194.
14. Collins AJ, Kasiske B, Herzog C, et al. Excerpts from the United States renal data system 2003 annual data report: atlas of end-stage renal disease in the United States. Am J Kidney Dis 2003;42:A5–A7.
15. Schwenger V, Mussig C, Hergesell O, Zeier M, Ritz E. Incidence and clinical characteristics of renal insufficiency in diabetic patients. Dtsch Med Wochenschr 2001;126:1322–1326.
16. Koch M, Thomas B, Tschope W, Ritz E. Survival and predictors of death in dialysed diabetic patients. Diabetologia 1993;36:1113–1117.
17. Koch M, Kutkuhn B, Trenkwalder E, et al. Apolipoprotein B, fibrinogen, HDL cholesterol, and apolipoprotein(a) phenotypes predict coronary artery disease in hemodialysis patients. J Am Soc Nephrol 1997;8:1889–1898.
18. Wanner C, Krane V, Ruf G, Marz W, Ritz E. Rationale and design of a trial improving outcome of type-2 diabetics on hemodialysis. Die Deutsche Diabetes Dialyse Studie Investigators. Kidney Int Suppl 1999;71:S222–S226.
19. Dikow R, Adamczak M, Henriquez DE, Ritz E. Strategies to decrease cardiovascular mortality in patients with end-stage renal disease. Kidney Int 2002;64:5–10.
20. Dikow R, Ritz E. Cardiovascular complications in the diabetic patient with renal disease: an update in 2003. Nephrol Dial Transpl 2003;18:1993–1998.

21. Iseki K, Tozawa M, Iseki C, Takishita S, Ogawa Y. Demographic trends in the Okinawa dialysis study (OKIDS) registry (1971–2000). Kidney Int 2002;61:668–675.
22. Gilbertson DT XJL, Collins AJ. The increasing burden of diabetes in United States ESRD patients. J Am Soc Nephrol 13:646a, 2002.
23. Chantrel F, Enache I, Bouiller M, et al. Abysmal prognosis of patients with type-2 diabetes entering dialysis. Nephrol Dial Transpl 1999;14:129–136.
24. Schwenger V, Hofmann A, Khalifeh N, et al. Uremic patients—late referral, early death. Dtsch Med Wochenschr 2003;128:1216–1220.
25. Stack AG, Bloembergen WE. A cross-sectional study of the prevalence and clinical correlates of congestive heart failure among incident US dialysis patients. Am J Kidney Dis 2001;38:992–1000.
26. Levin A, Djurdjev O, Barrett B, et al. Cardiovascular disease in patients with chronic kidney disease: getting to the heart of the matter. Am J Kidney Dis 2001;38:1398–1407.
27. Foley RN, Culleton BF, Parfrey PS, et al. Cardiac disease in diabetic end-stage renal disease. Diabetologia 1997;40:1307–1312.
28. Hypolite IO, Bucci J, Hshieh P, et al. Acute coronary syndromes after renal transplantation in patients with end-stage renal disease resulting from diabetes. Am J Transpl 2002;2:274–281.
29. Herzog CA, Ma JZ, Collins AJ. Poor long-term survival after acute myocardial infarction among patients on long-term dialysis. N Engl J Med 1998;339:799–805.
30. Shlipak MG, Fried LF, Crump C, et al. Cardiovascular disease risk status in elderly persons with renal insufficiency. Kidney Int 2002;62:997–1004.
31. Foley RN, Parfrey PS, Sarnak MJ. Epidemiology of cardiovascular disease in chronic renal disease. J Am Soc Nephrol 1998;9:S16–S23.
32. Standl E, Schnell O. A new look at the heart in diabetes mellitus: from ailing to failing. Diabetologia 2000;43:1455–1469.
33. Amann K, Ritz E. Microvascular disease—the Cinderella of uraemic heart disease. Nephrol Dial Transplant 2000;15:1493–1503.
34. Aviles RJ, Askari AT, Lindahl B, et al. Troponin T levels in patients with acute coronary syndromes, with or without renal dysfunction. N Engl J Med 2002;346:2047–2052.
35. Mallamaci F, Zoccali C, Parlongo S, et al. Troponin is related to left ventricular mass and predicts all-cause and cardiovascular mortality in hemodialysis patients. Am J Kidney Dis 2002;40:68–75.
36. Manske CL, Wang Y, Rector T, Wilson RF, White CW. Coronary revascularisation in insulin-dependent diabetic patients with chronic renal failure. Lancet 1992;340:998–1002.
37. Herzog CA, Ma JZ, Collins AJ. Long-term outcome of dialysis patients in the United States with coronary revascularization procedures. Kidney Int 1999;56:324–332.
38. Herzog CA, Ma JZ, Collins AJ. Comparative survival of dialysis patients in the United States after coronary angioplasty, coronary artery stenting, and coronary artery bypass surgery and impact of diabetes. Circulation 2002;106:2207–2211.
39. Zuanetti G, Maggioni AP, Keane W, Ritz E. Nephrologists neglect administration of betablockers to dialysed diabetic patients. Nephrol Dial Transpl 1997;12:2497–2500.
40. Cice G, Ferrara L, D'Andrea A, et al. Carvedilol increases two-year survivalin dialysis patients with dilated cardiomyopathy: a prospective, placebo-controlled trial. J Am Coll Cardiol 2003;41:1438–1444.
41. Tschope W, Koch M, Thomas B, Ritz E. Serum lipids predict cardiac death in diabetic patients on maintenance hemodialysis. Results of a prospective study. The German Study Group Diabetes and Uremia. Nephron 1993;64:354–358.
42. Liu Y, Coresh J, Eustace JA, et al. Association between cholesterol level and mortality in dialysis patients: role of inflammation and malnutrition. JAMA 2004;291:451–459.
43. Foley RN, Herzog CA, Collins AJ. Smoking and cardiovascular outcomes in dialysis patients: The United States Renal Data System Wave 2 Study. Kidney Int 2003;63:1462–1467.
44. Wu MS, Yu CC, Yang CW, et al. Poor pre-dialysis glycaemic control is a predictor of mortality in type II diabetic patients on maintenance haemodialysis. Nephrol Dial Transpl 1997;12:2105–2110.
45. Morioka T, Emoto M, Tabata T, et al. Glycemic control is a predictor of survival for diabetic patients on hemodialysis. Diabetes Care 2001;24:909–913.
46. Yusuf S, Sleight P, Pogue J, Bosch J, Davies R, Dagenais G. Effects of an angiotensin-converting-enzyme inhibitor, ramipril, on cardiovascular events in high-risk patients. The Heart Outcomes Prevention Evaluation Study Investigators. N Engl J Med 2000;342:145–153.
47. Brenner BM, Cooper ME, de Zeeuw D, et al. Effects of losartan on renal and cardiovascular outcomes in patients with type-2 diabetes and nephropathy. N Engl J Med 2001;345:861–869.
48. Lewis EJ, Hunsicker LG, Bain RP, Rohde RD. The effect of angiotensin-converting-enzyme inhibition on diabetic nephropathy. The Collaborative Study Group. N Engl J Med 1993;329:1456–1462.

49. Lewis EJ, Hunsicker LG, Clarke WR, et al. Renoprotective effect of the angiotensin-receptor antagonist irbesartan in patients with nephropathy due to type-2 diabetes. N Engl J Med 2001;345:851–860.
50. Palmer BF. Renal dysfunction complicating the treatment of hypertension. N Engl J Med 2002;347: 1256–1261.
51. Wolf G, Ritz E. Diabetic nephropathy in type-2 diabetes prevention and patient management. J Am Soc Nephrol 2003;14:1396–1405.
52. Kalantar-Zadeh K, Block G, Humphreys MH, Kopple JD. Reverse epidemiology of cardiovascular risk factors in maintenance dialysis patients. Kidney Int 2003;63:793–808.
53. Bosman DR, Winkler AS, Marsden JT, Macdougall IC, Watkins PJ. Anemia with erythropoietin deficiency occurs early in diabetic nephropathy. Diabetes Care 2001;24:495–499.
54. Thomas MC, MacIsaac RJ, Tsalamandris C, et al. Anemia in patients with type-1 diabetes. J Clin Endocrinol Metab 2004;89:4359–4363.
55. Ishimura E, Nishizawa Y, Okuno S, et al. Diabetes mellitus increases the severity of anemia in non-dialyzed patients with renal failure. US J Nephrol 1998;11:83–86.
56. Dikow R, Schwenger V, Schomig M, Ritz E. How should we manage anaemia in patients with diabetes? Nephrol Dial Transpl 2002;17(1):67–72.
57. Friedman EA, L'Esperance FA, Brown CD, Berman DH. Treating azotemia-induced anemia with erythropoietin improves diabetic eye disease. Kidney Int Suppl 2003;S57–S63.
58. Sinclair SH, DelVecchio C, Levin A. Treatment of anemia in the diabetic patient with retinopathy and kidney disease. Am J Ophthalmol 2003;135:740–743.
59. Hassan K, Simri W, Rubenchik I, et al. Effect of erythropoietin therapy on polyneuropathy in predialytic patients. J Nephrol 2003;16:121–125.
60. Wakeen M, Zimmerman SW. Association between human recombinant EPO and peripheral vascular disease in diabetic patients receiving peritoneal dialysis. Am J Kidney Dis 1998;32:488–493.
61. Spaia S, Pangalos M, Askepidis N, et al. Effect of short-term rHuEPO treatment on insulin resistance in haemodialysis patients. Nephron 2000;84:320–325.
62. Rigalleau V, Blanchetier V, Aparicio M, et al. Erythropoietin can deteriorate glucose control in uraemic non-insulin-dependent diabetic patients. Diabetes Metab 1998;24:62–65.
63. Goldsmith D, Ritz E, Covic A. Vascular calcification: a stiff challenge for the nephrologist: does preventing bone disease cause arterial disease? Kidney Int 2004;66:1315–1333.
64. Procopio M, Borretta G. Derangement of glucose metabolism in hyperparathyroidism. J Endocrinol Invest 2003;26:1136–1142.
65. Kuhlmann A, Haas CS, Gross ML, et al. 1,25-Dihydroxyvitamin D3 decreases podocyte loss and podocyte hypertrophy in the subtotally nephrectomized rat. Am J Physiol Renal Physiol 2004;286: F526–F533.
66. Block GA, Martin KJ, de Francisco AL, et al. Cinacalcet for secondary hyperparathyroidism in patients receiving hemodialysis. US N Engl J Med 2004;350:1516–1525.
67. Konner K, Nonnast-Daniel B, Ritz E. The arteriovenous fistula. J Am Soc Nephrol 2003;14:1669–1680.
68. Konner K. Primary vascular access in diabetic patients: an audit. Nephrol Dial Transpl 2000;15: 1317–1325.
69. Dixon BS, Novak L, Fangman J. Hemodialysis vascular access survival: upper-arm native arteriovenous fistula. Am J Kidney Dis 2002;39:92–101.
70. Gefen JY, Fox D, Giangola G, Ewing DR, Meisels IS. The transposed forearm loop arteriovenous fistula: a valuable option for primary hemodialysis access in diabetic patients. Ann Vasc Surg 2002;16:89–94.
71. Yeager RA, Moneta GL, Edwards JM, et al. Relationship of hemodialysis access to finger gangrene in patients with end-stage renal disease. J Vasc Surg 2002;36:245–249; discussion 249.
72. Daugirdas JT. Pathophysiology of dialysis hypotension: an update. Am J Kidney Dis 2001;38:S11–S17.
73. Karnik JA, Young BS, Lew NL, et al. Cardiac arrest and sudden death in dialysis units. Kidney Int 2001;60:350–357.
74. Joy MS, Cefalu WT, Hogan SL, Nachman PH. Long-term glycemic control measurements in diabetic patients receiving hemodialysis. Am J Kidney Dis 2002;39:297–307.
75. Ritz E, Koch M. Morbidity and mortality due to hypertension in patients with renal failure. Am J Kidney Dis 1993;21:113–118.
76. Malmberg K, Norhammar A, Ryden L. Insulin treatment post myocardial infarction: the DIGAMI study. Adv Exp Med Biol 2001;498:279–284.
77. van den Berghe G, Wouters P, Weekers F, et al. Intensive insulin therapy in the critically ill patients. N Engl J Med 2001;345:1359–1367.
78. Okuno S, Ishimura E, Kim M, et al. Changes in body fat mass in male hemodialysis patients: a comparison between diabetics and nondiabetics. Am J Kidney Dis 2001;38:S208–S211.

79. Saraheimo M, Teppo AM, Forsblom C, Fagerudd J, Groop PH. Diabetic nephropathy is associated with low-grade inflammation in Type-1 diabetic patients. Diabetologia 2003;46:1402–1407.
80. Suliman ME, Stenvinkel P, Heimburger O, Barany P, Lindholm B, Bergstrom J. Plasma sulfur amino acids in relation to cardiovascular disease, nutritional status, and diabetes mellitus in patients with chronic renal failure at start of dialysis therapy. Am J Kidney Dis 2002;40:480–488.
81. Cano NJ, Roth H, Aparicio M, et al. Malnutrition in hemodialysis diabetic patients: evaluation and prognostic influence. Kidney Int 2002;62:593–601.
82. Sehgal AR, Leon JB, Siminoff LA, Singer ME, Bunosky LM, Cebul RD. Improving the quality of hemodialysis treatment: a community-based randomized controlled trial to overcome patient-specific barriers. JAMA 2002;287:1961–1967.
83. Heaf JG, Lokkegaard H, Madsen M. Initial survival advantage of peritoneal dialysis relative to haemodialysis. Nephrol Dial Transpl 2002;17:112–117.
84. Winkelmayer WC, Glynn RJ, Mittleman MA, Levin R, Pliskin JS, Avorn J. Comparing mortality of elderly patients on hemodialysis versus peritoneal dialysis: a propensity score approach. J Am Soc Nephrol 2002;13:2353–2362.
85. Suzuki H, Kanno Y, Sugahara S, Okada H, Nakamoto H. Effects of an angiotensin II receptor blocker, valsartan, on residual renal function in patients on CAPD. Am J Kidney Dis 2004;43:1056–1064.
86. Nevalainen PI, Lahtela JT, Mustonen J, Pasternack A. Subcutaneous and intraperitoneal insulin therapy in diabetic patients on CAPD. Perit Dial Int 1996;16(1):S288–S2291.
87. Wolfe RA, Ashby VB, Milford EL, et al. Comparison of mortality in all patients on dialysis, patients on dialysis awaiting transplantation, and recipients of a first cadaveric transplant. N Engl J Med 1999;341:1725–1730.
88. Mieghem AV, Fonck C, Coosemans W, et al. Outcome of cadaver kidney transplantation in 23 patients with type-2 diabetes mellitus. Nephrol Dial Transpl 2001;16:1686–1691.
89. Manske CL, Thomas W, Wang Y, Wilson RF. Screening diabetic transplant candidates for coronary artery disease: identification of a low risk subgroup. Kidney Int 1993;44:617–621.
90. Kelly WD, Lillehei RC, Merkel FK, Idezuki Y, Goetz FC. Allotransplantation of the pancreas and duodenum along with the kidney in diabetic nephropathy. Surgery 1967;61:827–837.
91. Tyden G, Bolinder J, Solders G, Brattstrom C, Tibell A, Groth CG. Improved survival in patients with insulin-dependent diabetes mellitus and end-stage diabetic nephropathy 10 years after combined pancreas and kidney transplantation. Transplantation 1999;67:645–648.
92. Solders G, Tyden G, Tibell A, Persson A, Groth CG. Improvement in nerve conduction 8 years after combined pancreatic and renal transplantation. Transplant Proc 1995;27:3091.
93. Hathaway DK, Abell T, Cardoso S, Hartwig MS, el Gebely S, Gaber AO. Improvement in autonomic and gastric function following pancreas–kidney versus kidney-alone transplantation and the correlation with quality of life. Transplantation 1994;57:816–822.
94. Kahl A, Bechstein WO, Frei U. Trends and perspectives in pancreas and simultaneous pancreas and kidney transplantation. Curr Opin Urol 2001;11:165–174.
95. Hariharan S, Pirsch JD, Lu CY, et al. Pancreas after kidney transplantation. J Am Soc Nephrol 2002;13:1109–1118.
96. Rooney DP, Robertson RP. Hepatic insulin resistance after pancreas transplantation in type-I diabetes. Diabetes 1996;45:134–138.
97. Tyden G, Reinholt FP, Sundkvist G, Bolinder J. Recurrence of autoimmune diabetes mellitus in recipients of cadaveric pancreatic grafts. N Engl J Med 1996;335:860–863.
98. Luzi L, Perseghin G, Brendel MD, et al. Metabolic effects of restoring partial beta-cell function after islet allotransplantation in type 1 diabetic patients. Diabetes 2001;50:277–282.
99. Shapiro AM, Lakey JR, Ryan EA, et al. Islet transplantation in seven patients with type-1 diabetes mellitus using a glucocorticoid-free immunosuppressive regimen. N Engl J Med 2000;343:230–238.

25 Diabetic Renal and Related Heart Disease

ACE Inhibitors and/or Angiotensin Receptor Blockers: Does It Matter?

Carl Erik Mogensen, MD
and Niels Holmark Andersen, MD, PhD

Contents

INTRODUCTION

Several factors are important in determining the rate of progression of diabetic renal disease always starting from microalbuminuria *(1)*, and elevated blood pressure (BP) seems to be a major factor, both in types 1 and 2 diabetes *(1–3)*. This was confirmed in a new analysis in the follow-up studies of proteinuric patients conducted by Steno Diabetes Center *(2,3)*. Although the prognosis for diabetic nephropathy has improved in the last two decades, it is clear that proteinuric patients still have a poor prognosis *(1)*. For type 1 diabetes, this analysis *(2)* showed that elevated BP, glycemic control, and albuminuria were major factors in the progression. Serum cholesterol level also seemed to play some role. The rate of progression in patients with albuminuria and type 2 diabetes is quite similar *(3)*, although it should be noted that patients with type 2 diabetes and proteinuria most often die from cardiovascular (CV) disease before progression to end-stage renal disease (ESRD), even more than patients with type 1 diabetes and albuminuria.

Thus, there can be no doubt that high BP is a major factor in progression of diabetic nephropathy in the two types of diabetes *(1–3)*. Agents that block the renin–angiotensin system (RAS), angiotensin converting enzyme (ACE) inhibitor, or angiotensin receptor blocker (ARB) now dominate antihypertensive treatment in these patients *(4)*. The main purpose with this chapter is to analyze which treatment strategy is optimal in all

From: *Contemporary Diabetes: The Diabetic Kidney*
Edited by: P. Cortes and C. E. Mogensen © Humana Press Inc., Totowa, NJ

these patients. Here not only renal prognosis including decline in glomerular filtration rate (GFR) should be considered, but also other CV end points, also in the heart failure treatment. Obviously, also cost–benefit considerations must be taken into account. It should also be considered whether the so-called dual blockade may further improve the prognosis compared with single blockade of RAS *(4)*. Another important question remains to be answered: Is traditional antihypertensive treatment inferior to agents that block the RAS in inhibiting progression of diabetic nephropathy? The emerging role of aldosterone antagonism should also be taken into consideration *(5)*. In addition, a study of type 2 diabetes it was also shown that the degree of diabetic retinopathy and anemia was important. Anemia was a significant risk factor, although not very strong, and this was also the case for cigarette smoking, emphasizing the multifactorial risk profile *(1–3)*, including a low GFR. Therefore, it can be concluded that there is not a substantial difference between risk factors and progression promoters in the two types of diabetes, and the same strategy for treatment seems warranted, but early treatment is essential *(1,6,7)*.

RENAL DISEASE

ACE Inhibitors vs β-Blockers/Diuretics

In the paper by Hovind et al., a summary was also made on studies and clinical trials related to diabetic nephropathy in type 1 diabetic patients with or without antihypertensive treatment, including patients in placebo or control groups. In the analysis it was observed the decline of GFR with normotension was low *(2)*. The mean arterial BP in many other patients studied was much higher than in the present strategy of treatment, resulting with high pressure in rapid decline in GFR. Some studies suggested that ACE inhibitors were more efficient in reducing progression of diabetic nephropathy, but this was not the case in all studies, for example, not in the randomized trial by Elving et al. nor by Tarnow et al. *(2)*. In the observational study by Hovind, there seems to be no major difference between renal progression as far as a fall in GFR is concerned between non-ACE inhibition. However, new studies document that in microalbuminuric patients with type 1 diabetes mellitus, ACE inhibition clearly reduce progression of albuminuria compared with placebo administration *(6)*. Further arguments for using ACE inhibition in patients with type 1 are the fewer side effects seen in this type of treatment as compared with β-blockers, where hypoglycaemia unawareness maybe a serious problem. Therefore it can be concluded that treatment of choice of type 1 diabetes is usually ACE inhibition, although other antihypertensive agents are efficient. Indeed, the first studies in micro- and macroalbuminuric patients document that β-blockers are quite efficient in reducing albuminuria *(2,7)*.

Prevention of Diabetes: ACE Inhibitor and ARB?

In the treatment of hypertension in nondiabetic individuals, great care should be taken to select agents that do not confer an increased risk for the development of new diabetes. The aim should be to use agents that may at least be neutral, or even better to some extent protective against, the development of glucose intolerance. Hypertensive patients have a risk of developing diabetes of 1–2% per year *(8–10)*. It should also be noted that apart from glucose intolerance hyponatriaemia and hypokalemia may be a serious clinical problem, especially in elderly patients treated with thiazide diuretics.

A number of studies have shown that both ACE inhibitors and ARBs seem to confer an antidiabetic effect, at least when compared with diuretics and β-blockers. The

Table 1
Comparative Incidence of New-Onset Diabetes With ACE Inhibitor, ARBs, Diuretics, β-Blockers and Calcium Channel Blockers (CCBs) in Clinical Trials

Study	*Treatments*	*Duration (yr)*	*New-onset diabetes (%)*	*p*
CAPPP	ACE inhibitor vs β-blocker/diuretic	6.1	6.5 vs 7.3	<0.05
HOPE	ACE inhibitor vs placebo	4.5	3.6 vs 5.4	<0.001
LIFE	ARB vs β-blocker	4.8	6 vs 8	<0.001
SCOPE	ARB vs diuretic	3.7	4.9 vs 6	0.09
ALLHAT	ACE inhibitor vs CCB vs diuretic	4.9	8.1 vs 9.8 vs 11.6	< 0.05
ALPINE	ARB vs diuretic/β-blocker	1	0.5 vs 4.1	<0.05
CHARM	ARB vs conventional therapy	1.6	6 vs 7	<0.02
VALUE	ARB vs CCB	5.5	13.1 vs 16.4	<0.0001

Modified from ref. *8* (*see also* refs. *9* and *10*).

recently published Valsartan Antihypertensive Long-term Use Evaluation (VALUE) study *(11)* also showed that the ARB, valsartan, confers benefits in protecting against diabetes in comparison with the calcium channel blocker (CCB), amlodipine, with a highly significantly reduced risk of developing new type 2 diabetes during 5 yr of follow-up. A summary of evidence from clinical trials evidence to date is provided in Table 1.

Thus, a strong argument can already be made for the initial selection of these agents rather than diuretics or β-blockers alone, and now even CCBs *(11)*. This applies particularly to patients with CV disease and hypertension, and probably also to individuals with uncomplicated hypertension.

However, the issue is not completely settled. First of all, we may need a more definitive study, such as the ongoing diabetes reduction approaches with ramipril and rosiglitazone medications (dream) study, which will assess the effects of ramipril and rosiglitazone in patients at high risk of developing diabetes. We also need more information on the mechanisms of action of antihypertensives because details are not yet clearly understood.

Preventing Microalbuminuria in Diabetes

Patients with normoalbuminuria have been examined, first in type 2 diabetes, with an ACE inhibitor by Ravid and coworkers *(12)*. The ACE inhibitor prevented development of microalbuminuria. Kvetny et al. *(13)* showed the same for type 1 diabetes using Perindopril. The Bergamo Nephrologic Diabetes Complications Trial (BENEDICT) was recently published *(14)*. Indeed, it is important to distinguish between normo- and microalbuminuria and renal insufficiency, as confirmed by Adler and coworkers in the United Kingdom Prospective Diabetes Study (UKPDS) *(15)*. Clearly, patients with normoalbuminuria have the best prognosis and there is strong evidence showing that preventing progression is associated with a much better prognosis, which was also documented in the recent paper by Gaede and coworkers from the Steno Diabetes Center. They showed that remission to normoalbuminuria is associated with much better preservation of renal function in terms of GFR fall, which is stabilized *(16)*.

The most recent and comprehensive documentation regarding primary prevention, meaning that microalbuminuria can be prevented in type 2 diabetes, comes from the BENEDICT study group in Bergamo *(14)*. This is the largest study so far conducted, and very interestingly, this study also compares an ACE inhibitor with a calcium blocker, verapamil.

This was a large study in northern Italy, comprising 1204 patients randomly designated to 3 yr of treatment with trandolapril alone, trandolapril + verapamil, verapamil alone, and placebo *(14)*. Interestingly, hypertension was defined as low as a BP above 130/85 or ongoing antihypertensive treatment. The primary end point was development of persistent microalbuminuria with an overnight albumin excretion rate higher than 20 mg/min on two consecutive occasions.

The primary outcome was seen in 6% of the patients treated with the ACE inhibitor alone and in 10% of the patients receiving placebo, and there was a clearly significant difference ($p - 0.01$). Treatment with verapamil alone was not different from placebo. The authors also estimated the so-called acceleration factors, which were clearly in favor of the use of the ACE inhibitor. There were only minor differences of BP between the treatment arms, but this may still have played a role for the positive results with ACE inhibitor. There were few serious events in the two treatment groups. The conclusion was clear: in patients with type 2 diabetes and hypertension (above 130/85), but with normoalbuminuria, treatment with an ACE inhibitor was clearly beneficial in preventing development of microalbuminuria, which is the first sign of renal damage in these patients. Microalbuminuria is a major risk factor for vascular events, and obviously, also for advanced renal disease and death *(1,15)*.

In conclusion, there is now fairly good evidence from clinical trials that treatment with an ACE inhibitor should be started early in patients with type 2 diabetes and normoalbuminuria. Treatment should be initiated when systolic BP is more than 130 systolic mm/Hg. Systolic BP elevation is very common in patients with type 2 diabetes and metabolic syndrome. This means that most type 2 diabetes mellitus patients would qualify for this type of treatment. These patients also often show sodium retention and therefore a combination with an ACE inhibitor and diuretics seems to be most effective in reducing microalbuminuria and BP *(1)*. Now there seems to be a very good foundation for substantial improvements of the prognosis for patients with type 2 diabetes *(1,14)* and early treatment of hypertension leads to better prognosis, as does, but maybe to a lesser extent, improved euglycemic control *(16)*. Clearly treatment with statins is also important, as documented in many studies, among others the Steno-2 study *(16)*. Now we have apparently completed the paradigm shift: it is essential to normalize glycemia, BP, and dyslipedimia in all patients with type 2 diabetes. Further studies are ongoing *(17)*. Genetic factors (as previously commonly believed in the United States) have not yet been documented to play any significant role *(18)*, but there is clearly much more available room for intensified clinical care in patients with type 2 diabetes.

ACE Inhibitor or ARBs in Early Nephropathy

Furthermore, although it is evident that both classes of drugs, inhibiting the RAS, appear to be beneficial, an important question remains: Is one class superior for the prevention of the development of CV and renal disease? This particular issue has now been addressed by the Diabetics Exposed to Telmisartan and Enalapril (DETAIL) trial *(19)*.

DETAIL was a much-needed, long-term study comparing an ACE inhibitor with an ARB in a diabetic population. The 5-yr, prospective, multicenter, double-blind study directly compared the ACE inhibitor, enalapril, with the ARB, telmisartan, in patients with type 2 diabetes, hypertension and evidence of early nephropathy, and in many cases microalbuminuria. DETAIL was also the first study of its kind to monitor the progression of kidney disease by directly measuring the GFR, now recognized as the best indicator of overall kidney function and ESRD.

The fall in GFR at 5 yr—the main endpoint—was the same in patients treated with either drug, with changes in GFR from baseline of approx –17 mL/min/1.73m^2 in the telmisartan group and –15 mL/min/1.73m^2 in the enalapril group. Analysis of the secondary endpoint of the yearly change in GFR revealed an initial steep decline in GFR in both groups, of approx –8 mL/min/1.73m^2, which then stabilized to approx –2 mL/min/1.73m^2 beyond 3 yr.

BP was lowered to a comparable degree in each treatment group, and CV mortality was much lower than would be expected at 5 yr, with three and five CV-related deaths in the telmisartan and enalapril groups, respectively. Other adverse event rates were similar between the two groups, as ACE inhibitor-intolerant patients were excluded from the study. There were no cases of ESRD in either group.

Other shorter studies have indicated that the ACE inhibitors and ARBs exert similar effects as far as albuminuria and BP are concerned *(20–22)*. Furthermore, dual blockade using a drug of each class is a possible approach in patients who do not respond well to single blockade *(22,23)*, especially in microalbuminuric patients *(22)*.

Thus, with the latest results from DETAIL in mind, the clinician may choose either an ACE inhibitor or an ARB, or even the two in combination *(23)*. However, questions remain regarding the longer term in advanced nephropathy. The strong endpoint studies, namely the Reduction of endpoints in NIDDM with the Angiotensin II Antagonist Losartan (RENAAL) study and the Irbesartan type 2 Diabetic Nephropathy Trial (IDNT) study, in patients with type 2 diabetes and overt nephropathy, should be considered *(24,25)*. The results of these studies would favor the use of ARBs, and yet as there are no similar studies comparing ACE inhibitors with ARBs to provide further information in this patient group. Indeed, compared with advanced disease intervention in microalbuminuric patients may prove much more effective *(1,6,7,16,19–22)*.

The Effect of ACE Inhibitor and ARBs on Renal Outcomes and Mortality: Studies in Diabetic Nephropathy

During the oral presentation in San Francisco of the important studies on ARBs and overt diabetic nephropathy (type 2 diabetes) *(25)*, one of the dedicated physicians in the audience asked one of the principal investigators: Why did you not compare ACE inhibitors with ARBs, because we know that ACE inhibitors are quite effective in type 1 and 2 diabetes according to many studies? The principal investigators became slightly disturbed, but clearly this question was very relevant, and an important review article on this issue was recently published in the *British Medical Journal (26)*. It is an interesting meta-analysis conducted in a very systematic way.

The question put forward in this chapter was relevant and clear: when considering all papers dealing with ACE inhibitor and ARBs on renal outcomes and all-cause mortality in patients with diabetic nephropathy—is there a difference? The data sources were solid: Medline, EM-base, and Cochrane Central Register for controlled clinical and contacts to investigators. Patients with all stages of disease were included, which may be a drawback.

The data extracted concerned mortality and renal outcomes, which were:

1. Prevention of progression of micro- and macroalbuminuria as well as regression to normoalbuminuria.
2. Doubling of serum creatinine concentration.
3. ESRD, and the final outcome in all studies: mortality.

All the relevant papers were identified on the date of submission, comprising about 7500 patients. A major interest in this area is ESRD, and renal dysfunction.

Importantly, both agents had similar effect on both renal outcomes, also when confounders were taken into consideration. Directly comparing ACE inhibitor directly with ARBs was at that time difficult, but results from the DETAIL study are now available *(19)*.

The important point here is that ACE inhibitor had a significant effect on over all mortality, mainly driven by the Microalbuminuria Cardiovascular and Renal Outcomes in the Heart Outcomes Prevention Evaluation (MICRO-HOPE) study *(1,26)*. The test for the over all-effect on mortality had a $p =$ of 0.04. In contrast, the ARBs had no significant effect on mortality, with a $p = 0.95$ (but on ESRD). This is important because patients with renal disease may not die from ESRD (they undergo dialysis), the cause of death, especially in type 2 diabetes, is primarily cardiac mortality. A similar result is seen in a large Chinese study *(27)*.

Another impressing finding is that there was a very significant effect on regression from microalbuminuria to normoalbuminuria by ACE inhibitors—an effect, which has been observed earlier for type 1 diabetes *(6)*.

The authors *(26)* finally point out the need for more comparative trials. For instance, the ARB, losartan, was compared positively with a β-blocker in hypertensive diabetic (and nondiabetic) patients with left ventricular hypertrophy in the Losartan Intervention for Endpoint reduction in hypertensin (LIFE) study *(27)*. In addition, the authors conclude that combination therapy—including the use of diuretics—is important. Combining ACE inhibitor with ARBs also seems interesting especially in nondiabetic disease, as reported in the COOPORATE trials *(28)*. New studies are however highly needed, also within this area, and works are in progress *(29)*.

It is well known that ACE inhibitors have an effect on accumulation of bradykinin *(4)*, which may be beneficial and relevant to the main results of the meta-analysis. Thus, the pendulum may now be swinging in favor of ACE inhibition, but generally there is a positive effect of blocking the RAS, as seen in Table 2. Dual blockade is still being investigated with positive results *(30,31)* (Table 2). No substantial arguments against the BENEDICT study and the detail study have been presented *(32–38)*, but economic issues were also discussed *(34)*.

CONGESTIVE HEART FAILURE

ACE Inhibitor or ARBs in Heart Failure

ACE inhibition is a well-established part of heart failure treatment, but the role of the Angiotensin II receptor blocker in heart failure treatment has not yet been fully established.

The Losartan Heart Failure Survival Study (ELITE-II), Optimal Trial in Myocardial Infarction with Angiotensin II Antagonist Losartan (OPTIMAAL), and Valsartan Heart Failure Trial (VALHEFT) trials all failed to show superiority of the Angiotensin II receptor blocker compared with ACE inhibition in heart failure patients.

Retrospectively, some might suggest that these findings were mostly owing to dosing of the ARB, and it is worthwhile noticing that these studies were planned in the early 1990s, when knowledge was limited.

It was surprising, however, that the VALHEFT trial, which was a comprehensive heart failure study using the ARB valsartan added to concomitant heart failure medication showed that patients treated with both an ACE inhibitor and an Angiotensin II receptor blocker did not benefit from this treatment, and it was indeed unexpected that patients

Table 2
Evidence for Good Blood Pressure-Lowering Strategies

Before diabetes	*Normoalbuminuria*	*Microalbuminuria*	*Microalbuminuria, including diuretics treatment (1)*
Opie *(9)*	Ravid *(12)*	Mogensen *(1)*	PREMIER *(1)*
Lindholm *(10)*	Kvetny *(13)*	Barnett *(19)*	Several guidelines *(1)*
Padwal *(8)*	BENEDICT *(14)*	Gaede *(16,65)*	Mogensen *(1)*

treated with both ACE inhibitor, β-blocker, and valsartan had an increased risk of the combined endpoint of all-cause mortality and morbidity *(39)*.

The study was not designed to investigate dual blockade in heart failure and the mentioned results were based on subgroup analysis and should be interpreted with caution, but it was brought to attention whether some precautions should be taken using this drug combination in heart failure patients. This observation has not been found since the VALHEFT study, not even in the Ephesus study where Eplerenone was given to patients treated with the same dosage regimen *(40)*. The VALHEFT trial results also stand in clear contrast to several small dual blockade studies in heart failure patients, which all have shown promising results.

Several small experimental studies found beneficial effect on the neurohumeral activation in the failing heart *(41–43)*, and a few clinical trials support these observations. The V-HEFT trail found beneficial effect on BP, neurohumeral, and hemodynamics in a small short-term placebo-controlled study in 83 heart failure patients treated with varying dosages of valsartan added to concomitant ACE inhibitor treatment *(44)*.

Hamroff and colleagues found exercise capacity in a treadmill exercise significantly improved over a 6-mo follow-up period, when 50 mg of Losartan was added to the maximal recommended or tolerated doses of ACE inhibitor in a placebo-controlled study including 33 patients with heart failure *(45)*. In a larger study (the randomized evaluation of strategies for left ventricular dysfunction [RESOLVD] pilot trial), 768 heart failure patients (New York Heart Association [NYHA] II–IV) were randomized to either candesartan (up to 8 mg) or enalapril, or candesartan and enalapril in combination. The combination of candesartan and enalapril was more effective in preventing left ventricular remodeling than both candesartan and enalapril alone. Levels of brain natriuretic peptide were also significantly reduced during the 43-wk follow-up period *(46)*. The CHARM-added *(47)* and the Valsortan in Acute Myocardial Infarction Trial (VALIANT) are the only large dual blockade in heart failure trial available and their results point in either direction.

Stable Congestive Heart Failure

The CHARM-added study included 2548 patients with NYHA class II–IV heart failure and a left ventricular ejection fraction of 40% or lower. The main purpose was to investigate whether dual blockade with candesartan added to concomitant ACE inhibition would reduce the combined end point of CV death, myocardial infarction (MI), coronary intervention, hospitalization for heart failure, and stroke.

The patients had to have an admission to a hospital owing to cardiac conditions, and were on a stable dose of ACE inhibitor for 30 d before entering the study. Approximately 36% of the patients in the candesartan group were on an optimum dose of ACE inhibitor (investigators opinion) compared with 42% in the placebo group. A once-daily candesartan dose was then added mainly titrated from 4 mg to a mean daily dose after 6 mo of 24 mg. After a mean follow-up of 41 mo, a significant endpoint reduction of adding candesartan to an ACE inhibitor was found. In the candesartan group, 38% of the patients experienced an event and 42% in the placebo group experienced the primary outcome, which was significant (p = 0.011) *(47)*.

These results implicate that there might be an effect of dual blockade on stable heart failure patients, but there has been some controversy in this regard. The major point of criticism was the rather low prevalence of patients on a recommended dose of ACE inhibitor upon entrance in the study. It is unclear whether a further titration of the ACE inhibitor could have provided the same result as seen in the Assessment of Treatment with Lisinoptil and Survival (ATLAS) study *(48)*. This issue remains unsolved.

Post-MI Heart Failure Patients

However, in newly diagnosed post-MI heart failure patients, the issue regarding dual blockade seems clear. There does not seem to be any place for combining the ACE inhibitor and the ARB.

The recently published VALIANT study did not find any benefit in this particular kind of heart failure patients, except for significant BP reduction in the dual blockade arm, but instead the side effects were significantly higher *(49)*.

The VALIANT study enrolled 14,808 patients with acute MI and either clinical or radiological signs of heart failure or evidence of left ventricular systolic dysfunction (echocardiography or ventriculargraphy). The patients were titrated with valsartan, captopril, or the combination to a target dose of either 160 mg of valsartan, or 80 mg of valsartan and 50 mg of captopril, or finally 50 mg of captopril three times daily. During a 24.7-mo follow-up, there was an expectedly high event rate (approx 3000 deaths), equally distributed between the three treatment arms, which overall fell out to be negative with equal results with all three regimens.

Regarding the dual blockade arm, there was a significantly better BP control, which did not provide additional benefit for this population. In contrast, there was a significantly higher rate of some adverse events (hypotension, renal causes), but surprisingly not hyperkalemia. The rather modest results with dual blockade derived from the VALIANT and VALHEFT studies are probably owing to the cause of death in a post-MI heart failure population. The death causes are obviously most likely reinfarction and arrhythmia, of which inhibition of the RAS only plays a minor part.

The inclination for using dual blockade in the stable heart failure patient seems more robust from a "CHARM point of view." However, a large trial including a head-to-head comparison with a once-a-day up-titrated ACE inhibitor would settle this matter.

Nevertheless, it is questionable whether the issue of benefit from dual blockade in congestive heart failure ever will be settled, since no large trials using the combination of an ARB and an ACE inhibitor are underway. The closest we will get is the Ongoing Telmisartan Alone and in Combination with Ramipril Global Endpoint Trial (ONTARGET), which will further elucidate whether dual blockade has any influence on hard endpoints. This is a large, long-term study (23,400 patients, 5.5 yr). It will compare the benefits of ACE inhibitor treatment, ARB treatment, and treatment with an ACE inhibitor and ARB together, in a study population with established coronary artery disease, stroke, peripheral vascular disease, or diabetes with end-organ damage *(50)*.

In conclusion, the CHARM data do indicate that there might be a benefit form adding an ARB to patients with heart failure already treated with an ACE inhibitor for some time. However there seems no rationale for the use of dual blockade in post-MI heart failure patients. Table 3 provides an overview of the mentioned studies.

Table 3
Dual Blockade in Congestive Heart Failure Patients

Study	*Medication*	*N*	*Follow-up*	*Effect parameters*	*Results*
V-heft	Valsartan 80–160 mg Lisinopril	83	6 mo	Exercise capacity Blood pressure reduction	Improved exercise capacity significant systolic blood pressure reduction
Hamroff et al.	Losartan High dose ACE inhibitor	33	6 mo	Exercise capacity NYHA Class	Improved exercise capacity and NYHA class
RESOLVD	Candesartan 4–8 mg Enalapril	768	9.5 mo	Exercise capacity BNP-levels	Improved exercise capacity and reduced BNP levels with combination
VALHEFT	Valsartan ACE inhibitor	5010	27 mo	Combined end point of death, MI, admission for heart failure, and so on	Nonsignificant Increased risk of achieving endpoint with ACE, ARB, and BB
VALIANT	Valsartan Captopril Valsartan/captopril combo	14,808	24.7 mo	Combined end point of death, MI, admission for heart failure, and so on	Nonsignificant Increased side effects
CHARM	Candesartan ACE inhibitor	2548	41 mo	Combined end point of death, MI, admission for heart failure, and so on	Significant endpoint reduction

ACE Inhibitor or ARBs and MI

Recent controversy has emerged regarding whether the ARBs increase the risk, or at least seem less protective, in preventing MI when compared with other antihypertensive agents, especially ACE inhibitors and calcium antagonists *(51)*.

This postulate has been presented in an editorial primarily based on the findings in the VALUE study *(52)*, the two CHARM substudies, CHARM-preserved *(53)* and CHARM-alternative *(54)*, but also with reference to the metaanalysis by Strippoli et al. *(26)*, which concluded that the ARB actually did not exert any CV protection in trials on diabetic nephropathy compared with the ACE inhibitor where the cardioprotective abilities were evident.

Some caution should be taking before stating that the ARB actually increases the risk of MI, but especially the CHARM-alternative study gives some reason to speculate. In this trial, the purpose was to examine the role of candesartan vs placebo in ACE intolerant patients with reduced ejection fraction. This was done in a fashion analogous to the SOLVD trial *(55)* and the overall result was nonsignificant *(54)*. Unfortunately, a subgroup analysis in the CHARM-alternative trial uncovered a significant increase in MIs in the candesartan treated patients (unadjusted hazard ratio =1.52 [1.06–2.18] $p = 0.025$ *(54)*.

This was far from what had been observed with Enalapril in the SOLVD trial *(55)* or with Ramipril in the APRES study *(56)* and the HOPE trial *(57)*, where significant reductions the MI occurrence were seen with the ACE inhibitor.

Until a head-to-head comparison between an ACE inhibitor and an ARB has been published *(50)* the accusations regarding the ARBs and MI are solely speculative. However, when it comes to MI risk reduction it seems safe to state that: "an ARB is not an ACE inhibitor without the cough."

CONCLUSIONS

The basic abnormality responsible for diabetic nephropathy is elevated blood glucose, which over the years produces the abnormal functional and structural changes in the kidney and the heart. However, elevated BP also is important—in type 2 diabetes often at the clinical diagnosis, in type 1 diabetes typically with development of microalbuminuria or proteinuria. Elevated BP is a main risk factor for progression in both microalbuminuric and in proteinuric patients, and although any type of BP reduction seems important, it is now clear that blocking the RAS is the most important antihypertensive treatment strategy, both in type 1 and 2 diabetes, indeed, the basis for BP-lowering treatment. Many other agents can be used on top, especially diuretics, that are also a cornerstone in the treatment strategy. Indeed, aldosterone antagonists seem to be an increasingly important part in the management, especially of heart failure. There is still a discussion of whether ARBs or/and ACE inhibitor provide the same benefit. The most recent results suggest that there is no major difference between the two classes of drugs blocking the RAS as far as progression of kidney disease is concerned, although with advanced nephropathy in type 2 diabetes, ARBs may be advantageous because important studies have only been carried out with this class of drugs, namely the RENAAL study and the IDNT study.

The same conclusion can be drawn regarding diabetic (and nondiabetic) patients with left ventricular hypertrophy where Losartan was compared with a β-blocker with positive results. Even a minor increase in BP is of importance, also in normoalbuminuric patients, where progression to microalbuminuria can be inhibited by the use of ACE inhibitor, which is not well documented by the use of ARBs. Clearly, the glycemic control is important for the development of renal lesions, and treatment with agents that block the RAS may to some extent inhibit the development of type 2 diabetes.

Regarding heart failure, ACE inhibition is a well-established part of heart failure treatment, but the role of angiotensin receptor blockers is not fully established. However, there seems to be a benefit from adding an ARB in patients with heart failure already treated with an ACE inhibitor for some time. Conversely, there seems no rationale for the use of dual blockade in post-MI heart failure patients. Aldosterone antagonists seem also to play an important role in heart failure.

In conclusion: ACE inhibitor has been longest on the stage and is very well documented to be beneficial for renal disease and heart disease. ARBs have so far a weaker profile and it is difficult to argue that they are better than ACE inhibitor, except for better documentation in advanced renal disease in type 2 diabetes and in terms of the side effects, especially cough.

FINAL REMARKS

Regression of Albuminuria—Important Clinical Significance: A New Paradigm Shift (By ACE Inhibitor and ARBS and AHT Treatment)

It is well known to all diabetologists that patients with "proteinuria" or "albuminuria" carry a poor prognosis. The same is the case for microalbuminuria, but to a lesser extent. Indeed, the higher the level of albuminuria, the greater the risk of renal progression and the risk of all complications including early mortality. These results derive from studies of the so-called natural history of diabetic nephropathy, both in type 1 and 2. The next question is, of course, to ask whether regression or remission of albuminuria is of clinical relevance. Is it really associated with better prognosis? Blocking the RAS as well as dual blockade should be considered *(1,22,23)* along with BP lowering.

This question was discussed in a recent article in Kidney International by Hovind and coworkers *(58,59)*, who analyzed whether remission of nephrotic-range albuminuria is associated with a better prognosis. This, indeed, seems to be the case. It is now clear also from other studies that remission of albuminuria *(60–64)* is signifies a good prognosis, also in microalbuminuric patients. The results from the LIFE-study *(64)*, including diabetic patients *(64)*, and the RENAAL study *(24)*, clearly document that reduction of albuminuria and microalbuminuria really indicates a good prognosis.

Thus, it is obvious that it is important to screen for microalbuminuria, but now also to do a followup on the degree of albuminuria. Physicians should look for reduction by means of better BP control, especially ACE inhibition or other blockade of the RAS. This is indeed a second paradigm shift. The first paradigm shift was to screen for microalbuminuria, and the next is now to follow up on the level of albuminuria.

It is not difficult to screen for microalbuminuria. In our unit we use the first morning urine sample. This is used for screening using the albumin excretion ratio, which is a good parameter very well associated with excretion rate, both short term and 24 h. They are good and reliable reference values *(1)*. It could be argued that the classification normo-, macro- and microalbuminuria is somewhat artificial because albuminuria—like many other parameters (glycemic control and BP as well as cholesterol)—is a continuous variable. However, it is practical in the screening process to classify according to these entities. Early studies show that microalbuminuria is not only associated with progression to renal disease, but also to early mortality.

How can it be explained that reduction in albuminuria/microalbuminuria translates into better prognosis? Part of the explanation is reduction of BP and treatment with agents that block the RAS, but this may not be the whole story. Reduction in albuminuria means that the pressure over the glomerular membrane is specifically reduced, and there is good evidence to indicate that pressure-induced damage is an important factor for the deterioration in renal function observed in diabetic patients with proteinuria. Patients with microalbuminuria usually have well-preserved renal function, and thus, by reducing microalbuminuria by better treatment, both glycemic and antihypertensive treatment translate into better preservation of GFR *(65)*, and in this situation, preservation of renal function before the decline in GFR. With proteinuria there is normally a decline in GFR, which is related to a traditional risk factors, namely elevated BP, microalbuminuria, and HbA1c—risk markers that are clearly modifiable.

It is quite clear that early antihypertensive treatment has improved the prognosis for diabetic patients dramatically, and the prognosis may further improve with early screening for microalbuminuria and follow-up to monitor whether microalbuminuria is reduced. On the other hand, it may seem a paradox that we still have an increase in the number of patients developing end-stage renal failure owing to diabetes. However, this is explained by the fact that many more patients develop type 2 diabetes, and that these patients have a longer period of survival, because of better CV management, but further studies are needed *(66)*.

The very good news is that the total number of patients with ESRD entering dialysis or transplantation is now declining in Denmark. Obviously, further observation is needed, but this is anyway a very promising sign, even if the patients are becoming older and older. However, in most parts of the world, especially in the United States, more than 50% of the patients with ESRD have diabetes as the background. It is interesting to note that screening for microalbuminuria is primarily used in Europe. However, this has already for several years been proposed in guidelines from the American Diabetes Association *(67)*.

REFERENCES

1. Mogensen CE. Microalbuminuria and hypertension with focus on type 1 and type 2 diabetes. JIM 2003;254:45–66.
2. Hovind P, Rossing P, Tarnow L, Smidt UM, Parving HH. Progression of diabetic nephropathy. Kidney Int 2001;59:702–709.
3. Rossing K, Christensen PK, Hovind P, Tarnow L, Rossing P, Parving HH. Progression of nephropathy in type 2 diabetic patients. Kidney Int 2004;66:1596–1605.
4. Wolf G, Ritz E. Combination therapy with ACE inhibitors and angiotensin II receptor blockers to halt progression of chronic renal disease: pathophysiology and indications. Kidney Int 2005;67:799–812.
5. Rachmani R, Slavachevsky I, Amit M, et al. The effect of spironolactone, cilazapril, and their combination on albuminuria in patients with hypertension and diabetic nephropathy is independent of blood pressure reduction: a randomized controlled study. Diabetes Med 2004;21:471–475.
6. ACE Inhibitors in Diabetic Nephropathy Trialist Group. Should all patients with type 1 diabetes mellitus and microalbuminuria receive angiotensin-converting-enzyme inhibitors? A meta-analysis of individual patient data. Ann Intern Med 2001;134:370–379.
7. Christensen CK, Mogensen CE. Effect of Antihypertensive Treatment on Progression of Incipient Diabetic Nephropathy. Hypertension 1985;7(6 Part 2):II109–II113.
8. Opie LH, Schall R. Old antihypertensives and new diabetes. J Hypertens 2004;22:1453–1458.
9. Scheen AJ. Renin–angiotensin system inhibition prevents type 2 diabetes mellitus. Part 1. A meta-analysis of randomised clinical trials. Diabetes Metab 2004;30:487–496.

10. Scheen AJ. Renin–angiotensin system inhibition prevents type 2 diabetes mellitus. Part 2. Overview of physiological and biochemical mechanisms. Diabetes Metab 2004;39:498–505.
11. Julius S, Kjeldsen SE, Weber M, et al. Outcomes in hypertensive patients at high cardiovascular risk treated with regimens based on valsartan or amlodipine: the VALUE randomised trial. Lancet 2004;363:2022–2031.
12. Ravid M, Brosh D, Levi Z, Bar-Dayan Y, Ravid D, Rachmani R. Use of enalapril to attenuate decline in renal function in normotensive, normoalbuminuri patients with type 2 diabetes mellitus. A randomized, controlled trial. Ann Intern Med 1998;128:982–988.
13. Kvetny J, Gregersen G, Pedersen RS. Randomized Placebo-controlled trial of perindopril in normotensive, normoalbuminuric patients with type 1 diabetes mellitus. QJM 2001;94(2):89–94.
14. Ruggenenti P, Fassi A, Ilieva AP, et al. Preventing Microalbuminuria in Type 2 Diabetes. NEJM 2004;351(19);1941–1951.
15. Adler AI, Stevens RJ, Manley SE, et al. Development and progression of nephropathy in type 2 diabetes: the United Kingdom Prospective Diabetes Study. Kidney Int 2003;63:225–232.
16. Gæde P, Vedel P, Larsen N, Jensen GV, Parving HH, Pedersen O. Multifactorial intervention and cardiovascular disease in patients with type 2 diabetes. N Engl J Med 2003;348:383–393.
17. Mauer M, Zinman B, Gardiner R, et al. ACE-I and ARBs in early diabetic nephropathy. J Renin Angiotensin Aldosterone Syst 2002;3:262–269.
18. On behalf of the Family Investigation of Nephropathy and Diabetes Research Group. The Family Investigation of Nephropathy and Diabetes (FIND) Design and methods. J Diabetes Complications 2005;19:1–9.
19. Barnett AH, Bain SC, Bouter P, et al. Angiotensin-Receptor Blockade versus Converting-Enzyme Inhibition in Type 2 Diabetes and Nephropathy. N Engl J Med 2004;351:1952–1961.
20. Lacourciére Y, Bélanger A, Godin C, et al. Long-term comparison of losartan and enalapril on kidney function in hypertensive Type 2 diabetics with early nephropathy. Kidney Int 2000;58:762–769.
21. Muirhead N, Feagan BF, Mahon J, et al. The effects of valsartan and captopril on reducing microalbuminuria in patients with Type 2 Diabetes Mellitus: a placebo-controlled trial. Curr Therapeutic Res 1999;60:650–660.
22. Mogensen CE, Neldam S, Tikkanen I, et al. Randomised controlled trial of dual blockade of renin-angiotensin system in patients with hypertension, microalbuminuria, and non-insulin dependent diabetes: the candesartan and lisinopril microalbuminuria (CALM) study. BMJ 2000;321:1440–1444.
23. Andersen NH, Poulsen PL, Knudsen ST, et al. Long-term dual blockade with candesartan and lisinopril in hypertensive patients with diabetes mellitus. The CALM II Study. Diabetes Care 2005;48:273–277.
24. Brenner BM, Cooper ME, de Zeeuw D, et al. Effects of losartan on renal and cardiovascular outcomes in patients with type 2 diabetes and nephropathy. N Engl J Med 2001;345:861–869.
25. Lewis EJ, Hunsicker LG, Clarke WR, et al. Renoprotective effect of the angiotensin-receptor antagonist irbesartan in patients with nephropathy due to type 2 diabetes. N Engl J Med 2001;345:851–860.
26. Strippoli GFM, Craig M, Deeks JJ, Schena FP, Craig JC. Effects of angiotensin converting enzyme inhibitors and angiotensin II receptor antagonists on mortality and renal outcomes in diabetic nephropathy: systematic review. BMJ 2004;329(7470):1–12.
27. So WY, Ozaki R, Chan NN, et al. Effect of Angiotensin-converting Enzyme inhibition on Survival in 3773 Chinese Type 2 Diabetic Patients. Hypertension 2004;44:294–299.
28. Nakao N, Yoshimura A, Morita H, Takada M, Kayano T, Ideura T. Combination treatment of angiotensin-II receptor blocker and angiotensin-converting enzyme inhibitor in non-diabetic renal disease (COOPERATE): a randomised controlled trial. Lancet 2003:361:177–224.
29. Strippoli GFM, Jonathan CC. Combined treatment with angiotensin-converting enzyme inhibitors and angiotensin-receptor blockers to prevent end-stage kidney disease in patients who do not have diabetes. Med J Aust 2004;181:450, 451.
30. Izzo JL, Weinberg MS, Hainer JW, et al. Antihypertensive Efficacy of Candesartan-Lisinopril in Combination of Lisinopril: The AMAZE Trials. J Clin Hypertens 2004;6(9):485–493.
31. Fujisawa T, Ikegami H, Ono M, et al. Combination of Half Doses of Angiotensin Type 1 Receptor Antagonisk and Angiotensin-Converting Enzyme Inhibitor in Diabetic Nephropathy. Am J Hypertens 2005;18:13–17.
32. Asgari AA, Sarvghadi F, Zahed N. Telmisartan vs. Enalapril in Type 2 Diabetes. N Engl J Med 2005;352(8):835.
33. Parving H-H, Hovind P, Rossing P. Telmisartan vs. Enalapril in Type 2 Diabetes. N Engl J Med 2005;352(8):835.
34. Loewenstein JE. Telmisartan vs. Enalapril in Type 2 Diabetes. N Engl J Med 2005;352(8):836.

35. Bain SC, Barnett A. Telmisartan vs. Enalapril in Type 2 Diabetes. N Engl J Med 2005;352(8):836.
36. Zandi-Nejad K, Brenner BM. Preventing Microalbuminuria in Type 2 Diabetes. Telmisartan vs. Enalapril in Type 2 Diabetes. N Engl J Med 2005;352(8):833.
37. Mauer M, Fioretto P. Enalapril in Type 2 Diabetes. N Engl J Med 2005;352(8):834.
38. Ruggenenti P, Perna A, Remuzzi G. Enalapril in Type 2 Diabetes. N Engl J Med 2005;352(8):834.
39. Cohn JN, Tognoni G: A randomized trial of the angiotensin-receptor blocker valsartan in chronic heart failure. N Engl J Med 2001;345:1667–1675.
40. Pitt B, Remme W, Zannad F, et al. Eplerenone, a selective aldosterone blocker, in patients with left ventricular dysfunction after myocardial infarction. N Engl J Med 2003;348:1309–1321.
41. Koji T, Onishi K, Dohi K, et al. Addition of Angiotensin II Receptor Antagonist to an ACE Inhibitor in Heart Failure Improves Cardiovascular Function by a Bradykinin-Mediated Mechanism. J Cardiovasc Pharmacol 2003;41:632–639.
42. Nakamura Y, Yoshiyama M, Omura T, et al. Beneficial effects of combination of ACE inhibitor and angiotensin II type 1 receptor blocker on cardiac remodeling in rat myocardial infarction. Cardiovasc Res 2003;57:48–54.
43. Krombach RS, Clair MJ, Hendrick JW, et al. Angiotensin converting enzyme inhibition, AT1 receptor inhibition, and combination therapy with pacing induced heart failure: effects on left ventricular performance and regional blood flow patterns. Cardiovasc Res 1998;38:631–645.
44. Baruch L, Anand I, Cohen IS, Ziesche S, Judd D, Cohn JN: Augmented short- and long-term hemodynamic and hormonal effects of an angiotensin receptor blocker added to angiotensin converting enzyme inhibitor therapy in patients with heart failure. Vasodilator Heart Failure Trial (V-HeFT) Study Group. Circulation 1999;99:2658–2664.
45. Hamroff G, Katz SD, Mancini D, et al. Addition of angiotensin II receptor blockade to maximal angiotensin-converting enzyme inhibition improves exercise capacity in patients with severe congestive heart failure. Circulation 1999;99:990–992.
46. McKelvie RS, Yusuf S, Pericak D, et al. Comparison of candesartan, enalapril, and their combination in congestive heart failure: randomized evaluation of strategies for left ventricular dysfunction (RESOLVD) pilot study. The RESOLVD Pilot Study Investigators. Circulation 1999;100:1056–1064.
47. McMurray JJ, Ostergren J, Swedberg K, et al. Effects of candesartan in patients with chronic heart failure and reduced left-ventricular systolic function taking angiotensin-converting-enzyme inhibitors: the CHARM-Added trial. Lancet 2003;362:767–771.
48. Ryden L, Armstrong PW, Cleland JG, et al. Efficacy and safety of high-dose lisinopril in chronic heart failure patients at high cardiovascular risk, including those with diabetes mellitus. Results from the ATLAS trial. Eur Heart J 2000;21:1967–1978.
49. Pfeffer MA, McMurray JJ, Velazquez EJ, et al. Valsartan, captopril, or both in myocardial infarction complicated by heart failure, left ventricular dysfunction, or both. N Engl J Med 2003;349:1893–1906.
50. Yusuf S. From the HOPE to the ONTARGET and the TRANSCEND studies: challenges in improving prognosis. Am J Cardiol 2002;89:18A–25A.
51. Verma S, Strauss M: Angiotensin receptor blockers and myocardial infarction. BMJ 2004;329: 1248–1249.
52. Julius S, Kjeldsen SE, Weber M, et al. Outcomes in hypertensive patients at high cardiovascular risk treated with regimens based on valsartan or amlodipine: the VALUE randomised trial. Lancet 2004;363:2022–2031.
53. Yusuf S, Pfeffer MA, Swedberg K, et al. Effects of candesartan in patients with chronic heart failure and preserved left-ventricular ejection fraction: the CHARM-preserved trial. Lancet 2003;362:777–781.
54. Granger CB, McMurray JJ, Yusuf S, et al. Effects of candesartan in patients with chronic heart failure and reduced left-ventricular systolic function intolerant to angiotensin-converting-enzyme inhibitors: the CHARM-Alternative trial. Lancet 2003;362:772–776.
55. Effect of enalapril on survival in patients with reduced left ventricular ejection fractions and congestive heart failure. The SOLVD Investigators. N Engl J Med 1991;325:293–302.
56. Kjoller-Hansen L, Steffensen R, Grande P: The angiotensin-converting enzyme inhibition post revascularization study (APRES). J Am Coll Cardiol 2000;35:881–888.
57. Dagenais GR, Yusuf S, Bourassa MG, et al. Effects of ramipril on coronary events in high-risk persons: results of the heart outcomes prevention evaluation study. Circulation 104:522–526, 2001.
58. Hoving P, Tarnow L, Rossing P, Carstensen B, Parving HH. Improved survival in patients obtaining remission of nephrotic range albuminuria in diabetic nephropathy." Kidney Int 2004;66:1180–1186.
59. Hovind P, Rossing P, Tarnow L, Toft H, Parving J, Parving HH. Remission of nephrotic-range albuminuria in type 1 diabetic patients. Diabetes Care 2001;24:1972–1977.

60. Mogensen CE, Poulsen PL. Microalbuminuria, glycemic control, and blood pressure predicting outcome in diabetes type 1 and type 2. Kidney Int 2004;66(S92):S40, S41.
61. de Zeeuw D, Remuzzi G, Parving HH, et al. Proteinuria, a therapeutic target for cardiovascular protection in type 2 diabetic patients with nephropathy. Circulation 2004;110:921–927.
62. Yuyun MF, Dinnesen SF, Edwards OM, Wood E, Wareham NJ. Absolute level and rate of change of albuminuria over 1 year independently predict mortality and cardiovascular events in patients with diabetic nephropathy. Diabet Med 2003;20:277–282.
63. Spoelstra-de Man AM, Brouwer CB, Stehouwer CD, Smulders YM. Rapid progression of albumin excretion is an independent predictor of cardiovascular mortality in patients with type 2 diabetes and microalbuminuria. Diabetes Care 2001;24:2097–2101.
64. Ibsen H, Olsen MH, Wachtell K, et al. Does albuminuria predict cardiovascular outcomes on treatment with losartan versus atenolol in patients with diabetes, hypertension, and left vendtricular hypertrophy? Diabetes Care, In press.
65. Gaede P, Tarnow L, Vedel P, Parving HH, Pedersen O. Remission to normoalbuminuria during multifactorial treatment preserves kidney function in patients with type 2 diabetes and microalbuminuria. Nephrol Dial Transplant 2004;19(11):2784–2788.
66. Abraira C, Duchworth W, McCarren M, et al. Design of the cooperative study on glycemic control and complications in diabetes mellitus type 2 Veterans Affairs Diabetes Trial. J Diabetes Complications 2003;17:314–322.
67. American Diabetes Association: Clinical Practice Redommendations 2005. Diabetes Care 2005;28 (S1).

26 Management of Diabetic End-Stage Renal Disease With Dialysis

Ploumis S. Passadakis, MD
and Dimitrios G. Oreopoulos, MD, PhD, FRCPC, FACP

CONTENTS

INTRODUCTION

The management of diabetic patients with end-stage renal disease (ESRD) by either dialysis treatment (peritoneal dialysis [PD] or hemodialysis [HD]) is more complicated than in nondiabetic patients, mainly because of the presence of advanced comorbid conditions associated with the long-term course of diabetes. During the last two decades, improvements in dialysis modalities resulted in longer survival rates in diabetic patients. HD is the most commonly used therapy, whereas the role of PD in renal replacement therapy (RRT) in patients with diabetic nephropathy (DN) is well established. The decision regarding the choice for treatment options (PD vs HD) must be individualized as survival and rehabilitation data among the two modalities are comparable, at least for the first 5 yr after initiation. However, the best outcome of diabetic ESRD patients may be obtained by integrated care, starting with PD and switching to HD if problems arise, and keeping suitable patients on the renal or renal–pancreas transplantation waiting list.

From: *Contemporary Diabetes: The Diabetic Kidney*
Edited by: P. Cortes and C. E. Mogensen © Humana Press Inc., Totowa, NJ

Table 1
Potential Advantages of Peritoneal Dialysis in the Treatment of Diabetic Patients

No need for vascular access
No need for systemic anticoagulation
Continuous therapy
Gradual ultrafiltration
Fewer episodes of hypotension
Better preservation of renal function
Better blood pressure control
Better control of anemia
More liberal diet
Intraperitoneal administration of insulin
Lifestyle advantages

succeeded surviving for a maximum of 6 mo. At that time, initiation of HD in diabetic patients was almost absolutely contraindicated because it appeared very unlikely that they might benefit even for a short period of time since it had been experienced that dialysis treatment was accompanied by an excessive morbidity and mortality. Consequently, in the 1970s, the 2-yr mortality for diabetic patients in HD programs was distressingly high, ranging between 60 and 75% *(6,7)*. Also during the 1980s, reports from both Europe and the United States described that only one in every three diabetic patients on HD, mainly of type 1 diabetes, survived on dialysis therapy for 2–3 yr *(8)*.

Ten years later in 1977, the introduction of continuous ambulatory PD (CAPD) was considered more favorable for ESRD patients with diabetes because of several benefits inherent in that therapy (Table 1). As these patients were often debilitated, malnourished, and/or hemodynamically unstable, the simplicity of the PD offered the advantage of its continuous slow therapy without any need for highly trained personnel or for complex apparatus and requirements of systemic anticoagulation. Therefore, among the two main modes of RRT, many clinicians have favored CAPD for the treatment of diabetic patients.

However, several improvements in technology and in the area of vascular access, advances in the management of coronary artery disease (CAD), and critical care medicine, and the tendency for earlier initiation of dialysis have resulted in a progressive decrease in mortality rates among diabetic patients undergoing dialysis. Furthermore, there have been important changes in dialysis equipment, including a shift from cellulosic to synthetic HD membranes, a better control of ultrafiltration (UF), as well as improved connection devices for PD.

Subsequently, first-year HD mortality for diabetic patients in the United States decreased from 40.4 deaths per 100 patient per year in 1986 to 23.2 deaths per 100 patients per year in 1996 *(9)*, whereas during the same decade a similar improvement was observed at Toronto for diabetic patients undergoing CAPD *(10)*. Also first- and second-year death rates for US diabetic HD patients decreased between 1989 and 1998 by 12.8 and 9.29%, respectively, whereas the corresponding values of PD diabetic patients were better by 26.6 and 19.9%, respectively *(9)*. In addition, according to data from 10 European national registries, between 1991 and 2000, there was a marked reduction in the age- and gender-adjusted mortality during the first 2 yr of dialysis therapy among diabetic patients, mainly those with type 2 diabetes *(4)*. The

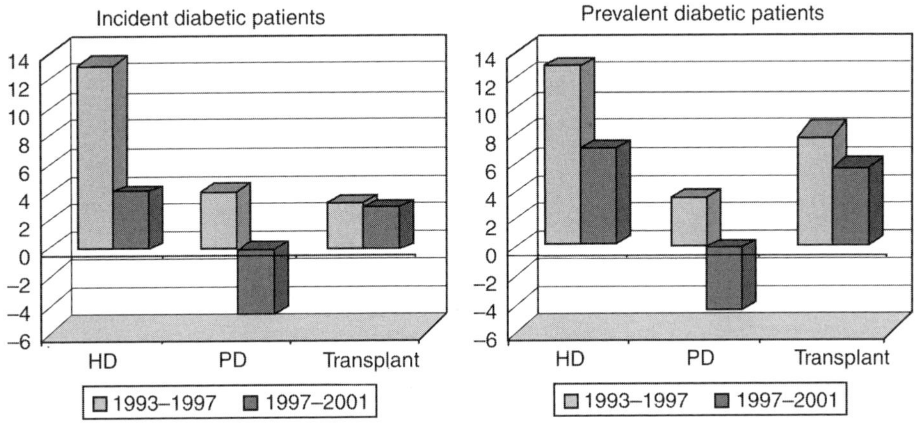

Fig. 3. The graphics show the changes in the average annual percent in rates per million for the incident and prevalent US diabetic patients, between the years 1993 and 2001 *(1)*.

lower patients mortality rates together with the increased acceptance of diabetic and older patients, has lead to the increase in the prevalence of diabetic ESRD population over the recent years *(1)*.

In diabetic patients, several complications such as retinopathy, glaucoma, cataracts, CAD, cardiomyopathy, cerebrovascular disease (CVD), peripheral vascular disease (PVD) limb amputation, motor neuropathy, sensory neuropathy, autonomic dysfunction (diarrhea, vomiting, postural hypotension), myopathy, and depression persist or progress during ESRD, and are already present at the initiation of RRT. Macrovascular disease, particularly CAD is accelerated in patients with diabetic ESRD and it is the most common cause of death in these patients. Early cardiac evaluation in all diabetic patients as well as vigorous treatment of hypertension is the key component in the management of DN.

Diabetes is now the primary cause of ESRD in new patients starting RRT modalities, 44.7% of those starting HD, 43.6% of those starting PD, and 15.1% of those receiving a preemptive kidney transplant, whereas the corresponding values of patients with ESRD owing to hypertension are 27.4, 19.4, and only 4.8%, respectively *(1)* The annual changes for the incident and prevalent US diabetic patients by modality between the years 1993 and 2001 are shown in Fig. 3. However, acceptance rates for RRT, as well as practice pattern differ among various countries as has been shown by the Dialysis Outcomes and Practice Pattern study *(11)*.

Despite important developments of RRT and the increasing acceptance rate of diabetic patients, the overall mortality in these patients remains two to three times higher than that of nondiabetic dialysis patients; cardiovascular and cerebrovascular diseases account for approximately two-thirds of deaths in the diabetic dialysis population *(12)*.

FACTORS AFFECTING THE CLINICAL OUTCOMES OF DIABETIC PATIENTS ON DIALYSIS

The presence of a variety of comorbid conditions at the initiation of dialysis (Table 2) may adversely affect the clinical outcome and thus the success of any chronic dialysis program on RRT, by increasing the morbidity and mortality of the dialysis population with the DN.

Table 2
Factors Affecting Outcome of Diabetic Patients With ESRD on Dialysis

Comorbidity at initiation of dialysis	Peripheral vascular disease Cerebrovascular disease Anemia Hypoalbuminemia–malnutrition infection Hyperparathyroidism
Patient's personality	Age Volume status Residual renal function
Dialysis characteristics	Dialysis complications (peritonitis) Adequacy of dialysis dose Ultrafiltration (UF failure)

Cardiovascular Disease

The risk of cardiovascular disease is higher in patients with diabetic kidney disease than in diabetic patients without kidney disease *(13)* and diabetes has been recently considered as "coronary equivalent," as diabetic patients without previous myocardial infarction (MI) were found to have as high a risk of MI as nondiabetic patients with a previous MI *(14)*. Also, the prevalence of significant (>50% stenosis) CAD in patients with diabetes who are starting treatment for ESRD is estimated to be 45–55%, and diabetic patients may have asymptomatic myocardial ischemia-induced angina, owing to diabetes-associated neuropathy. Hence, morbidity and mortality from cardiovascular disease are two to five times higher in patients with diabetes compared with nondiabetics and cardiac disease is the most frequent cause of death among diabetics, accounting for more than one-half of cases (Figs. 4 and 5) *(12,15)*.

Furthermore, diabetic ESRD patients experience an increased rate of strokes and transient ischemic attacks; deaths related to CVD are approximately twice as common in patients without diabetes once ESRD has occurred.

Age

Advanced age represents the most important predictor of survival in diabetic patients and correlates inversely with survival *(16)*. Also, advanced age and the presence of diabetes are strong risk factors for CAD and cardiac death in HD patients *(17)*.

Protein-Energy Malnutrition

Protein-energy malnutrition, is common among diabetic dialysis patients and many of them are already malnourished when they begin dialysis, which may be the result of the decreased protein intake, altered metabolism, and coexisting conditions such as uremia, intercurrent illness, gastroparesis, as well as poor socioeconomic conditions and depression. On the other hand, diabetes accelerates the synthesis and tissue deposition of advanced glycosylated endproducts (AGEs), compounds that normally are excreted by the kidney but accumulate in patients with renal failure, and exert their main pathological effect through abnormal permeability of blood vessels *(18)*.

Regarding dialysis dose, it has been shown in uncontrolled studies *(19)* that by increasing clearances, a marked improvement in survival could be achieved and thus it was emphasized that adequate dialysis prescriptions should be provided in this vulnerable dialysis diabetic population. However, the ADEMEX study *(20)* (a prospective randomized

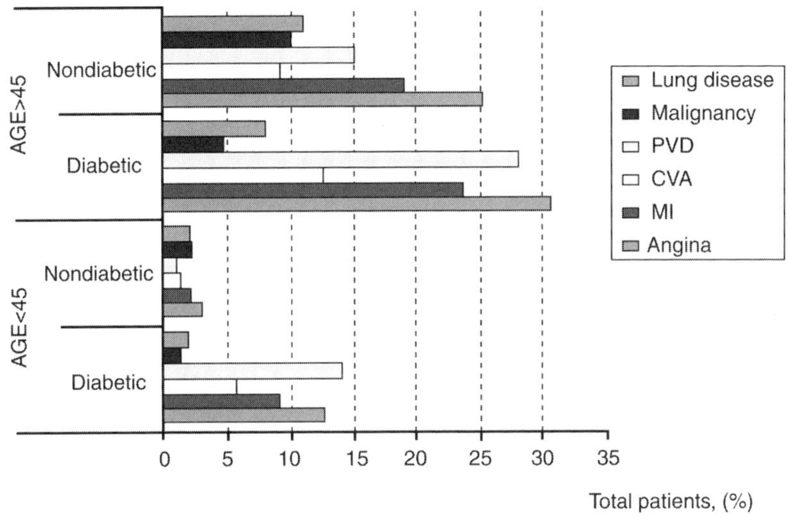

Fig. 4. Comorbidity among registered patients by age and diabetes status, Canada 1988–1994. PVD, peripheral vascular disease; CVA, cerebrovascular accident; MI, myocardial infarction.

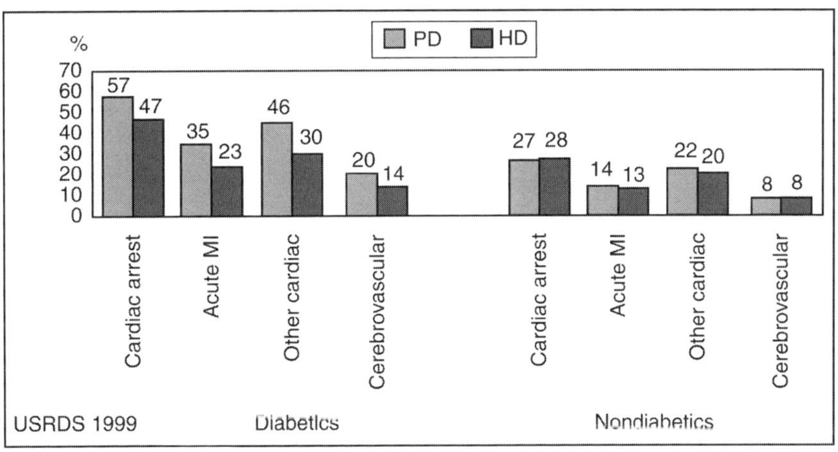

Fig. 5. Cause-specific death rates for diabetic dialysis patients aged 45–64 by modality, 1995–1997, from ref. *1*. Death rates (total deaths/1000 patient years at risk) for diabetic patients on PD and HD are 282 vs 205 respectively, whereas in nondiabetics these rates are 146 vs 141 for PD and HD, respectively.

controlled study) showed that in PD ESRD patients (42% diabetic) increases in peritoneal small-solute clearances within the National Kidney Foundation-Dialysis Outcomes Quality Initiative targets *(21)* have no effect on patient survival, even after controlling for a variety of factors (age, diabetes mellitus, serum albumin levels, normalized protein equivalent of total nitrogen appearance, and anuria) known to affect survival. Thus, it challenges us to focus on treating the entire patient to achieve optimal outcomes, including fluid control and nutrition management. Similarly, the Hemodialysis (HEMO) study concluded that patients undergoing HD three times a week appear to have no major benefit from a higher dialysis dose than that recommended by current guidelines or from the use of a high-flux membrane *(22)*. Current efforts are being focused on, improving phosphate control, and lowering traditional and nontraditional risk factors for adverse cardiovascular events in these patients *(23)*.

Consequently, diabetic dialysis patients commonly require preemptive, aggressive, and multidisciplinary management to ameliorate the devastating complications related to end-organ and system complications that are present in long-term diabetes.

CHOICE OF MODALITY IN DIABETIC ESRD PATIENTS: EARLY NEPHROLOGY REFERRAL

One of the most interesting parts of the RRT application is to choose the right modality for each diabetic patient. This is partially dependent (as with nondiabetic patients) on the same factors that include comorbid conditions, independence, and motivation of the patient, home, and social situation, and the patient's hemodynamic stability. The presence of autonomic neuropathy may result in the patient's inability to tolerate volume shifts predisposing to hypotensive episodes during HD sessions. In that situation, CAPD, by the more gradual fluid removal, may be the method of choice if there is no any other contraindication for its application. In the study by Stack et al. *(24),* HD was preferred over PD because it was associated with a survival advantage in diabetic patients with larger body mass index (BMI >30 kg/m^2). We believe that the final decision regarding the treatment choice of CAPD vs HD must be highly individualized and left up to patient, as there is no survival and rehabilitation advantage of one dialysis modality over another.

In Western countries, the majority of dialysis patients with DN are treated with HD, and CAPD is used by less than one-fifth of the patients, whereas there is an astonishing international variation in modality distribution. Although in centers, HD has poor survival and rehabilitation profile, the sickest, most debilitated patients with the highest number of comorbid conditions tend to be referred for this therapeutic modality. Still, the majority of clinical studies have concluded that survival on RRT has continued to improve. Several comparative studies of diabetic and nondiabetic patients on maintenance HD had shown that diabetics have inferior survival than nondiabetics *(25)*; however, over the years, survival of diabetics on maintenance HD has improved by better control of blood pressure and blood glucose, whereas home HD reported to have the highest survival rates *(26)*. Comparing technique survival rates, technique failure on CAPD is significantly higher than that of HD mainly because of infectious complications.

Regardless of modality selection, early nephrology referral as well as early start of RRT (creatinine clearance 15–20 mL/min) may provide adequate time either to create an autologous arterio-venous fistulae (AVF) several months before starting HD or to place a suitable peritoneal catheter at least 2–4 wk or even longer before starting PD *(21,27)*. Early nephrology referral before starting dialysis of diabetic ESRD patients has been associated with longer survival by either HD *(28)* or PD *(29)*. Despite this, 25–30% of diabetic type 2 patients starting RRT in Europe were referred to a nephrologist less than 1 mo before initiation of dialysis *(30)*.

HEMODIALYSIS-RELATED COMPLICATIONS IN DIABETIC DIALYSIS PATIENTS

Because diabetic patients are commonly subjected to various micro- and macrovascular complications and to a wide range of comorbidities, HD has not been considered to be the most appropriate replacement therapy. This is mainly owing to the difficulties in AVF creation, the presence of CAD, the patients' hemodynamic instability, and the requirements of systemic anticoagulation. However, HD is still the most commonly used therapy among diabetic patients worldwide, regardless of the following complications.

Table 3
Factors Contributing to Dialysis-Associated Hypotension in Diabetic Patients

Classification	*Causes/Contributors*
Autonomic neuropathy	Diabetic complication Uremic complication
Reduced myocardial ejection fraction	Atherosclerotic coronary artery disease Angina pectoris Consequence of myocardial infarction
Diastolic dysfunction	Diabetic cardiomyopathy
Anemia	Reduced blood viscosity Peripheral vascular resistance May precipitate dialysis-related angina
Hypoalbuminemia	Malnutrition Theory of thermal amplification

Table 4
Managing Intradialytic Hypotension in Diabetics

Use bicarbonate dialysate
High sodium (140–145 mmol/L) dialysate with linear sodium modeling
Reduce the rate of ultrafiltration–sequential ultrafiltration
Increase dialysis time
Maintain hematocrit ≥30% with rHu-EPO
No antihypertensive medications on morning of dialysis
Prime dialysis circuit with hypertonic albumin
Decrease dialysate temperature (particularly near end of dialysis)
Medications: α-agonists (midodrine)

Hypotension

During HD sessions, diabetic patients have 20% increased frequency of hypotension episodes *(12)*, owing to multifactorial causes (Table 3) and often associated with nausea and vomiting. Hypotension occasionally occurs in the presence of clinical volume overload or/and edema. Recurrent episodes of intradialytic hypotension may contribute to the increased mortality in diabetic patients *(31)*. Long-standing diabetes and autonomic neuropathy may suppress the increase in heart rate and peripheral vascular resistance, the two compensatory mechanisms to prevent hypotension.

Atherosclerotic CAD may also contribute to intradialytic hypotension in diabetic HD patients, by reducing myocardial ejection fraction *(32)*, whereas anemia may partially precipitate dialysis-related angina or may affect the ability to sustain UF by reducing blood viscosity and peripheral vascular resistance *(33)*. Miles et al. *(12)* reported some commonly used approaches for the management of dialysis-related hypotension (Table 4).

Hypertension

Hypertension is more commonly seen in diabetic than in nondiabetic HD patients, and may contribute to their increased cardiovascular morbidity and mortality. Regarding its pathogenesis, hypertension in most diabetic patients is principally volume-dependent, and therefore it may be corrected when dry weight is attained. Conversely, hypertension episodes may appear during or at the end of a dialysis session, which might be owing to acute activation of the renin–angiotensin system because of the UF-induced decline in intravascular fluid volume. In these cases, the use of angiotensin-converting enzyme inhibitors usually controls this problem.

The importance of achieving very low target blood pressure values has been well documented in predialysis diabetic patients both in the Hypertension Optimal Treatment (HOT) study *(34)* and in the UK Prospective Diabetes Study (PDS) *(35)*. In the latter, a difference of blood pressures of less than 10/5 mmHg reduced the risk of death from diabetes-related causes by 32%. However, as with nondialysis diabetic patients, angiotensin receptor antagonists regress left ventricular hypertrophy (LVH) associated with DN in dialysis patients. Actually, LVH is frequently found at the initiation of dialysis therapy for diabetic and hypertensive patients, and is highly predictive of future cardiac morbidity and mortality *(36)*.

Higher Weight Gain Between HD Sessions and Volume Overload

Diabetic patients were reported to gain 30–50% more interdialytic weight than nondiabetics *(12)*, and increased interdialytic weight has been independently associated with decreased survival of diabetic ESRD patients treated with HD *(37)*. The underlying mechanism is unclear and it might be correlated with the degree of hyperglycemia *(38)* or a higher intracellular sodium content producing increased thirst and further water intake *(39)*. The resulting volume overload requires further UF, which results in both hypotensive episodes and painful muscle cramps.

Vascular Access in Diabetic Hemodialysis Patients

Native AVFs are the preferred option both in the young patients with type 1 diabetes, as well as in older type 2 diabetic patients, because either grafts or central venous catheters (CVC) are subject to infectious and thrombotic complications. However, creation of an endogenous fistula in diabetic patients is not always feasible because of advanced PVD, presence of atherosclerotic lesions, destruction of veins owing to previous injuries by repeated intravenous injections or catheter insertions as well as medial calcinosis *(40)* factors that may lead to arterial vascular destruction and to the need of a synthetic, usually polytetrafluoroethylene, graft.

In older, mainly type 2 diabetics, calcifications may hinder the maturation of distal (wrist) vascular access, preventing the hypertrophy of the feeding artery, and thus it has been suggested *(41)* that the primary choice of an elbow AVF in general avoids frustrating attempts at the wrist, especially when late referral requires dialysis to be started rapidly. Also, many skilled surgical technical variations are possible in these patients because the increasing use of CVC for dialysis is a matter of concern. Rodriguez et al. *(42)* reported a prevalence of 79.6% of native vascular access in diabetics, with an 11% prevalence of CVC. Careful preoperative planning should allow examining the presence of adequate peripheral vessels and detection of suitable diabetic patients for a successful AVF and those at high risk of distal ischemia and steal syndrome.

PERITONEAL DIALYSIS-RELATED COMPLICATIONS IN DIABETIC PATIENTS

Because CAPD offers several advantages as a home dialysis treatment that allows flexibility and enables patients to enjoy most of their activities, it has become increasingly popular among diabetic patients with ESRD. However, peritonitis and exit-site infections and protein loss with the accompanying malnutrition are some of the shortcomings of PD. Furthermore, long-term studies in PD patients with DN have demonstrated that the micro- and macrovascular disease of diabetes continue to progress after initiation of CAPD, leading to ongoing problems with cardiovascular disease, malnutrition, autonomic neuropathy, retinopathy, and PVD *(43)*.

Peritonitis

Peritonitis remains the major cause of drop out for CAPD patients, whereas there is no evidence that diabetics are at increased risk for peritonitis as initially considered. Although catheter infection rates were 17% higher in the diabetics, there was no difference in time-to-first-catheter-infection between diabetics and nondiabetics ($p = 0.6$), whereas rates of peritonitis, peritonitis associated with catheter infections, multiple catheter infection, and catheter removal were also similar among the diabetics and controls *(44)*. Also, despite the initial thoughts that intraperitoneal administration of insulin in diabetics on CAPD would increase the frequency of peritonitis, reported experience of many centers indicates that the incidence of peritonitis among diabetics using intraperitoneal insulin is similar to that of nondiabetics *(45)*.

Peritonitis is also the most common complication and the major cause of hospitalization, whereas recurrent episodes of peritonitis were the leading cause in two-thirds of the permanent transfers to HD and the main cause of catheter replacement in two-thirds of all cases *(10)*. On the other hand, frequent severe peritonitis episodes may contribute to peritoneal membrane permeability alterations and UF loss, which in association with the higher incidence of comorbid factors, may result in a shortened CAPD longevity.

Malnutrition

Diabetic patients have an increased risk for developing malnutrition on CAPD and this contributes to morbidity and mortality *(46)*. Anorexia owing to underdialysis, metabolic acidosis, hyperglycemia, gastroparesis, the feeling of fullness owing to the presence of dialysis solution in the abdomen, and the loss of residual renal function may contribute to malnutrition in CAPD diabetic patients *(47)*.

Increased glucose absorption from the dialysis fluid may also decrease appetite, which adds to the complexity of this problem, whereas autonomic dysfunction with severe orthostatic hypotension, and bladder and bowel dysfunction, constitutes a real challenge to those treating diabetic patients. Gastroparesis and the associated nausea and vomiting, is a most frustrating complication of diabetes.

Ultrafiltration Failure

In relation to the UF changes, early studies *(48,49)* showed that the peritoneal permeability characteristics are well maintained overtime on PD, but current data would suggest that there is a tendency toward increasing permeability and UF failure in long-term PD patients. However, in patients with low rates of peritoneal inflammation, it has been estimated that after 5–11 yr, the human peritoneum shows functional stability (solute diffusion and water transport) *(49)*.

Actually, increased peritoneal capillary permeability has been described in studies of diabetic rats and in clinical studies *(50)*, an observation that resembles the leakage of albumin across capillary walls, which is characteristic of diabetic microvascular disease. Also, high peritoneal permeability has been related to the higher morbidity and mortality seen in high peritoneal transporters *(51)*. Besides, high peritoneal permeability may also result in low serum albumin concentration, a powerful indicator of mortality *(52)*. Moreover, Krediet's team analyzing the differences in fluid and solute transport between diabetic and nondiabetic patients suggested that the changes in capillary wall aquaporins observed in diabetic patients prior to CAPD are similar to those observed in nondiabetics after long-term exposure to high glucose concentrations in the dialysate *(53)*. Also, increased peritoneal expression of vascular endothelial growth factor, transforming growth factor-β_1 and excessive accumulation of AGEs may be involved in the progressive increase in membrane permeability, loss of UF, and peritoneal fibrosis *(54)*.

UF failure commonly results from rapid peritoneal transport of glucose, whereas occasionally a high peritoneal lymphatic absorption also might be responsible. Diabetics with frequent hyperglycemia episodes may develop fluid retention because of both increased fluid consumption, stimulated by thirst, and by reduced transperitoneal osmotic gradient. Nevertheless, there are no differences with nondiabetics and UF failure is not a frequent cause of technique failure or discontinuation of CAPD in diabetics *(42)*.

Peritonitis and conventional PD solutions containing high glucose and glucose-degradation products are implicated in PD technique failure *(54)*, whereas PD solutions without glucose or solutions containing low glucose degradation products may prevent or delay peritoneal membrane alterations and allow its long-time function in both diabetic and nondiabetic patients during long-term PD.

TECHNIQUE AND PATIENT SURVIVAL

The introduction of technological developments in HD treatment, the advent of volumetric HD machines, high-flux and high-efficiency dialyzers, along with computerization of the dialysis sessions have all contributed to better care for ESRD diabetic patients. Similarly, in PD treatment technological improvements such as the Y-set disconnect system have substantially decreased the incidence of peritonitis and improved CAPD technique survival, but still it is inferior to HD technique survival *(55)*. Furthermore, during the last decade, there was a great effort toward improving the quality of care, under the development of clinical practice guidelines, focusing at adequacy of treatment, and patient outcomes. Additionally, there is now effective treatment of the anemia of CKD, which improves survival, *(56)* decreases morbidity, *(57)* and increases quality of life *(58)*. Marcelli et al. *(59)* found that PD technique survival in diabetic patients, unadjusted for pretreatment prognostic differences, was 91% at 1 yr, 73% at 3 yr, and 61% at 5 yr, lower than the HD technique survival of 94, 80, and 75%, respectively.

Investigation of survival rates of diabetic patients on dialysis requires careful interpretation because the various relative studies commonly involve dissimilar patient groups with regards to age, race, diabetes type, factors of comorbidity and their severity, various complications, and degree of metabolic control. Thus, from reported diabetic patient survival data obtained mainly from retrospective multicenter or single-center studies for varying follow-up periods up to 18 yr, we found that mean survival rates for PD for the first, third, and fifth years were 85, 51, and 39%, respectively (Fig. 6) *(60)*. Similar results have been reported for diabetic patients on HD, 86.5% at 1 yr, 52% at 3 yr, and 34% at 5 yr *(59)*. Furthermore, several studies with varying proportions of diabetic patients, attempted to compare long-term clinical outcomes of the two RRT modalities. Despite the disparity of results, most medium- and long-term studies have

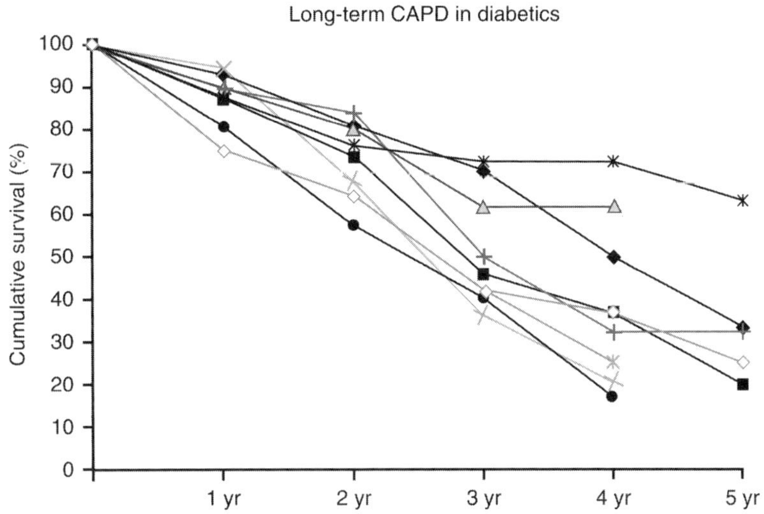

Fig. 6. Long-term survival of CAPD patients with diabetes mellitus *(60)*.

concluded that the differences between the overall survival rates of diabetic patients undergoing PD and HD are not statistically significant *(59,61–64)*, whereas other studies favor HD *(65,66)* and others favor PD *(67–69)*. Whenever a study made an adjustment for comorbid factors, the comparison among modes of dialysis either showed no statistically significant difference or favored CAPD. Table 5 summarizes the mortality relative risk (RR) for diabetic patients undergoing CAPD or HD. According to the more recent USRDS data *(1)*, diabetic patients continue to have the lowest probabilities of survival, with 27% of those on HD, and 23% of PD patients expected to survive 5 yr after initiation.

After adjusting for statistical differences, Vonesh and Moran *(64)* found that among diabetic patients, the PD-to-HD death rate ratio varied significantly according to gender and age. The average male diabetic patient had little or no difference in risk between PD and HD from 1989 to1993, whereas diabetic patients under the age of 50 yr treated with PD had a significantly lower risk of death than those treated with HD.

Also, incident Medicare patients treated between 1994 and 1996 were evaluated by Collins et al. *(69)* using Poisson regression and compared death rates, adjusting for age, gender, race, and primary renal diagnosis. They showed that patients undergoing CAPD/continous cycle (CC) PD have outcomes comparable with or significantly better than those undergoing HD, although results varied with time on dialysis. Cox regression analysis showed a lower PD-to-HD mortality ratio in diabetic CAPD/CCPD patients younger than 55 yr. In contrast, the risk of all-cause death for female diabetic patients aged 55 yr and older was 1.21 for CAPD/CCPD, and the risk of death was lower (1.03) in men over 55 yr.

However, more recent data *(70)* regarding the gender effect on mortality rate for HD and PD patients starting dialysis between 1990 and 1998 in Canada found that for HD patients there was no difference in adjusted mortality rate ratio (RR) among genders irrespective of diabetic status, whereas females 65 yr or older on PD had significantly higher adjusted mortality rates than males. Moreover, diabetic females on PD had significantly higher mortality rates than males in both age groups.

Table 5
Mortality RR for CAPD/CCPD vs HD in Diabetic Patients

Source (ref.)	*HD*	*CAPD*	*p-Value*
Bloembergen et al. *(25)*			
	1.00	1.38	<0.001
Age <55 yr	1.00	1.00	>0.05
Age >55 yr	1.00	RR > 1.00	<0.05
Held et al. *(66)*			
	1.00	1.26	0.03
Age <58 yr[a]	1.00	1.11	>0.05
Age ≥58 yr	1.00	1.25	<0.05
Age ≥63 yr	1.00	1.34	<0.01
Nelson et al. *(67)*			
Age 20–52 yr	1.00	0.40–0.70[b]	
Fenton et al. *(68)*[c]			
Age 0–64 yr	1.00	0.73 (0.62–0.87)	<0.01
Age over 65 yr	1.00	0.88	>0.05
Serkes et al. *(61)*			
	1.00	0.90	>0.05
Vonesh et al. *(64)*			
Average male			
1989–1991	1.00	1.02	>0.05
1990–1992	1.00	1.05	>0.05
1991–1993	1.00	1.08	<0.01
<50 yr:1989–1993	1.00	0.84–0.89	<0.05
>50 yr:1989–1993	1.00	1.28–1.30	<0.001
Female: 1989–1993	1.00	1.18–1.19	<0.001
Collins et al. *(69)*[d]			
Women <55	1.00	0.88	
Women >55	1.00	1.21	
Men <55	1.00	0.86	
Men >55	1.00	1.03	

[a]Age at onset of ESRD.
[b]This relative mortality risk was lowest for younger diabetics and statistically significant ($p \leq 0.05$) for ages 20–52 yr (0.40, 0.48, 0.58, 0.7 for 20–29, 30–39, 40–48, and 50–59 yr, respectively); also among diabetic patients, mortality rates rose significantly faster ($p = 0.03$) in CAPD-treated patients (RR = 1.37 per 10 yr of age) rather than HD-treated patients (RR = 1.14 per 10 yr).
[c]RR controlled for age, predialysis comorbid conditions, and center size.
[d]These values of RR reported to be significantly lower.

Despite these discrepancies, improvements in dialysis modalities during the last two decades resulted in longer survival rates in diabetic dialysis patients, but still lower than that of nondiabetic patients undergoing RRT. Worse outcomes have been mainly attributed to the increasing incidence of older diabetic patients with a rising occurrence of serious comorbid conditions, largely resulting from diabetic complications. This reflects the requirement for a rigorous predialysis care, an early nephrology referral, and an early dialysis initiation of the most appropriate treatment modality. On the other hand, an integrated care approach starting with PD and switching to HD if problems arise *(71)*, and keeping suitable patients on the renal or renal–pancreas transplantation waiting list, may offer the best outcome of the diabetic ESRD patients.

REFERENCES

1. US Renal Data System, USRDS 2003 Annual Data Report: Atlas of End-Stage Renal Disease in the United States, National Institutes of Health, National Institute of Diabetes, and Digestive and Kidney Diseases, Bethesda, MD, 2003.
2. Neel JV, Weder A. Julius S. Type II diabetes, essential hypertension, and obesity as "syndromes of impaired genetic homeostasis," the "thrifty genotype" hypothesis enters the 21st century. Perspecl Biol Med 1998;42:44–74.
3. Nishimura R, Dorman, JS, Bosnyak Z, Tajima N. Incidence of ESRD and survival after renal replacement therapy in patients with type 1 diabetes: A report from the allegheny county registry. Am J Kidney Dis 2003;42:117.
4. Van Dijk PC, Jager KJ, Stengel B, Gronhagen-Riska C, Feest TG, Briggs JD. Renal replacement therapy for diabetic end-stage renal disease: data from 10 registries in Europe (1991–2000). Kidney International 2005;67(4):1489–2005.
5. Avram MM. Use of special hemodialysis methods in diabetic uremia. New York: National Union Catalogue 1966;15–16.
6. Ghavamian M, Gulch CF, Kopp KF, et al. The sad truth about hemodialysis in diabetic nephropathy. JAMA 1972;222:1386–1389.
7. Comty CM, Kjellsen D, Shapiro FL. A reassessment of the prognosis of diabetic patients treated by chronic hemodialysis. Trans Am Soc Artif Intern Organs 1976;22:404.
8. Jacobs C, Broyer M, Brunner FP, et al. Combined report on regular dialysis and transplantation in Europe, XI, 1980. Presented at the 17th Congress of the European Dialysis and Transplantation Association, Paris, July 5–8, 1981.
9. U.S. Renal Data System, USRDS 2001 Annual Data Report: Atlas of End-Stage Renal Disease in the United States, National Institutes of Health, National Institute of Diabetes and Digestive and Kidney Diseases, Bethesda, MD, 2001.
10. Passadakis P, Oreopoulos DG. Continuous Ambulatory Peritoneal Dialysis in 224 diabetics with end stage renal disease: evidence of improved survival over the past 10 years. In: Eli A. Friedman, Francis A. L'Esperance, eds. Diabetic Renal-Retinal syndrome, 21st Century Management Now. Kluwer Academic Publishers, London, Great Britain, 1998, pp. 89–115.
11. Young EW, Goodkin DA, Mapes DL, et al. The Dialysis Outcomes and Practice Patterns Study (DOPPS): an international hemodialysis study. Kidney Int 2000;57(74):S74–S81.
12. Miles AM. Hemodialysis in patients with diabetes mellitus. In: Eli A. Friedman, Francis A. L'Esperance, eds. Diabetic Renal-Retinal syndrome, 21st Century Management Now. Kluwer Academic Publishers, London, Great Britain, 1998, pp. 89–115.
13. National kidney foundation. K/DOQI clinical practice guidelines for chronic kidney disease: evaluation, classification and stratification. Am J Kidney Dis 2002;39(1):S1–S266.
14. Haffner SM, Lehto S, Ronnemaa T, Pyorala K, Laakso M. Mortality from coronary heart disease in subjects with type 2 diabetes and in nondiabetic subjects with and without prior myocardial infarction N Engl J Med 1998;339(4):229–234.
15. Schaubel D, Fenton SSA. Diabetes and Renal Failure. Section 6. Canadian Organ Replacement Register. Annual report 1996. Canadian Institute of Health Information, Ottawa, Ontario March 1996.
16. Locatelli F, Pozzoni P, Del Vecchio L. Renal replacement therapy in patients with diabetes and end-stage renal disease. J Am Soc Nephrol 2004;15(1):S25.
17. Toriyama T, Yokoya M, Nishida Y, Kawajiri K, Takahashi H, Kawahara H. Increased incidence of coronary artery disease and cardiac death in elderly diabetic nephropathy patients undergoing chronic hemodialysis therapy J Cardiol 2000;36(3):165–171.
18. Brownlee M, Cerami A, Vlassara H. Advanced glycosylation end products in tissue and the biochemical basis of diabetic complication. N Engl J Med 1988;18:1315–1321.
19. Keshaviah P, Ma J, Thorpe K, Churchill D, Collins A. Comparison of 2 year survival on hemodialysis (HD) and peritoneal dialysis (PD) with dose of dialysis matched using the peak concentration hypothesis. J Am Soc Nephrol 1995;6:540.
20. Paniagua R, Amato D, Vonesh E, et al. Mexican Nephrology Collaborative Study Group. Effects of increased peritoneal clearances on mortality rates in peritoneal dialysis: ADEMEX, a prospective, randomized, controlled trial. J Am Soc Nephrol. 2002;13(5):1307–1320.
21. II. NKF-K/DOQI clinical practice guidelines for peritoneal dialysis adequacy: update 2000. Am J Kidney Dis. 2001;37(1 Suppl 1):S65–S136.
22. Eknoyan G, Beck GJ, Cheung AK, et al. Hemodialysis (HEMO) Study Group. Effect of dialysis dose and membrane flux in maintenance hemodialysis. N Engl J Med 2002;347(25):2010–2019.

23. Himmelfarb J. The HEMO study—where do we go from here? Curr Opin Nephrol Hypertens. 2003;12(6):587–591.
24. Stack AG, Murthy BV, Molony DA. Survival differences between peritoneal dialysis and hemodialysis among "large" ESRD patients in the United States. Kidney Int 2004;65(6):2398–2408.
25. Bloembergen WE, Port FK, Mauger EA, Wolfe RA. A comparison of mortality between patients treated with hemodialysis and peritoneal dialysis J Am Soc Nephrol 1995;6(2):177–183.
26. Perneger TV, Brancati FL, Whelton PK, Klag MJ. End-stage renal disease attributable to diabetes mellitus. Ann Intern Med 1994;121(12):912–918.
27. Wavamunno MD, Harris DC. The need for early nephrology referral. Kidney Int Suppl 2005;(94): S128–S132.
28. Lin CL, Wu MS, Hsu PY, Huang CC. Improvement of clinical outcome by early nephrology referral in type II diabetics on hemodialysis. Ren Fail 2003;25(3):455–464.
29. Wu MS, Lin CL, Chang CT, Wu CH, Huang JY, Yang CW. Improvement in clinical outcome by early nephrology referral in type II diabetics on maintenance peritoneal dialysis. Perit Dial Int 2003;23(1):39–45.
30. Ritz E. Consequences of late referral in diabetic renal disease. Acta Diabetol 2002;39:(1):S3–S8.
31. Collins AL, Liao A, Umen A, Hanson G, Keshaviah P. Diabetic hemodialysis patients treated with a high Kt/V have a lower risk of death than standard Kt/V. J Am Soc Nephrol 1991;2:318.
32. Nakamoto M. The mechanism of intradialytic hypotension in diabetic patients. Nippon Jinzo Gakkai Shi. Jap J Nephrol 1994;36:374–381.
33. Daugirdas JT. Dialysis hypotension: a hemodynamic analysis. Kidney Int 1991;39:223–246.
34. Hansson L, Zanchetti A, Carruthers SG, et al. Effects of intensive blood-pressure lowering and low-dose aspirin in patients with hypertension: principal results of the Hypertension Optimal Treatment (HOT) randomised trial. HOT Study Group Lancet 1998;351:1755–1762.
35. UK Prospective Diabetes Study Group. Tight blood pressure control and risk of macrovascular and microvascular complications in type 2 diabetes: UKPDS 38. Br Med J 1998;317:703–713.
36. Kanno Y, Kaneko K, Kaneko M, et al. Angiotensin receptor antagonist regresses left ventricular hypertrophy associated with diabetic nephropathy in dialysis patients. J Cardiovasc Pharmacol 2004;43(3):380–386.
37. Kimmel PL, Varela MP, Peterson RA, et al. Interdialytic weight gain and survival in hemodialysis patients: effects of duration of ESRD and diabetes mellitus. Kidney Int 2000;57(3);1141–1151.
38. Ifudu O, Dulin A, Lundin AP, et al. Diabetics manifest excess weight gain on maintenance hemodialysis. Am Soc Artif Intern Org 1992;21:85.
39. Jones R, Poston R, Hinestrota A, et al. Weight gain between dialysis in diabetics. Possible significance of raised intracellular sodium content. Br Med J 1980;1:153,154.
40. Konner K. Primary vascular access in diabetic patients: an audit. Nephrol Dial Transplant 2000;15: 1317–1325.
41. Bonucchi D. http://ndt.oupjournals.org/cgi/content/full/17/1/20-FN1, Cappelli Gand Albertazzi A. Which is the preferred vascular access in diabetic patients? A view from Europe. Nephrol Dial Transplant 2002;17:20–22.
42. Rodriguez JA, Lopez J, Montse Cleries, Vela E. Renal Registry Committee. Vascular access for haemodialysis—an epidemiological study of the Catalan Renal Registry. Nephrol Dial Transplant 1999;14:1651–1657.
43. Zimmerman S. The diabetic ESRD patient: Specific needs. Perit Dial Int 1997;17:(3):S9–S11.
44. Holley J, Bernardini J, Piraino B. Catheter infections in insulin-dependent diabetics on continuous ambulatory peritoneal dialysis. Perit Dial Int 1991;11(4):347–350.
45. Khanna R, Oreopoulos DG. Peritoneal dialysis in diabetic end-stage renal disease. J Diabet Complications 1989;1:12–17.
46. Espinosa A, Cueto-Manzano AM, Velazquez-Alva C, et al. Prevalence of malnutrition in Mexican CAPD diabetic and nondiabetic patients. Adv Perit Dial 1996;12:302–306.
47. Passadakis P, Thodis E, Vargemezis V, Oreopoulos DG. Nutrition in diabetic patients undergoing continuous ambulatory peritoneal dialysis. Perit Dial Int 1999;19(2):S248–S254.
48. Hallett MD, Charlton B, Farrell PC. Is the peritoneal membrane durable indefinitely? Adv Perit Dial 1990;6:197–201.
49. Selgas R, Fernandez-Reyes M, Bosque E, et al. Functional longevity of the human peritoneum. How long is CAPD possible? Results of a prospective medium long-term study. Am J Kidney Dis 1994;23(1):64–73.
50. Kriedet RT, Zuyderhoudt FMJ, Boeschoten EW, Arisz L. Peritoneal permeability to proteins in diabetic and non-diabetic continuous ambulatory peritoneal dialysis patients. Nephron 1986;42:133–140.

51. Fried L. Higher membrane permeability predicts poorer patient survival. Perit Dial Int 1997; 17: 387–389.
52. Lowrie EG, Huang WH, Lew NL. Death risk predictors among peritoneal dialysis and hemodialysis patients: a preliminary comparison. Am J Kidney Dis 1995;26:220–228.
53. Serlie MJ, Struijk DG, de Blok K, Krediet RT. Differences in fluid and solute transport between diabetic and nondiabetic patients at the onset of CAPD. Adv Perit Dial 1997;13:29–32.
54. Lee HB, Chung SH, Chu WS, Kim JK, Ha H. Peritoneal dialysis in diabetic patients. Am J Kidney Dis. 2001;38(4 Suppl 1):S200–S203.
55. Maiorca R, Vonesh E, and Cavalli PL, et al. A multi-centre, selection adjusted comparison of patient and technique survivals on CAPD and hemodialysis. Peritoneal Dialysis Int 1991;11:118–127.
56. Mocks J, Franke W, Ehmer B, Scigalla P, Quarder O. Analysis of safety database for long-term epoetin-beta treatment. A meta-analysis covering 3697 patients. In: Koch KM, Stein G, eds. Pathogenetic and Therapeutic Aspects of Chronic Renal Failure 12, Marcel Dekker, New York, 1997, pp. 163–79.
57. Consensus Development Conference Panel: morbidity and mortality of renal dialysis: an NIH consensus conference statement. Ann Intern Med 1994;121:62–70.
58. Delano BG: Improvements in quality of life following treatment with r-HuEPO in anemic hemodialysis patients. Am J Kidney Dis 1989;14:14–18.
59. Marcelli D, Spotti D, Conte F, et al. Survival oI diabetic patients on peritoneal dialysis or hemodialysis. Perit Dial Int 1996;16:S283–S287.
60. Passadakis P, Thodis E, Vargemezis V, Oreopoulos D. Long-term survival with peritoneal dialysis in ESRD due to diabetes. Clin Nephrol 2001;56:257–270.
61. Serkes KD, Blagg CR, Nolph KD, Vonesh EF, Shapiro F. Comparison of patient and technique survival in continuous ambulatory peritoneal dialysis (CAPD) and hemodialysis: a multicenter study. Perit Dia Int 1990;10:15–19.
62. Gentil MA, Carriazo A, Pavon MI, et al. Comparison of survival in continuous ambulatory peritoneal dialysis and hospital haemodialysis: a multicentric study. Nephrol Dial Transplant 1991;6:444–451.
63. Maiorca R, Cancarini GC, Zubani R, et al. CAPD viability: a long-term comparison with hemodialysis. Perit Dial Int 1996;16(3):276–287.
64. Vonesh EF, Moran J. Mortality in end-stage renal disease: a reassessment of differences between patients treated with hemodialysis and peritoneal dialysis. J Am Soc Nephr 1999;10(2):354–365.
65. US Renal Data System. USRDS 1991 Annual Data Report, the National Institute of Diabetes and Digestive and Kidney Diseases. Am J Kidney Dis 1991;18(2):49–60.
66. Held PJ, Port FK, Turenne N, Gaylin DS, Hamburger RJ, Wolfe RA. Continuous ambulatory peritoneal dialysis and hemodialysis: comparison of patient mortality with adjustment for comorbid conditions. Kidney Int 1994;45:1163–1169.
67. Nelson CB, Port FK, Wolfe RA, Guire KE. Comparison of continuous ambulatory peritoneal dialysis and hemodialysis patient survival with evaluation of trends during the 1980s. J Am Soc Nephrol 1992;3:1147–1155.
68. Fenton SS, Schaubel DE, Desmeules M, et al. Hemodialysis versus peritoneal dialysis: a comparison of adjusted mortality rates. Am J Kidney Dis 1997;30(3):334–342.
69. Collins AJ, Hao W, Xia H, et al. Mortality risks of peritoneal dialysis and hemodialysis. Am J Kidney Dis 1999;34(6):1065–1074.
70. Krishnan M, Schaubel D, Bargman JM, Oreopoulos DG, Fenton SA. Gender Differences in Outcome for Patients on HD and PD: a Canadian Perspective. J Am Soc Nephrol 2001;12:218A.
71. Van Biesen W, Vanholder RC, Veys N, Dhondt A, Lameire NH. An evaluation of an integrative care approach for end-stage renal disease patients. J Am Soc Nephrol. 2000;11(1):116–125.

II

Clinical Aspects of Diabetic Nephropathy

D. Related Abnormalities

27 Diabetic Retinopathy and Nephropathy

Ronald Klein, MD, MPH

Contents

INTRODUCTION

Over a nearly 25-yr period beginning in 1979, four "diabetic renal–retinal syndrome" meetings were held in New York City. They were led by Eli Friedman and Francis L'Esperance, who brought together epidemiologists, bench scientists, clinicians, nephrologists, and ophthalmologists involved in research and clinical care of persons with diabetic retinopathy and nephropathy *(1–4)*. The renal–retinal syndrome was defined in these meetings as "coincident kidney and eye diseases resulting from diabetic microvasculopathy in retinal and glomerular arterioles and capillaries" *(3)*. Data from clinical trials over this 25-yr period demonstrated the efficacy of panretinal and focal photocoagulation preventing visual loss owing to proliferative retinopathy and clinically significant macular edema and of intensive glycemic and blood pressure control preventing progression of retinopathy, nephropathy, and other vascular complications associated with diabetes *(4–10)*. Despite this, both retinopathy and nephropathy remain prevalent and are important causes of loss of function and quality of life *(11–14)*.

Prevention of retinopathy and nephropathy requires their early detection and the development of new treatments to complement glycemic and blood pressure control. The purpose of this chapter is to examine the epidemiological interrelationships between diabetic retinopathy and nephropathy. After a description of the natural history, pathogenesis, and epidemiology of diabetic retinopathy, the relationship of nephropathy as a risk factor for retinopathy and retinopathy as a risk indicator for nephropathy will be examined.

From: *Contemporary Diabetes: The Diabetic Kidney*
Edited by: P. Cortes and C. E. Mogensen © Humana Press Inc., Totowa, NJ

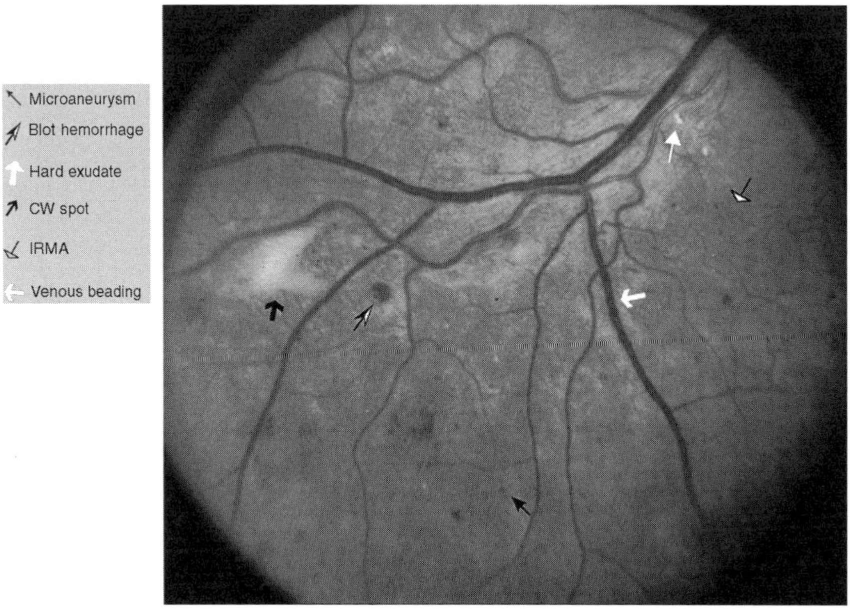

Fig. 1. Fundus photograph in a person with diabetes showing various signs of nonproliferative retinopathy.

NATURAL HISTORY OF DIABETIC RETINOPATHY

Retinopathy

The natural history of diabetic retinopathy has been well described *(15)*. The earliest clinically apparent change detected in the fundus using ophthalmoscopy is the retinal microaneurysm (Fig. 1) *(16)*. These are seen at time of diagnosis in approx 20–30% of persons with type 2 diabetes but are unusual in persons with type 1 diabetes of less than 3–5 yr duration *(17,18)*. The retinal microaneurysm is an outpouching of the weakened retinal capillary wall and appears as a round red dot, ranging in size from 20 to 200 μm in diameter. Eyes that manifest only retinal microaneurysms are classified as having minimal nonproliferative diabetic retinopathy (NPDR).

Retinal microaneurysms have abnormal permeability to lipoproteins and red blood cells *(16)*. By themselves, retinal microaneurysms are not a threat to vision. However, as retinopathy progresses, there may be extravasations of blood from retinal capillaries or microaneurysms into the inner nuclear layer of the retina leading to the appearance of blot hemorrhages (Fig. 1). Retinal hard exudates may result if there is leakage of lipoprotein material from retinal microaneurysms or capillaries (Fig. 1). Hard exudates appear as sharply defined, yellow, and variable deposits that may be aggregated, scattered, or "ring-like" in their distributions. Eyes with only retinal microaneurysms and blot hemorrhages and/or hard exudates are classified as having mild NPDR. If the foveal area is not involved by these abnormalities, the vision is usually normal.

These exudative changes are often accompanied by ischemia owing to closure of the retinal capillaries and arterioles. Microinfarcts of the nerve fiber layer of the retina appear as whitish or grayish swellings and are called "cotton-wool spots" or "soft exudates" (Fig. 1). Other manifestations seen in areas of focal retinal ischemia include dilated retinal capillaries (intraretinal microvascular abnormalities), large dark intraretinal

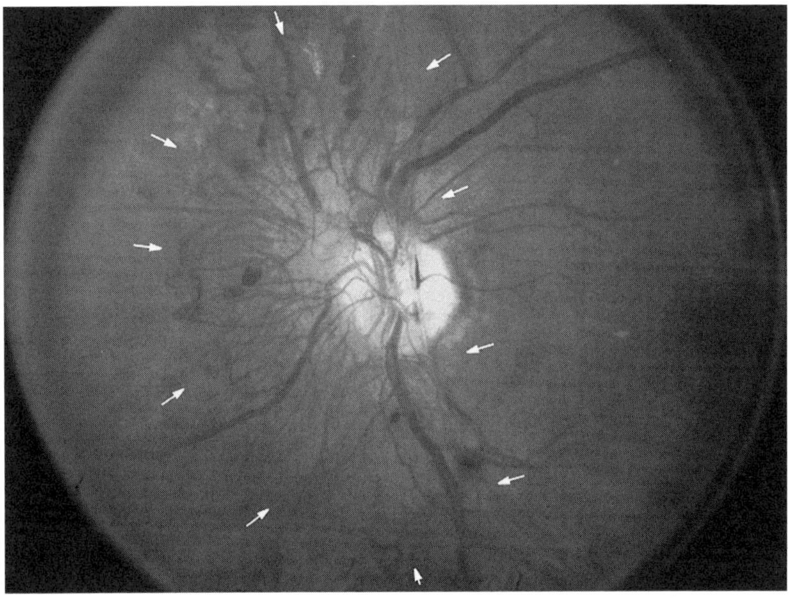

Fig. 2. Large area of retinal new vessels (outline by white arrows) is seen in area of optic nerve head in a left eye with proliferative diabetic retinopathy (PDR).

hemorrhages, and venous beading and duplication (Fig. 1). These changes have been called the "preproliferative phase" and are a warning sign of impending growth of abnormal new retinal vessels. These eyes are classified as having moderate to severe NPDR.

The appearance of abnormal new blood vessels and fibrous tissue usually originating near or from retinal venules or from the optic nerve head define the onset of the proliferative phase of diabetic retinopathy (Fig. 2). These vessels are prone to hemorrhage into the vitreous gel anterior to the retina and are often associated with fibrous tissue. Contraction of this fibrovascular tissue may result in a traction detachment of the retina and visual loss, if it involves the macular area. These eyes are classified as having proliferative diabetic retinopathy (PDR).

Macular Edema

Increased permeability of retinal capillaries and microaneurysms may result in the accumulation of extracellular fluid and thickening of the normally compact macular tissue. This is often associated with deposition of hard exudates, in rings, clumps, or large deposits. Accumulation of exudate is often gradual, and spontaneous resolution may occur in time. If macular edema involves the fovea, visual acuity may drop. It is thought that macular edema is a result of both increased leakage of fluid into the retina owing to breakdown of the blood–retinal barrier and impaired removal of the fluid by the retinal pigment epithelium *(19)*.

Pathogenesis

Almost all hypothesized pathogenetic mechanisms include hyperglycemia as having a critical role in initiating the retinopathy process. This is supported by data from animal models of experimental diabetes in which hyperglycemia results in retinopathy *(20)*, in epidemiological studies that demonstrate strong dose–response relationships of the incidence and progression of diabetic retinopathy to hyperglycemia *(21)*, and in randomized controlled clinical trials such as the Diabetes Control and Complications Trial (DCCT) and UK Prospective Diabetes Study (UKPDS) *(7,8)* that have demonstrated that intensive treatment of hyperglycemia results in a reduction of the incidence and progression of retinopathy. The pathogenetic mechanisms for diabetic retinopathy may be arbitrarily grouped in various categories (e.g., biochemical, physiological, rheological, growth factor changes, and so on). There has been recent speculation that hyperglycemia may increase reactive oxygen species (ROS) production and that ROS may serve as a possible causal link by activating some of these pathways (e.g., aldose reductase, protein kinase C) and inducing others (e.g., advanced glycation endproduct formation) *(22)*. The development and progression of retinopathy is likely secondary to a complex interplay of a number of these factors that may vary from person to person. It is likely that different mechanisms are operative and more important at different stages of retinopathy. Glycosylation, aldose reductase, protein kinase pathways, and increased retinal blood flow may be more important early in the course of diabetes before the development of microaneurysms than in later stages of retinopathy, such as during the progression of severe NPDR to PDR. Angiogenesis factors, such as vascular endothelial growth factor (VEGF) and growth hormone insulin-like growth factor-I are more likely to be important later in the course of the disease before the development of PDR. In addition, inter- and intraindividual variations of biochemical or physiological responses to hyperglycemia may exist among people at different stages of diabetes. This may explain why some diabetic patients have minimal retinopathy present despite years of severe hyperglycemia and hypertension, whereas others develop severe retinopathy over a shorter period of time despite relatively good glycemic and blood pressure control. Similar variation in response to hyperglycemia and other pathogenetic factors may occur among different tissues, partly explaining variations in retinopathy and nephropathy severity in the same individual.

Epidemiology of Retinopathy

The epidemiology of diabetic retinopathy has been well described elsewhere *(15)*. The Wisconsin Epidemiologic Study of Diabetic Retinopathy (WESDR) has provided epidemiological data on diabetic retinopathy, visual loss, and associated risk factors *(17,18,23–27)*.

Prevalence of Retinopathy

Persons with type 1 diabetes have higher frequencies of retinopathy, PDR, and clinically significant macular edema than those with type 2 diabetes (Table 1). Using pooled data from recently studied cohorts of persons 40 yr of age or older with type 2 diabetes, it was estimated that the crude prevalence of diabetic retinopathy was 40%, and the crude prevalence of severe retinopathy (preproliferative and proliferative retinopathy or macular edema) was 8% *(11)*. Projection of these proportions to the diabetic population 40 yr of age or older in the United States resulted in an estimate of 4 million persons with retinopathy, of whom 900,000 have signs of vision-threatening retinopathy (defined by the presence of either PDR and/or clinically significant macular edema).

Incidence and Progression of Retinopathy

In the WESDR, the 4-yr incidence (59% vs 39%) and progression of retinopathy (44 vs 30%) was higher in those with type 1 diabetes compared with those with type 2 diabetes *(24,25)*. Based on the WESDR data, it is estimated nationwide that there were

Table 1
Prevalence of any Retinopathy, PDR, and Clinically Significant Macular Edema by Type 1 and 2 Diabetes in the Wisconsin Epidemiologic Study of Diabetic Retinopathy, 1980–1982

	Type 1		*Type 2*	
Endpoint	*No.*	*Percentage*	*No.*	*Percentage*
Any diabetic retinopathy	996	71.8	1365	49.8
PDR	996	22.8	1365	5.7
Clinically significant macular edema	954	5.9	1318	5.2

PDR, proliferative diabetic retinopathy.

approx 63,000 new cases annually of PDR, 29,000 of whom developed PDR with Diabetic Retinopathy Study (DRS) high-risk characteristics for severe visual loss. In addition, there were 50,000 new cases of macular edema a year in the United States. These figures probably overestimate the actual incidence and progression of retinopathy because achievement of glycemic and blood pressure control is better than when the WESDR cohort was first studied 25 yr ago. Data from a Danish study showed a decrease in the cumulative incidence of diabetic retinopathy in persons with type 1 diabetes over a 35-yr period attributed to improved glycemic control, lower blood pressure levels, and reductions in smoking *(28)*.

Risk Factors for Diabetic Retinopathy

Race/Ethnicity

Retinopathy appears to be more frequent in Mexican Americans, Native Americans, and African Americans than in non-Hispanic whites with type 2 diabetes *(29–36)*. Poorer glycemic and blood pressure control is thought to explain the higher frequency of retinopathy in African Americans than in non-Hispanic whites *(33)*. Once these factors are controlled for, the differences in retinopathy frequency disappear. However, poorer control of glycemia and blood pressure in Mexican Americans did not explain differences in retinopathy rates with non-Hispanic whites.

Genetics

The severity and onset of retinopathy are similar among concordant identical twins, suggesting that the tendency to develop diabetic retinopathy and possibly its progression are influenced by genetic factors *(37)*. Data from the DCCT showed an increased risk of severe retinopathy among relatives of retinopathy-positive vs retinopathy-negative DCCT participants at baseline (odds ratio [OR] 3.1, 95% confidence interval [CI] 1.2, 7.8) *(38)*. Data from recent studies have shown associations between retinopathy and mitochondrial DNA mutations *(39)*, and polymorphisms of the aldose reductase gene *(40,41)*, *tumor necrosis factor (TNF)-β gene, NcoI gene (42)*, ε4 allele of apolipoprotein E gene *(43)*, paraoxonase (an enzyme that prevents oxidation of low-density lipoprotein [LDL]-cholesterol) gene *(44)*, endothelial nitric oxide synthase gene *(45)*, intercellular adhesion molecule-1 *(46)*, $\alpha_2\beta_1$ integrin gene (involved with platelet function) *(47)*, and cytokine VEGF gene *(48)*. With the advent of new cost-efficient methodologies to determine thousands of genetic polymorphisms, it will now be feasible to examine genetic factors for specific pathways for retinopathy, such as genes associated with aldose reductase activity, collagen formation, inflammatory processes, protein kinase activity, glycosylation, and hypertension.

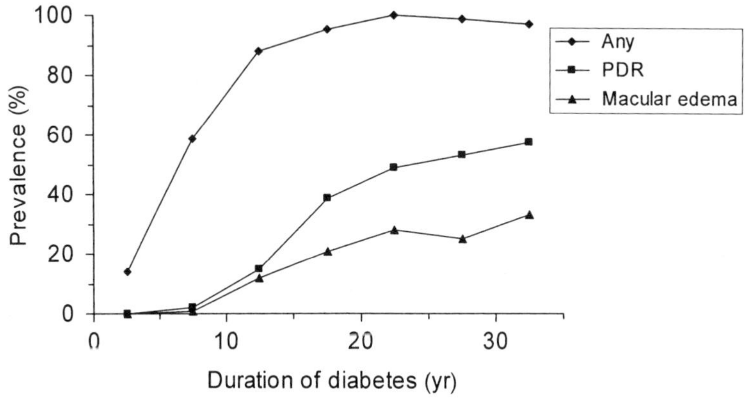

Fig. 3. The prevalence of any retinopathy, proliferative retinopathy, and macular edema in persons with younger onset (<30 yr of age at time of diagnosis of diabetes) type 1 diabetes in the Wisconsin Epidemiologic Study of Diabetic Retinopathy, 1980–1982.

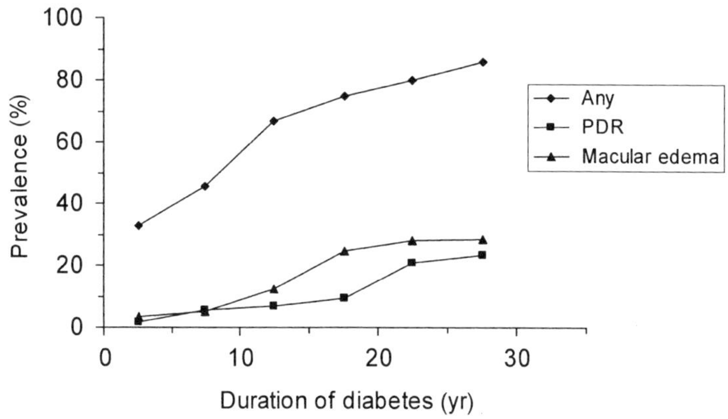

Fig. 4. The prevalence of any retinopathy, proliferative retinopathy, and macular edema in persons with older onset (30 yr of age or older at time of diagnosis of diabetes) in the Wisconsin Epidemiologic Study of Diabetic Retinopathy, 1980–1982.

Diabetes-Related Risk Factors

Duration of Diabetes

The prevalences of retinopathy, macular edema, and PDR increase with longer duration of diabetes (Figs. 3 and 4) *(34–36,49–51)*. In the WESDR, in those with type 1 diabetes, retinopathy was present in only 8%, and PDR and macular edema were not present during the first 3 yr of diabetes, whereas in those with type 2 diabetes, retinopathy occurred in 29%, PDR in 2%, and macular edema in 3% at the time of diagnosis of diabetes. These differences reflect, in part, the longer period between onset and diagnosis of diabetes in persons with type 2 diabetes compared with type 1 diabetes.

Glycemia

Understanding the role of glycemic control in reducing the incidence and progression of diabetic retinopathy is a rather late phenomenon. Although retinopathy was first described in 1860s shortly after the invention of the ophthalmoscope, as of 1978, West

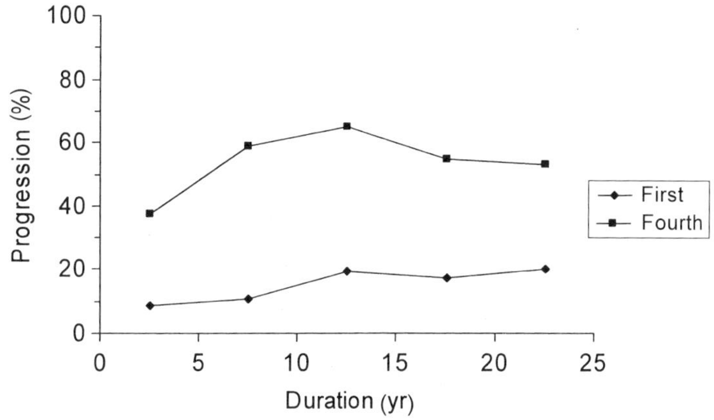

Fig. 5. The 4-yr progression of retinopathy by duration of diabetes by persons with good glycemic control (first quartile of glycosylated hemoglobin, 5.6–9.4%) vs those with poor glycemic control (fourth quartile of glycosylated hemoglobin, 12.1–19.5%) at baseline in persons with younger onset type 1 diabetes in the Wisconsin Epidemiologic Study of Diabetic Retinopathy, 1980–1982 to 1984–1986.

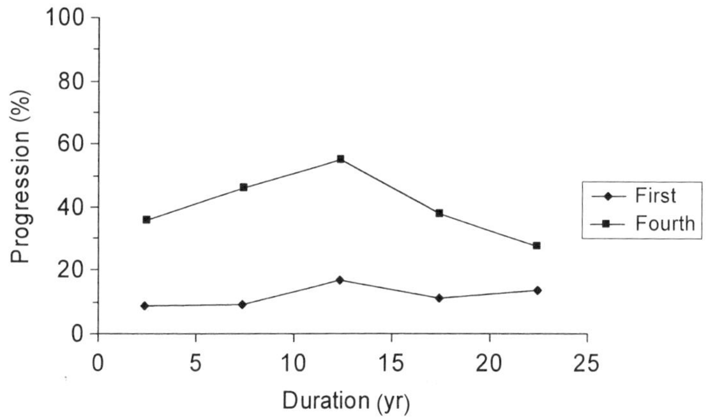

Fig. 6. The 4-yr progression of retinopathy by duration of diabetes by persons with good glycemic control (first quartile of glycosylated hemoglobin, 5.4–8.1%) vs those with poor glycemic control (fourth quartile of glycosylated hemoglobin, 10.9–20.8%) at baseline in persons with older onset type 2 diabetes in the Wisconsin Epidemiologic Study of Diabetic Retinopathy, 1980–1982 to 1984–1986.

wrote: "The extent to which hyperglycemia determines the risk of retinopathy is not at all clear. This is the most important issue at hand and deserves high priority in epidemiologic research" *(49)*. Over the next 25 yr, data from epidemiological studies consistently demonstrated an association between glycemic control and the incidence and progression of diabetic retinopathy *(21,29–32,50–60)*. Data from the WESDR showed that lower glycosylated hemoglobin at any stage of retinopathy before the proliferative phase and at any duration of diabetes was associated with lower 4-yr incidence and progression of retinopathy (Figs. 5–8) *(21,27,60)*. However, randomized clinical trials were necessary because epidemiological studies could not assess whether the underlying severity of the diabetes independently led to both poorer glycemic control and more severe retinopathy.

Data from the DCCT, a large randomized controlled clinical trial of more than 1400 patients with type 1 diabetes showed that those assigned to intensive glycemic control

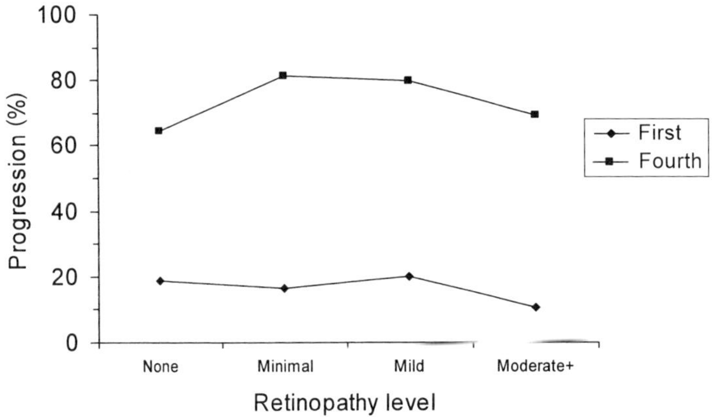

Fig. 7. The 4-yr progression of retinopathy by retinopathy severity at baseline in persons with younger onset type 1 diabetes in the Wisconsin Epidemiologic Study of Diabetic Retinopathy, 1980–1982 to 1984–1986. Minimal denotes eyes with nonproliferative retinopathy consisting of only retinal microaneurysms, mild eyes with nonproliferative retinopathy consisting of retinal microaneurysms and blot hemorrhages or hard exudates, and moderate + eyes with nonproliferative Retinopathy consisting of more severe signs of retinopathy such as intraretinal microvascular abnormities, large amounts of retinal blot hemorrhages, venous beading.

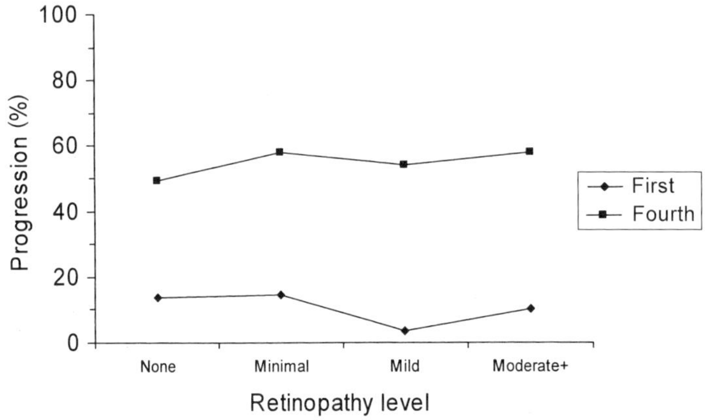

Fig. 8. The 4-yr progression of retinopathy by retinopathy severity at baseline in persons with older onset diabetes in the Wisconsin Epidemiologic Study of Diabetic retinopathy, 1980–1982 to 1984–1986. Minimal denotes eyes with nonproliferative retinopathy consisting of only retinal microaneurysms, mild eyes with nonproliferative retinopathy consisting of retinal microaneurysms and blot hemorrhages or hard exudates, and moderate + eyes with nonproliferative retinopathy consisting of more severe signs of retinopathy such as intraretinal microvascular abnormities, large amounts of retinal blot hemorrhages, venous beading.

had a 34% reduction in the progression of retinopathy, a 46% reduction in the incidence of PDR, a 22% reduction in the incidence of macular edema, and a 54% reduction in laser photocoagulation treatment compared with the group assigned to conventional insulin treatment *(7)*. The DCCT results demonstrated a causal relationship between glycemic control and the incidence and progression of retinopathy as well as other microvascular complications and suggested that lowering blood sugar, even modestly, may significantly reduce the incidence of these complications. Four years of additional follow-up of the DCCT cohort after the study was stopped revealed that despite convergence of glycosylated hemoglobin levels in the intensive and conventional groups, the protective effect of glycemic control was maintained in the intensive group *(61)*.

The UKPDS was a randomized controlled clinical trial involving 3867 newly diagnosed patients with type 2 diabetes *(8,62,63)*. After 12 yr of follow-up, there was a reduction in rate of progression of diabetic retinopathy of 21% and reduction in the need for laser photocoagulation of 29% in the intensive vs the conventional glycemic control treatment group. Based on the results of the DCCT and the UKPDS, the American Diabetes Association developed guidelines that stated a target goal of glycosylated hemoglobin A1c of 7.0% for persons with diabetes *(64)*. However, data from the National Health and Nutrition Examination Study (NHANES) III *(65)* and the WESDR *(66)* suggest that few persons with diabetes reach this targeted level of glycemic control.

Blood Pressure

Elevations in blood pressure have been postulated as having a role in the pathogenesis of diabetic retinopathy *(67)*. High blood pressure, through an effect on blood flow, has been thought to damage the capillary endothelial cells, possibly contributing to the development or progression of retinopathy *(68)*. Data from epidemiological studies on the relationship of blood pressure to the incidence and progression of retinopathy have been conflicting *(69–71)*. However, data from several recent clinical trials have demonstrated the efficacy of intensive treatment of blood pressure in lowering the incidence and progression of retinopathy *(9,10,72,73)*.

The EURODIAB-Controlled trial of Lisinopril in Insulin-Dependent diabetes mellitus (EUCLID) study examined the role of an angiotensin-converting enzyme (ACE) inhibitor, lisinopril, in reducing the incidence and progression of retinopathy in a group of largely normotensive type 1 diabetic patients of whom 85% did not have microalbuminuria at baseline *(72)*. This study showed a statistically significant 50% reduction in the progression of retinopathy in those taking lisinopril over a 2-yr period after adjustment for glycemic control. Progression to PDR was also reduced, although the relation was not statistically significant. There was no significant interaction with blood glucose control.

The UKPDS sought to determine whether lowering blood pressure was beneficial in reducing macrovascular and microvascular complications associated with type 2 diabetes *(9)*. The aim in the group randomized to "tight" control of blood pressure (by the standards at the beginning of the clinical trial) was to achieve blood pressure values <150/<85 mmHg. (This would be considered poor control by today's standards.) If these goals were not met with maximal doses of a β-blocker or ACE inhibitor, additional medications were prescribed, including a loop diuretic, a calcium channel blocker, and a vasodilator. The aim in the group randomized to less tight control was to achieve blood pressure values of <180/<105 mmHg. Tight blood pressure control resulted in a 35% reduction in retinal photocoagulation compared with conventional control owing to a lower incidence of macular edema *(73)*. After 7.5 yr of follow-up, there was a 34% reduction in the rate of progression of retinopathy and a 47% reduction in the deterioration of visual acuity by three lines or more using the Early Treatment Diabetic Retinopathy Study (ETDRS) charts (e.g., a reduction in vision from 20/30 to 20/60 or worse on a Snellen chart). Atenolol and captopril were equally effective in reducing the risk of developing these microvascular complications suggesting that blood pressure reduction was more important than the type of medication used to reduce it. The effects of blood pressure control were independent of those of glycemic control. These findings support the recommendations for blood pressure control in patients with type 2 diabetes as a means of preventing visual loss from diabetic retinopathy.

Data from another randomized controlled clinical trial, the Appropriate Blood Pressure Control in Diabetes (ABCD) trial did not demonstrate a significant reduction in the 5-yr incidence or progression of retinopathy in type 2 diabetes subjects treated with intensive antihypertensive treatment (the mean blood pressure achieved was 132/78 mmHg) compared with those in the moderate control group (mean blood pressure of 138/86 mmHg) *(74)*. The authors concluded that the lack of efficacy in their study compared with the UKPDS might have resulted from the shorter time period of the ABCD trial (5 vs 9 yr on average for the UKPDS), lower average blood pressure control in the ABCD trial (144/82 vs 154/87 mmHg in the UKPDS), and poorer glycemic control in the ABCD trial than in the UKPDS *(8,9)*.

However, results from a second ABCD clinical trial showed a benefit of intensive blood pressure control in normotensive (blood pressure <140/90 mmHg) type 2 diabetic patients at baseline *(10)*. Over the 5-yr period, the intensive blood pressure control group showed less progression of diabetic retinopathy (34% vs 46%, $p = 0.019$) than the moderate therapy group with no difference whether enalapril or nisoldipine was used as the initial antihypertensive agent. The authors concluded that "over a 5-yr follow-up period, intensive (approx 128/75 mmHg) control of blood pressure in normotensive type 2 diabetic patients decreased the progression of diabetic retinopathy." They concluded that the specific initial agent used (calcium channel blocker vs ACE inhibitor) appears to be less important than the achievement of the lower blood pressure values in normotensive type 2 diabetic patients.

Serum Lipids and Lipid Lowering

Epidemiological data have suggested a possible role of lipids in the development of diabetic macular edema with hard exudates. In the WESDR, higher total serum cholesterol was associated with higher prevalence of retinal hard exudates *(75)*. In the ETDRS, higher levels of serum lipids (triglycerides, LDLs, and very LDLs) at baseline were associated with an increased risk of developing hard exudates in the macula and decreased visual acuity *(76)*. In the DCCT, while controlling for treatment assignment, glycosylated hemoglobin, and other risk factors, high total- to high-density lipoprotein-cholesterol ratio and LDL predicted the development of clinically significant macular edema and hard exudates *(77)*.

In a study of Mexican patients with type 2 diabetes, Santos et al. *(43)* showed the frequency of severe retinal hard exudates was higher in those with ε4 allele polymorphism of the apolipoprotein E gene. To date, there have been no definitive clinical trial data showing the efficacy of control of lipids in preventing the incidence and progression of retinopathy.

Inflammation and Endothelial dysfunction

Inflammatory processes have been hypothesized to be involved in the pathogenesis of diabetic retinopathy and nephropathy *(78)*. Elevations in the level of markers of inflammation, such as serum fibrinogen, tumor necrosis factor-α, and C-reactive protein found in persons with diabetes have been attributed to hyperglycemia, elevations in advanced glycation endproducts, and increased body mass index *(79,80)*. However, there are few data regarding the role of inflammation in the progression of diabetic retinopathy in persons with diabetes *(81–85)*. In two case–control studies, diabetic subjects with macular edema *(84)* or PDR *(83)* had higher levels of VEGFs and cytokines in their vitreous than those without macular edema or PDR. In a cross-sectional study of normotensive persons with type 1 diabetes, serum C-reactive protein and fibrinogen levels were positively associated with diabetic retinopathy severity *(81)*.

Endothelial dysfunction may result in increased vascular permeability, alteration of blood flow, oxidative stress, and angiogenesis, and has been postulated to play a role in the pathogenesis of diabetic retinopathy *(45,86–92)*. There have been inconsistencies in the findings among studies that have examined the relationship of markers of endothelial injury and dysfunction with the prevalence, severity, and incidence of diabetic retinopathy *(45–53,81)*. Homocysteine and von Willebrand factor, two markers of endothelial dysfunction, have been inconsistently found to be associated with an increased incidence of retinopathy and nephropathy in clinical and population-based studies *(93–101)*. Fewer data are available about potentially protective factors such as serum folate and vitamins B_{12} and B_6 levels for progression of retinopathy and the incidence of proliferative retinopathy in persons with diabetes *(95–98)*.

Smoking

Most epidemiological data show no relationship between cigaret smoking and the incidence or progression of diabetic retinopathy *(32,52,56,58,102–105)*. This is despite the fact that smoking is known to cause tissue hypoxia by inducing vasoconstriction of the small blood vessels, increasing blood carbon monoxide levels *(106)* and increasing platelet aggregation and adhesiveness *(107)*, all factors hypothesized to be involved in the pathogenesis of diabetic retinopathy.

Anemia

Anemia, through hypoxia, has been hypothesized to be a risk factor for diabetic retinopathy *(108)*. Anemia, defined by a hemoglobin of less than 12 g/dL, has been found to be associated with the presence of retinopathy; more severe anemia was associated with more severe retinopathy *(109)*. In the ETDRS, there was a 50% increase in the odds of developing PDR in anemic compared with nonanemic persons *(110)*. There are reports of stabilization or regression of retinopathy after treatment of anemia in diabetic persons with nephropathy *(111)*.

Summary

Data from the WESDR and other population-based studies have shown associations of glycosylated hemoglobin, blood pressure, and serum total cholesterol with the incidence and progression of retinopathy and other micro- and macrovascular complications *(21,27,33,34,60,69,75)*. However, these factors only explain a small proportion of the incidence of PDR. Moreover, although glycemic control is associated with less severe retinopathy, there are people with diabetes who appear to be relatively protected despite poor control. This was corroborated in the experience of the DCCT *(7)*. Because hyperglycemia is difficult to control, there has been a search for other nontraditional risk factors (e.g., markers of inflammation and endothelial dysfunction) that could be treated and would prevent or delay the progression of diabetic retinopathy.

Table 2
Prevalence of Retinopathy and CSME by Microalbuminuria in the Wisconsin Epidemiologic Study of Diabetic Retinopathy, 1984–1986

Microalbuminuria status	*No.*	*None (%)*	*Early NPDR (%)*	*Mod-Sev NPDR (%)*	*PDR (%)*	*No.*	*CSME (%)*
Younger onset							
Absent	421	20.0	54.6	13.1	12.4	414	2.7
Present	167	7.8	40.1	24.0	28.1	164	6.1
				$p < 0.0001$		$p = 0.05$	
Older onset							
Absent	459	42.0	42.7	8.1	7.2	441	3.0
Present	204	25.0	50.5	12.8	11.8	195	5.1
				$p < 0.0001$		$p = 0.17$	

NPDR, nonproliferative diabetic retinopathy; PDR, proliferative diabetic retinopathy; CSME, clinically significant macular edema.

RELATIONSHIP OF DIABETIC NEPHROPATHY TO RETINOPATHY

Microalbuminuria and Diabetic Retinopathy

Diabetic nephropathy may lead to lipid, platelet, and rheological abnormalities, all of which have been hypothesized to be pathogenetic factors for the development of diabetic retinopathy *(112,113)*. Therefore, it is not surprising that, independent of blood pressure level, many studies have found an association between microalbuminuria and gross proteinuria and the presence and severity of diabetic retinopathy *(32,53,56,114–116)*. In the WESDR, both younger and older onset diabetic persons with microalbuminuria were more likely to have signs of PDR. Microalbuminuria was associated with clinically significant macular edema in the younger but not the older onset group (Table 2). While controlling for duration of diabetes, glycosylated hemoglobin, and diastolic blood pressure, persons with microalbuminuria were more likely to have retinopathy present (OR 1.9, 95% CI 0.95, 3.78 for younger onset and OR 1.80, 95% CI 1.22, 2.65 for older onset persons). In multivariable analyses, microalbuminuria remained statistically significantly associated with PDR in the younger (OR 2.14, 95% CI 1.27, 3.61) but not the older onset group (OR 1.05, 95% CI 0.56, 1.96). While controlling for other risk factors, the relationship of microalbuminuria to clinically significant macular edema was not statistically significant in either the younger (OR 2.05, 95% CI 0.81, 5.17, $p = 0.13$) or the older onset group (OR 1.26, 95% CI 0.52, 3.06, $p = 0.62$).

Early nephropathy has also been related to incident retinopathy in some studies. In Danish patients with type 1 diabetes, the annual incidence of PDR in persons with early nephropathy was 10–15% compared with only 1% in patients without signs of nephropathy *(117)*. In another clinical study of 82 patients with type 1 diabetes, of the 13 who developed a progressive increase in their albumin excretion rate and persistent microalbuminuria during the study period, 62% (8/13) developed macular edema or proliferative retinopathy compared with 7% (5/69) who remained normoalbuminuric *(118)*. In the population-based Epidemiology of Diabetes Complication (EDC) study, higher albumin excretion rate in persons with type 1 diabetes was related to the incidence of PDR but not incident NPDR or progression of retinopathy *(119,120)*. In a clinical study in persons with type 2 diabetes, microalbuminuria at baseline was associated with incidence of NPDR (OR 3.9, 95% CI 1.3–12.0) *(121)*. In the WESDR, persons with microalbuminuria had a higher 6-yr incidence of PDR but not clinically significant macular edema (Table 3). However, controlling for other factors at baseline, microalbuminuria status was not associated with the incidence of retinopathy, its progression to clinically significant macular edema, or the incidence of PDR. These data suggest that other factors, such as glycemic and blood pressure control, are the likely determinants of both outcomes. Alternatively, the lack of a finding of microalbuminuria as an independent risk factor for incident retinopathy in the WESDR may be owing to selective survival, i.e., persons with microalbuminuria who develop severe diabetic retinopathy are more likely to die and not be examined at follow-up compared with those with microalbuminuria who did not develop severe retinopathy. In addition, microalbuminuria in the absence of retinopathy in persons with type 2 diabetes may be owing to nondiabetic causes.

Gross Proteinuria and Diabetic Retinopathy

In the WESDR, persons with diabetes with trace or gross proteinuria were more likely to have signs of any retinopathy, PDR, or clinically significant macular edema at baseline than those without gross proteinuria (Table 4). While controlling for other factors, the odds of having PDR present when gross proteinuria was present varied from 4.58 (95% CI 3.77, 10.15) in those with younger onset type 1 diabetes to 2.71 (95% CI 1.64, 4.49) in those with older onset type 2 diabetes compared with those without gross proteinuria; for clinically significant macular edema the odds were 2.42 (95% CI 1.20, 4.88) and 1.47 (95% CI 0.83, 1.47) in type 1 and 2 diabetes, respectively. These findings are also consistent with other epidemiological and clinical studies. In Hispanics, gross proteinuria was cross-sectionally related to diabetic retinopathy (OR 11.14, 95% CI 1.2, 103) but not in non-Hispanic whites *(122)*. In a cross-sectional analysis of 982 Danish patients with type 1 diabetes, the prevalence of PDR and vision loss increased with increasing levels of albuminuria, being 12 and 1.4%, respectively, in persons with normoalbuminuria, 28 and 5.6% in those with microalbuminuria, and 58 and 10.6% in those with gross proteinuria *(123)*.

The cumulative 5-yr incidence of NPDR and PDR in Danish type 1 diabetic patients with gross proteinuria was 93 and 74%, respectively, and it was 37 and 14%, respectively in those without *(124)*. In the WESDR, the presence of gross proteinuria was associated with the 10-yr incidence of PDR in type 1 diabetes; otherwise, gross proteinuria was not associated with the progression of retinopathy or incidence of clinically significant macular edema (Table 5). The lack of an association in the WESDR may have been due, in part, to the high risk of persons with gross proteinuria who develop severe retinopathy dying and not being seen at follow-up.

Renal Failure and Macular Edema

There are anecdotal reports that treatment of renal failure will reduce macular edema in patients who have both *(125)*. However, hemodialysis failed to reduce fluorescein leakage in the eyes of type 2 diabetic patients with renal failure and macular edema *(126)*. There are no epidemiological studies or clinical trials that have demonstrated that reduction of microalbuminuria and prevention of overt diabetic nephropathy manifest by clinical proteinuria will result in reduction of risk of retinopathy. This may be a moot point because most treatments aimed at poor

Table 3
6-Year Incidence of any Retinopathy, Progression of Retinopathy, Incidence of PDR, and Incidence of CSME by Microalbuminuria Status in the Wisconsin Epidemiologic Study of Diabetic Retinopathy, 1984–1986 to 1990–1992

Microalbuminuria status	*No. at risk*	*Incidence of any retinopathy*	*No. at risk*	*Progression of retinopathy*	*No. at risk*	*Incidence of PDR*	*No. at risk*	*Incidence of CSME*
Younger onset								
Absent	68	72.1	344	55.5	344	17.2	329	9.4
Present	12	83.3	109	63.3	109	28.4	113	11.5
p-Values		0.41		0.15		0.01		0.52
Older onset								
Absent	116	50.0	288	47.2	288	9.4	258	9.3
Present	18	61.1	89	46.1	89	16.8	69	13.0
p-Values		0.38		0.85		0.05		0.36

CSME, clinically significant macular edema.

Table 4
Prevalence and Severity of Retinopathy and CSME by Dipstick Gross Proteinuria or Dialysis/Renal Transplant Status in the Wisconsin Epidemiologic Study of Diabetic Retinopathy, 1980–1982

Urine protein status	*No. at Risk*	*None (%)*	*Early NPDR (%)*	*Mod-sev NPDR (%)*	*PDR %*	*No. at risk*	*CSME %*
Younger onset							
None	652	35.9	43.7	10.3	10.1	639	3.8
Trace	93	20.4	49.5	14.0	16.1	91	2.2
Gross	183	8.7	24.6	10.9	55.7	168	14.3
Dialysis or renal transplant	27	0	0	0	100.0	18	11.1
p-Values				<0.0001		<0.0001	
Older onset							
None	953	47.6	37.2	8.9	6.3	919	6.1
Trace	145	40.0	42.1	9.0	9.0	136	8.1
Gross	192	25.0	37.0	19.3	18.8	178	14.0
Dialysis or renal transplant	3	0	33.3	33.3	33.3	2	50.0
p-Values				< 0.0001		<0.0001	

CSME, clinically significant macular edema

glycemic and blood pressure control have been shown to be beneficial to both conditions.

Common Risk Factors for Retinopathy and Nephropathy

In the preceding discussion, a number of risk factors and their associations with retinopathy were reviewed. Three of them— hyperglycemia, hypertension, and dyslipidemia— have been also shown to be related to the incidence of diabetic nephropathy. Other risk factors, such as high levels of markers of inflammation *(127)*, endothelial dysfunction, oxidative stress, and hypercoagulability have also been shown in some studies to be related to both retinopathy and nephropathy *(128)*. However, these factors explain only a small amount of the variance for each of these complications, and they do not explain why despite high levels of some risk factors some persons do not develop retinopathy, others do not develop nephropathy, and some do not get either complication. For this, genetic susceptibility has been postulated. However, few studies have examined the associations of familial and genetic factors in the codevelopment of both complications.

In one of these studies, diabetic retinopathy and nephropathy clustering in families of 372 subjects with type 1 diabetes participating in the DCCT were examined *(38)*. Statistically significant correlations were found for severity of retinopathy for all family members, parent–offspring, father–child, and mother–child but not sibling–sibling relationships, whereas none of the correlations for these relationships for nephropathy were statistically significant.

A few studies have examined the aldose reductase gene and diabetic microvascular complications *(129,130)*. In one such study, the associations of aldose reductase gene polymorphisms with diabetic nephropathy and retinopathy were investigated in Chinese

Table 5
10-Year Incidence of any Retinopathy, Progression of Retinopathy, Incidence of Proliferative Retinopathy, and Incidence of CSME by Dipstick Gross Proteinuria or Dialysis/Renal Transplant Status in the Wisconsin Epidemiologic Study of Diabetic Retinopathy 1980–1982 to 1990–1992

Urine/Protein status	*No. at risk*	*Incidence of any retinopathy*	*No. at risk*	*Progression of retinopathy*	*No. at risk*	*Incidence of PDR*	*No. at risk*	*Incidence of CSME*
Younger onset								
None	218	90.8	549	76.6	549	27.4	521	13.3
Trace	17	94.1	68	69.9	68	27.4	62	13.5
Gross	15	83.3	75	78.3	75	49.7	80	15.4
Dialysis or renal transplant	–	–	–	–	–	–	3	100.0
p-Values	0.92		0.80		0.0003		0.41	
Older onset								
None	360	69.6	689	58.6	689	15.4	595	12.2
Trace	44	76.7	93	70.0	93	19.1	81	15.6
Gross	28	75.9	89	60.2	89	14.2	75	12.7
Dialysis or renal transplant	–	–	1	100.0	1	100.0	–	–
p-Values	0.98		0.41		0.18		0.32	

CSME, clinically significant macular edema.

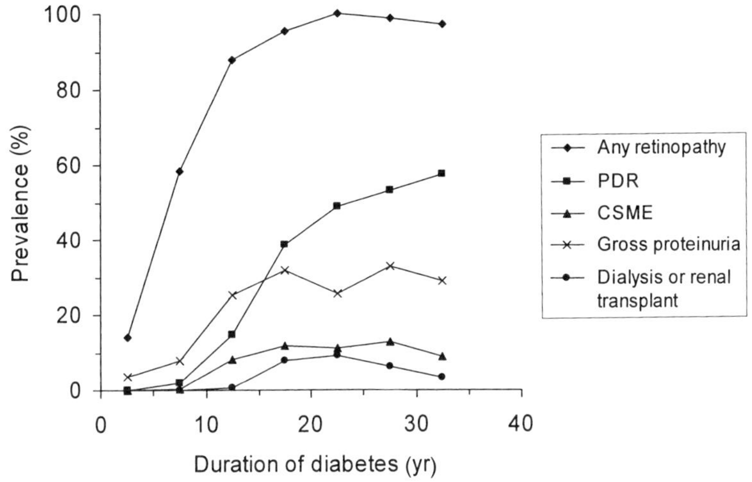

Fig. 9. The prevalence of retinopathy and nephropathy severity by duration of diabetes in younger onset type 1 diabetes group in the Wisconsin Epidemiologic Study of Diabetic Retinopathy, 1980–1982. CSME, clinically significant macular edema.

persons with type 2 diabetes; 291 free of diabetes complications, 159 with diabetic nephropathy only, 66 with diabetic retinopathy only, and 121 with both complications *(129)*. Associations of two aldose reductase gene (ALR2) polymorphisms (z-2 of a [CA] (*n*) microsatellite and T allele of C/T polymorphism at the 5′ region) with diabetic nephropathy and retinopathy were found. Data from another study suggested a genetic heterogeneity in diabetic microvascular complications *(44)*. In 372 adolescents with type 1 diabetes, polymorphisms of paraoxonase, a serum enzyme that prevents oxidation of LDL by lipid peroxide hydrolysis, were shown to be associated with retinopathy (PON1-leu/leu) and microalbuminuria (PON2-ser/ser).

RELATIONSHIP OF DIABETIC RETINOPATHY AS A MARKER OF DIABETIC NEPHROPATHY

Retinopathy is usually detected by direct observation using ophthalmoscopy. Grading of fundus photography offers an objective semiquantitative method of describing the presence and severity of various anatomic measures of retinopathy severity manifest by presence of retinal microaneurysms, hard and soft exudates, intraretinal microvascular abnormalities, venous beading, and thickening of the retina. The presence and severity of diabetic nephropathy is usually clinically characterized by functional changes such as increased albumin excretion and decreased creatinine clearance. Renal anatomical changes, sometimes advanced, can occur in the absence of renal functional abnormalities in persons with diabetes. This may account, in part, for the fact that signs of retinopathy are usually more frequently found than are signs of diabetic nephropathy and renal failure (Figs. 9 and 10). In one study in persons with type 1 diabetes, approx 35% of those with PDR had no detectable signs of nephropathy *(131)*. About one-third of patients with type 1 diabetes and PDR have been reported to have no signs of clinical nephropathy *(132)*.

Most attempts to examine correlations between retinal and renal changes have been done in patients with severe manifestations of these complications *(133–137)*. In one such study, 86 persons with type 1 diabetes were being evaluated for pancreatic transplant

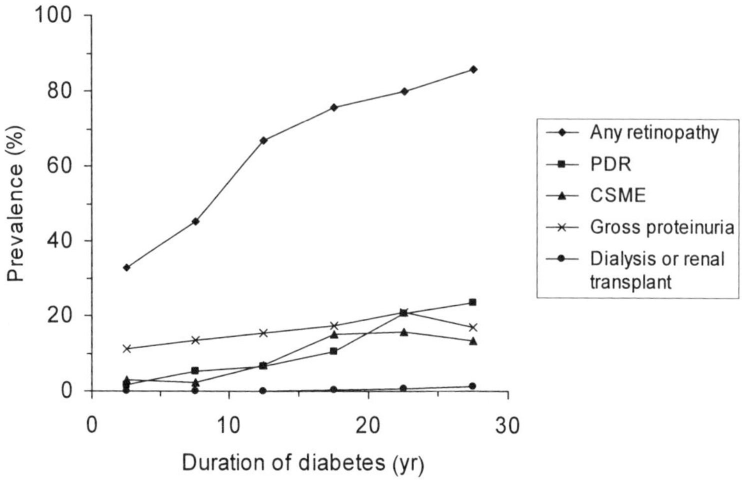

Fig. 10. The prevalence of retinopathy and nephropathy severity by duration of diabetes in older onset group in the Wisconsin Epidemiologic Study of Diabetic Retinopathy, 1980–1982. CSME, clinically significant macular edema.

alone. All subjects had retinopathy of whom 70% had PDR and 73% had clinical nephropathy defined as persistent microalbuminuria or overt proteinuria but without advanced renal insufficiency (GFR ≥ 102 ± 30 mL/min/1.73 m^2) *(134)*. More severe retinopathy was associated with advanced nephropathy as defined by increased mesangial fractional volume and decreased peripheral glomerular basement membrane surface density on biopsy. However, in the few subjects without clinical nephropathy or with minimal microalbuminuria, there was marked discordance between measures of retinopathy and anatomical measures of nephropathy.

There are few epidemiological data regarding the correlation of anatomic measures of diabetic retinopathy and nephropathy, especially early in the disease processes. The association of severity of diabetic retinopathy with histological measures of diabetic nephropathy was examined in 285 normoalbuminuric patients with type 1 diabetes mellitus in the Renin–Angiotensin System Study (RASS), a multicenter diabetic nephropathy primary prevention trial *(138)*. Participants were 16 yr of age or older and had 2–20 yr of type 1 diabetes with normal baseline renal function measures. Diabetic retinopathy was determined by masked grading of 30° color stereoscopic fundus photographs of seven standard fields using the ETDRS severity scale. Baseline renal structural parameters (e.g., mesangial fractional volume [Vv(Mes/glom)] and glomerular basement membrane [GBM] width) were assessed by masked electron microscopic morphometric analyses of research percutaneous renal biopsies. No retinopathy was present in 36%, mild NPDR in 53%, moderate to severe NPDR in 9%, and PDR in 2% of the cohort. Retinopathy was not related to albumin excretion rate, blood pressure, serum creatinine, or glomerular filtration rate. All renal anatomical endpoints were associated with increasing severity of diabetic retinopathy while controlling for other risk factors (Tables 6 and 7). The strong associations between retinopathy findings and renal biopsy measures could be useful in assessing renal risk in patients with type 1 diabetes. Patients who are normoalbuminuric despite long-standing type 1 diabetes are still at risk of progression to microalbuminuria. However, the results of this

Table 6
Renal Structural Characteristic by Diabetic Retinopathy Severity

Renal characteristic	*Diabetic retinopathy severity* No DR	Early NPDR	Moderate to severe NPDR and PDR	*p*
n	89	136	27	
Structure				
GBM width (nm)	430 ± 80	496 ± 83	527 ± 116	<0.0001
Mesangial fractional volume/ glomerulus	0.20 ± 0.04	0.21 ± 0.04	0.25 ± 0.05	<0.0001
Mesangial matrix fraction volume/glomerulus	0.11 ± 0.03	0.12 ± 0.03	0.14 ± 0.03	<0.0001
Vv(MC/glom)	0.07 ± 0.02	0.07 ± 0.02	0.09 ± 0.02	0.002
Peripheral GBM surface density/glomerulus	0.134 ± 0.021	0.127 ± 0.020	0.118 ± 0.021	0.001
Glomerulopathy index	53.6 ± 9.1	61.5 ± 9.7	66.8 ± 11.6	<0.0001

Data are means ± SD. DR, diabetic retinopathy; GBM, glomerular basement membrane.

Table 7
Multivariate Association of Diabetic Retinopathy With Renal Anatomic Characteristics Controlling for Age, Duration of Diabetes, Sex, HbA1c, Mean Arterial Blood Pressure, and BMI

Renal Characteristic	*Diabetic retinopathy severity* Early NPDR	Moderate to Severe NPDR and PDR	*P*
n	136	27	
GBM width (nm)	48.0	64.8	<0.0002
Mesangial fractional volume	0.0048	0.0257	0.03
Mesangial matrix fraction volume	0.0067	0.0170	0.04
Mesangial cell fraction volume	–0.0029	0.0063	0.06
Peripheral GBM surface density	–0.0043	–0.0095	0.15
Glomerulopathy index	5.5	8.2	0.0001

Values represent the change in renal characteristic at the diabetic retinopathy severity level compared with no retinopathy ($n = 89$). GBM, glomerular basement membrane.

cross-sectional study suggest that retinopathy findings may possibly serve a predictive role for progression from normoalbuminuria to microalbuminuria; however, a firm conclusion must await longitudinal study of the RASS cohort. This will be possible because all patients will undergo an end of study renal biopsy as well as retinal fundus photography.

The relation between retinopathy as a marker for nephropathy in those with type 2 diabetes may be more difficult because of the finding of lesions other than diabetic glomerulopathy in such patients. In one study by Richards et al. *(139)* although 19 of 22 type 1 diabetic patients had signs of diabetic glomerulopathy on biopsy, 22 of 46 type 2 diabetic patients were found to have an alternative diagnosis. There are no comparable studies to the RASS examining the relationship of retinopathy to glomerular anatomic changes for patients with type 2 diabetes without overt diabetic nephropathy or hypertension.

CONCLUSIONS

Results of the DCCT and UKPDS suggest that if intensive glycemic control can be achieved, there will be a reduction in the progression of both diabetic retinopathy and nephropathy. Epidemiological data and some clinical trial data suggest that blood pressure control might also be an effective approach to reducing both complications. There are some recent findings suggesting that inflammation, oxidative stress and coagulability may also have an affect on both complications. Both retinopathy and nephropathy are linked together as "microvascular" in origin and share similar risk factors. However, after long duration of disease, most individuals will develop retinopathy but about two-thirds will develop clinical signs of nephropathy. This suggests possible genetic differences making susceptibility to damage of each system different for a given level of exposure of blood pressure, glycemia, and other risk factors. Identification of genetic polymorphisms associated with risk for one or both complications may lead to newer preventive treatments in diabetic persons at risk of developing the earlier preclinical stages of the disease.

ACKNOWLEDGMENT

This chapter was supported by grants R010EY3083 and R01EY016379 from the National Eye Institute.

REFERENCES

1. Friedman EA, L'Esperance FA, Jr. Diabetic renal-retinal syndrome. Grune & Stratton, New York, 1980.
2. Friedman EA, L'Esperance FA, Jr. Diabetic renal-retinal syndrome. Prevention and management. Grune & Stratton, New York, 1982.
3. Friedman EA, L'Esperance FA, Jr. Diabetic renal-retinal syndrome. Therapy. Grune & Stratton, New York, 1986.
4. Friedman EA, L'Esperance FA, Jr. Diabetic renal-retinal syndrome. Pathogenesis and management update 2002. Kluwer Academic Publishers, Boston, 2002.
5. The Diabetic Retinopathy Study Research Group. Photocoagulation treatment of proliferative diabetic retinopathy. Clinical application of Diabetic Retinopathy Study (DRS) findings, DRS Report Number 8. Ophthalmology 1981;88:583–600.
6. Early Treatment Diabetic Retinopathy Study Research Group. Photocoagulation for diabetic macular edema. Early Treatment Diabetic Retinopathy Study report number 1. Arch Ophthalmol 1985;103:1796–806.
7. The Diabetes Control and Complications Trial Research Group. The effect of intensive treatment of diabetes on the development and progression of long-term complications in insulin-dependent diabetes mellitus. N Engl J Med 1993;329:977–986.
8. UK Prospective Diabetes Study (UKPDS) Group. Intensive blood-glucose control with sulphonylureas or insulin compared with conventional treatment and risk of complications in patients with type 2 diabetes (UKPDS 33). Lancet 1998;352:837–853.
9. UK Prospective Diabetes Study Group. Tight blood pressure control and risk of macrovascular and microvascular complications in type 2 diabetes: UKPDS 38. Brit Med J 1998;317:703–713.
10. Schrier RW, Estacio RO, Esler A, Mehler P. Effects of aggressive blood pressure control in normotensive type 2 diabetic patients on albuminuria, retinopathy and strokes. Kidney Int 2002;61:1086–1097.

11. Kempen JH, O'Colmain BJ, Leske MC, et al. The prevalence of diabetic retinopathy among adults in the United States. Arch Ophthalmol 2004;122:552–563.
12. Klein BE, Klein R, Moss SE. Self-rated health and diabetes of long duration: The Wisconsin Epidemiologic Study of Diabetic Retinopathy. Diabetes Care 1998;21:236–240.
13. Klein R, Moss SE, Klein BE, Gutierrez P, Mangione CM. The NEI-VFQ-25 in people with long-term type 1 diabetes mellitus: The Wisconsin Epidemiologic Study of Diabetic Retinopathy. Arch Ophthalmol 2001;119:733–740.
14. Harris MI, Cowie CC, Stern MP, Boyko EJ, Reiber GE, Bennett PH. Diabetes in America. Springfield, VA: NTIS Accession No. PB-95-1468;1985.
15. Klein R, Klein BE. Epidemiology of eye disease in diabetes. In: Flynn HWJr, Smiddy WE, eds. Ophthalmology monographs 14. Diabetes and ocular disease: past, present, and future therapies. IV Series. American Academy of Ophthalmology, San Francisco, 2000; pp. 19–67.
16. Bresnick GH. Diabetic retinopathy. In: Peyman GA, Sanders DR, Goldberg MF, eds. Principles and practice of ophthalmology. Saunders, Philadelphia, 1977.
17. Klein R, Klein BE, Moss SE, Davis MD, DeMets DL. The Wisconsin Epidemiologic Study of Diabetic Retinopathy. II. Prevalence and risk of diabetic retinopathy when age at diagnosis is less than 30. Arch Ophthalmol 1984;102:520–526.
18. Klein R, Klein BE, Moss SE, Davis MD, DeMets DL. The Wisconsin Epidemiologic Study of Diabetic Retinopathy. III. Prevalence and risk of diabetic retinopathy when age at diagnosis is 30 or more years. Arch Ophthalmol 1984;102:527–532.
19. Bresnick GH. Diabetic maculopathy. A critical review highlighting diffuse macular edema. Ophthalmology 1983;90:1301–1317.
20. Engerman RL, Kern TS. Progression of incipient diabetic retinopathy during good glycemic control. Diabetes 1987;36:808–812.
21. Klein R, Klein BE, Moss SE, Davis MD, DeMets DL. Glycosylated hemoglobin predicts the incidence and progression of diabetic retinopathy. JAMA 1988;260:2864–2871.
22. Nishikawa T, Edelstein D, Brownlee M. The missing link: a single unifying mechanism for diabetic complications. Kidney Int Suppl 2000;77:S26–S30.
23. Klein R, Klein BE, Moss SE, DeMets DL, Kaufman I, Voss PS. Prevalence of diabetes mellitus in Southern Wisconsin. Am J Epidemiol 1984;119:54–61.
24. Klein R, Klein BE, Moss SE, Davis MD, DeMets DL. The Wisconsin Epidemiologic Study of Diabetic Retinopathy. IX. Four-year incidence and progression of diabetic retinopathy when age at diagnosis is less than 30 years. Arch Ophthalmol 1989;107:237–243.
25. Klein R, Klein BE, Moss SE, Davis MD, DeMets DL. The Wisconsin Epidemiologic Study of Diabetic Retinopathy. X. Four-year incidence and progression of diabetic retinopathy when age at diagnosis is 30 years or more. Arch Ophthalmol 1989;107:244–249.
26. Klein R, Klein BE, Moss SE, Cruickshanks KJ. The Wisconsin Epidemiologic Study of Diabetic Retinopathy. XIV. Ten-year incidence and progression of diabetic retinopathy. Arch Ophthalmol 1994;112:1217–1228.
27. Klein R, Klein BE, Moss SE, Cruickshanks KJ. The Wisconsin Epidemiologic Study of Diabetic Retinopathy. XVII. The 14-year incidence and progression of diabetic retinopathy and associated risk factors in type 1 diabetes. Ophthalmology 1998;105:1801–1815.
28. Hovind P, Tarnow L, Rossing K, et al. Decreasing incidence of severe diabetic microangiopathy in type 1 diabetes. Diabetes Care 2003;26:1258–1264.
29. Haffner SM, Fong D, Stern MP, et al. Diabetic retinopathy in Mexican Americans and non-Hispanic whites. Diabetes 1988;37:878–884.
30. Hamman RF, Mayer EJ, Moo-Young GA, Hildebrandt W, Marshall JA, Baxter J. Prevalence and risk factors of diabetic retinopathy in non-Hispanic whites and Hispanics with NIDDM. San Luis Valley Diabetes Study. Diabetes 1989;38:1231–1237.
31. Rabb MF, Gagliano DA, Sweeney HE. Diabetic retinopathy in blacks. Diabetes Care 1990;13:1202–1206.
32. West KM, Erdreich LJ, Stober JA. A detailed study of risk factors for retinopathy and nephropathy in diabetes. Diabetes 1980;29:501–508.
33. Harris MI, Klein R, Cowie CC, Rowland M, Byrd-Holt DD. Is the risk of diabetic retinopathy greater in non-Hispanic blacks and Mexican Americans than in non-Hispanic whites with type 2 diabetes? A U.S. population study. Diabetes Care 1998;21:1230–1235.
34. West SK, Munoz B, Klein R, et al. Risk factors for Type II diabetes and diabetic retinopathy in a Mexican-American population: Proyecto VER. Am J Ophthalmol 2002;134:390–398.

35. Varma R, Torres M, Pena F, Klein R, Azen SP. Prevalence of diabetic retinopathy in adult Latinos: the Los Angeles Latino Eye Study. Ophthalmology 2004;111:1298–1306.
36. Roy MS, Klein R, O'Colmain BJ, Klein BE, Moss SE, Kempen JH. The prevalence of diabetic retinopathy among adult type 1 diabetic persons in the United States. Arch Ophthalmol 2004;122:546–551.
37. Leslie RD, Pyke DA. Diabetic retinopathy in identical twins. Diabetes 1982;31:19–21.
38. The Diabetes Control and Complications Trial Research Group. Clustering of long-term complications in families with diabetes in the Diabetes Control and Complications Trial. Diabetes 1997;46: 1829–1839.
39. Fukuda M, Nakano S, Imaizumi N, et al. Mitochondrial DNA mutations are associated with both decreased insulin secretion and advanced microvascular complications in Japanese diabetic subjects. J Diabetes Complications 1999;13:277–283.
40. Demaine A, Cross D, Millward A. Polymorphisms of the aldose reductase gene and susceptibility to retinopathy in type 1 diabetes mellitus. Invest Ophthalmol Vis Sci 2000;41:4064–4068.
41. Yamamoto T, Sato T, Hosoi M, et al. Aldose reductase gene polymorphism is associated with progression of diabetic nephropathy in Japanese patients with type 1 diabetes mellitus. Diabetes Obes Metab 2003;5:51–57.
42. Kankova K, Muzik J, Karaskova J, et al. Duration of non-insulin-dependent diabetes mellitus and the TNF-beta NcoI genotype as predictive factors in proliferative diabetic retinopathy. Ophthalmological 2001;215:294–298.
43. Santos A, Salguero ML, Gurrola C, Munoz F, Roig-Melo E, Panduro A. The epsilon4 allele of apolipoprotein E gene is a potential risk factor for the severity of macular edema in type 2 diabetic Mexican patients. Ophthalmic Genet 2002;23:13–19.
44. Kao Y, Donaghue KC, Chan A, Bennetts BH, Knight J, Silink M. Paraoxonase gene cluster is a genetic marker for early microvascular complications in type 1 diabetes. Diabet Med 2002;19:212–215.
45. Taverna MJ, Sola A, Guyot-Argenton C, et al. eNOS4 polymorphism of the endothelial nitric oxide synthase predicts risk for severe diabetic retinopathy. Diabet Med 2002;19:240–245.
46. Kamiuchi K, Hasegawa G, Obayashi H, et al. Intercellular adhesion molecule-1 (ICAM-1) polymorphism is associated with diabetic retinopathy in type 2 diabetes mellitus. Diabet Med 2002;19: 371–376.
47. Matsubara Y, Murata M, Maruyama T, et al. Association between diabetic retinopathy and genetic variations in alpha2beta1 integrin, a platelet receptor for collagen. Blood 2000;95:1560–1564.
48. Yang B, Cross DF, Ollerenshaw M, Millward BA, Demaine AG. Polymorphisms of the vascular endothelial growth factor and susceptibility to diabetic microvascular complications in patients with type 1 diabetes mellitus. J Diabetes Complications 2003;17:1–6.
49. West KM. Epidemiology of diabetes and its vascular lesions. Elsevier, New York, 1978.
50. Dorf A, Ballintine EJ, Bennett PH, Miller M. Retinopathy in Pima Indians. Relationships to glucose level, duration of diabetes, age at diagnosis of diabetes, and age at examination in a population with a high prevalence of diabetes mellitus. Diabetes 1976;25:554–560.
51. King H, Balkau B, Zimmet P, et al. Diabetic Retinopathy in Nauruans. Am J Epidemiol 1983;117: 659–667.
52. Ballard DJ, Melton LJ3, Dwyer MS, et al. Risk factors for diabetic retinopathy: A Population-based study in Rochester, Minnesota. Diabetes Care 1986;9:334–342.
53. Knuiman MW, Welborn TA, McCann VJ, Stanton KG, Constable IJ. Prevalence of diabetic complications in relation to risk factors. Diabetes 1986;35:1332–1339.
54. Sjolie AK. Ocular complications in insulin treated diabetes mellitus. An epidemiological study. Acta Ophthalmol Suppl 1985;172:1–77.
55. Teuscher A, Schnell H, Wilson PW. Incidence of diabetic retinopathy and relationship to baseline plasma glucose and blood pressure. Diabetes Care 1988;11:246–251.
56. Jerneld B. Prevalence of diabetic retinopathy. A population study from the Swedish island of Gotland. Acta Ophthalmol Suppl 1988;188:3–32.
57. McLeod BK, Thompson JR, Rosenthal AR. The prevalence of retinopathy in the insulin-requiring diabetic patients of an English country town. Eye 1988;2:424–430.
58. Kostraba JN, Klein R, Dorman JS, et al. The Epidemiology of Diabetes Complications Study IV. Correlates of diabetic background and proliferative retinopathy. Am J Epidemiol 1991;133: 381–391.
59. Fujimoto W, Fuduka M. Natural history of diabetic retinopathy and its treatment in Japan. In: Baba S, Goto Y, Fukui I, eds. Diabetes mellitus in Asia. Excerpta Medica, Amsterdam, 1976:225–231.
60. Klein R, Klein BE, Moss SE, Cruickshanks KJ. Relationship of hyperglycemia to the long-term incidence and progression of diabetic retinopathy. Arch Intern Med 1994;154:2169–2178.

61. The Diabetes Control and Complications Trial/Epidemiology of Diabetes Interventions and Complications Research Group. Retinopathy and nephropathy in patients with type 1 diabetes four years after a trial of intensive therapy. N Engl J Med 2000;342:381–389.
62. UK Prospective Diabetes Study (UKPDS) Group. Effect of intensive blood-glucose control with metformin on complications in overweight patients with type 2 diabetes (UKPDS 34). Lancet 1998;352:854–865.
63. United Kingdom Prospective Diabetes Study Group. Gray A, Raikou M, McGuire A, et al. Cost effectiveness of an intensive blood glucose control policy in patients with type 2 diabetes: economic analysis alongside randomised controlled trial (UKPDS 41). BMJ 2000;320:1373–1378.
64. American Diabetes Association. Standards of medical care for patients with diabetes mellitus. Diabetes Care 1994;17:616–623.
65. Harris MI. Health care and health status and outcomes for patients with type 2 diabetes. Diabetes Care 2000;23:754–758.
66. Klein R, Klein BE, Moss SE, Cruickshanks KJ. The medical management of hyperglycemia over a 10-year period in people with diabetes. Diabetes Care 1996;19:744–750.
67. Davis MD. Diabetic retinopathy, diabetes control, and blood pressure. Transplant Proc 1986;18: 1565–158.
68. Kohner EM. Diabetic retinopathy. Br Med Bull 1989;45:148–173.
69. Klein R, Klein BE, Moss SE, Davis MD, DeMets DL. Is blood pressure a predictor of the incidence or progression of diabetic retinopathy? Arch Intern Med 1989;149:2427–2432.
70. Klein BE, Klein R, Moss SE, Palta M. A cohort study of the relationship of diabetic retinopathy to blood pressure. Arch Ophthalmol 1995;113:601–606.
71. Adler AI, Stratton IM, Neil HA, et al. Association of systolic blood pressure with macrovascular and microvascular complications of type 2 diabetes (UKPDS 36): prospective observational study. BMJ 2000;321:412–419.
72. Chaturvedi N, Sjolie AK, Stephenson JM, et al. Effect of lisinopril on progression of retinopathy in normotensive people with type 1 diabetes. The EUCLID Study Group. EURODIAB controlled trial of lisinopril in insulin-dependent diabetes mellitus. Lancet 1998;351:28–31.
73. Matthews DR, Stratton IM, Aldington SJ, Holman RR, Kohner EM. Risks of progression of retinopathy and vision loss related to tight blood pressure control in type 2 diabetes mellitus: UKPDS 69. Arch Ophthalmol 2004;122:1631–1640.
74. Estacio RO, Jeffers BW, Gifford N, Schrier RW. Effect of blood pressure control on diabetic microvascular complications in patients with hypertension and type 2 diabetes. Diabetes Care 2000;23(2):B54–B64.
75. Klein BE, Moss SE, Klein R, Surawicz TS. The Wisconsin Epidemiologic Study of Diabetic Retinopathy. XIII. Relationship of serum cholesterol to retinopathy and hard exudate. Ophthalmology 1991;98:1261–1265.
76. Chew EY, Klein ML, Ferris FL, III, et al. Association of elevated serum lipid levels with retinal hard exudate in diabetic retinopathy. Early Treatment Diabetic Retinopathy Study (ETDRS) report 22. Arch Ophthalmol 1996;114:1079–1084.
77. Miljanovic B, Glynn RJ, Nathan DM, Manson JE, Schaumberg DA. A prospective study of serum lipids and risk of diabetic macular edema in type 1 diabetes. Diabetes 2004;53:2883–2892.
78. Adamis AP. Is diabetic retinopathy an inflammatory disease? Br J Ophthalmol 2002;86:363–365.
79. Lechleitner M, Koch T, Herold M, Dzien A, Hoppichler F. Tumour necrosis factor-alpha plasma level in patients with type 1 diabetes mellitus and its association with glycaemic control and cardiovascular risk factors. J Intern Med 2000;248:67–76.
80. Schmidt AM, Hori O, Chen JX, et al. Advanced glycation endproducts interacting with their endothelial receptor induce expression of vascular cell adhesion molecule-1 (VCAM-1) in cultured human endothelial cells and in mice. A potential mechanism for the accelerated vasculopathy of diabetes. J Clin Invest 1995;96:1395–403.
81. Schram MT, Chaturvedi N, Schalkwijk C, et al. Vascular risk factors and markers of endothelial function as determinants of inflammatory markers in type 1 diabetes: the EURODIAB prospective complications study. Diabetes Care 2003;26:2165–2173.
82. Schalkwijk CG, Chaturvedi N, Twaafhoven H, van Hinsbergh VW, Stehouwer CD. Amadori-albumin correlates with microvascular complications and precedes nephropathy in type 1 diabetic patients. Eur J Clin Invest 2002;32:500–506.
83. Powell ED, Field RA. Diabetic retinopthy and rheumatoid arthritis. Lancet 1964;41:17,18.
84. Yuuki T, Kanda T, Kimura Y, et al. Inflammatory cytokines in vitreous fluid and serum of patients with diabetic vitreoretinopathy. J Diabetes Complications 2001;15:257–259.

85. Funatsu H, Yamashita H, Ikeda T, Mimura T, Shimizu E, Hori S. Relation of diabetic macular edema to cytokines and posterior vitreous detachment. Am J Ophthalmol 2003;135:321–327.
86. Poston L, Taylor PD. Glaxo/MRS Young Investigator Prize. Endothelium-mediated vascular function in insulin-dependent diabetes mellitus. Clin Sci (Lond) 1995;88:245–255.
87. Frank RN. Diabetic retinopathy. N Engl J Med 2004;350:48–58.
88. Shibuki H, Katai N, Yodoi J, Uchida K, Yoshimura N. Lipid peroxidation and peroxynitrite in retinal ischemia-reperfusion injury. Invest Ophthalmol Vis Sci 2000;41:3607–3614.
89. Hartnett ME, Stratton RD, Browne RW, Rosner BA, Lanham RJ, Armstrong D. Serum markers of oxidative stress and severity of diabetic retinopathy. Diabetes Care 2000;23:234–240.
90. Tilton RG, Chang KC, LeJeune WS, Stephan CC, Brock TA, Williamson JR. Role for nitric oxide in the hyperpermeability and hemodynamic changes induced by intravenous VEGF. Invest Ophthalmol Vis Sci 1999;40:689–696.
91. Papapetropoulos A, Garcia-Cardena G, Madri JA, Sessa WC. Nitric oxide production contributes to the angiogenic properties of vascular endothelial growth factor in human endothelial cells. J Clin Invest 1997;100:313–319.
92. Fukumura D, Gohongi T, Kadambi A, et al. Predominant role of endothelial nitric oxide synthase in vascular endothelial growth factor-induced angiogenesis and vascular permeability. Proc Natl Acad Sci USA 2001;98:2604–2609.
93. Agardh CD, Agardh E, Andersson A, Hultberg B. Lack of association between plasma homocysteine levels and microangiopathy in type 1 diabetes mellitus. Scand J Clin Lab Invest 1994;54:637–641.
94. Hoogeveen EK, Kostense PJ, Eysink PE, et al. Hyperhomocysteinemia is associated with the presence of retinopathy in type 2 diabetes mellitus: the hoorn study. Arch Intern Med 2000;160:2984–2990.
95. Looker HC, Fagot-Campagna A, Gunter EW, et al. Homocysteine as a risk factor for nephropathy and retinopathy in type 2 diabetes. Diabetologia ER 2003;46:766–772.
96. Vaccaro O, Perna AF, Mancini FP, et al. Plasma homocysteine and microvascular complications in type 1 diabetes. Nutr Metab Cardiovasc Dis 2000;10:297–304.
97. Chiarelli F, Pomilio M, Mohn A, et al. Homocysteine levels during fasting and after methionine loading in adolescents with diabetic retinopathy and nephropathy. J Pediatr 2000;137:386–392.
98. Hultberg B, Agardh E, Andersson A, et al. Increased levels of plasma homocysteine are associated with nephropathy, but not severe retinopathy in type 1 diabetes mellitus. Scand J Clin Lab Invest 1991;51:277–282.
99. Hultberg B, Agardh CD, Agardh E, Lovestam-Adrian M. Poor metabolic control, early age at onset, and marginal folate deficiency are associated with increasing levels of plasma homocysteine in insulin-dependent diabetes mellitus. A five-year follow-up study. Scand J Clin Lab Invest 1997;57: 595–600.
100. Gaede P, Vedel P, Parving HH, Pedersen O. Elevated levels of plasma von Willebrand factor and the risk of macro- and microvascular disease in type 2 diabetic patients with microalbuminuria. Nephrol Dial Transplant 2001;16:2028–2033.
101. Lip PL, Belgore F, Blann AD, Hope-Ross MW, Gibson JM, Lip GY. Plasma VEGF and soluble VEGF receptor FLT-1 in proliferative retinopathy: relationship to endothelial dysfunction and laser treatment. Invest Ophthalmol Vis Sci 2000;41:2115–2119.
102. Lee ET, Lee VS, Kingsley RM, et al. Diabetic retinopathy in Oklahoma Indians with NIDDM incidence and risk factors. Diabetes Care 1992;15:1620–1627.
103. Klein R, Klein BE, Davis MD. Is cigarette smoking associated with diabetic retinopathy? Am J Epidemiol 1983;118:228–238.
104. Moss SE, Klein R, Klein BE. Association of cigarette smoking with diabetic retinopathy. Diabetes Care 1991;14:119–126.
105. Moss SE, Klein R, Klein BE. Cigarette smoking and ten-year progression of diabetic retinopathy. Ophthalmology 1996;103:1438–1442.
106. Goldsmith JR, Landaw SA. Carbon monoxide and human health. Science 1968;162:1352–1359.
107. Hawkins RI. Smoking, platelets and thrombosis. Nature 1972;236:450–452.
108. Sinclair SH. Macular retinal capillary hemodynamics in diabetic patients. Ophthalmology 1991;98: 1580–1586.
109. Qiao Q, Keinanen-Kiukaanniemi S, Laara E. The relationship between hemoglobin levels and diabetic retinopathy. J Clin Epidemiol 1997;50:153–158.
110. Davis MD, Fisher MR, Gangnon RE, et al. Risk factors for high-risk proliferative diabetic retinopathy and severe visual loss: Early Treatment Diabetic Retinopathy Study report no. 18. Invest Ophthalmol Vis Sci 1998;39:233–252.

111. Sinclair SH, DelVecchio C, Levin A. Treatment of anemia in the diabetic patient with retinopathy and kidney disease. Am J Ophthalmol 2003;135:740–743.
112. Borch-Johnsen K, Kreiner S. Proteinuria: value as predictor of cardiovascular mortality in insulin dependent diabetes mellitus. Br Med J (Clin Res Ed) 1987;294:1651–1654.
113. Winocour PH, Durrington PN, Ishola M, Anderson DC, Cohen H. Influence of proteinuria on vascular disease, blood pressure, and lipoproteins in insulin dependent diabetes mellitus. Br Med J (Clin Res Ed) 1987;294:1648–1651.
114. Nielsen NV. Diabetic retinopathy II. The course of retinopathy in diabetics treated with oral hypoglycaemic agents and diet regime alone. A one year epidemiological cohort study of diabetes mellitus. The Island of Falster, Denmark. Acta Ophthalmol (Copenh) 1984;62:266–273.
115. Biswas G, Dutta S, Mandal S, Biswas MC, Banerjee S, Saha SJ. Association of diabetic maculopathy with diabetic nephropathy—a study. J Indian Med Assoc 2002;100:567,568.
116. Zander E, Herfurth S, Bohl B, et al. Maculopathy in patients with diabetes mellitus type 1 and type 2: associations with risk factors. Br J Ophthalmol 2000;84:871–876.
117. Jensen T, Deckert T. Diabetic retinopathy, nephropathy and neuropathy. Generalized vascular damage in insulin-dependent diabetic patients. Horm Metab Res Suppl 1992;26:68–70.
118. Gilbert RE, Tsalamandris C, Allen TJ, Colville D, Jerums G. Early nephropathy predicts vision-threatening retinal disease in patients with type I diabetes mellitus. J Am Soc Nephrol 1998;9:85–89.
119. Lloyd CE, Klein R, Maser RE, Kuller LH, Becker DJ, Orchard TJ. The progression of retinopathy over 2 years: the Pittsburgh Epidemiology of Diabetes Complications (EDC) study. J Diabetes Complications 1995;9:140–148.
120. Lloyd CE, Orchard TJ. Diabetes complications: the renal-retinal link. An epidemiological perspective. Diabetes Care 1995;18:1034–1036.
121. Wirta O, Pasternack A, Mustonen J, Laippala P, Lahde Y. Retinopathy is independently related to microalbuminuria in type 2 diabetes mellitus. Clin Nephrol 1999;51:329–334.
122. Estacio RO, McFarling E, Biggerstaff S, Jeffers BW, Johnson D, Schrier RW. Overt albuminuria predicts diabetic retinopathy in Hispanics with NIDDM. Am J Kidney Dis 1998;31:947–953.
123. Parving HH, Hommel E, Mathiesen E, Skott P. Prevalence of microalbuminuria, arterial hypertension, retinopathy, and neuropathy in patients with insulin dependent diabetes. Brit Med J 1988;296: 156–160.
124. Kofoed-Enevoldsen A, Jensen T, Borch-Johnsen K, Deckert T. Incidence of retinopathy in type I (insulin-dependent) diabetes: association with clinical nephropathy. J Diabet Complications 1987;1:96–99.
125. Aiello LM, Rand LI, Briones JC, Weiss JN, Wafai MZ. Nonocular clinical risk factors in the progression of diabetic retinopathy. In: Little HL, Jack RL, Patz A, Forsham PH, eds. Diabetic retinopathy Thieme-Stratton, New York, 1983:21–32.
126. Tokuyama T, Ikeda T, Sato K. Effects of haemodialysis on diabetic macular leakage. Br J Ophthalmol 2000;84:1397–1400.
127. Tong PC, Lee KF, So WY, et al. White blood cell count is associated with macro- and microvascular complications in chinese patients with type 2 diabetes. Diabetes Care 2004;27:216–222.
128. Looker HC, Fagot-Campagna A, Gunter EW, et al. Homocysteine as a risk factor for nephropathy and retinopathy in Type 2 diabetes. Diabetologia ER 2003;46:766–772.
129. Ng PK, Chia KS, Koh D. Phenotypic heterogeneity and associations of two aldose reductase gene polymorphisms with nephropathy and retinopathy in type 2 diabetes: response to Wang et al. Diabetes Care 2004;27:289–290.
130. Chung SS, Chung SK. Genetic analysis of aldose reductase in diabetic complications. Curr Med Chem 2003;10:1375–1387.
131. Agardh E, Tallroth G, Bauer B, Cavallin-Sjoberg U, Agardh CD. Retinopathy and nephropathy in insulin-dependent diabetics: an inconsistent relationship? Diabet Med 1987;4:248–250.
132. Lovestam-Adrian M, Agardh E, Agardh CD. The incidence of nephropathy in type 1 diabetic patients with proliferative retinopathy: a 10-year follow-up study. Diabetes Res Clin Pract 1998;39:11–17.
133. Chavers BM, Mauer SM, Ramsay RC, Steffes MW. Relationship between retinal and glomerular lesions in IDDM patients. Diabetes 1994;43:441–446.
134. Schwartz MM, Lewis EJ, Leonard-Martin T, Lewis JB, Batlle D. Renal pathology patterns in type II diabetes mellitus: relationship with retinopathy. The Collaborative Study Group. Nephrol Dial Transplant 1998;13:2547–2552.
135. Kanauchi M, Kawano T, Uyama H, Shiiki H, Dohi K. Discordance between retinopathy and nephropathy in type 2 diabetes. Nephron 1998;80:171–174.

136. Williamson JR, Tilton RG, Chang K, Kilo C. Basement membrane abnormalities in diabetes mellitus: relationship to clinical microangiopathy. Diabetes Metab Rev 1988;4:339–370.
137. Silverstein JH, Fennell R, Donnelly W, et al. Correlates of biopsy-studied nephropathy in young patients with insulin-dependent diabetes mellitus. J Pediatr 1985;106:196–201.
138. Klein R, Zinman B, Gardiner R, et al. The relationship of diabetic retinopathy to preclinical diabetic glomerulopathy lesions in type 1 diabetic patients: the Renin-Angiotensin system study. Diabetes 2005;54:527–533.
139. Richards NT, Greaves I, Lee SJ, Howie AJ, Adu D, Michael J. Increased prevalence of renal biopsy findings other than diabetic glomerulopathy in type II diabetes mellitus. Nephrol Dial Transplant 1992;7:397–399.

28 Hypertension and Cardiovascular Disease

Adam Whaley-Connell, DO, *Kurt Sowers,* MD, *and James R. Sowers,* MD

Contents

INTRODUCTION

Type 2 diabetes mellitus (DM) is increasing exponentially; more than 18 million Americans are currently diagnosed, of which more than approx 73% have concomitant hypertension (HTN) *(1)*. Notably, at the time of diagnosis of diabetes, HTN is present in 50% of diabetic patients *(2)*. The presence of diabetic nephropathy (DN) and its clinical hallmark, microalbuminuria (MAU), with concommittant HTN accelerates progression to renal and cardiovascular disease (CVD). CVD risk progresses as DN progresses into chronic kidney disease (CKD) and finally end-stage renal disease (ESRD) requiring renal replacement therapy. Thus, it is then imperative to understand the close relationship that progressive DN has with HTN and concomitant advancing CVD risk. Primary preventive strategies are important to not only prevent DN, but to slow progression once it is present.

Only a subset of the DM population develops DN. Recent data suggests that inflammatory and oxidative stress in the glomerulus and the glomerular endothelium may parallel that in the vasculature in DM *(3)*. Accordingly, the pathogenesis of CVD in DM closely follows the development of diabetic glomerulosclerosis and MAU. Insulin resistance, MAU, and other components of the cardiometabolic syndrome (CMS) are risk factors for both diabetic atherosclerosis and glomerulosclerosis. Understanding the pathophysiology of these entities increases our potential for the

From: *Contemporary Diabetes: The Diabetic Kidney*
Edited by: P. Cortes and C. E. Mogensen © Humana Press Inc., Totowa, NJ

development of early prevention and treatment strategies that can delay/decrease associated CVD and glomerulosclerosis.

Modifying CVD and renal risk factors is a major goal in the interdisciplinary management of diabetes. In an effort to lower blood pressure (BP) and prevent progression of DN, initial therapy integrates lifestyle measures and medical therapy. An angiotensin-converting enzyme inhibitor (ACEI) or an angiotensin receptor blocker (ARB) combined with a thiazide diuretic or calcium antagonists provides significant reno- and CVD protective properties as first-line therapy in diabetic patients *(4)*. The development of diabetic glomerulosclerosis can complicate the management of HTN as well as accelerate CVD outcomes. CVD in patients with DM is compounded by insulin resistance. Managing CVD and renal risk factors in diabetic persons is challenging, especially with increasing duration of DM.

Diabetic Glomerulosclerosis

DN is the most common cause of progression of CKD to ESRD *(1)*, as well as morbidity and mortality in patients with DM. DN is characterized early by glomerular hemodynamic abnormalities that will eventually lead to glomerular hyperfiltration and then to glomerular structural changes (*see* Fig. 2) *(5–8)*. These changes progress to MAU and an eventual CKD and CVD if preventative measures are not taken.

Renal morphological changes in the initial stages involve hyperfiltration that is evidenced by glomerular basement thickening, mesangial extracellular matrix (ECM) expansion, and mesangial cell (MC) proliferation *(5–8)*. A major pathology in diabetic glomerulosclerosis involves ECM deposition and MC expansion and proliferation leading to associated dysfunctional filtration *(5)*. The abnormal filtration may be partly caused by an increase in the expression of growth factors and cytokines such as angiotensin (Ang)-II, aldosterone, tumor necrosis factor (TNF)-α, endothelin-1 (ET-1), interleukins (ILs), and vascular endothelial growth factor, all of which potentiate altered vascular flow and permeability *(5)*. Increased expression of fibrotic factors such as transforming growth factor (TGF)-β, connective tissue growth factor (CTGF), and vascular endothelial growth factor (VEGF) contribute to mesangial connective tissue deposition and expansion *(5,6)*.

Progression of DN and associated atherosclerosis are affected by many common factors including intraglomerular and systemic HTN, hyperglycemia, dysfunctional and activation of the renin–angiotensin–aldosterone system (RAAS), and various growth and inflammatory factors (*see* Fig. 1). There are several pathways that have been implicated in the increased production of metabolic toxins or increased rective oxygen species (ROS) and include excessive formation of advanced glycation endproducts (AGE), activation of protein kinase C (PKC), increased metabolism through the polyol pathways (*see* Fig. 2) *(5–19)*.

With hyperglycemia, there is an increased flux through the polyol pathway that converts glucose to fructose via two enzymes, aldose reductase and sorbitol dehydrogenase *(7)*. These enzymes use a cofactor, nicotinamide adenine dinucleotide phosphate (NADPH) and NAD^+, that when depleted, diminishes nitric oxide (NO) and vasodilatory prostaglandin production by endothelial cells (*see* Fig. 1). This may contribute to abnormal filtration and the associated increased NADPH/NAD^+ ratio, which reduces glycolytic pathway signaling resulting in increased oxidative stress, increased production of PKC, increased *de novo* diacylglycerol synthesis, and AGE *(5,8,9)*.

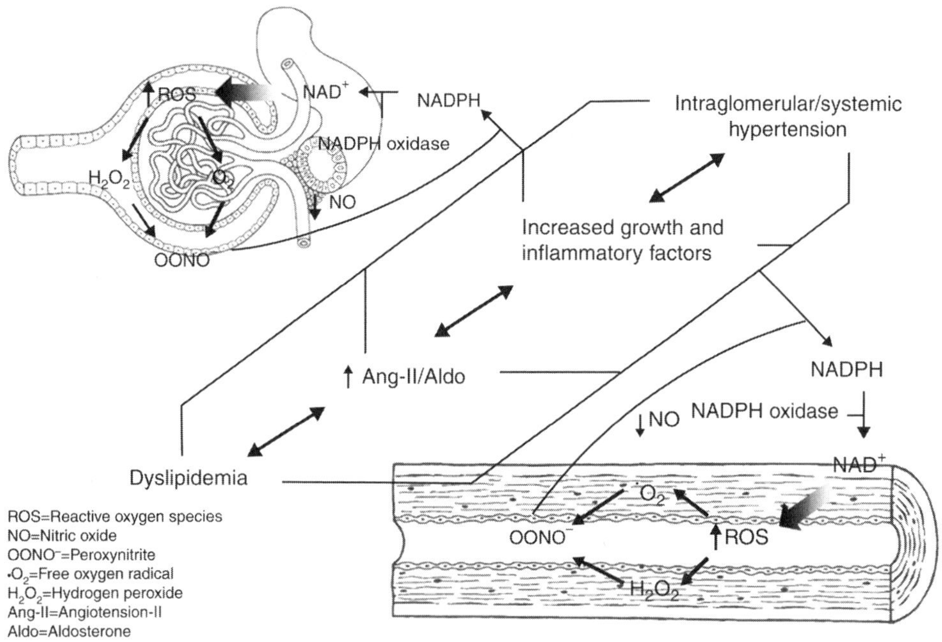

Fig. 1. Common diabetic glomerular and vascular atherosclerotic changes.

The concentration of AGE is increased in many vascular and renal tissues and is thought to be a major culprit in diabetic CVD complications *(10)*. Effects of AGE result from cell-surface binding to a receptor for AGEs (RAGE) and then subsequent accumulation in the ECM *(11)*. The AGE–RAGE complex has been implicated in alteration of cellular signaling pathway and subsequent metabolic deregulation. These pathways include p28 (ras)-extracellular signal-regulated protein kinases (Erk1/2), Jac2/Stat3, and transcription nuclear factor (NF)-$\kappa\beta$ signaling pathways *(12–14)*. This AGE–RAGE complex and its associated alteration of cell signaling has been shown to result in increased oxidative stress and activation of PKC and increased atherosclerosis and glomerulosclerosis *(16,17)*. The vascular MC activation results then in increased cytokine and growth factors, the aforementioned TGF-B, VEGF, and platelet-derived growth factor (PDGF) secretion leading to further vascular remodeling and mesangial expansion *(11–15)*.

Oxidative stress has been implicated as a major determinant in the CVD and renal complications of DM (*see* Figs. 1–3). This stress results from the imbalance of the generation of ROS (i.e., superoxide, hydrogen peroxide, and hydroxyl radical formation) and the reduced antioxidant mechanisms (i.e., superoxide dismutase, catalase, and glutathione peroxidase) (*see* Fig. 3) *(19)*. When there is an imbalance (as in a state of insulin resistance, CKD, and HTN), the increased ROS alters basic cellular proteins causing cellular damage and reduced endothelial-derived NO *(20)*. Many of the pathways for formation of ROS are interrelated and are driven, in part, by PKC activation and enhanced NADPH oxidase activity, xanthine oxidase, and uncoupled NO synthase *(16,21)*.

NADPH oxidase as the main enzymatic source of ROS generation in MCs and vascular smooth muscle cells (VSMC), and markers of oxidative stress are activated in the diabetic rat glomeruli *(21,22)*. ROS can also create increased expression of cell-signaling pathways

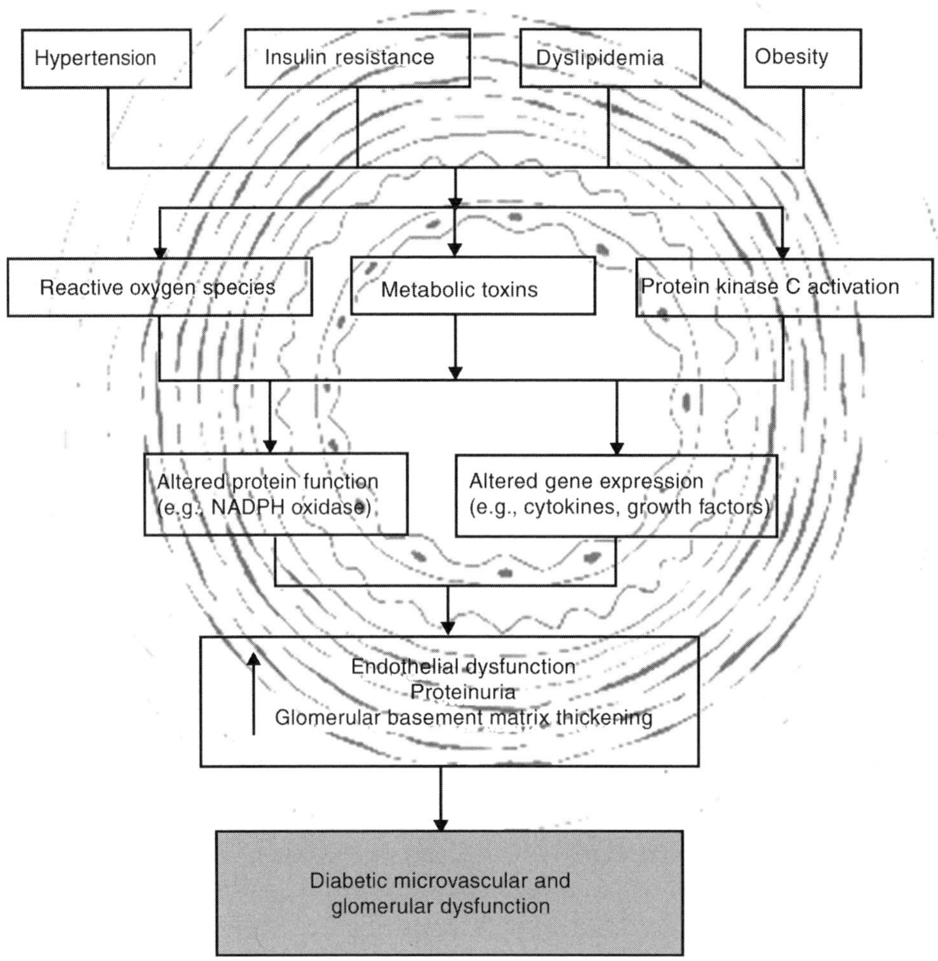

Fig. 2. Pathways for diabetic vascular dysfunction.

via a second messenger (i.e., responses to Ang-II or PDGF) that will then lead to overexpression of cytokines including TGF-β, TNF-α, monocyte chemoattractant protein-1, vascular cell adhesion molecule-1, IL-1, 6, and 8, and ECM proteins such as collagen IV *(23)*. Direct activation of NF-κβ and activator protein 1 by ROS are likely to play an important role as well in vascular cellular changes *(23)*.

The various PKC consitute a network of isoenzymes that act as intracellular signal transduction pathways for many hormones and cytokines. In diabetes, PKC activation may have effects on several intracellular signal transduction mechanism, including the previously mentioned Erk1/2, and NADPH oxidase *(24)*. PKC activation has also been implicated in increasing the actions of several cytokines, such as VEGF, PDGF-B, CTGF, and ET-1 *(25,26)*. Inhibition of PKC activity has shown to reduce elevated glomerular filtration rate (GFR), albuminuria, production of ECM proteins, expression of TGF-β, and CTGF, collagen deposition, and diabetic glomerulosclerosis *(25–28)*. Induced PKC inhibitor treatment in a hypertensive, insulin-resistant rat model with overexpression of rat renin gene, inhibited mesangial expansion and reduced proteinuria *(29,30)*. This would suggest that PKC inhibition could alter RAAS. In recent studies conducted in our laboratories, we have shown that increased tissue generation of ROS

Normal conditions

$$O_2 + e \longrightarrow O_2^{\underline{o}}$$

$$O_2^{\underline{o}} + O_2^{\underline{o}} + 2H^+ \xrightarrow{SOD} H_2O_2 + O_2$$

$$2H_2O_2 \xrightarrow{CAT} 2H_2O + O_2$$

*Under normal conditions superoxide formation is converted safety into water and molecular oxygen O_2, oxygen; e, electron; $O_2^{\underline{o}}$, superoxide; H^+, hydrogen; H_2O_2, hydrogen peroxide; CAT, catalase; H_2O, water.

Increased reactive oxygen species

$$H_2O_2 + O_2^{\underline{o}} \longrightarrow \cdot OH + OH^-$$

$$H_2O_2 + Cl^- + H^+ \xrightarrow{MPO} HOCL + H_2O$$

*In presence of excess superoxide, hydrogen peroxide can be converted to hydroxyl radicals, which are the most cytotoxic ROS known. As well, hydrogen peroxide can serve as a substrate for hypochlorous acid by myeloperoxidase, which is also a highly reactive ROS. H_2O_2, hydrogen peroxide; $O_2^{\underline{o}}$, superoxide; MPO, myeloperoxidase; OH, hydroxyl radical; OH^-, hydroxide; Cl^-, chloride anion; H^+, hydrogen cation; HOCL, hydrochlorous acid; H_2O, water.

Fig. 3. Formation of reactive oxygen species.

could also be corrected in this rodent model by angiotensin receptor-1 (AT_1R) blockade and by administration of tempol, a superoxide dismutase-1 mimetic *(29)*.

Role of RAAS in CVD and Renal Disease

HTN in DM is characterized by reduced NO-mediated vasorelaxation, reduced baroreflex sensitivity, and enhanced sympathetic activity, abnormalities that are promoted by aldosterone *(31)*. Changes in aldosterone secretion in response to changes in volume status or alteration in salt intake are mediated primarily by Ang-II. Although, patients with DM have usually normal Ang-II regulation of aldosterone and normal circulating levels of this hormone there may be increased tissue levels *(30)*. However, in diabetic patients with dysautonomia, usually associated with long-standing DM, there may be impaired conversion of the precursor of renin, prorenin, to renin by the diabetic kidney. This defect in the processing of renin may ultimately result in the syndrome of hyporenin–hypoaldosteronism (type 4 renal tubular acidosis), in which high levels of circulating prorenin are associated with unstimulatable renin, resulting in low aldosterone levels and a propensity to hyperkalemia *(31)*. Ang II and aldosterone are known to exert both genomic and nongenomic effects on the renal, systemic, and cerebral vasculature, that result in adverse CVD outcomes. Abrogation of the glomerular RAAS with AT_1R blockers, ACEI, and aldosterone antagonists likely decrease oxidative stress, one mechanism by which they decrease the progression of DN as well as vascular disease *(4,30–34)*.

Microalbuminuria

MAU is defined as albuminuria detected in urine at levels of 30–299 mg/d *(35–37)*. Albumin excretion exceeding these parameters is MAU, or overt proteinuria, and is a major independent risk factor for CVD *(33–35)*. MAU represents an increased permeability of the glomerulus, and has increasingly been shown to parallel vascular endothelial dysfunction in diabetic atherosclerosis (*see* Fig. 1) *(34)*. In fact, the presence of MAU is considered a marker for endothelial dysfunction *(35,36)*. There is also increasing evidence that it is an integral component of the metabolic syndrome associated with HTN *(37)*. Furthermore, the presence of albuminuria, alone or with decreased renal function, conveys increased CVD morbidity and mortality *(37–39)*. Patients who develop MAU are 20 times more likely to die from a CVD event *(40,41)*.

Unlike type 1 DM, in which HTN is often a consequence of renal disease *(41)*, MAU in type 2 DM is associated with insulin resistance, salt sensitivity, loss of nocturnal BP dipping, and left ventricular hypertrophy (LVH) *(32)*. Because MCs share many properties with VSMC, the appearance of MAU is related to endothelial dysfunction and other metabolic abnormalities that may lead to HTN. Conversely, HTN often antedates and likely contributes to the development of DN *(32)*.

Development of MAU or overt proteinuria often parallels the progression of CKD, typically progressing over 10–15 yr *(32–39)*. Once CKD develops, and the presence of either MAU or proteinuria, treatment is directed toward lowering BP to a goal of <130/80 mmHg and reducing proteinuria by at least 30–50% *(32–35)*. Medications that decrease both proteinuria and BP, such as ACEIs and ARBs are especially useful in these patients *(36–38)*.

Insulin Resistance/Hyperinsulinemia

The CVD risk that DN conveys is often compounded by the state of insulin resistance in DM *(3,42)*. Hyperinsulinemia/insulin resistance has been theorized as a potential cause of HTN and an additive CVD risk (e.g., the CMS). Insulin resistance is also increasingly recognized as a chronic, low-level, inflammatory state. Subclinical elevations of proinflammatory markers—IL-6, C-reactive protein (CRP), along with elevated white cell counts, PAI-1, fibrinogen levels, and uric acid are associated with the development of DM as well as CVD and renal disease in adults (*see* Table 1) *(43–46)*. This association is stronger in the obese *(43,44)*, and visceral fat accumulation is characterized by progressive infiltration of macrophages, which secrete proinflammatory molecules such as TNF-α, IL-6, and IL-1β *(45)*. These adipocytokines have been proposed to act through master proinflammatory regulators such as those of the nuclear factor-KB and the c-Jun NH2-terminal kinase (JNK)/AP-1 signaling pathways to modulate the expression of genes coding for many inflammatory proteins and to alter insulin signaling *(44)*. The central obesity characterizing the CMS is also associated with reduced adiponectin *(45–50)*. These actions have two basic consequences, first, to augment and perpetuate the proinflammatory diathesis, and second, to decrease insulin sensitivity *(43)*. Some adipocytokines have also been found to contribute to the development of hypertension through direct pressor actions and interactions with the RAAS *(46–50)*.

There is increasing data that suggests that Ang II, acting through the Ang-I receptor (AT_1R), inhibits the actions of insulin in vascular and skeletal muscle tissue *(29,42)*. This is mediated by insulin signaling through phosphatidylinositol 3-kinase (P13K) and protein kinase-B signaling pathways *(42)*. The inhibitory action of Ang-II is mediated by increased small-molecular-weight G proteins (i.e., RhoA) activity and oxidative stress *(46,47)*. This results in inhibition of P13K and protein kinase-B signaling thus decreasing endothelial cell production of NO, increased myosin light-chain

Table 1
Cardiovascular (CV) Risk Factors in Diabetics Linked to Vascular Dysfunction

- Central obesity
- Insulin resistance
- ↑ Triglycerides
- ↓ HDLC
- (Small dense LDL particles)
- Absent nocturnal drop in BP/HR
- Microalbuminuria
- Abnormal coagulation and fibroinolysis
- ROS generation
- Elevated CRP and other inflammatory markers
- Chronic kidney disease (estimated GFR < 60 mL/min)
- Increased uric acid
- Decreased diponectin

↑ CV oxidative stress/impaired endothelial function. HDLC, high-density lipoprotein cholesterol; LDL, low-density lipoprotein; ROS, reactive oxygen species; CRP, C-reactive protein; GFR, glomerular filtration rate. (Adapted from ref. *32*.)

activation with vasoconstriction, and reduced skeletal muscle glucose transport *(29,42,47–50)*.

Insulin is known to directly increase renal proximal tubular sodium reabsorption, thereby increasing extracellular volume and accounting for the fact that the HTN of DM is a volume-dependent, low-renin type, which is responsive to diuretic therapy in conjuction with RAAS blockers *(48)*. Insulin is also known to activate the RAAS and sympathetic nervous system *(49,50)*. Moreover, it causes an elevation of intracellular calcium concentration in VSMC and MCs, leading to vasoconstriction, VSMC proliferation, and increased vascular and glomerular fibrosis *(46,51)*.

ENDOTHELIAL DYSFUNCTION: ROLE IN VASCULAR AND GLOMERULAR DISEASE

In concert, insulin resistance, HTN, and DM, along with progression to MAU and CKD can lead to progressive endothelial dysfunction (ED) *(33,52)*. The vascular and glomerular endothelium will normally control VSMC and MC tone, and limits leukocyte adhesion, generation of ROS, and inflammatory activity. This is mediated in part by the actions of endothelial-derived factors such as NO, prostaglandins, endothelin, von Willebrand factor, as well as pro-thrombotic factors soluble thrombomodulin, soluble adhesion molecule and its inhibitors tissue-plasminogen activator and PAI-1 *(53)*. ED is present when these functions are altered and allow for the vascular endothelium to be more permeable to the proinflammatory modulators (cytokine-induced) and have increased interactions with leukocytes, adhesion molecules, and chemoattractants *(52,53)*. Once ED is present, this can initiate and allow for progression of atherosclerosis throughout the vasculature, whether it is in the kidney, heart, brain, or in the peripheral vasculature *(47)*.

We have reviewed how the progression of diabetic glomerulosclerosis and the development of MAU, combined with insulin resistance and DM produces a proinflammatory state to allow ED (both in the glomerular endothelium and the rest of the vasculature) to develop and progress to an overall risk for CVD. We will now review how therapy may reduce both microvascular and macrovascular complications.

TREATMENT STRATEGIES IN THE TREATMENT OF HYPERTENSION IN DIABETES

Current knowledge of the pathophysiological mechanisms of DN and advancing kidney disease occurring with insulin resistance and HTN in patients with diabetes will enable physicians to make rational choices in therapy. The initial evaluation of the hypertensive, diabetic patient should include a careful history and physical examination, focusing on his or her overall CVD risk. The degree of glucose control, presence of microvascular and macrovascular complications, and existence of end-organ damage from HTN will be emphasized.

Pharmacological Treatment

There is overwhelming evidence that the reduction of BP in patients with DM decreases the CVD mortality and the progression of diabetic renal disease. Clinical trials in hypertensive patients have shown that the reduction of BP decreases the incidence of stroke by 35–40%, myocardial infarction (MI) by 20–25%, and heart failure by 50% *(54)*. The Joint National Committee (JNC) VII recommends a goal BP of <130/80 mmHg in patients with DM *(54)*. This is also supported by the American Diabetes Association, World Health Organization/International Society of Hypertension, and the National Kidney Foundation *(55,56)*.

The Hypertension Optimal Treatment (HOT) trial demonstrated that diabetic patients had a 51% reduction of risk in cardiovascular events when their diastolic BP was treated to less than 80 mmHg, in comparison with those whose target was less than 90 mmHg *(57)*. Epidemiological analysis of the data from the UKPDS cohort has also shown a linear relationship between CVD risk and increasing systolic BP starting at 120 mmHg and above *(58)*. In addition, results from the Systolic Hypertension in the Elderly Program and Systolic Hypertension in Europe trials strongly support the aggressive antihypertensive treatment of diabetic patients with isolated systolic HTN *(59,60)*. A recent survey, utilizing the Framingham algorithm to evaluate coronary risk in National Health and Nutrition Examination Survey (NHANES) III individuals with the metabolic syndrome, estimated that controlling BP to normal levels (120–129/80–84 mmHg) would prevent 28.1% of coronary events in men and 12.5% of events in women *(61)*. It has also been shown that an average of 3.1 antihypertensive agents are required to reach a goal BP of less than 130/80 mmHg, and the addition of antihypertensive agents to current therapy should be based on their benefits in diabetic patients and their coexisting illnesses such as DN *(62)*. Furthermore, the Steno-2 trial showed that intervention on multiple cardiovascular risk factors (i.e., BP, glycemic, and lipid control) in patients with type 2 DM and MAU resulted in an absolute 20% reduction in CVD events *(63)*.

Angiotensin-Converting Enzyme Inhibitors

The RAAS plays a role in almost every step in the progression of atherosclerosis and HTN. Multiple clinical trials have demonstrated the pleiotropic effects of ACEIs and ARBs. In addition to being an effective antihypertensive, ACEIs have been proven to offer additional benefits in patients with DM. For example, of the 10,985 patients in the Captopril Prevention Project, 309 patients in the captopril group and 263 in the conventional therapy group were diabetic. Overall, captopril treatment markedly lowered the risk for fatal and nonfatal MI, stroke, and CVD deaths than in the conventional therapy group, which consisted of β-blocker or diuretic therapy *(64)*. The effects of the two regimens in the diabetic subpopulation showed a clear difference in the risk of developing a primary endpoint in favor of a captopril-based regimen *(65)*. The Heart Outcomes Prevention Evaluation (HOPE) trial studied 9541 patients, 3577 of whom were diabetic *(66)*. Ramipril use was associated with a significant 25% risk reduction in MI, stroke, or CVD death after a median follow-up period of 4.5 yr *(67)*. This benefit was independent of any BP-lowering effect.

In addition to the benefits of lowering the BP, ACEIs also decrease the membrane permeability to albumin and decrease intraglomerular pressure. By reducing MAU, ACEIs can help prevent the progression to DN. Meta-analyses have shown that this antiproteinuric effect is independent of the changes in BP. The Microalbuminuria, Cardiovascular, and Renal Outcomes in the Heart Outcomes Prevention Evaluation substudy also showed that ACEI therapy was associated with a decreased risk of development of overt DN in type-2 diabetic patients with MAU *(67)*. In type- I DM, ACEIs have been shown to prevent DN *(68)*. In type 2 DM, ACEIs have also been shown to slow the progression of DN in microalbuminuric, normotensive patients in comparison with other antihypertensives *(69–72)*. Recently, in a multicenter trial, ACEIs and ARBs were found to have equal reno-protective effects in patients with type 2 DM *(73)*.

Angiotensin Receptor Blockers

ARBs specifically block the AT_1R and offer a more complete blockade of the RAAS. It should be noted that ACEIs may not completely block the conversion of Ang I to Ang II owing to activation of alternate pathways *(74)*. The antihypertensive efficacy of ARBs are equivalent to ACEIs, and have been shown to have an improved side-effect profile. A comparison of irbesartan with enalapril in patients with severe HTN showed that irbesartan was associated with a significantly lower rate of coughing than with enalapril *(75)*. This may clinically translate to improved compliance with an ARB rather than an ACEI. Similar to ACEIs, the use of ARBs offer additional benefits in diabetic patients.

The Losartan Intervention for Endpoint Reduction in Hypertension trial showed a significant 13% reduction in cardiovascular death and MI, and a significant 25% reduction in the risk of stroke vs atenolol *(76)*. The subset of diabetic patients in this study had an even more significant reduction (24%) in the primary endpoint, as well as in CVD mortality (37%) and total mortality (39%) in comparison with atenolol *(76)*. However, the Irbesartan in Diabetic Nephropathy Trial, comparing irbesartan with a calcium antagonist, failed to show any significant difference between these two agents in terms of cardiovascular mortality *(77,78)*. In patients with LVH, heart failure, and post-MI, ARBs have been shown to be equal to ACEIs *(79)*.

Based on the current evidence and because of their tolerability, ARBs are recommended as first-line therapy for patients with DM, HTN, and significant proteinuria *(54)*. The Reduction of Endpoints in NIDDM with Ang-II Antagonist Losartan (RENAAL) and the Irbesartan in Diabetic Nephropathy Trial showed that ARBs reduce proteinuria, time to doubling of creatinine, and slow the progression of renal disease *(78,80)*. The Irbesartan in Microalbuminuria (IRMA) II and Microalbuminuria Reduction with Valsartan (MARVAL) trials also showed reduction in progression to nephropathy *(81,82)*. Again, the beneficial effects of ARB on nephropathy are shown to be independent of the changes in BP.

The Candesartan and Lisinopril Microalbuminuria trial showed greater reduction in albuminuria when both ARBs and ACEIs were used in combination, than when each was used alone *(83)*. In patients with nephrotic syndrome, combination therapy has been shown to reduce the proteinuria *(84)*. Although this appears promising, more data is needed before recommending the combination of these two agents to completely block the RAAS.

Thiazide Diuretics

Although diuretics have been shown to worsen insulin resistance, they have also consistently demonstrated their ability to reduce the CVD mortality in patients with DM. The Antihypertensive and Lipid-Lowering treatment to prevent Heart Attack Trial (ALLHAT), one of the largest antihypertension trials, concluded that thiazide diuretics comparably reduced all-cause mortality such as stroke, coronary artery disease (CAD), and heart failure *(85)*. This, along with the other studies on thiazide diuretics, has a short follow-up period of less than 10 yr; and the true impact of new-onset DM may not be fully appreciated on cardiovascular outcomes. Nevertheless, the electrolyte disturbances and the adverse effects on lipid and carbohydrate metabolism are uncommon with low-dose thiazide therapy *(35)*. Because the usefulness of chlorthalidone is controversial, hydrochlorthiazide has been widely accepted in clinical practice instead of the chlorthalidone. Diuretics continue to play an important role in the management of HTN in patients with DM, especially as an adjunct to ACEIs and ARBs.

Calcium Channel Blockers

Clinical studies have shown that at least 65% of hypertensive patients require two or more drugs to achieve the target BP of less than 130/80 *(86)*. Calcium channel blockers (CCBs) have been proven effective as second-line therapy as adjuncts to the above mentioned agents. CCBs are not only effective antihypertensive agents, they have also been shown to reduce insulin resistance or new-onset DM among people with cardiometabolic syndrome *(85,87–90)*. Both the ALLHAT and the RENAAL trials showed that the dihydropyridine calcium antagonists are reno-protective when used in combination with the agents that block the RAS *(85,91)*. Nondihydropyridine calcium antagonists, such as verapamil and diltiazem, have also been shown to have additional benefits of reducing proteinuria when used in combination with RAAS blockers *(92,93)*.

The Syst-Eur Trial with Netrendipine demonstrated that intensive antihypertensive therapy for older patients with type 2 DM and isolated systolic HTN eliminated the additional risk for CVD events and stroke associated with DM *(93)*. In the Hypertension Optimal Treatment trial, there was a reduction in major CVD events with diastolic BP control in patients with DM, when felodipine was used as first-line therapy *(58)*. It should be noted that in the ALLHAT study, CCBs had a significantly higher incidence of heart failure in comparison with diuretics *(85)*.

β-*Blockers*

The effectiveness of β-blockers in HTN, CAD and heart failure management have been proven beyond doubt in multiple clinical trials. Despite their adverse effects of the glucose tolerance and the peripheral vasculature, β-blockers have a significant role in HTN management in the diabetic population, especially in those with associated micro- and macro-vascular complications. In the UKPDS, atenolol was comparable to captopril in reducing BP and CVD outcomes *(58)*.

β-blockade can worsen the symptoms of peripheral vascular disease. However, selective β-blockers, such as carvedilol, have been shown to reduce CVD mortality and MAU without adversely affecting the glucose or lipid profiles *(94,95)*. When used with RAAS blockade, carvedilol and atenolol have also both been shown to reduce albuminuria *(96,97)*. In addition, carvedilol has been shown to slow the progression of nephropathy and to improve insulin sensitivity *(96–98)*.

In diabetic patients, β-blockers are used mostly in patients with coexisting CAD and congestive heart failure *(99)*. Despite their potential adverse metabolic effects, β-blockers have been proven to have significant favorable effects on CVD outcomes in hypertensive diabetic patients, especially in those with ischemic heart disease and congestive heart failure (CHF) *(35)*. Therefore, these agents should be included in the antihypertensive therapy in diabetic patients, specifically those with CAD and CHF.

CONCLUSIONS

The development of diabetic glomerulosclerosis and subsequent MAU in concert with insulin resistance creates a state of ED resulting from an overall proinflammatory state. This places patients at risk for CVD and increased CVD outcomes as well as progression of CKD. Treatment with traditional RAAS blockade cannot only reduce progression of DN, but can also improve CV outcomes. However, clinicians must note the beneficial effects on CV outcomes of diuretics, CCBs, and β-blockade in the management of HTN in patients with DN.

There is emerging a parallel of dysfunction between the glomerular endothelium and the rest of the vasculature that has yet to be definitively elucidated. However, the effects that hyperglycemia and insulin resistance have on the kidney are clear and the understanding of how the ROS, AGE, and activation of PKC all interact is critical to creating novel treatments for diabetes and preventing progression of DN.

REFERENCES

1. McFarlane S, Gizycki HV, Winer N, et al. Control of cardiovascular risk factors in patients with diabetes and hypertension at urban academic medical centers. Diabetes Care 2002;25:718–723.
2. American diabetes association national diabetes fact sheet. Accessed http://www.diabetes.org/diabetes-statistics/national-diabetes-fact-sheet.jsp on 3/14/05.
3. McFarlane SI, Banerji M, Sowers JR. Insulin resistance and cardiovascular disease. J Clin Endocrinol Metab 2001;86(2):713-718.
4. Couser WG, Johnson RJ. Mechanisms of progressive renal disease in glomerulonephritis. Am J Kidney Dis 1994;23:193–198.
5. Sheetz MJ, King GL. Molecular understanding of hyperglycemia's adverse effects for diabetic complications. J Am Med Assoc 2002;288:2579–2588.
6. Sharma K, Ziyadeh FN. Hyperglycemia and diabetic kidney disease. The case for transforming growth factor-beta as a key mediator. Diabetes 1995;44:1139–1146.
7. Brownlee M. Biochemistry and molecular cell biology of diabetic complications. Nature 2001;414: 813–820.
8. Setter SM, Campbell RK, Cahoon CJ. Biochemical pathways for microvascular complications of diabetes mellitus. Ann Pharmacother 2003;37:1858–1866.
9. Tilton RG. Diabetic Vascular Dysfunction: Links to glucose-induced reductive stress and VGEF. Microscopic Res Tech 2002;57:390–407.
10. Brownlee M, Cerami A, Vlassara H. Advanced glycosylation end products in tissue and the biochemical basis of diabetic complications. N Engl J Med 1988;318:1315–1321.
11. Doi T, Vlassara H, Kirstein M, et al. Receptor-specific increase in extracellular matrix production in mouse mesangial cells by advanced glycosylation end products is mediated via platelet-derived growth factor. Proc Natl Acad Sci USA 1992;89:2873–2877.
12. Lander HM, Tauras JM, Ogiste JS, et al. Activation of the receptor for advanced glycation end products triggers a p21(ras)-dependent mitogen activated protein kinase pathway regulated by oxidant stress. J Biol Chem 1997;272:17,810–17,814.

13. Sakaguchi T, Yan SF, Yan SD, et al. Central Role of RAGE-dependent neointimal expansion in arterial restenosis. J Clin Invest 2003;111:959–972.
14. Huttunen HJ, Fages C, Rauvala H. Receptor for advanced glycation end-products (RAGE)-mediated neurite outgrowth and activation of NK-kappaB require the cytoplasmic domain of the receptor but different downstream signaling pathways. J Biol Chem 1999;274:199,919–199,924.
15. Vasan S, Foiles P, Founds H. Therapeutic potential of breakers of advanced glycation end product-protein crosslinks. Arch Biochem Biophys 2003;282:F975–F980.
16. Sowers JR. Hypertension, Angiotensin II, and Oxidative Stress. N Engl J Med 2002;346:1999–2001.
17. Scivittaro V, Ganz MB, Weiss MF. AGE's induce oxidative stress and activate protein kinase C-beta (III) in neonatal mesangial cells. Am J Physiol Renal Physiol 2000;278:F676–F683.
18. Oldfield MD, Bach LA, Forbes JM, et al. Advanced glycation end products cause epithelial-myofibroblast transdifferentiation via the receptor for advanced glycation end products (RAGE). J Clin Invest 2001;108:1853–1863.
19. Frank JG. Oxygen, oxidative stress, hypoxia, and heart failure. J Clin Invest 2005;115:500–508.
20. Cai H, Harrison DG. Endothelial dysfunction in cardiovascular diseases: the role of oxidant stress. Circ Res 2000;87:84–844.
21. Kitada H, Tanaka M, Takemura Y, et al. Translocation of glomerular p47phox and p67phox by protein kinase C-beta activation is required for oxidative stress in diabetic nephropathy. Diabetes 2003;52: 2603–2614.
22. Jones SA, Hancock JT, Jones OT, et al. The expression of NADPH-oxidase components in human glomerular mesangial cells: detection of protein and mRNA for p47phox, p67phox, and p22phox. J Am Soc Nephrol 1995;5:1483–1491.
23. Tylicki L, Rutkowski B, Horl WH. Antioxidants: a possible role in kidney protection. Kidney Blood Press Res 2003;26:303–314.
24. Igashari M, Wakasaki H, Takahora N, et al. Glucose or diabetes activates p38 mitogen-activated protein kinase via different pathways. J Clin Invest 1999;103:185–195.
25. Kaya D, Jirousek MR, Lin YW, et al. Characterization of protein kinase C beta isoform activation on the gene expression of transforming growth factor-beta, extracellular matrix components, and prostanoids in the glomeruli of diabetic rats. J Clin Invest 1997;100:115–126.
26. Way KJ, Isshiki K, Suzama K, et al. Expression of connective tissue growth factor is increased in injured myocardium associated with protein kinase C beta2 activation and diabetes. Diabetes 2002;51:2709–2718.
27. Kaya D, Haneda M, Nakagawa H, et al. Amelioration of accelerated diabetic mesangial expansion by treatment with a PKC beta inhibitor in diabetic db/db mice, a rodent model for type 2 diabetes. FASEB J 2000;14:439–447.
28. Kelly DJ, Zhang Y, Hepper C, et al. Protein kinase C-beta inhibition attenuates the progression of experimental diabetic nephropathy in the presence of continued hypertension. Diabetes 2003;52:512–518.
29. Blendea MC, Jacobs D, Stump C, et al. Abrogation of oxidative stress improves insulin sensitivity in the Ren-2 rat model of tissue angiotensin II overexpression. Am J Physiol Endocrinol Metab 2005;288:E353–E359.
30. McFarlane SI, Sowers JR. Aldosterone function in diabetes mellitus: Effects on cardiovascular and renal disease. J Clin Endocrinol Metab 2003;88:516–523.
31. Sowers JR, Beck F, Waters D, et al. Studies of rennin activation and regulation of aldosterone and 18-hydroxycorticosterone biosynthesis in hyporeninemic, hypoaldosteronism. J Clin Endocrinol Metab 1985;61:60–67.
32. Sowers JR, Haffner S. Treatment of cardiovascular and renal risk factors in the diabetic hypertensive. Hypertension 2002;40:781–788.
33. Garg JP, Bakris GL. Microalbuminuria: marker of vascular dysfunction, risk factor for cardiovascular disease. Vasc Med 2002;7:35–43.
34. Sowers JR. Recommendations for special populations: diabetes mellitus and the metabolic syndrome. Am J Hypertens 2003;16(11):41S–45S.
35. Ljungman S, Wikstrand J, Hartford M, Berglund G. Urinary albumin excretion–a predictor of risk of cardiovascular disease. A prospective 10 year follow-up of middle-aged non-diabetic normal and hypertensive men. Am J Hypertens 1996;9:770–778.
36. Dineen SF, Gerstein HC. The association of microalbuminuria and mortality in non-insulin-dependent diabetes mellitus: a systematic overview of the literature. Arch Intern Med 1997;157:1413–1418.
37. Eknoyan G, Hostetter T, Bakris GL, et al. Proteinuria and other markers of Chronic Kidney Disease: a position statement of the National Kidney Foundation (NKF) and the national institute of Diabetes and digestive and kidney diseases (NIDDK). Am J Kidney Dis 2003;42:617–622.

38. K/DOQI clinical practice guidelines for chronic kidney disease: evaluation, classification, and stratification. Kidney disease outcome quality initiative. Am J Kidney Dis 2002;39:S1–S246.
39. Bakris GL, Walsh MF, Sowers JR. Endothelium/mesangium interactions: role of insulin-like growth factors. In: Sowers JR, ed. Endocrinology of the vasculature. Humana, Totowa NJ, 1996, pp. 341–356.
40. Arun CS, Stoddart J, Mackin P, et al. Significance of microalbuminuria in long-duration type 1 diabetes. Diabetes Care 2003;26:2144–2149.
41. Lewis EJ, Hunsicker LG, Clarke WR, et al. Renoprotective effect of the angiotensin-receptor antagonist irbesartan in patients with nephropathy due to type 2 diabetes. N Engl J Med 2001;345: 851–860.
42. Sowers JR. Insulin Resistance and Hypertension. Am J Physiol Heart Circ Physiol 2004;286(5): H1597–H1602.
43. Bianchi S, Bigazzi R, Quinones G, et al. Insulin Resisitance in microalbuminuric hypertension: sites and mechanisms. Hypertension 1995;57:1803–1817.
44. Duncan BB, Schmidt MI, Pankow JS, et al. Low-grade systemic inflammation and the development of diabetes: the atherosclerosis risk in communities study. Diabetes 2003;52:1799–1805.
45. Weisberg SP, McCann D, Desnai M, et al. Obesity is associated with macrophage accumulation in adipose tissue. J Clin Invest 2003;112:1796–1808.
46. Fernández-Real JM, Ricart W. Insulin resistance and chronic cardiovascular inflammatory syndrome. Endocr Rev 2003;24(3):278–301.
47. Tan A, Kuppuswamy S, Whaley-Connell A, Romayne L, Sowers JR. "Recommendations for Special Populations: the Treatment of Hypertension in Diabetes Mellitus." Endocrinologist 2004;6:368–381.
48. Stas S, El-Atat F, Sowers JR. Pathogenesis of Hypertension in Diabetes. Rev Endocr Metab Disord 2005;5:221–225.
49. Sowers JR, Frolich ED. Insulin and Insulin Resistance: impact on blood pressure and Cardiovascular Disease. Med Clin North Am 2004;88:63–82.
50. Sowers JR, Stump C. Insights into the biology of diabetic vascular disease: What's new? Am J Hypertens 2004;17(11):S2–S6.
51. Berne C, Fagius J, Pollare T, Hjemdahl P. The sympathetic response to euglycaemic hyperinsulinaemia. Diabetologia 1992;35:873–879.
52. Aras R, Sowers JR, Arora R. The Proinflammatory and Hypercoaguable State of Diabetes Mellitus. Rev Cardiovasc Med 2005;10(6):1–15.
53. Stehouwer CDA. Endothelial Dysfucntion in diabetic nephropathy: state of the art and potential significance for non-diabetic renal disease. Nephrol Dial Transplant 2004;19:778–781.
54. Chobanian AV, Bakris GL, Black HR, et al. Seventh Report of the Joint National Committee on Prevention, Detection, Evaluation, and Treatment of High Blood Pressure. JAMA 2003 289(19) 2560–2571.
55. Bakris GL, Williams M, Dworkin L, et al. Preserving renal function in adults with Hypertension and Diabetes: a consensus approach. National Kidney Foundation Hypertension and Diabetes Executive Committees Working Group. Am J Kidney Dis 2000;36:646–661.
56. World Health Organization, International society of Hypertension Writing Group.2003 World Health Organization (WHO)/International society of Hypertension (ISH) statement on management of hypertension. J Hypertens 2003;21(11):1983–1992.
57. Hansson L, Zanchetti A, Carruthers SG, et al. Effects of intensive blood pressure lowering and low-dose aspirin in patients with hypertension: principal results of the Hypertension Optimal Treatment (HOT) randomized trial. Lancet 1998;351:1755–1762.
58. Adler AI, Stratton IM, Neil HAW, et al. Association of systolic blood pressure with macrovascular and microvascular complications of type 2 diabetes (UKPDS 36): prospective observational study. Br Med J 2000;321:412–419.
59. Curb JD, Pressel SL, Cutler J, et al. Effect of diuretic-based antihypertensive treatment on cardiovascular risk in older diabetic patients with isolated systolic hypertension. JAMA 1996;276:1886–1892.
60. Tuomilehto J, Rastenyte D, Birkenhäger WH, et al. The Systolic Hypertension in Europe Trial investigators: effect of calcium-channel blockage in older patients with diabetes and systolic hypertension. N Engl J Med 199;340:677–684.
61. Wong ND, Pio JR, Franklin SS, et al. Preventing coronary events by optimal control of blood pressure and lipids in patients with the metabolic syndrome. Am J Cardiol 2003;91(12):1421–1426.
62. McFarlane S, Gizycki HV, Winer N, et al. Control of Cardiovascular Risk Factors in Patients With Diabetes and Hypertension at Urban Academic Medical Centers. Diabetes Care 2002;25:718–723.
63. Gaede P, Vedel P, Larsen N, et al. Multifactorial Intervention and Cardiovascular Disease in Patients with Type 2 Diabetes. N Engl J Med 2003;348(5):383–393.

64. Hansson L, Lindholm LH, Niskanen L, et al. Effect of angiotensin-converting-enzyme inhibition compared with conventional morbidity and mortality in hypertension: the Captopril Prevention Project (CAPPP) randomised trial. Lancet 1999;353:611–616.
65. Niskanen L, Hedner T, Hansson L, Lanke J, Niklason A. Reduced cardiovascular morbidity and mortality in hypertensive diabetic patients on first-line therapy with an ACE inhibitor compared with a diuretic/β-blocker–based treatment regimen: a subanalysis of the Captopril Prevention Project. Diabetes Care 2001;24:2091–2096.
66. Yosuf S, Sleight P, Pogue J, Bosch J, Davies R, Dagenais G. Effects of an angiotensin-converting-enzyme inhibitor, ramipril, on cardiovascular events in high-risk patients. The Heart Outcomes Prevention Evaluation Study Investigators. N Engl J Med 2000;342:145–153.
67. Heart Outcomes Prevention Evaluation Study Investigators. Effects of ramipril on cardiovascular and microvascular outcomes in people with diabetes mellitus: results of the HOPE study and MICRO-HOPE substudy. Lancet 2000;355:253–259.
68. Lewis EJ, Hunsicker LG, Bain RP, Rohde RD. The Effect Of Angiotensin-Converting-Enzyme Inhibition On Diabetic Nephropathy. The Collaborative Study Group. N Engl J Med 1993;329(20): 1456–1462
69. Euclid Study Group: randomised placebo-controlled trial of lisinopril in normotensive patients with insulin-dependent diabetes and normoalbuminuria or microalbuminuria. Lancet 1997;349:1787–1792.
70. Bakris GL, Smith AC, Richardson DJ, et al. Impact of ACE inhibitor and calcium antagonist on microalbuminuria and lipid subfractions in type 2 diabetes: a randomized, multi-center pilot study. J Hum Hypertens 2002;16:185–191.
71. Ravid M, Archmani R, Lishner M. Long-term renoprotective effect of angiotensin-converting enzyme inhibition in non-insulin dependent diabetes mellitus; A 7-year follow-up study. Arch Intern Med 1996;156:286–289.
72. Remenenti P, Fassi A, Parnova I, et al. Preventing microalbuminuira in type 2 diabetes. N Engl J Med 2004;351(19):1941–1951.
73. Barnett AH, Bain SC, Bouter P, et al. Angiotensin-Receptor Blockade versus Converting-Enzyme Inhibition in Type 2 Diabetes and Nephropathy. N Engl J Med 2004;351(19):1952–1961.
74. Deedwania PC. Hypertension and diabetes: New therapeutic options. Arch Intern Med 2000;160(11): 1585–1594.
75. Larochelle P, Clack JM, Marbury T, et al. Effects and tolerability of irbesartan versus enalapril in patients with severe hypertension. Am J Cardiol 1997;80:1613–1615
76. Lindholm LH, Ibsen H, Dahlof B, et al. Cardiovascular morbidity and mortality in patients with diabetes in the Losartan Intervention For Endpoint reduction in hypertension study (LIFE): a randomised trial against atenolol. Lancet 2002;359(9311):1004–10.
77. Zanchetti A, Ruilope LM. Antihypertensive treatement in patients with type-2 diabetes mellitus: what guidance from recent controlled randomized trials? J Hypertens 2002;20(11)2099–2110.
78. Lewis EJ, Hunsicker LG, Clarke WR, et al. Renoprotective effect of the angiotensin-receptor antagonist irbersartan in patients with nephropathy due to type 2 diabetes and nephropathy. N Engl J Med 2001;345:861–869.
79. Pfeffer MA, McMurray JJ, Velazquez EJ, et al. Valsartan, captopril or both in myocardial infarction complicated by heart failure, left ventricular dysfunction, or both. N Engl J Med 2001;349:1893–1906.
80. Bakris GL, Weir MR, Shanifar S, et al. Effects of blood pressure level on progression of diabetic nephropathy: results from the RENAAL study. Arch Intern Med 2003;163(13):1555–1565.
81. Parving HH, Lehnert H, Brochner-Mortensen J, et al. The effect of Irbesartan on the development of diabetic nephropathy in patients with type 2 diabetes. N Engl J Med 2001;345(12):870–878.
82. Viberti GC, Wheelden NM, for the MicroAlbuminuria Reduction With VALsartan (MARVAL) Study Inverstigators: Micoralbuminuira reduction with valsartan in patients with type 2 diabetes mellitus: a blood pressure-independent effect. Circulation 2002;106:672–678.
83. Mogensen CE, Neldam S, Tikkanen I, et al. Randomized controlled trial of dual blockade of rennin-angiotensin system in patients with hypertension, microalbuminuria, and non-insulin dependent diabetes: the candersartan and lisinopril microalbuminuria (CALM) study. BMJ 2000;321:1440–1444.
84. Ferrari P, Marti HP, Pfister M, Frey FJ. Additive antiproteinuric effect of combined ACE inhibition and angiotensin II receptor blockade. J Hypertens. 2002;20(1):125–130.
85. The ALLHAT Officers and Coordinators for the ALLHAT Collaborative Research Group. Major outcomes in high-risk hypertensive patients randomized to angiotensin-converting enzyme inhibitor or calcium channel blocker vs diuretic: the Antihypertensive and Lipid-Lowering Treatment to Prevent Heart Attack Trial (ALLHAT). J Am Med Assoc 2002;288(23):2981–2997.

86. Black HR, Elliot WJ, Neaton JD, et al. Baseline characteristics and early blood pressure control in the CONVINCE Trial. Hypertension 2001;37:12–18.
87. American Diabetes Association. Hypertension Management in Adults With Diabetes: clinical practice recommendations 2004. Diabetes Care 2004;27(1):S65–S67
88. Koyama Y, Kodama K, Suziki M, Harano Y. Improvement of insulin sensitivity by a long-acting nifedipine preparation (nifedipine-CR) in patients with essential hypertension. Am J Hypertens 2002;15:927–931.
89. Zanella MT, Kohlmann O, Ribero AB. Treatment of obesity hypertension and diabetes syndrome. Hypertension 2001,38:705–708.
90. Black HR, Elliott WJ, Grandits G, et al. Principal results of the controlled onset verapamil investigation of cardiovascular end points (CONVINCE) trial. J Am Med Assoc 2003;289(16):2073–2082.
91. Pepine CJ, Handberg EM, Cooper-DeHoff RM, et al. A calcium antagonist vs a non-calcium antagonist hypertension treatment strategy for patients with coronary artery disease. The International Verapamil-Trandolapril Study (INVEST): a randomized controlled trial. J Am Med Assoc 2003; 290(21):2805–2816.
92. Brenner Bm, Cooper ME, de Zeeuw D, et al. Effects of losartan on renal and cardiovascular outcomes in patients with type 2 diabetes and nephropathy. N Engl J Med 2001;345:861–869.
93. Birkenhager WH, Staessen JA, Gasowski J, de Leeuw PW. Effects of antihypertensive treatment on endpoints in the diabetic patients randomized in the Systolic Hypertension in Europe (Syst-Eur) trial. J Nephrol 2000;13(3):232–237.
94. Jacob S, Balletshofer B, Henriksen EJ, et al. Beta-blocking agents in patients with insulin resistance: effects of vasodialting beta-blockers. Blood Press 1999;8:261–268.
95. Giugliano D, Acampora R, Marfella R, et al. Metabolic and cardiovascular effects of carvedilol and atenolol in non-insulin-depenedent diabetes mellitus and hypertension. A randomised, controlled trial. Ann Intern Med 1997;126:955–959.
96. Fassbinder W, Quarder O, Waltz A. Treatment with Carvedilol is associated with a significant reduction in microalbuminuria: a multi-center, randomized study. Int J Clin Pract 1999;53:519–520.
97. Dargie HJ. Effect of carvedilol on outcome after myocardial infarction in patients with left-ventricular dysfunction: the CAPRICORN randomized trial. Lancet 2001;357:1385–1390.
98. Poole-Wilson PA, Swedberg K, Cleland JG, et al. Comparison of carvedilol and metoprolol on clinical outcomes in patients with chronic heart failure in the Carvedilol Or Metoprolol European Trial (COMET): a randomized controlled trial. Lancet 2003;362:7–13.
99. American Diabetes Association. Hypertension Management in Adults With Diabetes: clinical practice recommendations 2004. Diabetes Care 2004;27(1):S65–S67.

29 Endothelial Dysfunction

A Key to Understanding the Association Between Nephropathy and Vascular Disease in Individuals With and Without Diabetes

Coen D. A. Stehouwer, MD, PhD, *Maya S. P. Huijberts,* MD, PhD, *Alfons J. H. M. Houben,* PhD, *and Nicolaas C. Schaper,* MD, PhD

CONTENTS

INTRODUCTION

Much of the disease burden in diabetes occurs in patients with diabetic nephropathy (DN), as they have the highest chance of developing cardiovascular disease (CVD) as well as severe retinopathy and neuropathy. Two issues appear crucial in stemming the epidemic of DN and CVD. One is the prevention of diabetes and the solution here from a public health point of view lies in the prevention of obesity. The other is improved understanding of the pathogenesis of renal and vascular disease in diabetes. Here, endothelial dysfunction (ED) is thought to play a key role *(1)*. What is the state of the art regarding this hypothesis?

From: *Contemporary Diabetes: The Diabetic Kidney*
Edited by: P. Cortes and C. E. Mogensen © Humana Press Inc., Totowa, NJ

WHAT IS ENDOTHELIAL DYSFUNCTION?

The endothelium is an important site of control of vascular functions *(2)*. Vascular endothelium normally decreases vascular tone; limits leukocyte adhesion and, thus, inflammatory activity in the vessel wall; regulates vascular permeability to nutrients, macromolecules, and leukocytes; inhibits platelet adhesion and aggregation by producing prostacyclin, nitric oxide (NO) and ectonucleotidases; limits activation of the coagulation cascade by the thrombomodulin-protein C, heparin sulphate-antithrombin and tissue factor–tissue factor pathway inhibitor interactions; and regulates fibrinolysis by producing tissue-type plasminogen activator and its inhibitor, plasminogen activator inhibitor (PAI)-1. NO is a particularly important endothelium-derived mediator because of its vasodilator, anti-platelet, antiproliferative, anti-adhesive, permeability-decreasing, and anti-inflammatory properties.

ED can be considered present when endothelial properties have changed in a way that is inappropriate regarding the preservation of organ function. For example, basement membrane synthesis may be altered, which can contribute to arterial stiffening and increased microvascular permeability; vascular tone and permeability may increase, which contributes to increased blood pressure and atherogenesis; and the endothelium may lose its antithrombotic and profibrinolytic properties and may instead acquire prothrombotic and antifibrinolytic properties. Such alterations (endothelial dysfunctions) do not necessarily occur simultaneously and may differ according to the nature of the injury and the intrinsic properties of the endothelium (e.g., venous vs arterial vs microvascular). Endothelial activation designates one specific type of ED characterized by (usually, inflammatory cytokine-induced) increased interactions with blood leukocytes, in which adhesion molecules and chemoattractants are essential. ED can be conceptualized as a transducer of atherogenic risk factors and is thought to play an important role both in the initiation and the progression of atherosclerosis. In this view, risk factors, such as oxidatively modified low-density lipoprotein cholesterol, smoking, hypertension, angiotensin-II, and diabetes, initiate atherosclerosis through endothelial activation. The predilection to atherosclerosis of arterial branching points, bifurcations, and convexities is explained by the fact that blood flow there is nonlaminar or even turbulent with low or oscillatory shear stress. These conditions increase endothelial activation, effects that are enhanced by hypertension. These risk factors also have in common that NO availability is decreased through decreased production and (or) increased degradation, which furthers endothelial activation.

CAN ENDOTHELIAL DYSFUNCTION BE ASSESSED IN HUMANS?

Much of the above is based on experimental data. Testing these concepts in patients, above all, requires reliable measurements of endothelial function. Endothelial function cannot be measured directly in humans and, thus, indirect estimates are often used, which include endothelium-dependent vasodilation and plasma levels of endothelium-derived regulatory mediators, such as NO_x, endothelin, von Willebrand factor, soluble thrombomodulin, soluble adhesion molecules, tissue-type plasminogen activator, and PAI-1. But are these tests valid estimates of endothelial function? On the one hand, many cross-sectional studies have shown impaired endothelium-dependent vasodilation and high levels of endothelium-derived regulatory proteins in diseases that involve injury to the endothelium, such as atherothrombosis, pre-eclampsia and vasculitis, as well as in individuals with risk factors for atherothrombosis. Moreover, prospective studies have shown that individuals with impaired endothelium-dependent vasodilation and high levels of endothelium-derived regulatory proteins have an adverse cardiovascular prognosis *(3–6)*. Vice versa, there is evidence that interventions that lower cardiovascular risk factors, such as with statin therapy in individuals with hypercholesterolemia, result in an improvement of endothelium-dependent vasodilation and lowering of circulating endothelium-derived regulatory proteins *(7,8)*. On the other hand, the interpretation of these tests is not as straightforward as one would wish. First, tests intended to estimate NO-mediated endothelium-dependent vasodilation in part measure effects of other endothelial vasodilators, such as prostacyclin and endothelium-derived hyperpolarizing factor. This has two consequences, which are not often emphasized, namely:

- that quantitatively normal endothelium-dependent vasodilation does not guarantee normal endothelial function, as less NO might be compensated by more endothelium-derived hyperpolarizing factor, and
- that abnormal endothelium-dependent vasodilation in the presence of normal sodium nitroprusside-mediated vasodilation (i.e., normal vascular smooth muscle cell responsiveness to exogenous NO) does not guarantee impaired endothelial function, as this combination of findings is also compatible with an abnormal smooth muscle cell response to endothelium-derived vasodilators other than NO.

Second, the concept that high plasma levels of endothelium-derived mediators reflect ED in clinically relevant arteries (such as the coronary and carotid) requires:

- that other cell types are not an important source of these mediators,
- that synthesis of these mediators is more important than clearance regarding the determination of plasma levels, and
- that endothelial function in the microvasculature parallels that in large arteries, because microvascular endothelium, with its very large surface area and synthetic capacity, is the most important determinant of plasma levels of endothelium-derived mediators.

Information on the validity of these assumptions is scarce. In some cases, the assumptions are clearly invalid. For example, PAI-1 can be produced not only by endothelial cells, but also by hepatocytes, adipocytes, and vascular smooth muscle cells.

Clinical use of the concept of ED faces three major problems. First, the estimates that exist for assessing endothelial function in vivo in humans are reasonable but far from perfect. Second, there is a lack of markers for specific endothelial functions, such as large artery permeability. Third, specific interventions to improve endothelial function are not available. Statins, angiotensin-converting enzyme inhibitors, angiotensin-II receptor blockers, oestrogen, l-arginine, antioxidants, and folic acid have all been shown to improve some aspects of endothelial function, but these compounds have many other effects, so that it has not been possible to determine to what extent improvement of endothelial function explains clinical effects (e.g., statin-induced reduction of risk of myocardial infarction).

DOES ENDOTHELIAL DYSFUNCTION CAUSE (MICRO) ALBUMINURIA?

(Micro) albuminuria in type 1 and 2 diabetes is usually *(9,10)*, but perhaps not always *(11,12)*, accompanied by generalized ED: there is impairment of many aspects of endothelial function in many vascular beds. Importantly, this association between microalbuminuria and ED is also seen in nondiabetic individuals *(13–17)*. For example, a recent large population-based study of 645 individuals (mean age 68 yr; 248 with normal glucose metabolism, 137 with impaired glucose metabolism, and 260 with type 2 diabetes) showed that endothelial NO synthesis, as estimated from ultrasonically measured brachial artery endothelium-dependent, flow-mediated dilation, was impaired in individuals with diabetes as in comparison with those without, and was also impaired in individuals with (micro) albuminuria as in comparison with those without, regardless of whether they had diabetes *(17,18)*. Specifically, flow-mediated dilation of the brachial artery was 0.12 mm in the presence of (micro) albuminuria (defined as urinary albumin–creatinine ratio ≥2 mg/mmol) and 0.18 in its absence ($p = 0.002$). After adjusting ACR for age, sex, baseline arterial diameter, and other potential confounders, flow-mediated dilation was 0.038 mm (95% confidence interval, 0.001–0.075) lower in the presence of (micro) albuminuria ($p = 0.04$), and decreased linearly across (micro) albuminuria categories (by 0.027 mm [0.007–0.046]/category [<2, ≥2 to 5, ≥5 to 10, ≥10 mg/mmol] increase of (micro) albuminuria; $p = 0.007$). Endothelium-independent, nitroglycerin-induced vasodilation was similar in individuals with and without (micro) albuminuria. All results were similar in individuals without and with diabetes. In more advanced stages of nephropathy, endothelial function is progressively impaired, as was shown by measuring flow-mediated dilation of the brachial artery in patients with chronic kidney disease and patients with endstage renal disease on hemodialysis *(19)*. In patients with both end-stage renal disease and diabetes, endothelial dysfunction was more pronounced in diabetic than in nondiabetic individuals *(20)*.

These findings support the concept that impaired endothelial NO synthesis plays a role in the association of microalbuminuria with CVD risk whether or not diabetes is present. Such data, together with data showing that ED precedes and predicts the onset of microalbuminuria *(6,14,16,21,22)*, clearly raise the possibility that ED in (micro) albuminuria explains why (micro) albuminuria is a consistent marker of increased risk of atherothrombosis *(23,24)*. This in turn raises the question of how ED could cause (micro) albuminuria. Theoretically, ED could cause albuminuria both directly, by increasing glomerular pressure and glomerular basement membrane permeability, and indirectly, by influencing mesangial cell and podocyte function in a paracrine fashion (e.g., through inflammatory mechanisms). Importantly, the molecular pathways by which ED causes (micro) albuminuria have yet to be worked out. Alternatively, the link between ED and microalbuminuria could be explained by a common antecedent which causes both, but the association between ED and microalbuminuria remains when adjusted for example, common risk factors.

Diabetes is a state of chronic, low-grade inflammation *(4,25)*. Causes of inflammation in diabetes strongly resemble those of ED and include hyperglycemia, advanced glycation endproducts, adipokines (e.g., tumour necrosis factor-α), dyslipidemia, and hypertension. Regardless of the presence of diabetes, chronic, low-grade inflammation is associated with the occurrence and progression of (micro) albuminuria *(6,16,26)* and with risk of atherothrombotic disease *(6,16,27)*. In addition, chronic, low-grade inflammation can be both, the cause and consequence of ED *(2,6,25,28)* and the two are tightly linked. Figure 1 shows how conventional risk factors, ED, and inflammation may interact to cause CVD in diabetes. Finally, some studies suggest that insulin resistance is associated with microalbuminuria, possibly as a result of ED. Combined these two risk factors are very powerful predictors of CVD *(29)*.

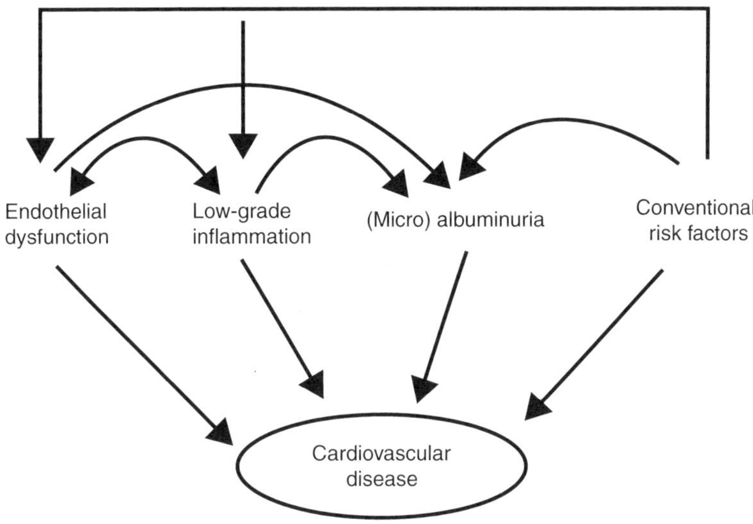

Fig. 1. Potential pathways leading to cardiovascular disease in diabetes.

WHEN DOES ENDOTHELIAL DYSFUNCTION OCCUR IN DIABETES?

In type 1 diabetes, ED precedes and may cause diabetic microangiopathy, but it is not clear whether hyperglycemia is a sufficient cause of ED *(30–36)*. In our view, it is more likely that hyperglycemia predisposes to the development of ED and that other factors, genetic or environmental, play a role in determining who among type 1 diabetic patients goes on to develop ED, nephropathy and aggressive angiopathy, and who does not. In type 2 diabetes, ED is present from the onset of the disease and is strongly related to adverse outcomes *(4,16)*. Type 2 diabetes mostly occurs in the setting of the metabolic syndrome, but ED in type 2 diabetes is not explained by hypertension, obesity, or dyslipidemia *(37)*. It is not clear whether this diabetes-specific ED is caused by hyperglycemia or other factors. An important potential determinant is increased inflammatory activity (Fig. 1). In addition, part of the ED in type 2 diabetes may be "primary," i.e., cause of diabetes rather than caused by diabetes (*see* the following section).

CAN ENDOTHELIAL DYSFUNCTION CAUSE HYPERTENSION, INSULIN RESISTANCE, AND TYPE 2 DIABETES?

The association between essential hypertension and insulin resistance is well established but presently unexplained. Compensatory hyperinsulinemia has been proposed to be the missing causal link explaining this association. However, this explanation has remained controversial, mostly because acute administration of insulin, despite its presumed prohypertensive effects on the sympathetic nervous system, transmembrane cation transport, and renal sodium reabsorption, leads to vasodilatation *(38,39)* rather than vasoconstriction, and even exerts a small blood pressure-lowering effect in patients with essential hypertension *(40)*. As an alternative, a connection between the two abnormalities can be envisioned at the level of the microcirculation (Fig. 2).

Recent research suggests that physical integrity and normal function of the arteriolar and capillary network are prerequisites for normal insulin action *(38)*. In addition, disturbances of the microcirculation may initiate the pathogenic sequence in primary

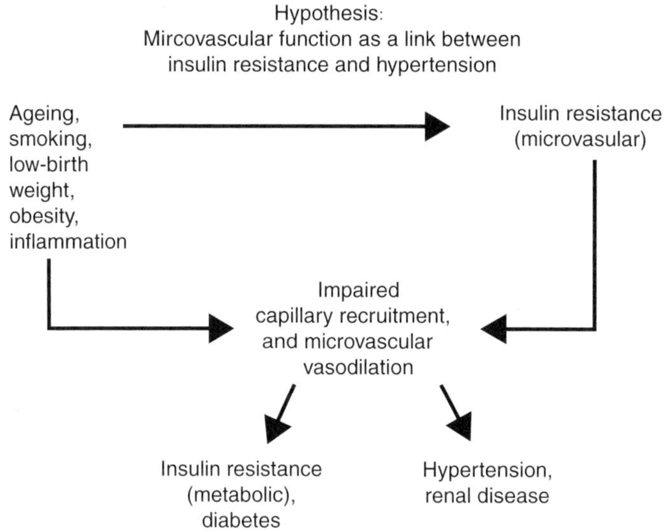

Fig. 2. Microvascular dysfunction as a potential link between common risk factors on the one hand and insulin resistance, type 2 diabetes, hypertension, and renal disease on the other.

hypertension *(41)* and thus explain, at least in part, the association between insulin resistance and hypertension. An important consequence of this concept is that any condition that impairs microvascular function *(42–48)* will predispose to both insulin resistance and hypertension (Fig. 2). Thus, if ED in large arteries, an early and prominent event in atherothrombosis, is paralleled by ED in resistance vessels and metabolically important capillary beds that contributes to the development of hypertension and insulin resistance (and later type 2 diabetes), then the association of insulin resistance, diabetes, hypertension, and atherosclerosis may in part have its roots in generalized ED of large and small vessels *(49)*.

What is the Evidence That Microcirculatory Dysfunction Can Contribute to Hypertension?

The established phase of human essential hypertension is characterized by a normal cardiac output and an elevation in peripheral vascular resistance. Peripheral vascular resistance is dictated primarily by resistance across vessels between 10 and 300 μm in luminal diameter, and the increase in total peripheral vascular resistance in essential hypertension is, therefore, likely to reflect changes in these vessels. Changes in the microcirculation of hypertensive patients include a reduction in the number of capillaries and arterioles, so-called rarefaction, in many tissues *(41,50)*. Microvascular rarefaction, similar in magnitude to the rarefaction observed in patients with established hypertension, can already be demonstrated in subjects with mild hypertension, and in normotensive subjects with a genetic predisposition to high blood pressure. This suggests that rarefaction is not solely secondary to sustained elevation of blood pressure, but may precede and thus be a causal component of high blood pressure. Indeed, capillary rarefaction in muscle has been shown to predict the increase in mean arterial pressure over two decades *(51)*. In addition, a smaller retinal arteriolar diameter has been shown to predict the occurrence and development of hypertension in a prospective, population-based study of normotensive middle-aged persons *(52)*. Calculations by mathematical modeling of in vivo microvascular networks predict an exponential relationship between capillary and arteriolar number, and vascular resistance *(41)*. Total vessel rarefaction up to 42% (within the range observed in hypertensive humans) can increase tissue vascular resistance by 21%. Thus, as seems likely, microvascular abnormalities can both result from and contribute to hypertension, and a "vicious cycle" may exist in which the microcirculation maintains or amplifies an initial increase in blood pressure. Because, according to the Borst-Guyton concept, chronic hypertension can occur only if renal function is abnormal, with a shift in the renal pressure–natriuresis relationship, subtle renal microvascular disease as well as a reduced number of nephrons *(53)* may reconcile the Borst-Guyton concept with the putative role of vessel rarefaction in the etiology of high blood pressure. This may also explain the relationship between salt sensitivity of blood pressure and insulin resistance *(53)*.

How Can Microcirculatory Dysfunction Impair Insulin-Induced Glucose Disposal?

Before insulin interacts with the receptor on the plasma membrane, insulin and glucose must be delivered to the muscle cells in normal amount and time course. Insulin and glucose delivery to muscle cells is a multistep process that involves the amount of insulin and glucose delivered to the tissue (i.e., the product of arterial insulin/glucose concentration times muscle blood flow), transendothelial transport, and the diffusion process within the interstitial fluid. Recently, there has been a surge of interest in these precellular steps, especially because insulin is known to be an endothelium-dependent vasodilator. Initially, it was therefore hypothesized that insulin-induced vasodilation and increase in limb blood flow would enhance access of insulin and glucose to muscle cells and thus contribute to insulin-induced glucose uptake. However, because the insulin-induced increase in glucose uptake precedes the insulin-induced increase in total limb blood flow, the latter cannot cause the former *(54)*. Next, Clark and colleagues introduced the concept that distribution of blood flow in nutritive in comparison with non-nutritive vessels, rather than total flow, may affect insulin-mediated glucose uptake *(38)*. Studies performed in the constant flow rat hindlimb model have shown that vasoconstriction that led to decreases in nutritive blood flow and metabolism also reduced insulin-mediated glucose uptake, resulting in acute insulin resistance. In addition, studies using contrast-enhanced ultrasound in the rat hindlimb have shown that insulin specifically increases microvascular blood volume and that these changes precede increases in total blood flow *(38)*.This has led to the hypothesis that insulin, possibly by reducing precapillary arteriolar tone and/or altering arteriolar vasomotion, redirects blood flow from non-nutritive vessels to nutritive capillary beds, resulting in an increased and more homogeneous overall capillary perfusion termed functional capillary recruitment. The latter would enhance the access of insulin and glucose to a greater mass of muscle for metabolism uptake. Indeed, muscle capillary density has been shown to be positively correlated with insulin sensitivity *(55)*, and the number of capillaries per fibre ratio is significantly associated with basal and insulin-stimulated blood flow *(56)*. In humans, it has recently been shown that insulin is capable of rapidly inducing microvascular dilation, including functional recruitment of capillaries, and of altering vasomotion *(57,58)*. This insulin-dependent capillary recruitment was associated with the number of capillaries recruited during post-occlusive reactive hyperaemia without insulin infusion, a measure of capillary recruitment which has been shown to be related to insulin-mediated whole body glucose uptake and to be decreased in insulin-resistant subjects *(43,44,47,59,60)*.

Thus, in an endothelium-dependent process termed capillary recruitment, insulin can redirect blood flow in skeletal muscle from non-nutritive capillaries (those that are not coupled to muscle cells) to nutritive capillaries (those that are) and, thus, increase glucose disposal even without increasing total blood flow. In this way, physical integrity and normal function of the arteriolar, and capillary endothelium are prerequisites for normal metabolic insulin action. Indeed, according to these concepts, ED can cause insulin resistance both when the microvascular endothelium is otherwise healthy but cannot react properly to insulin ("endothelial insulin resistance") and when the microvascular endothelium is injured through other mechanisms, such as age-related capillary drop-out ("rarefaction," i.e., reduced capillary density per volume of tissue). More generally, microvascular rarefaction and ED may provide a common pathway through which common risk factors, such as age, obesity, smoking and low birthweight, increase the risk of developing insulin resistance, hypertension and renal disease in diabetic and nondiabetic individuals (Fig. 2). Recent prospective studies showing that markers of microvascular structure and of endothelial dysfunction predict the occurrence of type 2 diabetes provide intriguing observational support for this concept *(61,62)*. Clearly, this hypothesis is far from proven, but it focuses attention on microvascular function as a potential treatment target.

CONCLUSIONS

The endothelium is an important locus of control of vascular functions, and reasonable but not perfect methods exist for assessing ED in vivo in humans. ED in diabetes complicated by (micro) albuminuria is generalized. The close link between (micro) albuminuria and ED is an attractive but unproven explanation for the fact that (micro) albuminuria is a risk marker for atherothrombosis. ED predicts the occurrence of (micro) albuminuria, but whether this is causal has not been determined. ED in diabetes is caused by hyperglycemia, advanced glycation endproducts, and the components of the metabolic syndrome. It is not clear whether hyperglycemia is sufficient to cause ED. In type 2 diabetes, ED occurs from the onset of the disease and is strongly related to adverse outcomes. Microvascular ED is closely associated with and may contribute to insulin resistance, hypertension and renal disease, regardless of the presence of diabetes. If this hypothesis is correct, then improvement of microvascular function should be considered an important target of treatment.

REFERENCES

1. Stehouwer CDA. Endothelial dysfunction in diabetic nephropathy: state of the art and potential significance for non-diabetic renal disease (editorial). Nephrol Dial Transpl 2004;19:778–781.
2. de Caterina R. Endothelial dysfunctions: common denominators in vascular disease. Curr Opin Lipidol 2000;11:9–23.
3. Schächinger V, Britten MB, Zeiher AM. Prognostic impact of coronary vasodilator dysfunction on adverse long-term outcome of coronary heart disease. Circulation 2000;101:1899–1906.
4. Jager A, van Hinsbergh VWM, Kostense PJ, et al. Von Willebrand factor, C-reactive protein and 5-year mortality in diabetic and nondiabetic subjects: the Hoorn Study. Arterioscler Thromb Vasc Biol 1999;19:3071–3078.
5. Jager A, van Hinsbergh VWM, Kostense PJ, et al. Increased levels of soluble vascular cell adhesion molecule 1 are associated with risk of cardiovascular mortality in type 2 diabetes. Diabetes 2000; 49:485–491.
6. Stehouwer CDA, Gall MA, Twisk JWR, Knudsen E, Emeis JJ, Parving HH. Increased urinary albumin excretion, endothelial dysfunction, and chronic low-grade inflammation in type 2 diabetes.

Progressive, interrelated, and independently associated with risk of death. Diabetes 2002; 51: 1157–1165.
7. Sakabe K, Fukuda N, Wakayama K, Nada T, Shinohara H, Tamura Y. Lipid-altering changes and pleiotropic effects of atorvastatin in patients with hypercholesterolemia. Am J Cardiol 2004;94: 497–500.
8. Davignon J, Ganz P. Role of endothelial dysfunction in atherosclerosis. Circulation 2004;109 (23 Suppl 1):III27–III32.
9. Stehouwer CDA, Lambert J, Donker AJM, van Hinsbergh VWM. Endothelial dysfunction and the pathogenesis of diabetic angiopathy. Cardiovasc Res 1997;34:55–68.
10. Houben AJHM, Schaper NC, Slaaf DW, Tangelder GJ, Nieuwenhuijzen Kruseman AC. Skin blood cell flux in insulin-dependent diabetic subjects in relation to retinopathy or incipient nephropathy. Eur J Clin Invest 1992;22:67–72.
11. Stehouwer CDA, Yudkin JS, Fioretto P, Nosadini R. How heterogeneous is microalbuminuria? The case for 'benign' and 'malignant' microalbuminuria. Nephrol Dial Transplant 1998;13:2751–2754.
12. Jager A, van Hinsbergh VWM, Kostense PJ, et al. Prognostic implications of retinopathy and a high plasma von Willebrand factor concentration in type 2 diabetic subjects with microalbuminuria. Nephrol Dial Transplant 2001;16:529–536.
13. Volpe M, Cosentino F, Ruilope LM. Is it time to measure microalbuminuria in hypertension? J Hypertens 2003;21:1213–1220.
14. Clausen P, Feldt-Rasmussen B, Jensen G, Jensen JS. Endothelial haemostatic factors are associated with progression of urinary albumin excretion in clinically healthy subjects: a 4-year prospective study. Clin Sci (Lond) 1999;97:37–43.
15. Clausen P, Jensen JS, Jensen G, Borch-Johnsen K, Feldt-Rasmussen B. Elevated urinary albumin excretion is associated with impaired arterial dilatory capacity in clinically healthy subjects. Circulation 2001;103:1869–1874.
16. Jager A, van Hinsbergh VWM, Kostense PJ, et al. C-reactive protein and soluble vascular cell adhesion molecule-1 are associated with elevated urinary albumin excretion but do not explain its link with cardiovascular risk. Arterioscler Thromb Vasc Biol 2002;22:593–598.
17. Henry RMA, Ferreira I, Kostense PJ, et al. Type 2 diabetes is associated with impaired endothelium-dependent, flow-mediated dilation, but impaired glucose metabolism is not. The Hoorn Study. Atherosclerosis 2004;174:49–56.
18. Stehouwer CDA, Henry RMA, Dekker JM, Nijpels G, Heine RJ, Bouter LM. Microalbuminuria is associated with impaired brachial artery, flow-mediated vasodilation in elderly individuals without and with diabetes: Further evidence for a link between microalbuminuria and endothelial dysfunction—The Hoorn Study. Kidney Int 2004;66(92):S42–S44.
19. Ghiadoni L, Cupisti A, Huang Y, et al. Endothelial dysfunction and oxidative stress in chronic renal failure. J Nephrol 2004;17:512–519.
20. Stewart J, Kohen A, Brouder D, et al. Non-invasive interrogation of microvasculature for signs of endothelial dysfunction in patients with chronic renal failure. Am J Physiol 2004;287(Heart Circ Physiol):H2687–H2696.
21. Stehouwer CDA, Nauta JJP, Zeldenrust GC, Hackeng WHL, Donker AJM, den Ottolander GJH. Urinary albumin excretion, cardiovascular disease, and endothelial dysfunction in non-insulin-dependent diabetes mellitus. Lancet 1992;340:319–323.
22. Stehouwer CDA, Fischer HRA, van Kuijk AWR, Polak BCP, Donker AJM. Endothelial dysfunction precedes the development of microalbuminuria in insulin-dependent diabetes mellitus. Diabetes 1995;44:561–564.
23. Jager A, Kostense PJ, Ruhé HG, et al. Microalbuminuria and peripheral arterial disease are independent predictors of cardiovascular and all-cause mortality, especially among hypertensive subjects. Five-year follow-up of the Hoorn Study. Arterioscler Thromb Vasc Biol 1999;19:617–624.
24. Gerstein HC, Mann JFE, Yi Q, et al. For the HOPE Study Investigators. Albuminuria and risk of cardiovascular events, death, and heart failure in diabetic and nondiabetic individuals. JAMA 2001;286: 421–426.
25. Schalkwijk CG, Poland DCW, van Dijk W, et al. Plasma concentration of C-reactive protein is increased in type I diabetic patients without clinical macroangiopathy and correlates with markers of endothelial dysfunction: evidence for chronic inflammation. Diabet 1999;42:351–357.
26. Schram MT, Chaturvedi N, Schalkwijk CG, Fuller JH, Stehouwer CDA. Markers of inflammation are cross-sectionally associated with microvascular complications and cardiovascular disease in Type 1 diabetes–the EURODIAB Prospective Complications Study. Diabet 2005;48:370–378.

27. Ridker PM. Clinical application of C-reactive protein for cardiovascular disease detection and prevention. Circulation 2003;107:363–369.
28. Schram MT, Chaturvedi N, Schalkwijk CG, et al. Vascular risk factors and markers of endothelial function as determinants of inflammatory markers in type 1 diabetes—The EURODIAB Prospective Complications Study. Diabetes Care 2003;26:2165–2173.
29. Yudkin JS. Hyperinsulinaemia, insulin resistance, microalbuminuria and the risk of coronary heart disease. Ann Med 1996;28:433–438.
30. Giugliano D, Marfella R, Coppola L, et al. Vascular effects of acute hyperglycemia in humans are reversed by l-arginine: evidence for reduced availability of nitric oxide during hyperglycemia. Circulation 1997;95:1783–1790.
31. Chan NN, Vallance P, Colhoun HM. Nitric oxide and vascular responses in type 1 diabetes. Diabet 2000;43:137–147.
32. Huvers FC, de Leeuw PW, Houben AJHM, et al. Endothelium-dependent vasodilation, plasma markers of endothelial function, and adrenergic vasoconstrictor responses in type 1 diabetes under near-normoglycemic conditions. Diabetes 1999;48:1300–1307.
33. Vervoort G, Wetzels JF, Lutterman JA, van Doorn LG, Berden JHM, Smits P. Elevated skeletal muscle blood flow in uncomplicated type 1 diabetes mellitus. Role of nitric oxide and sympathetic tone. Hypertension 1999;34:1080–1085.
34. O'Byrne S, Forte P, Roberts LJ, et al. Nitric oxide synthesis and isoprostane production in subjects with type 1 diabetes and normal urinary albumin excretion. Diabetes 2000;49:857–862.
35. Chiarelli F, Cipollone F, Romano F, et al. Increased circulating nitric oxide in young patients with type 1 diabetes and persistent microalbuminuria. Diabetes 2000;49:1258–1263.
36. Houben AJHM, Schaper NC, de Haan CHA, et al. Local hyperglycemia for 24 hours does not affect endothelium (in)dependent vasoreactivity in man. Am J Physiol 1996;270(Heart Circ Physiol 39): H2014–H2020.
37. Hogikyan RV, Galecki AT, Pitt B, Halter JB, Greene DA, Supiano MA. Specific impairment of endothelium-dependent vasodilation in subjects with type 2 diabetes independent of obesity. J Clin Endocrinol Metab 1998;83:1946–1952.
38. Clark MG, Wallis MG, Barrett E, et al. Blood flow and muscle metabolism: a focus on insulin action. Am J Physiol Endocrinol Metab 2003;284:E241–E258.
39. de Haan CHA, van Dielen FM, Houben AJHM, et al. Peripheral blood flow and noradrenaline responsiveness: the effect of physiological hyperinsulinemia. Cardiovasc Res 1997;34:192–198.
40. Heise T, Magnusson K, Heinemann L, Sawicki PT. Insulin resistance and the effect of insulin on blood pressure in essential hypertension. Hypertension 1998;32:243–248.
41. Levy BI, Ambrosio G, Pries AR, Struijker Boudier HAJ. Microcirculation in hypertension. A new target for treatment? Circulation 2001;104:735–740.
42. Serné EH, Gans ROB, Maaten JC ter, Tangelder GJ, Donker AJM, Stehouwer CDA. Impaired skin capillary recruitment in essential hypertension is caused by both functional and structural capillary rarefaction. Hypertension 2001;38:238–242.
43. Serné EH, Stehouwer CDA, ter Maaten JC, ter Wee PM, Donker AJM, Gans ROB. Birth weight relates to blood pressure and microvascular function in normal subjects. J Hypertens 2000;18:1421–1427.
44. IJzerman RG, van Weissenbruch MM, Voordouw JJ, Yudkin JS, Delemarre-van de Waal H, Stehouwer CDA. The association between birth weight and capillary recruitment is independent of blood pressure and insulin sensitivity: a study in prepubertal children. J Hypertens 2002;20:1957–1963.
45. IJzerman RG, Serné EH, Weissenbruch MM van, Jongh RT de, Stehouwer CDA. Cigarette smoking is associated with an acute impairment of microvascular function in humans. Clin Sci 2003;104:247–252.
46. IJzerman RG, Jongh RT de, Beijk MAM, et al. Individuals at increased coronary heart disease risk are characterized by an impaired microvascular function in skin. Eur J Clin Invest 2003;33:536–542.
47. Jongh RT de, Serné EH, IJzerman RG, Vries G de, Stehouwer CDA. Impaired microvascular function in obesity: implications for obesity-associated microangiopathy, hypertension and insulin resistance. Circulation 2004;109:2529–2535.
48. Jongh RT de, Serné EH, IJzerman RG, Vries G de, Stehouwer CDA. FFA levels modulate microvascular function: relevance for obesity-associated insulin resistance, hypertension and microangiopathy. Diabetes 2004;53:2873–2882.
49. Pinkney JH, Stehouwer CDA, Çoppack SW, Yudkin JS. Endothelial dysfunction: cause of the insulin resistance syndrome. Diabetes 1997;46(2):S9–S13.
50. Houben AJHM, Canoy MC, Paling HA, Derhaag PJ, de Leeuw PW. Quantitative analysis of retinal vascular changes in essential and renovascular hypertension. J Hypertension 1995;13:1729–1733.

51. Hedman A, Reneland R, Lithell HO. Alterations in skeletal muscle morphology in glucose-tolerant elderly hypertensive men: relationship to development of hypertension and heart rate. J Hypertension 2000;18:559–565.
52. Wong TY, Klein R, Sharrett AR, et al. For the Atherosclerosis Risk in Communities Study. Retinal arteriolar diameter and risk for hypertension. Ann Int Med 2004;140:248–255.
53. Johnson RJ, Herrera-Acosta J, Schreiner GF, Rodriguez-Iturbe B. Subtle acquired renal injury as a mechanism of salt-sensitive hypertension. N Engl J Med 2002;346:913–923.
54. Yki-Järvinen H, Utriainen T. Insulin-induced vasodilatation: physiology or pharmacology? Diabetologia 1998;41:369–379.
55. Lillioja S, Young AA, Culter CL, et al. Skeletal muscle capillary density and fiber type are possible determinants of in vivo insulin resistance in man. J Clin Invest 1987;80:415–424.
56. Utriainen T, Holmäng A, Björntorp P, et al. Physical fitness, muscle morphology, and insulin-stimulated limb blood flow in normal subjects. Am J Physiol 1996;270:E905–E911.
57. Serné EH, IJzerman RG, Gans ROB, et al. Direct evidence for insulin-induced capillary recruitment in skin of healthy subjects during physiological hyperinsulinemia. Diabetes 2002;51:1515–1522.
58. Jongh RT de, Clark ADH, IJzerman RG, Serné EH, Vries G de, Stehouwer CDA. Physiological hyperinsulinaemia increases intramuscular microvascular reactive hyperaemia and vasomotion in healthy volunteers. Diabet 2004;47:978–986.
59. Serné EH, Stehouwer CDA, ter Maaten JC, et al. Microvascular function relates to insulin sensitivity and blood pressure in normal subjects. Circulation 1999;99:896–902.
60. Serné EH, Gans ROB, Maaten JC ter, Wee PM ter, Donker AJM, Stehouwer CDA. Capillary recruitment is impaired in essential hypertension and relates to insulin's metabolic and vascular actions. Cardiovasc Res 2001;49:161–168.
61. Wong TY, Klein R, Sharrett AR et al. and the ARIC Investigators. Retinal arteriolar narrowing and risk of diabetes mellitus in middle-aged persons. JAMA 2002;287:2528–2533.
62. Meigs JB, Hu FB, Rifai N, Manson JE. Biomarkers of endothelial dysfunction and risk of type 2 diabetes mellitus. JAMA 2004;291:1978–1986.

30 Anemia and Diabetic Nephropathy

George Jerums, MBBS, MD, FRACP,
Richard MacIsaac, PhD, MD, FRACP,
Sianna Panagiotopoulos, PhD,
and *Merlin Thomas*, MB, CHB, PhD

CONTENTS

INTRODUCTION

Although anemia is a common problem in patients with chronic kidney disease (CKD), it is only in the last decade that an appreciation of its potential impact in patients with diabetes has emerged *(1,2)*. The prevalence of anemia in patients with diabetes is twice that seen in patients with nondiabetic renal disease and similar renal function. Approximately one in five patients with type 1 or 2 diabetes have hemoglobin (Hb) levels below the gender-specific normal range. Importantly, it is patients with vascular complications that are both at increased risk for anemia, and are most likely to suffer its adverse consequences.

This chapter will consider the relationship between anemia and diabetes in three parts. The first part will deal with the epidemiology and possible mechanisms associated with anemia, in the setting of diabetic nephropathy (DN). It will describe the prevalence of anemia in three Australian clinics and compare this with large community-based studies

From: *Contemporary Diabetes: The Diabetic Kidney*
Edited by: P. Cortes and C. E. Mogensen © Humana Press Inc., Totowa, NJ

of anemia, including National Health and Nutrition Education Survey-III. The role of "functional erythropoietin deficiency" in which erythropoietin levels are inappropriately low for the ambient Hb, will also be discussed.

The second part of this chapter will deal with the anemia associated with advanced DN, starting with epidemiological data from the US Renal Data System. This will include the emerging concept that anemia is not only a product of the process of renal impairment but also a contributor to the development of congestive heart failure (CHF) and increased cardiovascular mortality associated with end-stage renal disease (ESRD) in patients with diabetes. The frequent coexistence of CHF, renal impairment, and anemia has been called the cardio–renal–anemia syndrome, with the component of anemia offering a potential means of therapy *(3)*. The coexistence of two or more components of this syndrome appears to increase mortality and, interestingly, this may occur in the absence of overt renal disease.

The final section of this chapter will examine the potential role for correction of anemia in patients with diabetes, using iron and erythropoietin, and the difficulties experienced so far in interpreting cardiovascular and renal outcomes of intervention studies.

ERYTHROPOIETIN AND THE ANEMIA OF DIABETIC NEPHROPATHY

Although a number of mechanisms potentially contribute to the development of anemia in diabetes, damage to the renal mechanisms that normal control Hb levels appears to be an essential component. Consistent with this paradigm, at moderate levels of renal impairment, with glomerular filtration rate (GFR) in the range 30–60 mL/min/1.73 m^2, anemia is present in more than one-third of patients with diabetes. Once GFR is below 30 mL/min/1.73 m^2, anemia is more common, affecting up to half of all patients. For the same level of GFR, patients with increased levels of urinary albumin excretion (UAE) have an increased prevalence of anemia, such that those patients with macroalbuminuria are nearly 10-fold more likely to have anemia that those with normoalbuminuria and normal renal function.

The kidney has a central role in the control of hemopoiesis and hence the oxygen-carrying capacity of blood. Erythropoietin is produced predominantly in the kidneys in adults *(4)*, with smaller amounts made in the liver and other sites. Within the kidneys, erythropoietin is expressed in the cortical and outer medullary fibroblasts, located between capillaries and oxygen-consuming tubules *(5,6)*. There is a close correlation between hematocrit, renal erythropoietin gene expression, and serum erythropoietin levels. Increases in erythropoietin secretion result when the oxygen supply is reduced as a result of a decrease in Hb levels, a decrease in oxygen-carrying capacity of Hb, or a decrease in oxygen saturation of Hb. At a local level, erythropoietin synthesis is controlled via the induction of oxygen-sensing mechanisms including hypoxia-inducible factor (HIF)-1 *(7,8)*. HIF-1 increases exponentially as cellular oxygen tension decreases and activates the gene expression of erythropoietin *(9)*. HIF-1 also activates transcription of several hypoxia-inducible genes including vascular endothelial growth factor (VEGF) and several glycolytic enzymes involved in anerobic ATP generation *(10,11)*.

DN is associated with a reduced renal capacity to synthesize and secrete erythropoietin in response to anemia. Erythropoietin levels in diabetes are in the normal range and are not low, as would be consistent in a true deficiency state. However, in the setting of anemia, in which erythropoietin levels would normally rise exponentially, levels in patients with DN remain "inappropriately" in the normal range. DN therefore represents a state of functional erythropoietin deficiency and may consequently be responsive to supplementation. In our recent studies, erythropoietin levels were measured in 722 patients with diabetes *(12)*. In the 23% of the study population with anemia, 77% had erythropoietin levels inappropriately within the normal range. Although 55% of anemic patients had moderate renal impairment, erythropoietin levels were also inappropriately normal in 18 of 26 of anemic patients with normal renal function (GFR > 90 mL/min/1.73 m^2). However, 17 of these 26 patients had DN as reflected by an increase in albumin excretion rate (AER). It follows that failure to produce erythropoietin in response to a declining Hb level may be one of the earliest manifestations of DN *(2,12)*. In addition, the severity of erythropoietin deficiency, as a cause of anemia in patients with diabetes, is not always proportional to the degree of renal impairment.

The precise mechanisms by which diabetes impairs the renal erythropoietin response to reduced Hb remain to be established. Although "functional erythropoietin deficiency" is clearly linked to renal dysfunction in diabetes, the reduction in synthesis of erythropoietin in response to anemia appears to be greater than that seen in other renal (and particularly glomerular) diseases. Like anemia, tubulo-interstitial damage may be seen in diabetes, independent of and in advance of late changes of declining glomerular filtration. For example, thickening and reduplication of the tubular and epithelial basement membrane can be readily observed in the early diabetic kidney, even among normoalbuminuric patients *(13)*. It is conceivable that damage to the erythropoietin-producing cells in the cortical interstitium or disruption of the delicate interaction between tubule, peritubular fibroblast, and endothelium required for normal hemopoietic function in the kidney, may contribute to impaired erythropoietin release. In fact, endogenous erythropoietin production has been suggested as a possible marker of the severity of tubulo-interstitial damage in diabetes *(1)*.

Renal injury leads to a decrease in erythropoietin production and anemia. Although this may be partly mediated through the loss of erythropoietin-producing cells from the kidney, some patients with CKD are able to mount an appropriate increase in erythropoietin levels in response to hypoxia, suggesting that sensing rather than synthetic pathways are chiefly disrupted *(14)*. Although erythropoietin gene expression has been well documented in peritubular fibroblasts, it has so far not been demonstrated in cultured renal cells. This suggests that an interaction is necessary between proximal tubular epithelial cells and peritubular fibroblasts as a prerequisite for erythropoietin gene activation. Damage to this delicate interaction, as a result of interstitial fibrosis and cytoskeletal disorganization associated with renal injury, may also contribute to functional erythropoietin deficiency.

Renal injury also causes a transformation of peritubular fibroblasts into myofibroblasts. One hypothesis is that myofibroblasts can still generate erythropoietin but less well than fibroblasts *(11)*. This is of interest in relation to diabetic nephropathy, as advanced glycation endproducts (AGEs) have been shown to modulate myofibroblast transformation *(15)*. This may be one explanation for the occurrence of anemia in DN at an earlier stage than in nondiabetic renal disease with a similar degree of renal impairment.

Erythropoietin deficiency in diabetes may also be caused by autonomic dysfunction. Watkins et al. *(16)* originally demonstrated that patients with primary autonomic failure suffer from erythropoietin deficiency and anemia. A further study by his group showed a strong correlation between polyneuropathy and the development of anemia in patients with type 1 diabetes *(17)*. However, these patients also had coexisting nephropathy making it difficult to distinguish cause from association. In addition, denervated kidneys are still able to produce erythropoietin in response to anemia. Nonetheless, a key role for the sympathetic nervous system in impaired erythropoietin responsiveness should not be discounted.

Functional as well as structural changes may also contribute to impaired erythropoietin production. Increased metabolic demand in diabetic tubular cells and chronic hypoxia in the tubulo-interstitium may also be an important mediator of anemia in diabetes *(18)*. Oxidized nucleic acids, endogenous polyamines, and cobalt all inhibit the cellular release of erythropoietin in vitro, and are increased in diabetes. Each of these factors may contribute to a recalibration of the "set-point" for erythropoietin secretion, which can still be overcome with sufficient stimulation. This is phenomenologically similar to impaired glucose sensing in diabetic islets, which may respond normally to acute stimulation with arginine or tolbutamide but inappropriately to a physiological glucose stimulus *(19)*.

Urinary erythropoietin loss, associated with proteinuria in patients with diabetes has also been proposed as a mechanism for reduced circulating erythropoietin levels in patients with DN *(20)*. Patients with heavy proteinuria have substantial loss of erythropoietin in their urine. Our studies have demonstrated that patients with proteinuria have an increased prevalence of anemia, independent to renal function. However, neither the urinary excretion of erythropoietin nor its fractional excretion appears to be significantly increased in diabetes in the absence of heavy protein losses. In addition, erythropoietin deficiency may be observed in diabetes in the absence of proteinuria, although it is most commonly seen in this subgroup.

In our study of 722 patients with diabetes, anemia in association with increased erythropoietin levels (>30 mU/mL) was observed in 37 patients, representing approx 20% of the 165 patients with anemia *(12)*. A recent report has described the association of raised erythropoietin levels and anemia in the absence of nephropathy *(21)*. Anemia was present in 10 of 62 patients with type 2 diabetes. Serum erythropoietin levels increased appropriately with decreasing Hb, but in patients with anemia raised erythropoietin levels were not associated with the expected increase in reticulocyte count. This study raises the possibility that resistance to erythropoietin rather than impaired erythropoietin secretion may contribute to anemia in a subgroup of patients without overt renal disease.

ANEMIA AS A PROGRESSION PROMOTER IN DIABETIC NEPHROPATHY

Several studies have shown that anemia is an independent risk factor for progression in both diabetic and nondiabetic renal disease *(22)*. For example, in the Reduction of Endpoints in NIDDM with Angiotensin II Antagonist Losartan Study (RENAAL) study of patients with type 2 diabetes and nephropathy, anemia at the start of the study was a strong predictor of the rate of doubling of serum creatinine or development of ESRD *(23)*. Similarly, the Canadian multicenter cohort study of 313 predialysis patients with CKD showed that a decrease in baseline Hb of 5 g/L over a median follow-up of 2 yr was associated with a 13% shorter time to initiation of renal replacement *(24)*. The time to renal replacement shortened more than eightfold as Hb fell from 130 to less than 100 g/L.

However, it remains to be established whether patients with anemia simply have more severe renal disease. Anemia *per se* does not result in renal damage. As anemia may be considered a manifestation of renal injury, it is easy to imagine that damaged kidneys may be subject to more aggressive renal disease. Nonetheless, there are several potential mechanisms linking anemia with the progression of DN.

For instance, tissue hypoxia is a common mechanism for progression of various forms of renal disease in addition to high blood pressure and proteinuria *(14)*. Anemia may induce mitogenic and fibrogenic stimuli by lowering the partial oxygen tension in the renal cortex. This could be mediated by HIF-1 which regulates genes involved in angiogenesis (such as the prosclerotic mitogen, VEGF), vasomotor response (inducible nitric oxide synthase), heme oxygenase-1 and endothelins, glycolysis (the glucose transporter GLUT-1 and glycolytic enzymes), matrix metabolism (transforming growth factor-β_1, collagens, and matrix metalloproteinases), and cell survival, all pathways implicated in the pathogenesis of progressive renal disease.

A major consequence of anemia is an increase in oxidative stress *(25)*, a key mediator in the development and progression of diabetic renal disease. This may be mediated by the loss of antioxidant properties of erythrocytes including the enzymes superoxide dismutase, catalase, and other antioxidant proteins. In addition, renal anemia is associated with increased production of free radicals. It is conceivable that the combination of increased oxidative stress and tissue hypoxia associated with anemia may act to stimulate the production of extracellular matrix, increasing interstitial fibrosis and tubular apoptosis, and lead to tubular atrophy associated with progressive renal disease.

ANEMIA AND EXTRA-RENAL MICROVASCULAR DISEASE

Several lines of evidence suggest that anemia may influence the course of extrarenal microvascular disease in diabetes. Anemia is associated with an increased risk of background and proliferative retinopathy in patients with diabetes. Given that renal disease and retinopathy are closely associated, it is perhaps not surprising to see an increased prevalence of anemia in patients with more aggressive microvascular disease. However, anemia may also have a direct effect on the development and progression of diabetic retinal disease. Anemia may act to accelerate diabetic retinopathy by promoting retinal hypoxia and macularedema *(26)*. This may be mediated by VEGF, which is a potent stimulus to new vessel formation and increased capillary permeability *(27)*. Consistent with this hypothesis, a few small studies have demonstrated that correction of anemia in patients with diabetes may be associated with a reduction in macular hard exudates *(28,29)* and edema *(30)*. However, further interventional studies are required to determine if anemia is causally related to diabetic retinopathy.

Similar considerations apply to the association of anemia with DN. Endoneural hypoxia, owing to decreased microvascular blood flow and altered vascular permeability, is observed early in the course of diabetes and the resultant ischemia plays a role in the progressive DN. Factors that exacerbate hypoxia are known to accelerate nerve injury in diabetes and there is evidence that erythropoietin itself has neuroprotective and neurotrophic effects in experimental diabetes *(31)*. In diabetic patients with anemia and polyneuropathy, erythropoietin therapy has been associated with improvements in motor nerve conduction velocity but no correlation was found between the increase in Hb and improvement in nerve function *(32)*. This raises the possibility that erythropoietin may have a direct impact on microvascular complications, independent of red cell formation. For instance, erythropoietin has been shown to have proangiogenic properties *(33)* and also to protect vascular endothelial cells and smooth muscle cells against apoptosis *(34,35)*. It follows that the pleiotropic effects of erythropoietin may promote new vessel formation and limit vascular injury in peripheral nerves, kidneys, and the heart in addition to correcting anemia.

EPIDEMIOLOGY OF ANEMIA IN DIABETES: COMMUNITY AND CLINIC-BASED STUDIES

Diabetes is responsible for 45% of new patients entering ESRD programs in the United States, 36% in Germany, and 22% in Australia. The majority of these patients will have anemia, although this represents the tip of a much larger problem. Most patients with DN will not survive to reach ESRD, succumbing instead to comorbid vascular complications and infection. It is not yet clear how anemia contributes to their morbidity or mortality, as there have been comparatively few studies in early diabetes. Table 1 summarizes the studies of anemia in patients with diabetes and nephropathy before ESRD.

An early study documenting the presence of normochromic, normocytic anemia in overt DN was reported by Watkins' group in London *(2)*. Anemia was defined as Hb ≤115g/L for women and ≤120g/L for men. Of 27 patients with type 1 diabetes and nephropathy, 13 were anemic compared with none of 27 patients with glomerulonephritis with similar levels of proteinuria and serum creatinine. Serum creatinine levels were similar in the 13 patients with DN and anemia (mean 110, range 63–160 μ*M*) compared with the 14 patients without anemia (mean 88, range 64–133 μ*M*). The majority of patients with type 1 diabetes and anemia were shown to have inappropriately low erythropoietin levels *(1,2,36)*.

Two recent community-based studies from the United States have assessed the prevalence of anemia according to GFR. The Third National Health and Nutrition Examination Survey (NHANES-III), performed between 1988 and 1994, was a large, community-based study of the prevalence of anemia according to kidney function. In the study group as a whole (15,971 adults), a significant decrease in Hb was apparent in men with GFR (estimated as creatinine clearance) ≤70 mL/min and in women with GFR ≤50 mL/min *(37)*. It was estimated from NHANES-III data that 9.7 million adult women and 3.8 million adult men in the United States have a GFR ≤50 mL/min. When anemia was defined as Hb <110 g/L, it was estimated that 610,000 women and 230,000 men had anemia associated with impaired kidney function. When anemia was defined as Hb <120 g/L, the estimated burden of anemia associated with renal insufficiency in the United States was 1.2 million women and 390,000 men.

A further analysis of the NHANES-III data compared the prevalence of anemia, (Hb <120g/L), according to GFR in people with and without diabetes *(38)*. This analysis found that people with diabetes and moderate renal impairment had a higher prevalence of anemia when compared with people without diabetes and similar degrees of renal impairment (Fig. 1). In the GFR range of 60–30 mL/min/1.73 m^2, anemia was present in 6, 12, and 22% of nondiabetic subjects as GFR decreased from 60–50, to 50–40 and to 40–30 mL/min/1.73 m^2, respectively. By contrast, in the same categories of GFR in diabetic subjects, anemia was present in 16% ($p < 0.001$), 24% ($p < 0.01$) and 41% ($p < 0.04$), respectively *(38)*. This study confirmed that anemia was more prevalent in

Table 1
Anemia in Early Diabetic Nephropathy

Study	*Participants*	*Stage of diabetic nephropathy*	*Results*
Inomata (1997) *(1)*	Type 2 DM	N, Micro overt	– Hb and EPO both ↓ with advancing DN – ↓ initial serum EPO and ↓ [Hb × EPO] in six patients with decreasing GFR compared with seven patients with stable GFR over 26 mo
Bosman (2001) *(2)*	Type 1 DM overt DN ($n = 27$) vs glomerular nephritis ($n = 26$)	Overt DN TP 1086 mg/24 h serum creatinine ≤180 μ*M* Gl N TP 1874 mg/24 h	– 13 of 27 DN anemic, Hb 106 ± 9 g/L – 0 of 26 GLN anemic, Hb 137 ± 14 g/L – S EPO in DN failed to ↑ c/w nondiabetic microcytic anemia patients. Therefore anemia with ↓ EPO occurs in DN before advanced renal failure
Winkler (1999) *(69)*	Type 1 DM ($n = 15$) + AN vs Type 1 DM without AN ($n = 15$)	3 Micro, 12 overt serum creatinine <122 μ*M*	– Group with DN + AN had lower Hb (111 ± 12 vs 137 ± 7 g/l) – Results suggest AN as a cause of anemia but role of DN cannot be excluded
Bosman (2002) *(17)*	Type 1 DM + DN + AN ($n = 5$) vs nondiabetic CKD ($n = 4$)	Overt DN	– Diabetic group: inappropriately low EPO for severity of anemia, but normal EPO response to acute hypoxia
Astor (2002) *(38)* NHANES-III	Community survey (Total $N = 15{,}971$) (diabetic $n = 1195$)	EGFR Estimated by MDRD-4 formula	– Twofold ↑ prevalence of anemia (16–41%) in people with diabetes and moderate renal impairment (eGFR 30–60 mL/min/1.73 m^2) than in people without diabetes and similar renal function (6–22%)
Thomas (2003) *(41)*	Type 2 DM in one clinic ($n = 820$)	N, Micro or overt	– Anemia present in 23% – Prevalence two to three times greater than for patients with comparable renal function and iron stress on general population – Predictors of Hb: transferrin saturation, GFR, sex, AER, and HbA_{1c}

(Continued)

Table 1 *(Continued)*

Study	*Participants*	*Stage of diabetic nephropathy*	*Results*
Thomas (2004) *(44)*	Clinic survey Type 2 DM Three Australian Centers (*n* = 2125)	N, Micro or overt	– Anemia present in 20% – Anemia associated with ↓CC or ↑ AER in >75% of patients – Patients with CC 60–90 twice as likely to have anemia compared with CC > 90 mL/min/1.73 m^2
Thomas (2004) *(45)*	Cross-sectional survey Type 1 DM (*n* = 312)	N, Micro or overt	– Anemia present in 14% overall <8% of N, 24% of Micro, 52% of overt – Renal impairment associated with sixfold ↑ in anemia
El-Achkar (2005) *(39)* Kidney Early Evaluation Program	Community survey (*n* = 5380) Mean age 53 yr 27% with diabetes	eGFR using MDRD-4 formula 5% with serum creatinine > 1.4 (F) >1.5 (M) mg/dL 16% with GFR < 60 mL/min/1.73 m^2	– Anemia present in 12% of diabetic and 6% of nondiabetic participants – ↑ Prevalence of anemia with diabetes and eGFR 30–89 mL/min//1.73 m^2 – Prevalence of anemia similar in diabetic + nondiabetic for eGFR >90 or <30 mL/min/1.73 m^2

N, normoalbuminuria; DN, diabetic nephropathy; Micro, microalbuminuria; AN, autonomic neuropathy; CC, creatinine clearance; Overt, overt nephropathy.

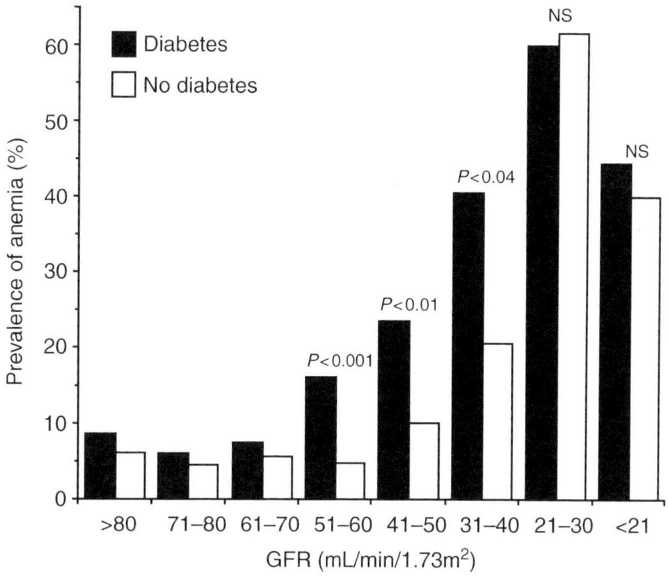

Fig. 1. Doubling of prevalence of anemia in diabetic compared with nondiabetic participants between GFR 30 and 60 mL/min/1.73 m^2 in NHANES-III *(38)*.

people with diabetes even when serum creatinine levels were still in the normal range. By the time that severe renal impairment developed at a GFR of <30 mL/min/1.73 m^2, the prevalence of anemia was nearly 60%. This was roughly that also seen in the nondiabetic population.

The Kidney Early Prevention Program (KEEP 2.0), organized by the National Kidney Foundation, studied 5380 individuals over 18 yr of age including 1769 men and 3611 women *(39)*. Anemia was defined as Hb < 120 g/L in men and women aged older than 51 yr and <110 g/L in women younger than 51 yr. GFR was calculated using the simplified Modification of Diet in Renal Disease (MDRD) formula. Diabetes and anemia were present in 25.7% and 7% of the cohort, respectively. In persons with diabetes, anemia prevalence increased from 6.4, 6.7, 16.5 to 57.1% as GFR decreased from >90, 89–60, 59–30 to <30 mL/min/1.73 m^2. In the GFR category 59–30 mL/min/1.73 m^2, anemia prevalence was significantly higher in persons with diabetes compared with persons without diabetes (16.5 vs 6.8%, $p < 0.001$). In addition, there was a greater risk of anemia among men with diabetes compared with women with diabetes when a gender-specific definition was used. Importantly, because most patients with DN have little overt renal impairment, the majority of patients with anemia are supervised by their primary care physician. In this context, anemia is usually unrecognized and almost always untreated.

In the KEEP 2.0 study *(39)*, there was no difference in the prevalence of anemia in patients with and without diabetes at GFR levels <30 mL/min/1.73 m^2. This is consistent with findings from the Predialysis Survey of Anemia Management (PRE-SAM) study of advanced kidney disease, which showed the prevalence of anemia appears to be similar in predialysis patients both with and without diabetes *(40)*. However, both these results may underestimate the impact of anemia, because of the premature death of diabetic patients with early anemia.

In our studies, we examined the prevalence and predictors of anemia in 820 patients from a single diabetes clinic in a tertiary referral center *(41)*. Eligibility for inclusion in the study was defined as patients having at least three estimations of AER, with at least one AER having been performed within the previous 2 yr *(41)*. The study included 458 men (56%) and 362 women who had been followed for a median of 4.8 yr (range 1–28). The mean age was 62.2 yr. Of the women in the study population 71% were aged older than 55 yr and were therefore likely to be postmenopausal. More than 95% were of Caucasian descent. The majority of participants had type 2 diabetes (80%), of whom 46% were receiving insulin. The mean HbA_{1c} was 7.9%. In a randomly selected subgroup of 330 patients (40%), a clinical history detailing the presence or absence of specific diabetes complications and treatment modalities was also obtained.

Many participants had experienced complications of diabetes, consistent with the mean known duration of diabetes of 16 yr *(41)*; 37% had evidence of retinopathy, 27% microalbuminuria, and 13% macroalbuminuria; 69% were receiving antihypertensive medication and 44% had evidence of macrovascular disease; 30% had moderate renal impairment defined by a GFR less than 60 mL/min/1.73 m^2. Interestingly, approx 20% of those with moderate renal impairment had normoalbuminuria. We found that in our population of 820 patients nearly one-fourth (23%) had anemia according to World Health Organization guidelines (men Hb < 130 g/L, women Hb < 120g/L). This was very similar to that found in the NHANES-III population with mild-to-moderate renal impairment *(38)*. That is, at every level of renal function in the GFR range of 30–60 mL/min/1.73 m^2 people with diabetes were twice as likely to have anemia (Fig. 2).

Univariate analysis revealed several predictors of anemia in people with diabetes including female gender, low GFR, increased age, low-iron stores, increased AER and, unexpectedly, low HbA_{1c}. Multiple regression revealed that five variables explained approx 42% of the Hb variance in the entire clinic population. Independent predictors for Hb were transferrin saturation, GFR, gender, AER, and HbA_{1c} level. Although gender was an important determinant of raw Hb levels, the most powerful predictors were transferrin saturation and GFR, accounting for 22 and 10% of the variance of Hb, respectively *(41)*. After adjusting for GFR age and all of the potential clinical determinants of anemia lost statistical significance. Although inflammation may cause anemia, no independent association was found between C-reactive protein and Hb.

Decreased transferrin saturation predicted low Hb levels at every level of renal impairment. However, decreased iron stores do not explain the increased rates of anemia in patients with diabetes. The rates of iron deficiency in our study population were the same or slightly lower than that seen in the general Australian population, and the overall iron stores are slightly higher than that seen in the general population *(42)*. There was an association between higher iron stores and worse glycemic control, consistent with studies by Fernandez-Real *(43)* showing that iron modulates insulin action so that to increase insulin resistance and oxidative stress. However, although reduced iron availability may predict the Hb level in people with diabetes, it is not the reason for the increased prevalence of anemia in people with diabetes and nephropathy.

The prevalence and predictors of anemia in long-term outpatients with type 2 diabetes from three large Australian clinical centers confirmed the findings reported earlier *(44)*. In a combined study population of 2125 patients, roughly one in five patients had anemia. Patients with mild renal impairment were twice as likely to have anemia as those with normal renal function, and patients with moderate renal impairment were twice as likely to have anemia as those with mild renal impairment.

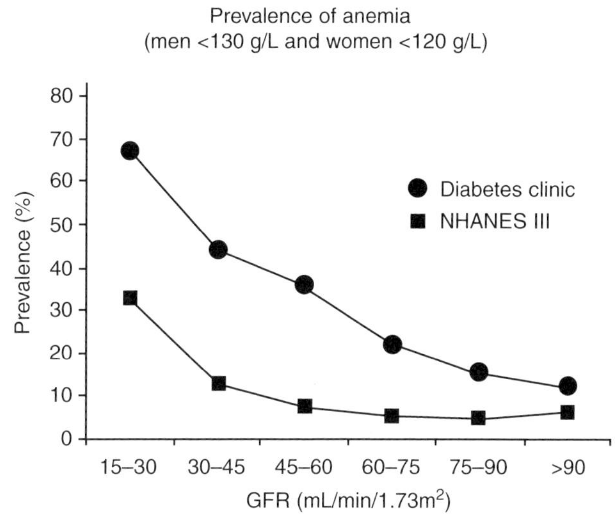

Fig. 2. Prevalence of anemia in an Australian Clinic setting *(41)* compared with NHANES-III *(37)*.

In a study population of 312 patients with type 1 diabetes from the same three centers, one in seven patients had anemia *(45)*. Patients at greatest risk were identified either by renal impairment or albuminuria. Patients with renal impairment were six times more likely to have anemia than those with normal renal function. Fifty-two percent of patients with macroalbuminuria had anemia compared with 24% of patients with microalbuminuria but less than 8% of normoalbuminuric patients.

Recent studies in the same cohort have examined the potential role of AGEs mediating the interaction between anemia and nephropathy. In this study, serum levels of low-molecular-weight fluorescent AGEs in 604 patients with type 2 diabetes were 34% higher than in nondiabetic subjects *(46)*. Notably, independent predictors of low-molecular-weight AGEs were low GFR and Hb. Whether AGEs contribute to anemia or are a marker of renal damage in diabetes will need to be determined by prospective studies.

ANEMIA, CARDIAC FAILURE, AND CARDIOVASCULAR OUTCOMES IN RENAL DISEASE

Patients with diabetes have an increased risk of cardiovascular events (Table 2) and heart failure (Table 3). Early in the course of diabetes, cardiac fibrosis and hypertrophy occur, leading to diastolic dysfunction, characterized by impaired relaxation and a stiff ventricle *(47,48)*. Anemia has the potential to exacerbate cardiac dysfunction in diabetes. In normal subjects, a fall in Hb from 140 to 40 g/L evokes an adaptive response in the heart. In the short term, oxygen extraction increases from 24 to 31% and cardiac output increases from 3 to 5.5 L/min/m^2 *(49)*. In the long term, these adaptive changes may lead to left ventricular hypertrophy (LVH), a known risk factor for adverse clinical outcomes. Several observational studies have demonstrated that anemia in combination with severe renal insufficiency *(50,51)* or cardiac failure *(52)* is an independent risk factor for worse cardiovascular outcomes (Table 2). For example, in a Canadian study of patients with ESRD, a decrease in Hb was associated with an increased risk of left ventricular dilatation, new and recurrent heart failure, and death but not with ischemic heart disease *(50)*. This was consistent with the concept that the long-term response to

Table 2
Observational Studies: Anemia and Cardiovascular and Renal Outcomes in Patients With Advanced Renal Disease

Study	*Participants*	*Duration*	*Results*
Foley (1996) *(50)*	ESRD ($n = 432$)	Prospective echo study 41 mo	– Each 10 g/L ↓ Hb independently associated with 46% ↑ risk of LV dilatation on repeat echo, 28% ↑ risk of new CHF and 20% ↑ risk of recurrent CHF – Each 10 g/L ↓ Hb associated with 14% increase in mortality
Madore (1997) *(56)*	H-Dialysis + EPO if indicated ($n = 21{,}899$)	Multiple linear regression	– Hb < 100–110 g/L associated with ↓ survival – Hb > 110 g/L not associated with further improvements in survival – Fe stores albumin, dialysis dose predicts Hb level
Levin (1999) *(54)*	Early CKD ($n = 246$)	Prospective multicenter echo study Baseline vs 12 mo comparison of LV growth	– LV mass index ↑ in 25% over 12 mo – After adjusting for baseline LVMI, ↓ Hb, and ↑ SBP were independent predictors of LV growth
Levin (2001) *(24)*	Early CKD, mean CC 36 mL/min mean age 56 yr 30% diabetic ($n = 313$)	Canadian multicenter cohort study 23 mo	– Pre-existing CVD 4in 6%, independent of severity of kidney dysfunction – 20% incidence of new or worsening CV events – Best predictors of new CVD: diabetes (OR 5.35), age (OR 1.26) – Progression of existing CVD mediated by low DBP (OR 0.72) and ↑ triglycerides (OR 1.48) – ↓ Hb by 5 g/L predicts shorter time to dialysis (OR 0.87)
Ofsthun (2003) *(59)*	H-Dialysis for at least 6 mo + EPO if indicated ($n = 44{,}500$)	First 6 mo (baseline) vs second 6 mo	– Risk of death + hospitalization inversely associated with Hb, no additional risk with Hb > 120 g/L 84% survival if baseline Hb < 90 g/L 94% survival if baseline Hb ≥ 130 g/L

Table 3

Observational Studies of Anemia and Cardiovascular Outcomes in Patients With Cardiac Failure and Early CKD

Study	*Participants*	*Design/duration*	*Results*
Al-Ahmad (2001) *(70)*	CHF (ACE_1 vs placebo) ($n = 6000$)	5 yr Retrospective analysis of SOLVD database	– 2% lower Hct and 10 mL/min/1.73 m^2 lower eGFR each independently associated with 6% ↑ in mortality
Horwich (2002) *(52)*	CHF (NYHA class III or IV) and LVEF < 40% ($n = 1061$)	Retrospective cohort study 1 yr	– Anemia associated with ↓ GFR – Hb associated with more severe CHF – Survival 55.6% with Hb < 123 g/L 74.4% with Hb > 148 g/L
McClellan (2002) *(71)*	CHF (+ CKD in 38%) Admitted to community hospitals $N = 665$ (mean age 76 yr)	Retrospective cohort study 1 yr	– Mortality 44.9% with CKD, 31.4% without CKD – Mortality 31.2% with Hct ≥ 40%, 33.8% with Hct 36–39%, 36.7% with Hct 30–35% and 50% with Hct 30–35%
Ezekowitz (2003) *(53)*	New onset CHF Discharged from community hospitals, Canada $N = 12{,}065$ (median age 78 yr)	Retrospective cohort study 5 yr	– Anemia present in approx 30% women, 17% men (defined as Hb < 120 g/L in women, Hb < 130 g/L in Men) – ↓ survival if anemia present
Collins (2003) *(72)*	CHF Diabetic + nondiabetic ($N = 665$) Medicare beneficiaries	Observational 2 yr	– CKD (RR 2.0), anemia (RR 2.0), diabetes (RR 1.5) and CHF (RR 2.9) are independent risk factors for mortality – Combination of risk factors increase mortality: diabetes + CHF (RR 3.7), diabetes + CKD (RR 2.4), CKD + anemia (RR 3.7)

CHF frequently leads to plasma volume expansion, which could itself falsely lower Hb concentration. In a study of plasma volume in 37 patients with CHF and low haematocrit (Hct), haemodilution, and true anemia were present in equal proportions *(76)*.

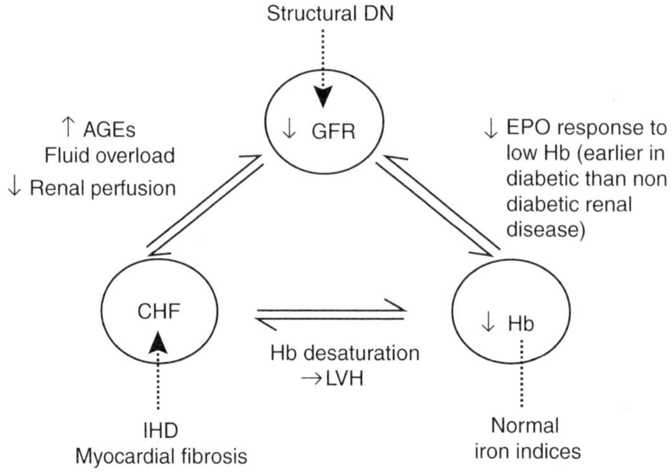

Fig. 3. Contributing factors and interrelationships in cardio–renal anemia *(60)*.

anemia involves a cardiomyopathic rather than an ischaemic mechanism *(49)*. Similarly, in a study of survival of patients with heart failure, the Hb at the time of initial diagnosis of heart failure was a significant predictor of survival *(53)*. Another cross-sectional study in patients with early renal disease showed that left ventricular mass index (LVMI) increased by 33% for every 5 g/L decrease in Hb and for every 15 mmHg increase in systolic blood pressure *(54)*. The extent of risk associated with anemia was, therefore, similar to traditional risk factors such as hypertension and dyslipidemia.

The prognosis of heart failure is significantly worse in patients with diabetes than in nondiabetic patients. It is conceivable that anemia may contribute to this risk, as part of the "cardio–renal–anemia syndrome," a triad of complications that often occur in the one patient *(3)* (Fig. 3). Two recent epidemiological studies have suggested that cardiovascular outcomes appear to worsen in patients with two or more components of this triad when compared with patients with only one component. For example, the atherosclerosis risk in communities study showed a twofold higher risk of coronary heart disease in patients with elevated serum creatinine levels, but this was evident only in the presence of anemia *(19)*. Another study of 2000 patients with heart failure showed that anemia has a high prognostic impact. Each 1% drop in hematocrit below normal was associated with a 2% increase in mortality over 12 mo *(55)*.

The association of anemia with cardiovascular and other outcomes has also been studied in patients with ESRD as part of the US Renal Data System, which included a database of 66,671 patients of which more than 40% had diabetes. A Hb < 110 g/L predicted increased risk of death after adjustment for clinical and laboratory parameters *(56)*. Another study of incident hemodialysis patients showed that a hematocrit of 36–39%, approximately equivalent to a Hb of 130 g/L, was associated with a 22% lower risk of admission to hospital when compared with patients with a hematocrit in the range of 33–36% *(57)*.

In patients with renal disease, anemia is also a risk factor for cerebrovascular disease. The Atherosclerosis Risk in Community study assessed the risk of incident stroke in a middle-aged population *(58)*. Patients with renal insufficiency alone had an increased hazard ratio for cerebrovascular accident of 1.81 (1.26–2.02, 95% confidence interval [CI]), but the hazard ratio increased to 5.48 (2.04–14.41, 95% CI) in patients with renal insufficiency and anemia. A large observational study of 44,000 patients receiving hemodialysis has been performed recently in the United States *(59)*. All participants had survived 6 mo of dialysis and erythropoietin therapy, with 6 mo of follow-up. Patients with Hb >120 g/L had a reduced mortality compared with patients with Hb <110 g/L. For every decile of Hb from 90 to more than 130 g/L, there was a graded increase in the proportion of surviving patients *(59)*.

Caution should be taken in extrapolating data in patients with ESRD, to patients with diabetes and earlier stages of renal disease. Although the mechanism of anemia may be similar, a number of risk factors work in different ways in these two settings. For example, elevated lipid levels are associated with an increased risk of adverse outcomes in patients with diabetes and early nephropathy, whereas in ESRD elevated levels of cholesterol and obesity are associated with improved outcomes. Further prospective studies are required to address the role of anemia in pre-ESRD patients with diabetes.

In summary, renal impairment worsens heart function and compromises its therapy, heart failure worsens renal function and anemia worsens prognosis in people with combined cardiac and renal disease *(60)*. It remains to be seen if diabetes-specific pathogenetic links such as AGEs modulate the prevalence and expression of this syndrome in diabetic nephropathy.

THE POTENTIAL UTILITY OF ANEMIA CORRECTION IN PATIENTS WITH DIABETES

Although there is a clear rationale for the use of supplemental erythropoietin in diabetic patients with "functional erythropoietin deficiency," there is no conclusive evidence that correcting anemia significantly improves clinical outcomes in patients with CKD, apart from quality-of-life indices (Table 4). Because of difficulties in separating cause-and-effect in observational studies, several studies have attempted to determine if correction of anemia ameliorates cardiovascular and/or renal outcomes in patients with ESRD. Two early studies were performed in cardiac patients with the aim of normalizing Hb. The US Normalized Hematocrit trial in patients with overt cardiac failure *(61)* showed no overall benefit, a trend to reduced survival in the intervention group, and a high incidence of vascular access thrombosis. However, a posthoc subgroup analysis in each treatment group showed that higher Hb levels conferred a survival advantage. The Canadian Normal Hemoglobin study in patients with asymptomatic LVH found that erythropoietin treatment conferred no benefit in regressing LVH or in changing vascular access thrombosis *(50)*.

A controlled but not randomized study was performed in 153 hemodialysis patients who received anemia therapy with erythropoietin as well as antihypertensive medication *(62)*. After a follow-up of 54 ± 37 mo, the mean Hb rose from 86 to 105 g/L and mean blood pressure fell from 169/90 to 146/78. In patients who showed a decrease in LVMI, survival was improved so that a 10% decrease in LVMI was associated with a 22% decrease in all-cause mortality *(62)*.

A randomized controlled trial of normalization of Hb was performed in 416 Scandinavian patients with renal disease. Participants were recruited in three categories: predialysis, peritoneal dialysis, and hemodialysis *(63)*. Participants from each category were randomly allocated to normalization of Hb or to a subnormal Hb group. Approximately 20% of participants had diabetes, which was a much lower prevalence

Table 4
Interventional Studies of Anemia in Advanced Renal Disease

Study	*Participants*	*Design/duration*	*Study groups*	*Results*
Kuriyama (1997) *(73)*	Predialysis, serum creatinine 2–4 mg/dL Hct < 30% (*n* = 108)	Prospective randomized end point: Doubling serum creatinine over 36 mo	Gp1—untreated anemia (*n* = 31) vs Gp 2—anemia treated with EPO (*n* = 42) vs Gp 3—untreated, nonanemic control (*n* = 35)	– Rate of doubling of serum creatinine significantly greater in untreated group (Gp 1–84%, Gp 2–52%, Gp 3–60%) – Anemia *per se* is a factor in progression of ESRD – Better survival rate in Gp 2 attributed to nondiabetic patients
Besarab (1998) *(61)* "Normal Hct Cardiac Trial"	H-Dialysis (+ EPO) With CHF or IHD Mainly diabetic (*n* = 1233)	Randomized prospective 14 mo (median)	"Normal" Hct, 42 ± 3% vs 'Low' Hct, 30 ± 3%	– Study terminated prematurely – Trend for ↑ deaths + ↑ non fatal MI in normal Hct gp (RR 1.3, CI 0.9 - 1.9) – *Post hoc* within-group analysis – ↑ survival with ↑ Hb levels
London (2001) *(62)*	H-Dialysis (+ EPO) (*n* = 153)	Pre vs post comparison 54 ± 37 mo LV mass estimated by echocardiogram	EPO, Fe and BP therapy for all SBP 169 → 146 mmHg Hb 86 → 105 g/L	– Overall mortality 58/153 – Every 10% ↓ LVMI reduced mortality by 22%, CV mortality by 28% – ↓ in LVMI correlated with ↑ Hb – Uncertainty regarding relative roles of anemia and BP control
Collins (2001) *(57)* USRDS	Incident H-dialysis (*n* = 66,671)	Before/after EPO/Fe 12 mo		– CV mortality rate in ESRD 20-40 times higher than in general population – Risk of hospitalisation 16-22% lower if Hct 36–39% compared with Hct 33–36%, but mortality not different

Furuland (2003) *(63)*	Three groups of CKD patients – Predialysis three groups of CKD patients – PD – Haemodialysis ($n = 416$) approx 20% diabetic	Randomized, controlled 48–76 wk	EPO, Fe therapy for all "Normal" Hb 135–160 g/L vs "Subnormal" Hb 90–120 g/L	– Overall mortality 13.4% N-Hb, 13.5 S-Hb – Primary analysis: improved quality of life in normal-Hb group – No difference in survival or hospitalization among groups – Sub-analysis: within each randomized group, ↑ mortality with lower Hb
Silverberg (2003) *(64)*	Severe resistant CHF + early CKD Diabetic ($n = 84$) + nondiabetic ($n = 95$)	Open, uncontrolled 12 mo	EPO, Fe therapy Diabetic Hb 104→ 131 g/L Nondiabetic Hb 105→ 129 g/L	Exercise capacity ↑ (NYHA class ↑ by 34.8% in diabetic ↑ by 32.4% in nondiabetic) ↓ diuretic use ↓ hospitalization Serum creatinine stable during intervention
Roger (2004) *(74)*	CKD (cc 15–20 mL/min) predialysis ($n = 155$)	Prospective, randomized end point change in LVMI 2 yr	Targets A = Hb 120–130 g/L vs B = Hb 90–100 g/L	– Achieved Hb A = 121 ± 14 g/L B = 108 ± 13 g/L – No difference in changes in LVMI or GFR between A and B
Gouva (2004) *(75)*	Nondiabetic predialysis serum creatinine 2–6 mg/dL Hb 90–116 g/L ($n = 88$)	Prospective, randomized primary end point: Doubling of serum creatinine, renal replacement or death (22.5 mo)	Early EPO ($n = 45$) vs late EPO ($n = 43$)	– Primary end point: Early EPO 13/45 ($p = 0.0078$) Late EPO 23/43 – Adjusted for baseline serum creatinine, relative hazard for primary end point early vs late = 0.37 ($p = 0.004$)
Strippoli (2004) *(65)*	19 trials Meta-analysis by random effects model	Randomized trial evidence from Cochrane registry, Medline embase	12 trials EPO vs placebo ($n = 638$) seven trials Higher vs lower Hb targets ($n = 2058$)	– Compared with Hb > 130 g/L, Hb < 120 g/L associated with lower all cause mortality (RR 0.84, CI 0.71–1.00) – Hb ≤ 100 g/L reduced hypertension by half but increased seizures fivefold

In CKD with CV disease, benefits associated with higher Hb (↓ seizures) are outweighed by ↑ risk of hypertension and death.

than in studies performed in the United States. In each of the three study groups, normalization of Hb was associated with improved quality of life after a follow-up of 48–76 wk but there were no differences in thrombosis, blood pressure, hospitalization, or survival. A *post hoc* analysis within the normalized and subnormal groups showed that the lower the Hb the lower the survival rate *(63)*.

Another study assessed the effects of correction of anemia with erythropoietin and intravenous iron in a mixed group of diabetic and nondiabetic patients with CHF and CKD *(64)*. As there was no concurrent control group, the study was based on before and after comparisons. The baseline serum creatinine was approx 200 μ*M*, corresponding to a GFR of between 10 and 20 mL/min/1.73 m^2. After 12 mo of therapy, Hb increased from 102 to 120 g/L. In both diabetic and nondiabetic patients left ventricular ejection fraction, hospital admission rates, and heart functional class all improved. In addition, self reported symptoms of heart failure and fatigue score improved in both groups. GFR was estimated by the Cockcroft-Gault formula (eGFR) in the 12 mo before intervention and during 12 mo of intervention. Serum creatinine levels remained unchanged from 0 to 12 mo, suggesting an apparent arrest of decline in eGFR *(64)*. However, the authors did not exclude the possibility that erythropoietin induced weight gain rather than a change in GFR was responsible for the apparent stabilization of eGFR.

In treating patients with anemia, any potential benefits need to be carefully balanced against the significant financial cost involved. Although exogenous erythropoietin or erythropoietin analogues are generally well tolerated, there is a potential for significant adverse events. The impact of hypertension, increased blood viscosity and peripheral resistance associated with increase Hb levels may offset any benefit arising from correction of anemia. Increasing the Hb level to the high normal range may also be associated with increased mortality. Correcting anemia via other means such as transfusion also carries associated risks including HLA sensitisation, which may render a patient ineligible for transplantation. Repletion of iron may also act to promote intracellular oxidative stress and impair insulin sensitivity.

In summary, the balance of risk and potential benefits form correcting anemia in patients with diabetes remains to be established. A recent meta-analysis of randomized controlled trials has addressed cardiovascular outcomes in intervention studies for the anemia of CKD *(65)*. This has shown that in CKD patients with existing cardiovascular disease, the benefits associated with higher Hb targets (reduced seizures) are outweighed by the harms (increased risk of hypertension and death). However, there are insufficient data to guide decisions in patients without existing cardiovascular disease or in patients with early diabetic renal disease.

At present, at least four ongoing trials (CREATE *[66]*, TREAT, CHOIR *[67]* and ACORD *[68]*) are addressing the potential vascular and renal impact of different Hb targets for erythropoietin therapy. Results of these studies should provide a definitive guide to the role of intervention for anemia in patients with overt diabetic nephropathy. However, additional diabetes-specific trials will be necessary to address the effects of correction of anemia on the progression of early renal and extrarenal diabetic microvascular disease.

CONCLUSION

Anemia is a common complication of diabetic renal disease, seen with a two to three times greater prevalence and earlier onset than in patients with renal impairment from other causes. At least one in five patients with type 1 or 2 diabetes in tertiary referral clinics have anemia, in which it constitutes a significant additional burden. In these patients, erythropoietin levels are normal but inappropriately low in the context of the subnormal Hb level (functional erythropoietin deficiency). This may be owing to the predominance of damage to cells and vascular architecture of the renal tubulo-interstitium associated with DN. These changes may be apparent, like albuminuria, before demonstrable changes in GFR. In addition, systemic inflammation, autonomic neuropathy, and reduced red cell survival may compound the effects of anemia in diabetes. In contrast to the inappropriately low erythropoietin levels in the majority of diabetic patients with anemia, a small subgroup of patients with anemia and normal renal function may have resistance to erythropoietin.

Although anemia may be considered a marker of diabetic kidney disease, reduced Hb levels, even within the normal range, identify diabetic patients with an increased risk of hospitalization and mortality. As with macrovascular disease, several observational studies indicate a worse outcome for diabetic retinopathy and neuropathy. Anemia may also be significant in determining the outcome of heart failure and hypoxia-induced organ damage in patients with diabetes as part of the cardiorenal anemia syndrome. Upcoming studies will determine whether correction of anemia will lead to improved outcomes in patients with diabetes.

REFERENCES

1. Inomata S, Itoh M, Imai H, Sato T. Serum levels of erythropoietin as a novel marker reflecting the severity of diabetic nephropathy. Nephron 1997;75:426–430.
2. Bosman DR, Winkler AS, Marsden JT, Macdougall IC, Watkins PJ. Anemia with erythropoietin deficiency occurs early in diabetic nephropathy. Diabetes Care 2001;24:495–499.
3. Silverberg D. Outcomes of anemia management in renal insufficiency and cardiac disease. Nephrol Dial Transplant 2003;18(2):ii7–ii12.
4. Koury ST, Koury MJ, Bondurant MC, Caro J, Graber SE. Quantitation of erythropoietin-producing cells in kidneys of mice by in situ hybridization: correlation with hematocrit, renal erythropoietin mRNA, and serum erythropoietin concentration. Blood 1989;74:645–651.
5. Lacombe C, Da Silva JL, Bruneval P, et al. Peritubular cells are the site of erythropoietin synthesis in the murine hypoxic kidney. J Clin Invest 1988;81:620–623.
6. Maxwell PH, Osmond MK, Pugh CW, et al. Identification of the renal erythropoietin-producing cells using transgenic mice. Kidney Int 1993;44:1149–1162.
7. Maxwell PH, Pugh CW, Ratcliffe PJ. Inducible operation of the erythropoietin 3′ enhancer in multiple cell lines: evidence for a widespread oxygen-sensing mechanism. Proc Natl Acad Sci USA 1993;90:2423–2427.
8. Wang GL, Semenza GL. General involvement of hypoxia-inducible factor 1 in transcriptional response to hypoxia. Proc Natl Acad Sci USA 1993;90:4304–4308.
9. Jiang BH, Rue E, Wang GL, Roe R, Semenza GL. Dimerization, DNA binding, and transactivation properties of hypoxia-inducible factor 1. J Biol Chem 1996;271:17,771–17,778.
10. Semenza GL, Agani F, Booth G, et al. Structural and functional analysis of hypoxia-inducible factor 1. Kidney Int 1997;51:553–555.
11. Eckardt KU. Biology of erythropoietin production. Nephrol Dial Transplant 1995;10:1572–1574.
12. Thomas MC, Cooper ME, Tsalamandris C, MacIsaac R, Jerums G. Anemia with impaired erythropoietin response in diabetic patients. Arch Intern Med 2005;165:466–469.
13. Thomas M, Burns W, Cooper M. Tubular changes in early diabetic nephropathy. Adv Chronic Kidney Dis 2005;12:177–186.
14. Fine LG, Bandyopadhay D, Norman JT. Is there a common mechanism for the progression of different types of renal diseases other than proteinuria? Towards the unifying theme of chronic hypoxia. Kidney Int Suppl 2000;75:S22–S226.
15. Oldfield MD, Bach LA, Forbes JM, et al. Advanced glycation end products cause epithelial-myofibroblast transdifferentiation via the receptor for advanced glycation end products (RAGE). J Clin Invest 2001;108:1853–1863.
16. Yoshida H, Kuriyama S, Atsumi Y, et al. Angiotensin I converting enzyme gene polymorphism in non-insulin dependent diabetes mellitus. Kidney Int 1996;50:657–664.

17. Bosman DR, Osborne CA, Marsden JT, Macdougall IC, Gardner WN, Watkins PJ. Erythropoietin response to hypoxia in patients with diabetic autonomic neuropathy and non-diabetic chronic renal failure. Diabet Med 2002;19:65–69.
18. Baba T, Nakajima S, Yajima Y. Beta3-adrenergic receptor gene polymorphism is not associated with hypertension in NIDDM patients without nephropathy. Horm Metab Res 1998;30:629–632.
19. Jurkovitz CT, Abramson JL, Vaccarino LV, Weintraub WS, McClellan WM. Association of high serum creatinine and anemia increases the risk of coronary events: results from the prospective community-based atherosclerosis risk in communities (ARIC) study. J Am Soc Nephrol 2003;14:2919–2925.
20. Thomas MC, Tsalamandris C, MacIsaac R, Jerums G. Anemia in diabetes: An emerging complication of microvascuar disease. Current Diabetes Reviews 2005;1:107–126.
21. Craig KJ, Williams JD, Riley SG, et al. Anemia and diabetes in the absence of nephropathy. Diabetes Care 2005;28:1118–1123.
22. Deicher R, Horl WH. Anemia as a risk factor for the progression of chronic kidney disease. Curr Opin Nephrol Hypertens 2003;12:139–143.
23. Keane WF, Lyle PA. Recent advances in management of type 2 diabetes and nephropathy: lessons from the RENAAL study. Am J Kidney Dis 2003;41:S22–S25.
24. Levin A, Djurdjev O, Barrett B, et al. Cardiovascular disease in patients with chronic kidney disease: getting to the heart of the matter. Am J Kidney Dis 2001;38:1398–1407.
25. Guest CS, Ratnaike S, Larkins RG. Albuminuria in aborigines and Europids of south-eastern Australia. Med J Aust 1993;159:335–338.
26. Sinclair SH. Diabetic macular edema: New concepts of pathology and treatment. Semin Ophthalmol 1999;14:197–199.
27. Aiello LP, Pierce EA, Foley ED, et al. Suppression of retinal neovascularization in vivo by inhibition of vascular endothelial growth factor (VEGF) using soluble VEGF-receptor chimeric proteins. Proc Natl Acad Sci USA 1995;92:10,457–10,461.
28. Friedman EA, L'Esperance FA, Brown CD, Berman DH. Treating azotemia-induced anemia with erythropoietin improves diabetic eye disease. Kidney Int Suppl 2003:S57–S63.
29. Berman DH, Friedman EA. Partial absorption of hard exudates in patients with diabetic end-stage renal disease and severe anemia after treatment with erythropoietin. Retina 1994;14:1–5.
30. Friedman EA, Brown CD, Berman DH. Erythropoietin in diabetic macular edema and renal insufficiency. Am J Kidney Dis 1995;26:202–208.
31. Bianchi R, Buyukakilli B, Brines M, et al. Erythropoietin both protects from and reverses experimental diabetic neuropathy. Proc Natl Acad Sci USA 2004;101:823–828.
32. Hassan K, Simri W, Rubenchik I, et al. Effect of erythropoietin therapy on polyneuropathy in predialytic patients. J Nephrol 2003;16:121–125.
33. Ribatti D, Presta M, Vacca A, et al. Human erythropoietin induces a pro-angiogenic phenotype in cultured endothelial cells and stimulates neovascularization in vivo. Blood 1999;93:2627–2636.
34. Carlini RG, Alonzo EJ, Dominguez J, et al. Effect of recombinant human erythropoietin on endothelial cell apoptosis. Kidney Int 1999;55:546–553.
35. Akimoto T, Kusano E, Inaba T, et al. Erythropoietin regulates vascular smooth muscle cell apoptosis by a phosphatidylinositol 3 kinase-dependent pathway. Kidney Int 2000;58:269–282.
36. Cotroneo P, Maria Ricerca B, Todaro L, et al. Blunted erythropoietin response to anemia in patients with Type 1 diabetes. Diabetes Metab Res Rev 2000;16:172–176.
37. Hsu CY, McCulloch CE, Curhan GC. Epidemiology of anemia associated with chronic renal insufficiency among adults in the United States: results from the Third National Health and Nutrition Examination Survey. J Am Soc Nephrol 2002;13:504–510.
38. Astor BC, Muntner P, Levin A, Eustace JA, Coresh J. Association of kidney function with anemia: the Third National Health and Nutrition Examination Survey (1988–1994). Arch Intern Med 2002;162:1401–1408.
39. El-Achkar TM, Ohmit SE, McCullough PA, et al. Higher prevalence of anemia with diabetes mellitus in moderate kidney insufficiency: The Kidney Early Evaluation Program. Kidney Int 2005;67:1483–1488.
40. Valderrabano F. Anemia management in chronic kidney disease patients: an overview of current clinical practice. Nephrol Dial Transplant 2002;17(1):13–18.
41. Thomas MC, MacIsaac RJ, Tsalamandris C, Power D, Jerums G. Unrecognized anemia in patients with diabetes: a cross-sectional survey. Diabetes Care 2003;26:1164–1169.
42. Thomas MC, MacIsaac RJ, Tsalamandris C, Jerums G. Elevated iron indices in patients with diabetes. Diabet Med 2004;21:798–802.
43. Fernandez-Real JM, Lopez-Bermejo A, Ricart W. Cross-talk between iron metabolism and diabetes. Diabetes 2002;51:2348–2354.

44. Thomas MC, MacIsaac RJ, Tsalamandris C, et al. The burden of anemia in type 2 diabetes and the role of nephropathy: a cross-sectional audit. Nephrol Dial Transplant 2004;19:1792–1797.
45. Thomas MC, MacIsaac RJ, Tsalamandris C, et al. Anemia in patients with type 1 diabetes. J Clin Endocrinol Metab 2004;89:4359–4363.
46. Thomas MC, Tsalamandris C, MacIsaac R, et al. Low-molecular-weight AGEs are associated with GFR and anemia in patients with type 2 diabetes. Kidney Int 2004;66:1167–1172.
47. Poirier P, Bogaty P, Garneau C, Marois L, Dumesnil JG. Diastolic dysfunction in normotensive men with well-controlled type 2 diabetes: importance of maneuvers in echocardiographic screening for preclinical diabetic cardiomyopathy. Diabetes Care 2001;24:5–10.
48. Sarnak MJ, Levey AS, Schoolwerth AC, et al. Kidney disease as a risk factor for development of cardiovascular disease: a statement from the American Heart Association Councils on Kidney in Cardiovascular Disease, High Blood Pressure Research, Clinical Cardiology, and Epidemiology and Prevention. Circulation 2003;108:2154–2169.
49. Weiskopf RB, Viele MK, Feiner J, et al. Human cardiovascular and metabolic response to acute, severe isovolemic anemia. JAMA 1998;279:217–221.
50. Foley RN, Parfrey PS, Harnett JD, Kent GM, Murray DC, Barre PE. The impact of anemia on cardiomyopathy, morbidity, and and mortality in end-stage renal disease. Am J Kidney Dis 1996;28: 53–61.
51. Mann JF. What are the short-term and long-term consequences of anemia in CRF patients? Nephrol Dial Transplant 1999;14(2):29–36.
52. Horwich TB, Fonarow GC, Hamilton MA, MacLellan WR, Borenstein J. Anemia is associated with worse symptoms, greater impairment in functional capacity and a significant increase in mortality in patients with advanced heart failure. J Am Coll Cardiol 2002;39:1780–1786.
53. Ezekowitz JA, McAlister FA, Armstrong PW. Anemia is common in heart failure and is associated with poor outcomes: insights from a cohort of 12,065 patients with new-onset heart failure. Circulation 2003;107:223–225.
54. Levin A, Thompson CR, Ethier J, et al. Left ventricular mass index increase in early renal disease: impact of decline in hemoglobin. Am J Kidney Dis 1999;34:125–134.
55. Kosiborod M, Smith GL, Radford MJ, Foody JM, Krumholz HM. The prognostic importance of anemia in patients with heart failure. Am J Med 2003;114:112–119.
56. Madore F, Lowrie EG, Brugnara C, et al. Anemia in hemodialysis patients: variables affecting this outcome predictor. J Am Soc Nephrol 1997;8:1921–1929.
57. Collins AJ, Li S, St Peter W, et al. Death, hospitalization, and economic associations among incident hemodialysis patients with hematocrit values of 36 to 39%. J Am Soc Nephrol 2001;12:2465–2473.
58. Abramson JL, Jurkovitz CT, Vaccarino V, Weintraub WS, McClellan W. Chronic kidney disease, anemia, and incident stroke in a middle-aged, community-based population: the ARIC Study. Kidney Int 2003;64:610–615.
59. Ofsthun N, Labrecque J, Lacson E, Keen M, Lazarus JM. The effects of higher hemoglobin levels on mortality and hospitalization in hemodialysis patients. Kidney Int 2003;63:1908–1914.
60. Silverberg DS, Wexler D, Blum M, Iaina A. The cardio renal anemia syndrome: correcting anemia in patients with resistant congestive heart failure can improve both cardiac and renal function and reduce hospitalizations. Clin Nephrol 2003;60(1):S93–S102.
61. Besarab A, Bolton WK, Browne JK, et al. The effects of normal as compared with low hematocrit values in patients with cardiac disease who are receiving hemodialysis and epoetin. N Engl J Med 1998;339:584–590.
62. London GM, Pannier B, Guerin AP, et al. Alterations of left ventricular hypertrophy in and survival of patients receiving hemodialysis: follow-up of an interventional study. J Am Soc Nephrol 2001;12:2759–2767.
63. Furuland H, Linde T, Ahlmen J, Christensson A, Strombom U, Danielson BG. A randomized controlled trial of haemoglobin normalization with epoetin alfa in pre-dialysis and dialysis patients. Nephrol Dial Transplant 2003;18:353–361.
64. Silverberg DS, Wexler D, Blum M, et al. The effect of correction of anemia in diabetics and nondiabetics with severe resistant congestive heart failure and chronic renal failure by subcutaneous erythropoietin and intravenous iron. Nephrol Dial Transplant 2003;18:141–146.
65. Strippoli GF, Craig JC, Manno C, Schena FP. Hemoglobin targets for the anemia of chronic kidney disease: a meta-analysis of randomized, controlled trials. J Am Soc Nephrol 2004;15:3154–3165.
66. Macdougall IC. CREATE: new strategies for early anemia management in renal insufficiency. Nephrol Dial Transplant 2003;18(2):ii13–ii16.

67. Reddan D, Tran L-L, Jollis L, Singh A. Anemia correction and left ventricular hypertrophy: an echocardiographic substudy of the Correction of Hemoglobin and Outcomes in Renal Insufficiency (CHOIR) study. J Am Soc Nephrol 2002;13:676A.
68. Laville M. New strategies in anemia management: ACORD (Anemia Correction in Diabetes) trial. Acta Diabetol 2004;41(1):S18–S22.
69. Winkler AS, Marsden J, Chaudhuri KR, Hambley H, Watkins PJ. Erythropoietin depletion and anemia in diabetes mellitus. Diabet Med 1999;16:813–819.
70. Al-Ahmad A, Rand WM, Manjunath G, et al. Reduced kidney function and anemia as risk factors for mortality in patients with left ventricular dysfunction. J Am Coll Cardiol 2001;38:955–962.
71. McClellan WM, Flanders WD, Langston RD, Jurkovitz C, Presley R. Anemia and renal insufficiency are independent risk factors for death among patients with congestive heart failure admitted to community hospitals: a population-based study. J Am Soc Nephrol 2002;13:1928–1936.
72. Collins AJ. The hemoglobin link to adverse outcomes. Adv Studies in Med 2003;3:S14–S17.
73. Kuriyama S, Tomonari H, Yoshida H, Hashimoto T, Kawaguchi Y, Sakai O. Reversal of anemia by erythropoietin therapy retards the progression of chronic renal failure, especially in nondiabetic patients. Nephron 1997;77:176–185.
74. Roger SD, McMahon LP, Clarkson A, et al. Effects of early and late intervention with epoetin alpha on left ventricular mass among patients with chronic kidney disease (stage 3 or 4): results of a randomized clinical trial. J Am Soc Nephrol 2004;15:148–156.
75. Gouva C, Nikolopoulos P, Ioannidis JP, Siamopoulos KC. Treating anemia early in renal failure patients slows the decline of renal function: a randomized controlled trial. Kidney Int 2004;66:753–760.
76. Androne AS, Katz SD, Lund L, et al. Hemodilution is common in patients with advanced heart failure. Circulation 2003;107:226–229.

INDEX

B

C